Clinical Textbook
of Dental Hygiene and Therapy

Companion Website

This book is accompanied by a website:

www.wiley.com/go/noble/dentalhygiene

The website includes:

- Multiple Choice Questions
- Figures from the book

Clinical Textbook of Dental Hygiene and Therapy

Second Edition

Edited by

Suzanne L. Noble
Director of the Birmingham School of Dental Hygiene & Therapy
The University of Birmingham
UK

WILEY-BLACKWELL

A John Wiley & Sons, Ltd., Publication

This edition first published 2012 © 2012 by John Wiley & Sons, Ltd.

Wiley-Blackwell is an imprint of John Wiley & Sons, formed by the merger of Wiley's global Scientific, Technical and Medical business with Blackwell Publishing.

Registered Office
John Wiley & Sons, Ltd, The Atrium, Southern Gate, Chichester, West Sussex, PO19 8SQ, UK

Editorial Offices
9600 Garsington Road, Oxford, OX4 2DQ, UK
The Atrium, Southern Gate, Chichester, West Sussex, PO19 8SQ, UK
111 River Street, Hoboken, NJ 07030-5774, USA

For details of our global editorial offices, for customer services and for information about how to apply for permission to reuse the copyright material in this book please see our website at www.wiley.com/wiley-blackwell.

The right of the author to be identified as the author of this work has been asserted in accordance with the UK Copyright, Designs and Patents Act 1988.

Library of Congress Cataloging-in-Publication Data

Clinical textbook of dental hygiene and therapy / edited by Suzanne Noble. – 2nd ed.
    p. ; cm.
  Rev. ed. of: Clinical textbook of dental hygiene and therapy / [edited by] Robert Ireland. 2006.
  Includes bibliographical references and index.
  ISBN 978-0-470-65837-6 (pbk. : alk. paper)
I. Noble, Suzanne.
[DNLM: 1. Tooth Diseases–Problems and Exercises.   2. Oral Health–Problems and Exercises.
WU 140]
  617.6'01076–dc23

2011044219

A catalogue record for this book is available from the British Library.

Wiley also publishes its books in a variety of electronic formats. Some content that appears in print may not be available in electronic books.

Set in 10.5/12.5pt Minion by SPi Publisher Services, Pondicherry, India

Printed in the UK

Contents

Companion Website

This book is accompanied by a website:

www.wiley.com/go/noble/dentalhygiene

The website includes:

- Multiple Choice Questions
- Figures from the book

Author biographies

Editor

Suzanne L. Noble BDS, MFGDP, MDentSci, FHEA
Director of the Birmingham School of Dental
Hygiene & Therapy
The University of Birmingham
Birmingham, UK

Suzanne Noble is the Director of the Birmingham School of Dental Hygiene and Therapy. Having qualified from Birmingham University in 1980, she obtained the MFGDP in 1992 and MDentSci in 1995. She has 25 years' experience teaching dental hygienists and 8 years teaching dental therapists. She is a fellow of the Higher Education Academy. She has lectured widely as the team approach to Management of Oral Disease and has co-developed a postgraduate training programme for dental hygienists and therapists in the West Midlands.

Chapter 1

Sheila Phillips EDT, EDH
Principal Dental Therapy and Dental Hygiene Lecturer
University of Portsmouth
Portsmouth, UK

Sheila Phillips is Principal Dental Therapy and Dental Hygiene Lecturer at the Dental Academy, University of Portsmouth. Sheila Phillips qualified as a dental therapist in 1981 and a dental hygienist in 1982. For the last 19 years she has been involved in the education and training of dental hygienists and dental therapists. She is a member of the Higher Education Academy.

Chapter 2

Henk S. Brand PhD
Assistant Professor
Academic Centre for Dentistry Amsterdam (ACTA)
Amsterdam, The Netherlands

Henk S. Brand studied biology at the Vrije Universiteit in Amsterdam. He was awarded his Master's degree in 1986 and his PhD in 1990. He is Assistant Professor at the Academic Centre for Dentistry Amsterdam (ACTA), with a research interest in the relation between systemic diseases and oral health. He lectures to both undergraduate and postgraduate students and has published over 90 research papers. He is editor of the international textbook *Local Anaesthesia in Dentistry* and a Dutch textbook for dental students, *General Pathology for Dentists*.

Arjan Vissink DDS, MD, PhD
Professor of Oral Medicine
Department of Oral and Maxillofacial Surgery
University Medical Center Groningen
Groningen, The Netherlands

Arjan Vissink graduated as a dentist at the University of Groningen, the Netherlands. In 1985, he defended his PhD thesis entitled 'Xerostomia. Development, properties and application of a mucin-containing saliva substitute'. Between 1987 and 1992 he was a fellow of the Dutch Royal Academy of Sciences. During this period he studied the mechanism and the prevention of irradiation-damage to salivary gland tissue. Thereafter, he became a resident in oral and maxillofacial surgery. Since 1996 he is employed as an oral and maxillofacial surgeon at the University Medical Center Groningen. In 1999 he graduated as a physician. In 2003 he was appointed as a professor in Oral Medicine at the University of Groningen. His research focuses on oral medicine (in particular the relation between systemic diseases and oral health), reconstructive preprosthetic surgery and implant dentistry. Arjan Vissink has (co) authored many scientific publications and books.

Chapter 3

Paula Farthing BSc, BDS, PhD, FDSRCS, FRCPath, FEA
Professor and Honorary Consultant in Oral & Maxillofacial Pathology
School of Clinical Dentistry
Sheffield, UK

Paula Farthing has extensive experience of undergraduate education for both dental hygiene and therapy students including curriculum innovation, development and implementation. She is a member of the Teachers Group of the British Society for Oral and Maxillofacial Pathology, a member of the Higher Education Academy and Director of Learning and Teaching in Sheffield. Her research interests lie in the area of mucosal immunology and include the diagnosis and pathogenesis of mucosal disease.

Chapter 4

Avijit Banerjee BDS, MSc, PhD (Lond), LDS FDS (Rest Dent), FDS RCS (Eng), FHEA
Professor of Cariology & Operative Dentistry & Hon. Consultant in Restorative Dentistry
Kings College, London, UK

After qualifying from Guy's Dental School in 1993, Professor Avijit Banerjee currently holds a chair in Cariology & Operative Dentistry and Hon. Consultant in Restorative Dentistry at the King's College London Dental Institute, King's Health Partners, London. He also holds a visiting Chair in Restorative Dentistry at the Oman Dental College as well as being a specialist practitioner in Restorative Dentistry, Periodontics and Prosthodontics in the UK. He is the primary author of the definitive text in his specialist area, *Pickard's Manual of Operative Dentistry* (9th edn, Oxford University Press) and is an internationally renowned researcher, lecturer and teacher in the subjects of caries, minimal intervention dentistry and adhesive dental materials.

Naveen Karir BDS, MFDS, RCS(Eng)
Registrar in Restorative Dentistry
Birmingham, UK

Naveen graduated from The Victoria University of Manchester in 2004. Having completed Vocational training on the Bedford scheme, he went on to work as an associate in general practice after which he completed a series of senior house officer jobs in Restorative dentistry, Periodontics, Prosthetics and Oral surgery. He obtained his membership of the faculty of dental surgery in 2006 and was appointed as a specialist registrar in Restorative dentistry at Birmingham in 2009, where he now works. He is an examiner for the MJDF examination and he is currently a council member for the British Society of Prosthodontics.

Chapter 5

Philip R. Greene BDS, FDSRCPS
Specialist Dental Practitioner
The Malt House Specialist Dental Centre
Manchester, UK

Philip Green qualified from the University of Liverpool in 1971. He was awarded the Fellowship in Dental Surgery from the Royal College of Surgeons of Glasgow in 1980 and was accepted on to the General Dental Council's Specialist List in Periodontics when it was established in 1998. He has taught in the Department of Restorative Dentistry at the University of Manchester Dental School where he also presents his '*Effective Periodontics*' practical seminar programme for the Department of Postgraduate Dentistry. He has been engaged in full-time specialist periodontal practice since 1995 and has published many papers in a wide variety of dental magazines and journals.

Maggie Jackson EDH, MPhil
Dental Hygienist
Manchester, UK

Maggie Jackson qualified as a dental hygienist in 1960, having trained in the WRAF.

She is a passionate believer in continuing education and has obtained dental health education and adult education qualifications. In 2003 she was awarded a Master of Philosophy in Dentistry from Leeds University. Currently she is working in specialist periodontal practices in Manchester and Essex. She has been an invited speaker at many hygienists' conferences, including being the first hygienist to lecture on Stafford Miller's 'Talking Points' road show.

Chapter 6

Jane M. Pratt MSc, BSc, DipDH, PGCert PSE, FAETC, FHEA, Cert HSC, BTEC Oral Health Promotion
Dental Hygienist Tutor
Birmingham School of Dental Hygiene and Therapy
Birmingham, UK

Jane Pratt has worked as a Dental Hygienist Tutor at the Birmingham School of Dental Hygiene and Therapy for over six years, as well as working in general dental practice. She teaches oral health promotion within the School and promotes oral health in nurseries, schools and hospitals. She has also informally mentored dental nurses for the NVQ and the Oral Health Education Post Certificate qualification and became a fellow of the Higher Education Academy in 2010.

Chapter 7

Suzanne L. Noble BDS, MFGDP, MDentSci, FHEA
Director of the Birmingham School of Dental Hygiene & Therapy
The University of Birmingham
Birmingham, UK

Suzanne Noble is the Director of the Birmingham School of Dental Hygiene and Therapy. Having qualified from Birmingham University in 1980, she obtained the MFGDP in 1992 and MDentSci in 1995. She has 25 years' experience teaching dental hygienists and 8 years teaching dental therapists. She is a fellow of High Education Academy. She has lectured widely as the team approach to Management of Oral Disease and has co-developed a postgraduate training programme for dental hygienists and therapists in the West Midlands.

Chapter 8

Mary J. O'Donnell RDN, FETC, MSc, PhD
Senior Experimental Officer in Applied Microbiology
Division of Oral Biosciences
Trinity College, University of Dublin
Dublin, Ireland

Mary O'Donnell qualified as a dental nurse in 1985 from the Dublin Dental University Hospital. She was appointed Senior Dental Nurse in 1990 and went on to take up the post of Dental Nurse Tutor at the Dublin Dental University Hospital in October 1992. She was awarded an MSc in applied microbiology with the Microbiology Research Unit at the Dublin Dental University Hospital in 2002. She was appointed Senior Experimental Officer with the Microbiology Research Unit in 2004 and was awarded a PhD in 2009. Her major research interests include the development of intelligent, automated and environmentally friendly methods of controlling microbial biofilms in dental unit waterlines and suction systems.

Denise MacCarthy BDS NUI, MA, MDentSci, FDS RCS (Edin)
Senior Lecturer-Consultant
Restorative Dentistry and Periodontology
Trinity College, University of Dublin
Dublin, Ireland

Denise MacCarthy qualified from University College Cork in 1977 and worked in general practice in the UK and Australia. She was awarded a Fellowship from the Royal College of Surgeons in Edinburgh in 1983 and an MDentSci from Trinity College, Dublin in 1991. She was appointed Senior Lecturer-Consultant in Restorative Dentistry and Periodontology in 1992 at the Dublin Dental University Hospital. She has worked in periodontology since 1981 and has developed the dental undergraduate programme in periodontology. She established the first teaching programme in dental hygiene in Ireland in 1992 and was Director for 15 years. In 1997 she set up a clinic for the dental management of head and neck cancer patients and currently manages the pre-radiotherapy assessments for these patients. Her main areas of current interest are periodontology, undergraduate education, and dental/oral care of the head and neck cancer patient.

David C. Coleman BA (Mod), PhD, FTCD, FRCPath
Professor of Oral and Applied Microbiology and
Director of the Microbiology Research Unit
Division of Oral Biosciences
Trinity College, University of Dublin
Dublin, Ireland

David Coleman graduated in microbiology at Trinity College, Dublin in 1979. He completed his PhD in microbial genetics in 1982 and was appointed Lecturer in Microbiology (1989), Senior Lecturer in Microbiology (1993), Associate Professor in Microbiology (1997) and Professor in Oral and Applied Microbiology (personal chair) (2006) at the Dublin Dental University Hospital. He was elected a fellow of Trinity College in 1994. His major research interests include the biology, and population structure of *Candida* species, the molecular epidemiology of methicillin-resistant *Staphylococcus aureus* (MRSA) and microbial biofilm formation and its management in dental chair waterlines and suction systems. He has published 154 peer-reviewed research papers in international journals and book chapters.

Chapter 9

Paul Franklin BDS, MDentSci, FHEA
Senior Clinical Teaching Fellow
Leeds Dental Institute
Leeds, UK

Paul Franklin qualified from Newcastle Dental School in 1989. He worked as a general practitioner until 1997 and then as a community dental officer. Following completion of an MDentSci in restorative dentistry from Leeds Dental Institute Paul took up the position of Senior Dental officer (Gerodontology) in the community Dental Service. In 2002 Paul joined Leeds Dental Institute as a lecturer in restorative dentistry and is currently working as a Senior Clinical Teaching Fellow with overall responsibility for the clinical skills courses.

Paul Brunton BChD, MSc, PhD, FDSRCS, FFGDP(UK)
Professor and Honorary Consultant in Restorative Dentistry
Leeds Dental Institute
Leeds, UK

Paul Brunton qualified at Leeds Dental Institute in 1984 and has worked in general practice, community practice and hospital dentistry. He was awarded an MSc in 1992 and a PhD in 1996. He is currently Professor and Honorary Consultant in Restorative Dentistry at Leeds Dental Institute. He is a council member for the British Society for Restorative Dentistry and serves on the editorial boards of *Operative Dentistry* and the *Journal of Dentistry*. Currently Paul is the President of the Section of Odontology of the Royal Society of Medicine and leads the e-Den project.

Chapter 10

Margaret Kellett BDS, PhD, MSc, FDSRCS (Eng)
Dean of School and Director
NHS Services at the Leeds Dental Institute
Leeds, UK

Margaret Kellett has had a career that spans both university-based academic dentistry and hospital-based specialist clinical service. With over 25 years experience of teaching and leading education in Dental Hygiene and Dental Therapy she has recently led an expansion of Dental Undergraduate education in Leeds alongside introduction of University based programmes in Dental Hygiene, Dental Therapy and Dental Technology. Margaret has championed the development of team based education and service delivery.

Chapter 11

Sarah Murray MA, Dip Dent Hygiene, Dip Dent Therapy, FHEA
Queen Mary, University of London
London, UK

Sarah Murray is Centre Lead at Barts and The London School of Medicine and Dentistry, Queen Mary, University of London. She qualified as a dental hygienist and therapist in 1990 from the London Hospital Medical College, and graduated with a Master's degree in Primary Health and Community Care from the University of Westminster. Her career has been focused on the development of dental hygienists and dental therapists at an undergraduate level, with her research interests being around the utilisation of dental hygienists and dental therapists in the area of prevention.

Baldeesh Chana Dip Dent Hygiene, Dip Dent Therapy, Diploma in Dental Health Education, City and Guilds FETC
President of The British Association of Dental Therapists
Barts and The London Hospital
London, UK

Baldeesh Chana is Deputy Principal, Dental Hygiene and Dental Therapy Tutor at Barts and The London, where she qualified in 1992. Before her appointment as President in 2010 she had held the position of Chair, she currently represents BADT on a number of boards. Bal is a DCP Inspector with the GDC and an internal and external examiner for The Diploma in Dental Hygiene and Therapy. She received the Dental Therapist of the Year award in 2006.

Chapter 12

Sharon M.G. Lee BDS, FDSRCS, FDS(PaedDent) RCSEdin
Consultant in Paediatric Dentistry
University of Liverpool Dental and Royal Liverpool Children's (Alder Hey) Hospitals
Liverpool, UK

Sharon Lee graduated from Liverpool in 1992 and was house officer at Liverpool for a short time before taking up senior house officer posts in Preston and Birmingham. Having gained her FDS, she began her specialist training as specialist registrar in paediatric dentistry at the Liverpool Dental and Royal Liverpool Children's (Alder Hey) Hospitals, which she completed in 2002. She was appointed to the post of Consultant in Paediatric Dentistry at the University of Manchester and Pendlebury Children's Hospitals and took up her present appointment at Liverpool in 2006.

George T.R. Lee BDS, MDS, FDSRCPS
Senior Lecturer in Paediatric Dentistry
The University of Liverpool
Liverpool, UK

George Lee graduated from Liverpool and, after a short time in general dental practice, returned to Liverpool, initially as research assistant and then as lecturer in paediatric dentistry. In 1982 he was appointed as Senior Lecturer and Honorary Consultant in Paediatric Dentistry and since 1995 he has been head of the clinical department at Liverpool. He has been a founder member of the Merseyside Branch of the British Society of Paediatric Dentistry and was national president of the society in 1996/7. He has also been an examiner for the National Examination Board for Dental Nurses for both the National Examination as well as for the Advanced Certificate in Dental Sedation.

Chapter 13

Ann C. Shearer PhD, MSc, BDS, FDS, MRD RCS(Ed)
Consultant and Honorary Senior Lecturer
in Restorative Dentistry
Dundee Dental Hospital and School
Dundee, UK

Ann Shearer qualified in Dundee in 1983. She held junior hospital posts in London, Newcastle and Bristol before being appointed as lecturer in Restorative Dentistry at the University of Manchester in 1985. While in Manchester she completed higher training in Restorative Dentistry, an MSc and a PhD. She was appointed as a Consultant in 1997 and was promoted to Senior Lecturer in 2001.

In September 2001 she moved to her current post in Dundee Dental Hospital and School where she is Director of the BSc course in Oral Health Sciences and also has responsibility for the teaching of integrated oral care to the final year BDS students.

She is a past secretary of the British Society for Restorative Dentistry and was President of the Society in 2009. She is Vice-Dean of the Dental Faculty of the Royal College of Surgeons of Edinburgh where she has also been Dental Examinations Convener and an elected member of Dental Council.

Chapter 14

Hazel J. Fraser EDT, EDH, CertEd, FETC
Dental Therapist in General Practice
Lecturer for Dental Nursing, West Cheshire College
Chester, UK

Hazel Fraser qualified from New Cross as a dental therapist, then from Edinburgh as a dental hygienist. She has worked in community dental service, further education, university, industry and general practice. She was awarded a Churchill Fellowship in Dentistry, was Principal Tutor in dental therapy at University of Liverpool and was President of the British Association of Dental Therapists. She is an Education Inspector for the GDC and sits on the Council of the General Dental Council.

Chapter 15

Fiona Sandom EDH, EDT
Dental Hygienist & Therapist Tutor for North Wales
Cardiff University Dental Postgraduate Education
Department
Bodelwyddan, UK

Fiona Sandom obtained the National Certificate in Dental Nursing in 1992. In 1993 she was awarded the Diploma in Dental Hygiene at Manchester University Dental Hospital and in 1999 the Diploma in Dental Therapy at the University of Liverpool. From 2000 to 2002 she was a part-time dental therapy tutor at the University of Liverpool Dental School. She is an examiner for the National Examining Board for Dental Nurses and is currently a dental hygienist/therapist tutor for North Wales under the auspices of Cardiff University Postgraduate Education Department.

Chapter 16

Lesley Longman BSc, BDS, FDSRCS (Ed), PhD
Senior Lecturer and Honorary Consultant in Restorative and Special Care Dentistry

School of Dentistry, The University of Liverpool
Liverpool, UK

Lesley Longman was appointed Lecturer in Restorative Dentistry at the University of Liverpool Dental School in 1984 and gained her FDS (Ed) in the same year. She was awarded a PhD in 1991 and appointed Consultant in Restorative Dentistry in 1997. She is on the specialist register for Prosthodontics, Restorative and Special Care Dentistry. She has contributed to national guidelines on dental prescribing, sedation and management of patients with latex allergy. She has also contributed to other books including *Tyldesley's Oral Medicine, Advanced Dental Nursing* and coauthored *The Management of Medical Emergences – A Guide for Dental Care Professionals* with Colette Balmer. She is actively involved with the teaching of medical emergencies to all members of the dental team.

Colette Balmer BSc, BChD, FDSRCS (Ed), PCTLCP, MA, Clin Ed FHEA
Consultant in Oral Surgery
Liverpool University Dental Hospital
Liverpool, UK

Colette Balmer gained a BSc honours degree in Microbiology in 1979, and then studied Dentistry at Leeds Dental School, qualifying in 1983. She gained her FDS (Edinburgh) in 1987 and followed a career in oral surgery and is currently a Consultant in Oral Surgery at Liverpool University Dental Hospital She has always been actively involved in the teaching of dental undergraduates, dental postgraduates and DCPs and has a Postgraduate Teaching Certificate, Diploma and Masters in Clinical Education, is a Fellow of the Higher Education Academy, an honorary clinical lecturer and Associate Postgraduate Dental Dean. She has a major interest in teaching medical emergency management and is an ALS instructor for the Resuscitation Council UK.

Chapter 17

Hilary R. Samways EDH, EDT
Tutor in Dental Hygiene and Therapy
Sheffield University Dental Hospital
Sheffield, UK

Hilary Samways qualified as a dental nurse in 1979 at Sheffield Dental Hospital. She gained her Diploma in Dental Hygiene in 1983, her Adult Education Teaching Certificate in 1985 and Certificate in Health Education in 1989, after which she worked as a dental tutor at the Health Sciences Institute, Muscat, Sultanate of Oman. In 2000 she obtained a Diploma in Dental Therapy at the University of Liverpool. She has worked in general dental practice, community dental service, further education, retail and university. She currently works as a dental hygienist and therapist tutor in the UK.

Chapter 18

Philip Wander BDS, MGDSRCS, DDFHom, FFHom (Hon)
General Dental Practitioner
Manchester, UK

Philip Wander qualified from the University of Liverpool in 1966 and obtained his MGDS from the Royal College of Surgeons in London in 1980. He is a founder and chairman of the British Homeopathic Dental Association, and obtained his Diploma in Dental Homeopathy in October 1994. He was recently awarded an honorary fellowship of the Faculty of Homeopathy. He lectures throughout the UK on Complementary Therapies in dentistry and has had numerous articles published on the topic. Phil coauthored the BDJ book *Dental Photography* and runs educational courses on this topic. In 2009 he was voted as one of the most influential dentists in the UK in a UK poll. He is currently consultant to NHS and private practices in the Manchester area.

Chapter 19

Sara Holmes MBE, MA, BSc
Director, University of Portsmouth Dental Academy & Honorary Senior Lecturer King's College London
The Dental Institute
London, UK

Sara Holmes started her career as a Dental Nurse and has worked in NHS, private, salaried and secondary care settings. On joining the University of Portsmouth in 1994 she led the development of the School for Dental Care Professionals and later the development of the Dental Academy. In 2010, she sat her viva for the Professional Doctorate in Education (EdD), University of Brighton, having previously obtained her BSc (Hons) in Health Promotion and Masters in Health Professional Education at the University of Portsmouth. In 2006, she was awarded Member of the Order of the British Empire for services to dental education.

Leanna Wynne EDH
Principal Lecturer and Course Leader
The University of Portsmouth
Portsmouth, UK

Leanna Wynne is Course Leader of the BSc (Hons) Hygiene and Therapy and Principal lecturer at the University of Portsmouth. Leanna completed a MA Learning and Teaching, with the research interest being feedback within the academic environment. Leanna is currently focused on making the ethos of team working a key component of the curriculum at the University of Portsmouth. The aim is to better prepare the student for employment and to be able to operate effectively as an integral part of the healthcare workforce

Preface

Since the first edition of this textbook was published in 2006 the education of Dental Hygienists and Therapists in the United Kingdom has continued to evolve and expand. The second edition has reflected changes in clinical practice protocols and legislation, together with changes in the regulation and delivery of dental care services. The authors and co-authors, many of whom contributed to the first edition have updated the text. There has been a significant contribution from Dental Hygienist and Dental Therapists bringing their experience of clinical practice and of teaching students into the text. All the chapters have a summary so the reader may see at a glance the chapter contents.

The attraction of the book is that is brings together the key skills of Dental Hygienists and Therapists under one cover for the enhancement of learning both for the undergraduate and also for those who are qualified. Each chapter includes guidance for further reading as inevitably the chapters have been limited by size.

Students in Higher Education Institutes can be confident that the contents reflect the learning outcomes published by the General Dental Council in *Outcomes for Registration 2011* where this is appropriate.

Suzanne L. Noble

Acknowledgements

The editor and authors would like to thank the following for their support in preparing the book and for permission to use their original work in the 2nd Edition.

Robert Ireland	Editor, 1st Edition
David Beighton	Chapter 4, 1st Edition
David Bartlett	Chapter 4, 1st Edition
Kathy Needs	Chapter 6, 1st Edition
Jan Postans	Chapter 6, 1st Edition
Charlotte Jeavons	Chapter 11, 1st Edition
John Cunningham	Chapter 20, 1st Edition

Dunja Przulj and Oliver West for help with Chapter 11.

Christine Taylor for the help with the preparation of the manuscript.

Section 1

Core Basic Science

1

Oral embryology, histology and anatomy

Sheila Phillips

Summary

This chapter covers:

- Oral embryology
- Early tooth development
- Development of the dental tissues
- Histology of oral tissues
- Histology of dental tissues
- Oral anatomy
- Tooth morphology

Introduction

A basic understanding of the development, structure and relationship of the tissues and structures which constitute the oral cavity and its associated environment is fundamental to the practice of clinical dentistry. It enables the clinician better to appreciate how subsequent pathology change may be influenced by adjacent anatomical structures or tissues and therefore helps to provide a better understanding of the rationale for potential treatment options.

Oral embryology

Development of the face

4 weeks of intrauterine life

The primitive oral cavity, which is known as the **stomodeum**, develops five facial swellings (Figure 1.1): one frontonasal process, two maxillary processes and two mandibular processes. The frontonasal process eventually develops to form the forehead, nose and philtrum; the two maxillary processes form the middle face and upper lip; and the two mandibular processes form the mandible and lower lip.

Development of the palate

5 weeks of intrauterine life

The frontonasal process produces the medial and lateral nasal processes. Failure of fusion of the maxillary and medial nasal processes produces a **cleft lip**.

6 weeks of intrauterine life

The primary nasal septum and primary palate are formed, both derived from the fronto-nasal process (Figure 1.2). Two lateral palatal shelves develop behind the primary palate from the maxillary process. A secondary nasal septum grows behind the primary nasal septum from the roof of the primitive oral cavity dividing the nasal cavity into two.

8 weeks of intrauterine life

The palatal shelves contact each other forming the secondary palate; the shelves also contact anteriorly with the primary palate dividing the oral and nasal cavities.

Development of the jaws

The mandible

6 weeks of intrauterine life

The mandible appears as a band of dense fibrous tissue known a **Meckel's cartilage**; this cartilage provides a framework around which the bone will form.

7 weeks of intrauterine life

Bone formation commences at the mental foramen area and begins to spread backwards, forwards and upwards outlining the future body of the mandible. As the bone

Clinical Textbook of Dental Hygiene and Therapy, Second Edition. Edited by Suzanne L. Noble.
© 2012 John Wiley & Sons, Ltd. Published 2012 by John Wiley & Sons, Ltd.

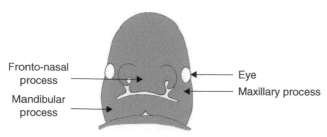

Figure 1.1 Facial development at 4 weeks of intrauterine life.

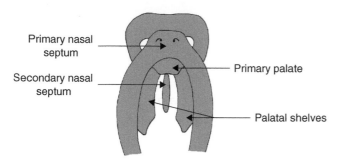

Figure 1.2 Palatal development at 6 weeks of intrauterine life.

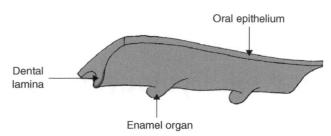

Figure 1.3 Dental lamina showing enamel organs. Reproduced by kind permission of R. Ireland.

- The ectodermal epithelium thickens in these areas and protrudes into the mesenchymal cells forming the primary epithelial band.

Development of the vestibular band and dental lamina

- At 7 weeks of intrauterine life.
- The primary epithelial band develops two processes the vestibular band and the dental lamina.
- The vestibular band forms buccally and will eventually form the vestibule, separating the lips and cheeks from the teeth and gingivae.
- The dental lamina forms lingually and develops into an arch shape band on which the tooth germs will develop (Figure 1.3).

Development of the tooth germ

The tooth germ develops in three stages: bud, cap and bell (Figure 1.4).

Bud

At 8 weeks of intrauterine life, clumps of mesenchymal cells induce the dental lamina to form swellings known as **enamel organs**. Each enamel organ will be responsible for the development of each tooth (Figure 1.4a).

Cap

As the enamel organs grow and increase in size, the inner aspect becomes concave resembling skull caps. By the late cap stage, at 12 weeks of intrauterine life, cells on the inner aspect of the enamel organ change from cuboidal to columnar forming the **inner enamel epithelium**. The outer layer of cells remains cuboidal and is known as the **outer enamel epithelium**. (Figure 1.4b)

Beneath the inner enamel epithelium the condensation of mesenchymal cells is termed the **dental papilla**; this will eventually become the pulp. A fibrous capsule surrounds each enamel organ and this is termed the **dental follicle**; this will eventually become the periodontal ligament.

grows backwards, two small secondary cartilages develop, which eventually form the **condyle** and **coronoid processes**. Anteriorly, the left and right mandibular plate of bone is separated by cartilage at the **mandibular symphysis**; these two plates eventually unite to form a single bone approximately 2 years after birth. The upward growth of bone increases the height of the mandible forming the alveolar process which will surround the developing tooth germ.

The maxilla

8 weeks of intrauterine life

Ossification of the maxilla commences at the area of the developing primary (deciduous) canines; from this area, bone formation spreads, developing the maxillary processes: palatal, zygomatic, frontal and alveolar. Growth of the maxilla occurs by remodelling of bone and by **sutural growth**. The stimulus for sutural bone growth is thought to be related to the tension produced by the displacement of bone. Growth carries the maxilla forwards and downwards as it increases in size.

Early tooth development

Development of primary epithelial band

- The first sign of tooth development occurs at the 6th week of intrauterine life.
- Underneath the oral ectodermal epithelium there is a condensation of mesenchymal cells in areas where teeth will eventually form.

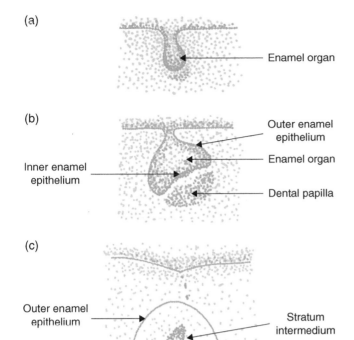

(a)

Enamel organ

(b)

Outer enamel epithelium

Enamel organ

Inner enamel epithelium

Dental papilla

(c)

Outer enamel epithelium

Stratum intermedium

Stellate reticulum

Dental follicle

Inner enamel epithelium

Herwig's root sheath

Dental papilla

Figure 1.4 Stages in the development of the tooth germ.

Bell

By 14 weeks of intrauterine life (Figure 1.4c) the enamel organ consists of the following:

- **Inner enamel epithelium:**
  - Cells lining the inner surface of the enamel organ which are columnar in shape.
  - The inner enamel epithelium defines the shape of the crown.
  - They will eventually differentiate into enamel forming cells (**ameloblasts**).
- **Stratum intermedium:**
  - Lies over the inner enamel epithelium.
  - Consists of two to three layers of cells.
  - Transports nutrients to and from the ameloblasts.
- **Stellate reticulum:**
  - Lies between the stratum intermedium and the outer enamel epithelium.
  - It consists of star-shaped cells that protect the underlying dental tissues.
  - It also maintains the shape of the tooth.
- **Outer enamel epithelium:**
  - Cells lining the outer surface of the enamel organ. They are cuboidal in shape.

- They maintain the shape of the enamel organ.
- The outer enamel epithelium meets with the internal enamel epithelium at the cervical loop.
- Eventually the inner and outer enamel epithelium grows downwards at the cervical loop forming **Hertwig's root sheath**, which maps out the shape of the root.

At the late bell stage the dental lamina disintegrates and is ready for the formation of dental hard tissue. Dentine formation always precedes enamel formation.

Development of the dental tissues

Dentine formation – (dentinogenesis)

- Late bell stage the inner enamel epithelium cells have mapped out the shape of the crown.
- The inner enamel epithelium cells induce cells at the periphery of the dental papilla to form columnar **odontoblast** cells (dentine-forming cells).
- Odontoblast cells begin to secrete an unmineralised dentine matrix.
- As more dentine matrix is deposited, the odontoblast cells retreat in the direction of the pulp leaving an elongated process known as the **odontoblast process**.
- The dentine matrix formed prior to mineralisation is termed **predentine**. A narrow layer of predentine is always present on the surface of the pulp.
- Mineralisation of dentine begins when the predentine is approximately 5 μm thick.
- Spherical zones of hydroxyapatite called **calcospherites** are formed within the dentine matrix.
- Mineralisation of the dentine matrix starts at random points and eventually these calcospherites fuse together to form mineralised dentine.
- Dentinal tubules form around each odontoblast process (Figure 1.5).
- The odontoblasts retreat in S-shaped curves towards the dental papilla.
- The first layer of mineralised dentine is called **mantle dentine** and the remaining bulk of the mineralised dentine is known as **circumpulpal dentine.**

Enamel formation (amelogenesis)

- Immediately after the first layer of dentine is formed, the inner enamel epithelium **ameloblast** cells (enamel forming cells).
- The ameloblast cell is columnar in shape with its base attached to cells of the stratum intermedium.
- At the secretory end of ameloblast cells is a pyramidal extension called the **Tomes' process** (Figure 1.6).
- The enamel matrix is secreted through the Tomes' process at the amelodentinal junction.

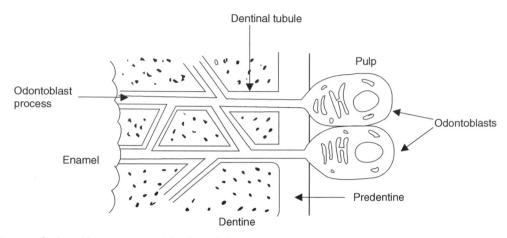

Figure 1.5 Diagram of odontoblast process and dentine tubules.

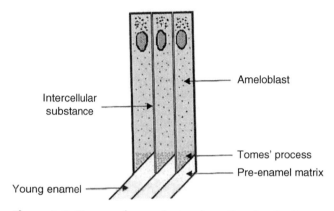

Figure 1.6 Diagram of enamel prism formation showing Tomes processes.

- Calcium and phosphate ions are secreted into the enamel matrix and mineralisation of enamel occurs immediately, forming hydroxyapatite crystallites.
- As more enamel matrix is secreted and mineralised, the ameloblast cells move away from the amelodentinal junction forming a pattern of crystallites, which are contained within enamel prisms.
- Enamel prisms are also known as enamel rods they run from the amelodentinal junction to the enamel surface.

Enamel maturation

- During maturation from pre-enamel to mature enamel, the enamel crystallites increase in size and the organic content is reduced.
- On completion of enamel formation the ameloblast cell loses the Tomes' process, flattens and becomes the **reduced enamel epithelium**.
- The reduced enamel epithelium protects the enamel during eruption and will eventually become the **junctional epithelium**.

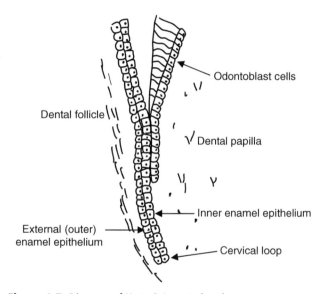

Figure 1.7 Diagram of Hertwig's root sheath.

Formation of the root

- Occurs when the crown has completed.
- The internal and external enamel epithelium grows downwards at the cervical loop to form a double layered epithelial wall – **Hertwig's root sheath** (Figure 1.7).
- The Hertwig's root sheath grows apically mapping out the shape of the root enclosing the dental papilla.
- The dental follicle lies external to the Hertwig's root sheath.

Cementum formation (cementogenesis)

- The Hertwig's root sheath induces the formation of odontoblast cells.

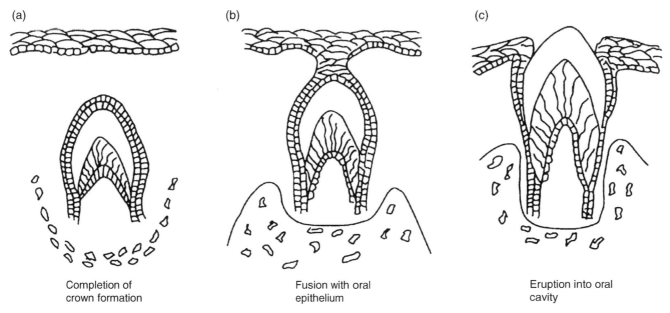

(a)   (b)   (c)

Completion of
crown formation

Fusion with oral
epithelium

Eruption into oral
cavity

Figure 1.8 Diagram showing phases of tooth eruption.

- When root dentine has formed, Hertwig's root sheath fragments allowing adjacent cells from the dental follicle to come into contact with the root dentine.
- These cells differentiate into **cementoblasts** (**cementum-forming cells**).
- Cementoblasts are cuboidal in shape and form a single layer on the surface of the root dentine.
- The cementoblasts secrete cementum matrix and crystallites of hydroxyapatite are deposited in this matrix and mineralisation occurs.
- During formation, a thin layer of unmineralised cementum is always present on the surface; this is known as **cementoid**.

Formation of the periodontal ligament

- Cells within the dental follicle give rise to **fibroblasts** that secrete collagen.
- Once cementum formation has begun, collagen fibres within the dental follicle orientate themselves into bundles, which are perpendicular to the root surface.
- These fibres will form the **principal fibres** of the periodontal ligament.
- The ends of these fibres become embedded in the developing cementum and alveolar bone and are known as **Sharpey's fibres**.

Tooth eruption

Tooth eruption is the bodily movement of a tooth from its development position into its functional position in the oral cavity. It can be broken down into two phases; the per-functional eruptive phase and the functional eruptive phase (Figure 1.8).

Prefunctional phase

- During the prefunctional phase, crown formation has completed.
- As root formation begins the developing tooth begins to erupt.
- The overlying alveolar bone is resorbed by **osteoclasts** and gradually the tooth moves in an axial direction towards the oral cavity.
- The enamel surface of the tooth is covered by the reduced enamel epithelium which fuses with the oral epithelium.
- The pressure from the tip of the tooth breaks down the oral epithelium allowing the tooth to emerge into the oral cavity without any rupturing of blood vessels.
- Once the tooth has emerged, the reduced enamel epithelium is known as the **epithelial attachment**.
- Tooth eruption continues until the tooth contacts (occludes with) the opposing tooth in the opposite jaw.

Functional eruptive phase

- The functional eruptive phase continues throughout life due to functional changes.
- The alveolar bone continuously remodels in response to tooth movement and enamel wear allowing teeth to maintain contact with each other and with opposing teeth.

Mechanisms of tooth eruption

The eruptive force of tooth eruption is unclear; however, several theories have been put forward although there is little evidence to support them. These are:

- Root growth generates a force beneath the tooth, elevating the tooth towards the oral cavity.

Table 1.1 Approximate dates of tooth development, eruption and exfoliation for the primary dentition.

Tooth (in order of eruption)	Approximate initial calcification date	Approximate eruption date	Approximate exfoliation date
Upper and lower primary central incisors (A's)	3–4 months *in utero*	6–8 months	6–7 years
Upper and lower primary lateral incisors (B's)	4½ months *in utero*	7–9 months	7–8 years
Upper and lower primary first molars (D's)	5 months *in utero*	12–14 months	9–11 years
Upper and lower primary canines C's	5 months *in utero*	16–18 months	9–12 years
Upper and lower primary second molars E's	6 months *in utero*	20–24 months	10–12 years

Table 1.2 Approximate dates of tooth development and eruption for the permanent dentition.

Tooth (in order of eruption)	Approximate initial calcification date	Approximate eruption date
Upper and lower permanent first molars (6's)	At birth	6–7 years
Upper and lower permanent central incisors (1's)	3–4 months	6–7 years
Upper and lower permanent lateral incisors (2's)	Upper 10–12 months Lower 3–4 months	7–8 years
Lower permanent canines (3's)	4–5 months	9–10 years
Upper and lower permanent first premolars (4's)	1–2 years	10–11 years
Upper and lower permanent second premolars (5's)	2–3 years	11–12 years
Upper permanent canines (3's)	4–5 months	11–12 years
Upper and lower permanent second molars (7's)	2–3 years	12–13 years
Upper and lower permanent third molars (8's)	7–10 years	18+ years

- Remodelling and deposition of the bone beneath the developing tooth pushes the tooth upwards.
- Traction of the periodontal fibres exerts an upward pull on the tooth.
- Cellular proliferation at the base of the pulp creates pressure that pushes the tooth from the dental follicle.
- An increase in tissue fluid or blood pressure generates an eruptive force on the tooth.

The approximate initial calcification and eruption dates are listed in Tables 1.1 and 1.2.

Histology of oral tissues

The three primary layers of an embryo are described as:

- **Ectoderm** (the outermost layer). This develops into structures such as the nervous system, the epidermis and epidermal derivatives and the lining of various body cavities such as the mouth.
- **Mesoderm** (the middle layer), which forms into many of the bodily tissues and structures such as bone, muscle, connective tissue and skin.
- **Endoderm** (the innermost layer), which develops to form the digestive tract and part of the respiratory system.

The oral mucosa

The surface of the oral mucosa consists of **epithelial tissue**. Epithelial tissue is first classified according to the shape of the cells as being squamous (flat cells), cuboidal (cube shaped) or columnar (tall, narrow cells) and second by the number of cell layers. A single layer of epithelial cells is called simple and where there are several layers it is called stratified.

The oral mucosa consists of:

- A surface layer of **stratified squamous epithelium**.
- Underneath this there is a layer of highly vascular connective tissue, the **lamina propria** (Figure 1.9).
- The mucous membrane is attached to underlying structures by connective tissue of varying thickness (the **submucosa layer**), which contains larger arteries, veins and nerves.

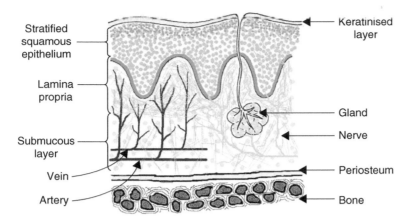

Figure 1.9 Diagram of the structure of the oral mucosa. Reproduced by kind permission of R. Ireland.

The structure of the mucous membrane varies in different parts of the oral cavity according to the variation in function. In areas subject to chewing such as the hard palate and the attached gingivae, the mucosa has a firm **keratinised epithelial layer** of fibrous protein (also found on the palms of the hands and soles of the feet). In other areas such as the cheeks and floor of the mouth that require more flexibility, this is reduced or absent. The cells of this keratin layer have no nuclei and no nerve supply.

Underneath the keratinised layer of cells is a non-keratinised layer of epithelial cells which have nuclei and act as cushion against mechanical forces. The deepest layer of these cells is known as the **basal layer** and is attached to the basal lamina.

The oral cavity is kept lubricated by mucus secretions from the major and minor salivary glands; this epithelium is sometimes termed mucous membrane.

There are three types of oral mucosa found in the oral cavity.

- **Lining mucosa:**
  - This covers the inside of the cheeks, lips, alveolar mucosa, soft palate, under surface of tongue and floor of the mouth.
  - This mucosa is non-keratinised and loosely attached.
  - It has a submucosa layer, which contains blood vessels and nerves.
  - Between the muscle layer and epithelium lay numerous minor salivary glands; sometimes these salivary ducts may become obstructed and a **mucocele** may develop.
- **Masticatory mucosa:**
  - This covers the hard palate and gingiva.
  - This mucosa has to withstand the friction of mastication; it is keratinised and firmly attached to the underlying bone.

  - A layer of connective tissue lies between the masticatory mucosa and bone and the submucosa layer is absent.
- **Specialised mucosa:**
  - This covers the dorsum of the tongue.
  - It is keratinised and contains special taste receptors.

Muscular tissue

Muscle develops from mesodermal tissue and is specialised tissue in that it has both the ability to contract and the ability to conduct electrical impulses. Muscles are classified both functionally as either voluntary or involuntary and structurally as either striated or smooth.

There are therefore three types of muscles:

- Smooth involuntary muscle (e.g. intestinal).
- Striated voluntary muscle (e.g. skeletal).
- Striated involuntary muscle (e.g. cardiac).

All the oral musculature consists of striated voluntary muscle. The cells are cylindrical, unbranched and multinucleate. They contain actin and myosin which are contractile proteins. The cells are arranged in bundles (fascicles) surrounded by connective tissue which also serves to anchor the muscle to bone in the form of a tendon.

Glandular tissue

The most important glands of the oral cavity are the salivary glands. The principal salivary glands are the **parotid** (situated buccal to the upper molars), **submandibular** and **sublingual** (located in the floor of the mouth). There are in addition a number of minor salivary glands on the surface of the tongue, the internal surfaces of the lips and in the buccal mucosa.

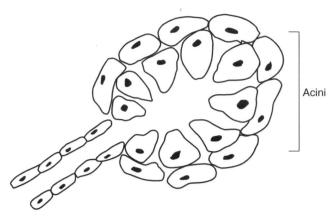

Figure 1.10 Diagram of secretory cells of salivary gland.

Production of saliva

- Each gland is made up of lobules, which resemble a bunch of grapes.
- The basic secretory units of salivary glands are clusters of cells called **acini** (Figure 1.10).
- These acinous epithelial cells consist of two types; serous cells which secrete a watery fluid low in mucous and mucous cells producing a glycoprotein (mucin) rich secretion.
- The serous cells are polyhedral in shape and produce a thin watery secretion.
- The mucous cells are cuboidal and produce a viscous secretion containing mucin.
- When mixed, the serous cells form a cap (demilune) around the periphery of the mucous cells.
- The parotid glands produce a serous secretion, the submandibular produce a mixture of serous and mucous and the sublingual glands produce a mainly mucous secretion.
- Secretion is under the control of the autonomic nervous system which controls both the volume and type of saliva produced.
- Saliva passes through the intercalated ducts, then the striated ducts and finally passes through the excretory ducts carrying the saliva to the oral cavity.

Constituents of saliva

The composition of saliva is subject to individual variation. It consists of 99.5% water and 0.5% dissolved substances that are made up of:

- **Salivary proteins**: these include:
  - **Glycoproteins (mucoids)**: lubricate oral tissues; the acquired pellicle provides tooth protection.
  - **Enzyme amylase**: converts starch to maltose.
  - **Lactoferrins**: ferric iron is an essential microbial nutrient; lactoferrins bind to ferric ions producing an antibacterial effect.
  - **Lysozomes**: attack the cell walls of bacteria protecting the oral cavity from invading pathogens.
  - **Silaloperoxidase (lactoperoxidase)**: controls established oral flora by controlling bacterial metabolism.
  - **Histatins**: inhibit *Candida albicans*.
  - **Statherin**: inhibits precipitation of calcium phosphates.
  - **Proline-rich proteins**: encourages adhesion of selected bacteria to the tooth surface. They inhibit precipitation of calcium phosphates.
  - **Salivary immunoglobulins**: produce protective antibodies which help to prevent infection.
- **Inorganic ions**: bicarbonate and phosphate ions provide a buffering action, which regulates the pH of the oral cavity. Calcium and phosphate ions maintain the integrity of teeth by providing minerals for newly erupted teeth, which helps with the posteruptive maturation of enamel and prevents tooth dissolution by enhancing the remineralisation of enamel. Small amounts of sodium, potassium, chloride, and sulphate can also be found in saliva.
- **Gases formed**: newly formed saliva contains dissolved oxygen, carbon dioxide and nitrogen.
- **Other additives**: urea is formed as a waste product. Saliva also contains a vast number of microorganisms and remnants of food substances.

Bone

Bone is a specialised form of dense connective tissue. Two types of bone can be distinguished:

- **Compact (cortical or lamellar) bone:** forms the outer layer of all bones and consists almost entirely of extracellular substance (**matrix**). It is built up of numerous vascular canals (**Haversian canals**) running along the long axis of the bone around which bone is deposited by **osteoblasts** in a series of concentric layers (**lamellae**) As the matrix is deposited, the osteoblasts become trapped in small hollows (**lacunae**) and cease to be active in laying down bone and become **osteocytes** (Figure 1.11). Osteocytes have several thin processes, which extend from the lacunae into small channels within the bone matrix (**canaliculi**).Compact bone is surrounded by a layer of dense connective tissue, the **periosteum**.
- **Trabecular bone (cancellous or spongy bone)**: consists of delicate bars and sheets of bone (trabeculae), which branch and intersect to form a sponge like network but there are no Haversian systems.

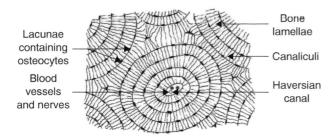

Figure 1.11 Cross-section of compact bone. Reproduced by kind permission of R. Ireland.

Bone is subject to constant remodelling by osteoblastic and osteoclastic (bone destroying) activity. The bone tissue of the maxilla is more vascular and less dense than that of the mandible.

Histology of dental tissues

Dentine

Physical characteristics of dentine

- Dentine is mineralised tissue forming the bulk of the tooth.
- It underlies the enamel in the crown area and is covered by the cementum in the root area.
- Dentine is pale yellow in colour and is harder than bone and cementum but not as hard as enamel.

Chemical composition of dentine

- 70% inorganic material (by weight) of which the main inorganic component is hydroxyapatite $[Ca_{10}(PO_4)_6(OH)_2]$.
- 20% organic material (by weight). The main organic component is collagen fibres embedded in amorphous ground substance.
- 10% water (by weight).

Structure of dentine

- Dentine consists of many dentinal tubules that run parallel to each other following a double curved course and extend from the pulp to the amelodentinal junction.
- Each dentinal tubule contains an odontoblast process surrounded by intercellular ground substance composed of fine collagenous fibrils.
- The odontoblast cells are a layer of closely arranged cells on the pulpal surface of the dentine with their nuclei situated at the basal (pulpal) end of each cell.

Features of dentine

The following features of dentine are significant:

- **Peritubular dentine**: this is highly mineralised dentine found within each dentinal tubule surrounding the odontoblast process and can be visualised as similar to 'furred' pipes.
- **Interglobular dentine**: these are areas of dentine that remain unmineralised.
- **Incremental lines**: these are produced due to the rhythmic pattern of dentinogenesis often referred as **contour lines of Owen**. These lines are seen when dentinogenesis is disrupted (as with amelogenesis).
- **Neonatal line**: this is only seen in primary teeth and first permanent molars as a line that marks dentine formation before and after birth.
- **Granular layer of Tomes**: this is a narrow layer of granular dentine found in root dentine immediately beneath the cementum.

Age changes in dentine

Secondary dentine

Dentine is a living tissue and with age more dentine continues to form slowly; this dentine is termed **secondary dentine**. Secondary dentine is laid down at the pulpal end of the primary dentine. As a result of this the pulp chamber reduces in size with age.

Peritubular dentine

Peritubular dentine tends to increase with age reducing the diameter of the dentinal tubules.

Translucent/sclerotic dentine

The tubules may also become completely obliterated and when this happens the dentine becomes more translucent; this is termed translucent or **sclerotic dentine**.

Reparative dentine

Reparative dentine or irregular secondary dentine is laid down on the pulpal surface of the dentine in response to an external stimulus, such as caries, cavity preparation or excessive wear. Following a severe stimulus, the odontoblast process may be destroyed and the contents of the tubule then necrose leaving the dentinal tubule empty; this is termed a **dead tract**.

Dentine hypersensitivity

There are many theories for the mechanism of dentine sensitivity. The principal current theories are:

- **Innervation theory**: the nerve fibres of the pulp pass into the dentinal tubules.
- **Odontoblast receptor theory**: the odontoblasts act as a receptor transmitting nerve impulses.
- **Brännström's hydrodynamic theory**: this suggests that there is movement of fluid within the dentinal tubules.

Enamel

Physical characteristics of enamel

- Enamel is highly mineralised and is the hardest tissue in the body.

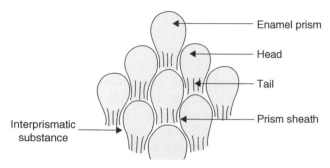

Figure 1.12 Diagram of magnified appearance of enamel prisms.

- Enamel covers the anatomical crown of the tooth and varies in thickness.
- It is semi-translucent and its colour can vary from bluish white to hues of yellow.

Chemical composition of enamel

- 96–97% inorganic material (by weight), the main inorganic component being hydroxyapatite.
- 1% organic material (by weight), the main organic component being protein.
- 2–3% water (by weight)

Structure of enamel

- Enamel is made up of millions of enamel prisms or rods, which run from the amelodentinal junction to the enamel surface.
- Each prism is made up of a large number of enamel crystallites.
- When viewed under a light microscope each prism resembles the rounded 'head' portion of a keyhole (Figure 1.12).
- The enamel crystallites run parallel to the long axis of the prism and in the 'tail' portion the enamel crystallites are inclined away from the long axis of the enamel prism.

Enamel is laid down in layers which produce **incremental growth lines**. After each successive layer the ameloblasts retreat so as not to be trapped within their matrix. Some growth lines mark daily deposits which are about 4 µm thick; these are called **cross striations**.

Features of enamel

The following features of enamel are significant:

- **Brown striae of Retzius:** these are brown lines indicating variations in weekly deposits that run obliquely from the amelodentinal junction towards the enamel surface. When the striae emerge onto the enamel surface a series of grooves may be seen; these are termed **perikymata** grooves.
- **Hunter–Schreger bands:** when viewed under a light microscope, broad dark and light bands can be seen

running obliquely from the amelodentinal junction to two-thirds of the thickness of the enamel. They are curved with the convexity of the curve always facing rootwards.

- **Neonatal line:** since this line marks the disruption in amelogenesis at birth, it can only be seen in primary teeth and first permanent molars. It can provide an important forensic landmark.
- **Enamel spindles:** this is when the dentinal tubules extend into the enamel and are found most frequently beneath cusps.
- **Lamellae:** these are sheets like faults that run vertically through the entire thickness of the enamel.
- **Enamel tufts:** these are pieces of incomplete mineralised enamel that resemble tufts of grass. They extend from the amelodentinal junction and follow the direction of the enamel prisms.
- **Amelodentinal junction:** the enamel and dentine meet at the amelodentinal junction; this junction has a scalloped appearance.

Cementum
Physical characteristics of cementum

- Cementum is a pale yellow calcified tissue covering the root dentine.
- It is softer than dentine and can easily be worn away resulting in exposure of the dentine.
- Its thickness varies according to location; it is thickest towards the apical third of the root and thinnest cervically.

Chemical composition of cementum

- 65% by weight inorganic (mainly hydroxyapatite).
- 23% organic (mainly collagen).
- 2% water.

Structure of cementum

Cementum has a similar structure to bone. It may be classified by the presence or absence of cells:

- **Acellular cementum:** it is the first cementum to form and is sometimes termed **primary cementum**. It covers the root dentine from the cement-enamel junction to near the root apex and does not contain cells.
- **Cellular cementum:** this is found as a thin layer at the apical third of the tooth. It is sometimes termed secondary cementum. As cellular cementum develops, the **cementoblasts** that have created the cementum become embedded within the cementum matrix and become inactivated; these cells are termed **cementocytes**. Cementocytes are contained in lacunae and their tiny processes spread along canaliculi to join up

with other cementocytes. Their processes are directed towards the periodontal ligament, from which they obtain nutrients.

Features of cementum

The following features of cementum are significant:

- **Cementoenamel junction**: this can be variable. In approximately 60% of teeth the cementum overlaps the enamel: in approximately 30% of teeth the cementum and enamel meet exactly and in approximately 10% of teeth the cementum and enamel do not meet thus leaving an area of dentine exposed.
- **Functional changes of cementum**: cementum formation continues throughout life. The attachment of the periodontal fibres in cementum can alter according to the functional needs of the tooth. Movement of teeth during orthodontic treatment or eruption can result in the periodontal fibres becoming re-arranged and re-attached in a new position.
- **Resorption of cementum**: resorption of the cementum is not fully understood; it can affect individual or groups of teeth. Resorption of cementum occurs when teeth are placed under excessive masticatory stress or orthodontic loading.
- **Hypercementosis:** hypercementosis is an increased thickening of cellular cementum. Chronic periapical inflammation around the apex of a root or excessive occlusal attrition may give rise to localised hypercementosis. Hypercementosis affecting all the teeth may be associated with Paget's disease.
- **Ankylosis**: ankylosis is a term used when the cementum of a tooth is fused with the alveolar bone of the tooth socket.
- **Concrescence: is** used to describe when two teeth are fused together by cementum.

Dental pulp

The dental pulp is what remains after dentine formation. It is surrounded by dentine and is contained in a rigid compartment.

Functions of pulp

The dental pulp has the following functions:

- At late bell stage the cells at the periphery of the pulp differentiate into odontoblasts forming dentine.
- It provides nutrients to the odontoblasts
- It acts as a sensory organ especially when dentine is exposed. The pulp rapidly responds to stimuli such as caries and attrition by laying down reparative or reactionary dentine.
- It mobilises defence cells when bacteria enter it.

- Cells proliferating in the pulpal tissue create pressure; this is thought to play a part in tooth eruption

Shape and form

Pulp is a soft vascular connective tissue occupying the centre of the tooth. The shape of the pulp approximately follows the shape of the outer surface of the tooth. The pulp is made up of a pulp chamber in the crown and root canals extending the length of the root. The shape and number of root canals can vary considerably. At the apex of each root is a foramen or foramina through which blood vessels, nerves and lymphatics pass. Small projections of the pulp are found under each cusp, these are known as pulp horns or **cornua**.

Cellular structure

- The pulp has a gelatinous consistency containing cells and intercellular substances.
- Odontoblasts can be found at the periphery of the pulp.
- At the time of eruption, a cell-free zone known as the **basal layer of Weil** often develops beneath the odontoblasts and deep to this zone can be found a cell-rich zone which contains a plexus of capillaries and nerves.
- Fibroblast cells are very numerous within the pulp and function to produce collagen. Defence cells (histiocytes) or fixed macrophages are the main defence cells found within the pulp.
- When the pulp is inflamed, histiocytes become free macrophages. Polymorphonuclear leucocytes can also be found in response to inflammation.

Intercellular substances

The intercellular substances consist of fibres and amorphous ground substance, blood vessels and nerves.

- Collagen fibres are scattered throughout the pulp and provide support to the pulpal tissue.
- The amorphous ground substance is a gelatinous substance that gives the pulp its shape.
- The pulp has a very rich supply of blood. Arterioles enter the pulp through the apical foramen and then ascend towards the crown area giving off several branches which anastomose (join together) with other arterioles. The arterioles terminate in a dense capillary plexus under the odontoblasts and drain into venules; these leave the pulp through the apical foramen.
- Both non-myelinated and myelinated nerve fibres enter the pulp through the apical foramen and generally follow the blood vessels.
- When the nerve fibres ascend towards the crown area they branch towards the periphery of the pulp and subdivide forming a network of fibres known as the **plexus of Raschkow** just beneath the cell free layer of

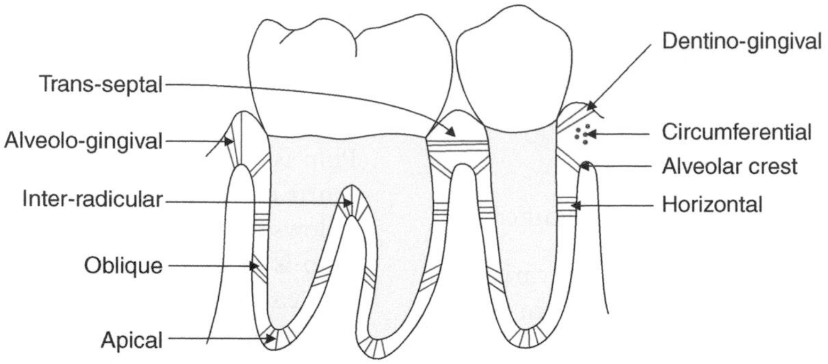

Figure 1.13 Gingival fibre groups of the periodontal membrane. Reproduced by kind permission of R. Ireland.

Weil. Some fibres cross the cell free layer of Weil passing through the odontoblasts and pre-dentine layer and enter the dentinal tubules.

Age changes

The primary changes are:

- A reduction in volume due to continuing dentine formation throughout life.
- A change in content resulting in more collagen, a reduced cellular content and a reduced nerve supply making the pulp less sensitive. Irregular calcifications (pulp stones) can be found but have little clinical significance except when undertaking root canal therapy.

Periodontal ligament

The periodontal ligament is a specialised fibrous connective tissue that surrounds the root area of the tooth. It consists mainly of collagenous fibres.

Function of the periodontal ligament

- It provides a support mechanism for the tooth; it cushions teeth against excessive occlusal forces preventing damage to the blood vessels and nerves at the root apex.
- It maintains the functional position of a tooth by keeping the teeth in contact and prevents the tooth from drifting or tilting
- The periodontal fibres undergo continuous change. Its cells form, maintain and repair the alveolar bone and cementum.
- Sensors in the periodontal ligament provide proprioceptive input, detecting pressures on the tooth
- The periodontal ligament has a rich supply of blood, which provides nutrients to the cementoblasts.

Structure of the periodontal ligament

- The predominant cells found within the periodontal ligament are fibroblasts. Cementoblasts cover the surface of the cementum and osteoblasts and osteoclasts cover the surface of alveolar bone.

- Remnants of the disintegrated Hertwig's root sheath remain into adult life and can be found between the collagen fibres of the periodontal ligament. They are known as the **epithelial cell rests of Malassez**.
- The blood supply runs along the long axis of the tooth close to the wall of the socket between the principal fibre bundles. Branches are given off forming a network of capillaries that encircles the tooth.
- The nerves follow the pathway of the blood vessels. Two types of nerve fibres are present: sensory nerve fibres responsible for pain and pressure and autonomic nerve fibres running alongside blood vessels and controlling the blood supply.

The periodontal ligament is made up of two groups of fibres, the gingival fibre groups and the principal fibre groups (Figure 1.13).

The gingival fibre groups of the periodontal ligament

- **Dentinogingival fibres** (free gingival fibres) are attached to the cementum and fan out into the gingival tissue.
- **Trans-septal fibres** run horizontally from the cervical area of one tooth to the adjacent tooth.
- **Alveologingival fibres** arise from the alveolar crest and run coronally into the attached and free gingiva.
- **Circumferential fibres** (**circular**) encircle the neck of the tooth.
- **Alveolar crest fibres** run from the cervical cementum to the alveolar crest.

The principal fibre groups of the periodontal ligament

These are:

- **Oblique fibres**, which run obliquely from alveolar bone to tooth.
- **Apical fibres**, which radiate from the apex of the tooth to the adjacent alveolar bone.

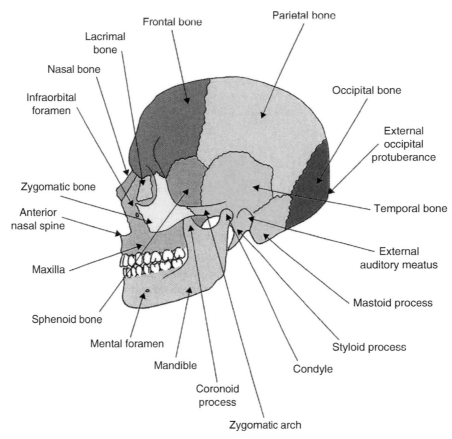

Figure 1.14 Bones of the skull. Reproduced by kind permission of R. Ireland.

Table 1.3 Bones of the cranium and facial region.

Cranium	Number	Facial region	Number
Frontal	1	Mandible	1
Ethmoid	1	Vomer	1
Occipital	1	Maxilla	2
Sphenoid	1	Palatal	2
Parietal	2	Zygomatic	2
Temporal	2	Nasal	2
		Lacrimal	2
		Inferior concha	2
Total	**8**	**Total**	**14**

- **Horizontal fibres**, which run horizontally from the cementum to the adjacent alveolar bone.
- **Inter-radicular fibres**, which are found between the roots of multi-rooted teeth and run from the root to the adjacent alveolar bone.

Oral anatomy

The skull

The skull consists of the bones of the cranium and the facial region (Figure 1.14).

Cranium

The **cranium** houses and protects the brain It consists of eight distinct bones which are joined together by sutures in the adult (Table 1.3).

Facial region

The **facial region** is made up of 14 separate bones, which include those that make up the jaws, cheeks and nose (Table 1.3).

The maxilla

The maxilla accommodates the upper dentition and forms the upper jaw. It is largely hollow because of the presence of the large **maxillary sinus** and consists of a roughly four-sided pyramidal body and four processes:

- The **frontal process** projects upwards and helps to form the lateral border of the nasal aperture and joins the frontal bone of the skull.
- The **zygomatic process** joins the zygomatic bone.
- The **horizontal palatine processes** from both maxillae form the anterior part of the hard palate. The horizontal plates of the palatine bone form the posterior part of the hard palate. The following foramina

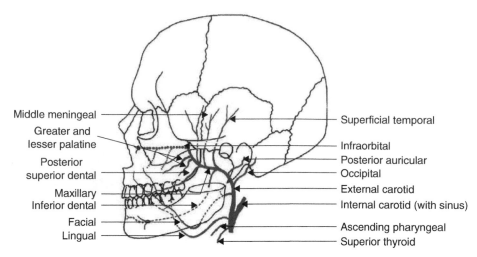

Middle meningeal
Greater and lesser palatine
Posterior superior dental
Maxillary
Inferior dental
Facial
Lingual

Superficial temporal
Infraorbital
Posterior auricular
Occipital
External carotid
Internal carotid (with sinus)
Ascending pharyngeal
Superior thyroid

Figure 1.15 The arterial supply to the anterior part of the head. Reproduced by kind permission of R. Ireland.

can be found on the hard palate – the incisive foramen located at midline behind the central incisors through which pass the nasopalatine nerve and artery, the greater and lesser palatine foramina can be found on the posterior part of the hard palate through which pass the greater and lesser palatine nerve and artery.

- The curved **alveolar process** projects downwards and contains the sockets of the maxillary teeth.

An orbital plate forms the base of the orbit. On the anterior surface below the lower border of the orbit is the **infraorbital foramen** through which passes the infraorbital nerve and artery.

The mandible

Outer surface of the mandible

- The mandible has a horseshoe shaped body which extends upwards and backwards into the ramus.
- The ramus has two processes; the posterior **condylar process** which forms part of the temporomandibular joint and the **anterior coronoid process** to which the temporal muscle is attached.
- Anteriorly there is a triangular prominence near the midline called the **mental protuberance**.
- The **mental foramen**, through which the mental nerve and artery pass, is located buccally between the first and second premolars.
- Just posterior to the mental foramen can be found the **external oblique line** which gives attachment to the buccinator muscle.

Inner surface of the mandible (lingual)

- Anteriorly at the midline close to the lower border is a roughened oval depression called the **digastric fossa**, which is the area of attachment of the anterior belly of the digastric muscle.

- Also at the midline can be found the superior genial tubules, which provide attachment for the genioglossus muscle and the inferior genial tubules, which provide attachment for the geniohyoid muscle.
- There is a crest, the **mylohyoid line**, on the lingual surface extending from the third molar diagonally downwards and forwards from which the mylohyoid muscle takes its origin,
- Just below the mylohyoid line is a depression called the submandibular fossa which accommodates the submandibular salivary gland.
- Above the mylohyoid line anteriorly is the sublingual fossa which accommodates the sublingual salivary gland.
- In the centre of the inner surface of the ramus is the **mandibular foramen**, into which the inferior dental (alveolar) nerve and artery enter the inferior dental canal.
- Anteriorly to the mandibular foramen is a small projection of bone called the lingula which gives attachment to the sphenomandibular ligament.

Arterial supply to the oral region

The right and left common carotid arteries form the main blood supply to the head and neck. They ascend to the thyroid cartilage where they divide into the internal and external carotid arteries (Figure 1.15).

The internal carotid artery

The internal carotid artery enters the cranium through the carotid canal to supply the eye and the brain.

The external carotid artery

This has the following branches:

- **Superior thyroid artery:** this is the first branch of the external carotid artery and supplies the thyroid gland.

- **Ascending pharyngeal artery**: this supplies the pharyngeal wall.
- **Lingual artery**: this branch is given off at the level of the mandible; it enters the base of the tongue and divides into the sublingual, the dorsal lingual and the deep lingual arteries. The sublingual artery supplies the lingual gingiva, floor of the mouth and the sublingual salivary gland. The dorsal lingual artery supplies the posterior aspect of the tongue, pharyngeal surface and palatine tonsil. The deep lingual artery supplies the tip of the tongue.
- **Facial artery**: this branches off above the lingual artery to supply the superficial structures of the face. The facial artery has seven branches:
  - **Ascending palatine artery**: this supplies the soft palate. After giving off this branch, the facial nerve passes forwards and upwards entering the submandibular salivary gland. It then hooks around part of this salivary gland and the lower border of the mandible to emerge onto the face. At this point it gives off the submental artery.
  - **Submental artery**: this supplies the submandibular and sublingual salivary glands, adjacent muscles and skin area. After giving off this branch the facial artery runs obliquely across the face up to the medial corner of the eye, giving off the following branches:
  - **Inferior labial artery**: this supplies the lower lip
  - **Superior labial artery**: this supplies the upper lip
  - **Lateral nasal artery**: this supplies the skin and muscles of the nose.
  - **Angular artery**: this supplies the eyelids
  - **Supraorbital artery**: this supplies the forehead area.
- **Occipital artery**: this supplies the occipital scalp area.
- **Posterior auricular artery**: this branch is given off at the level of the ear lobe and supplies the outer ear and adjacent scalp area.
- **Superficial temporal artery**: this branch originates within the parotid gland; it supplies the parotid gland, masseter and temporalis muscles and the outer ear.
- **Maxillary artery**: the superficial temporal artery and the maxillary artery are the terminal branches of the external carotid. The maxillary artery is the largest and most complex branch supplying the deep structures of the face. The following branches are relevant to the oral cavity:
  - **Middle meningeal artery**: this artery enters the cranium through the foramen spinosum to supply the dura mater.
  - **Inferior dental artery**: this follows the same course as the inferior dental nerve. It enters the mandibular foramen to supply the mandibular molars and premolars. Just before the inferior dental artery enters the mandibular canal it gives off the mylohyoid branch that supplies the mylohyoid muscle. At the mental foramen area the inferior dental artery branches into two, the mental and incisive branches. The **mental branch** supplies the labial gingiva of mandibular anterior teeth, mucosa and skin of the lower lip and the chin. The **incisive branch** continues in the inferior dental canal to supply the mandibular anterior teeth.
  - **Posterior superior dental artery**: this supplies the maxillary molar teeth and adjacent buccal gingiva and maxillary sinus.
  - **Infraorbital artery**: this has two branches; the **middle superior dental** branch supplies the maxillary premolar teeth and adjacent buccal gingiva. The **anterior superior dental** branch supplies the maxillary canine, lateral and central teeth and adjacent buccal gingiva.
  - **Greater and lesser palatine arteries**: the greater palatine artery supplies the hard palate and the palatal gingiva. The lesser palatine artery supplies the soft palate.
  - **Nasopalatine artery**: this branches off the sphenopalatine artery and passes through the incisive foramen to join the greater palatine artery.
  - **Masseteric artery**: this supplies the masseter muscle.
  - **Temporal artery**: this supplies the temporalis muscle.
  - **Medial and lateral pterygoid arteries**: these supply the medial and lateral pterygoid muscles.
  - **Buccal artery**: supplies the cheek and buccinator muscle.

Venous drainage of the oral region

The venous drainage of the head and neck is almost entirely by branches of the internal jugular vein. The pathways of the veins are much more variable than the arteries and therefore their location is much less predictable. In addition there are numerous anastomoses with different veins.

The veins of the face are divided into superficial and deep veins.

Superficial veins

The superficial **temporal** and **facial** veins drain the superficial areas of the face.

The superficial temporal vein descends through the parotid gland and is joined by the maxillary vein to form the **retromandibular vein**. The retromandibular vein divides into posterior and anterior branches. The **posterior retromandibular vein** joins with the **posterior auricular vein** forming the **external jugular vein**. The anterior branch joins the facial vein forming the **common facial vein** draining into the internal jugular vein, which empties into the brachiocephalic vein.

Deep veins

The pterygoid plexus is a dense network of veins situated within the infratemporal fossa close to the lateral pterygoid muscle. This plexus drains the oral and nasal cavities and empties into the maxillary vein. The pterygoid plexus has direct communication with the cavernous sinuses within the cranium. Misplaced block local analgesic injections can penetrate this plexus and may result in a haematoma (bleeding into the tissues). Infections from the oral cavity may also track to the brain via this route.

Nerve supply of the oral region

The nervous system of the body is made up of the central nervous system (CNS – the brain and spinal cord) and the peripheral nervous system (PNS). The PNS is further subdivided into the sensory–somatic nervous system, consisting of 12 pairs of cranial nerves and 31 pairs of spinal nerves, and the autonomic nervous system which has nerve fibres running between the CNS and various internal organs (e.g. heart, lungs and salivary glands). The autonomic nervous system is further subdivided into the sympathetic nervous system (prepares the body for flight or fright by the release of acetyl choline and norepinephrine (noradrenaline)) and the parasympathetic nervous system (reverses the changes induced by the sympathetic nervous system).

The 12 pairs of cranial nerves arise directly from the brain. They are either:

- **Sensory**: they contain sensory (afferent) nerve fibres, which transmit stimuli such as pain, smell or visual images to the brain, e.g. the optic and ophthalmic nerves.
- **Motor**: these contain motor (efferent) nerve fibres and pass nerve impulses from the brain to muscles, e.g. the hypoglossal nerve.
- **Mixed**: as their name implies, contain both sensory and motor nerve fibres, e.g. the trigeminal, facial and glossopharyngeal nerves.

The 12 cranial nerves are:

I	Olfactory
II	Optic
III	Oculomotor
IV	Trochlear
V	Trigeminal
VI	Abducent
VII	Facial
VIII	Vestibulocochlear
IX	Glossopharyngeal
X	Vagus
XI	Accessory
XII	Hypoglossal

The trigeminal nerve – Vth cranial nerve

The trigeminal nerve is the main source of innervation for the oral cavity; it is the largest cranial nerve arising from the **pons**. At the **semilunar ganglion**, the trigeminal nerve divides into three divisions: the ophthalmic, the maxillary and the mandibular. It is the maxillary and mandibular divisions that innervate the teeth and their surrounding tissues.

Maxillary division

The maxillary nerve leaves the cranium through the **foramen rotundum** and enters the pterygopalatine fossa where it subdivides into three main branches, the zygomatic nerve, the pterygopalatine nerves and the infraorbital nerve.

- The **zygomatic nerve** enters the orbit through the inferior orbital fissure to supply sensory fibres to the zygomatic area of the face.
- The pterygopalatine ganglion gives rise to the **pterygopalatine nerves**, the nasopalatine, the greater palatine and the lesser palatine nerve. They supply the sensory fibres to the palatal mucosa of the hard palate and palatal gingiva. The **nasopalatine nerve** passes through the incisive foramen to supply the anterior region and the **greater palatine nerve** passes through the greater palatine foramen to supply the posterior premolar and molar regions. The **lesser palatine nerve** passes through the lesser palatine foramen to supply the soft palate.
- **The infraorbital nerve** enters the orbit through the inferior orbital fissure and passes along the infraorbital canal from where it finally emerges onto the face through the infraorbital foramen to supply the lower eyelid, the side of the nose and the upper lip. The infraorbital nerve gives off the superior alveolar nerve branches. These are:
  - The **posterior superior alveolar nerve**: this branch is given off just before the infraorbital nerve enters the canal. It passes downwards onto the posterior surface of the maxilla and enters very small canals that run above the tooth roots to supply sensory fibres to the maxillary third and second molar teeth and the distobuccal and palatal roots of the maxillary first molar. This nerve also supplies sensory fibres to the adjacent buccal gingiva and maxillary sinus.
  - The **middle superior alveolar nerve**: this is not always present. When it is, it arises from the infraorbital nerve within the infraorbital canal. It passes down the wall of the maxillary sinus to supply sensory fibres to the mesiopalatal root of the maxillary first molar and the first and second premolar teeth. This nerve also supplies sensory

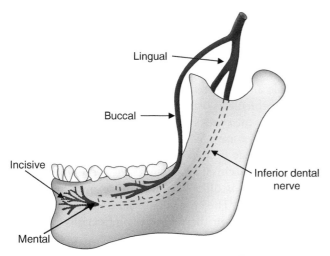

Figure 1.16 Diagram of the main branches of the mandibular nerve.

fibres to the adjacent buccal gingiva and maxillary sinus.

○ The **anterior superior alveolar nerve**: this arises from the infraorbital nerve just before it emerges through the infraorbital foramen. It passes downwards inside the maxillary antrum. It supplies sensory fibres to the maxillary central and lateral incisor and canine teeth and to the adjacent labial gingiva. It also supplies the maxillary sinus.

The branches of the superior dental nerves form a plexus above the apices of the maxillary teeth.

Mandibular division

The mandibular division is the largest division of the trigeminal nerve. It contains both motor and sensory fibres. It leaves the cranium through the **foramen ovale** and enters the infratemporal fossa, (deep to the lateral pterygoid muscle) where it gives off the following branches (Figure 1.16):

- **Nerves to the muscles of mastication**: these branches supply motor fibres to the masseter, temporalis and lateral pterygoid muscle.
- **Buccal nerve (long buccal)**: this nerve supplies sensory fibres to the mucosa and skin of the cheek and the buccal gingiva of the lower molar teeth.
- **Auriculotemporal nerve**: this branch supplies sensory fibres to the temporomandibular joint, the skin of the outer ear and temporal area. It also carries parasympathetic fibres derived from the glossopharyngeal nerve to the parotid gland.
- **Lingual nerve**: this branch supplies sensory fibres to the lingual gingiva of all the lower teeth, the anterior two-thirds of the tongue and the floor of the mouth. The chorda tympani branch of the facial nerve joins the

lingual nerve providing special taste fibres to the anterior two-thirds of the tongue. It also carries parasympathetic fibres to the submandibular ganglion to supply the submandibular and sublingual salivary glands.

- **Inferior dental (alveolar) nerve**: this nerve enters the inferior dental canal through the mandibular foramen. Just before it enters it gives off the **mylohyoid nerve** that supplies motor fibres to the mylohyoid muscle and the anterior belly of the digastric. Within the inferior dental canal, the inferior dental nerve gives off sensory fibres to the mandibular molars and premolars. At the mental foramen area the inferior dental nerve branches into the mental and incisive branch. The **mental branch** passes through the mental foramen to supply sensory fibres to the labial gingiva of mandibular anterior teeth, mucosa and skin of the lower lip and the chin. The **incisive branch** continues in the inferior dental canal to supply sensory fibres to the mandibular anterior teeth.

The facial nerve – VIIth cranial nerve

The facial nerve enters the internal auditory meatus and travels through the facial canal which is in the temporal bone. Within the facial canal it gives off the following branches (Figure 1.17):

- **Chorda tympani nerve**: this nerve joins the lingual nerve carrying special taste fibres to the anterior two-thirds of the tongue.
- **Greater petrosal nerve**: this nerve supplies parasympathetic fibres to the mucous membrane of the palate and nasal cavity.
- The facial nerve leaves the cranium through the stylomastoid foramen and gives off branches to the posterior belly of the digastric and stylohyoid muscle. It enters the parotid gland where it gives off five terminal branches: the **temporal, zygomatic, buccal, mandibular** and **cervical**. These branches supply motor fibres to the muscles of facial expression.

The glossopharyngeal nerve – IXth cranial nerve

The glossopharyngeal nerve leaves the cranium through the jugular foramen. It supplies sensory taste fibres to the posterior one-third of the tongue and sensory and motor fibres to the soft palate and pharynx. It also carries parasympathetic fibres to the auriculotemporal nerve and mandibular division of the trigeminal.

The hypoglossal nerve – XIIth cranial nerve

The hypoglossal nerve leaves the cranium through the hypoglossal canal. It supplies motor fibres to the intrinsic and extrinsic muscles of the tongue (except the palatoglossal muscle).

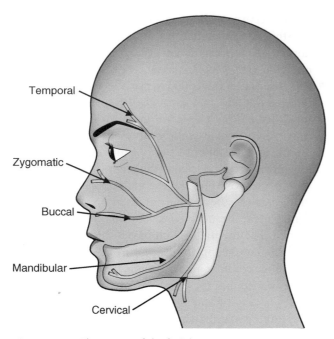

Figure 1.17 The course of the facial nerve.

Anatomy of the oral cavity

The oral cavity is bounded by the lips and cheeks anteriorly and it extends posteriorly to the palatoglossal and palatopharyngeal arches (pillars of the fauces). The hard palate forms the roof of the oral cavity and the floor of the mouth forms the floor, this space being occupied by the tongue. The oral cavity also contains the upper and lower alveolar ridges which house the teeth. The area between the lips and alveolar ridge and teeth is termed the **vestibular sulcus**.

The lips

The lips contain the orbicularis oris muscle. They are covered by skin externally and mucous membrane internally; where the external surface meets the internal surface a distinct line may be seen termed the **vermillion border**.

The external red border of the lips is termed the **vermillion zone**. A shallow depression extending from the midline of the nose to the centre of the upper lip is called the philtrum. The **nasolabial grooves** are shallow depressions extending from the corner of the nose to the corner of the lips. Between the lower lip and chin can be found a midline linear depression. This is called the **labiomental groove**.

The inner surface of the lip is tightly bound to connective tissue. At the midline, the upper and lower lips are attached to the alveolar ridges by a **labial fraenum**.

Cheeks

The bulk of the cheek is made up of the **buccinator muscle**, which is attached to the alveolar bone adjacent to the upper molar region, the external oblique line of the mandible and the **pterygomandibular raphe**; it inserts into the orbicularis oris muscle. The buccinator muscles give tone to the cheeks and play a part in mastication.

The cheeks are covered by skin externally and the internal surface is covered by non-keratinized mucosa, except at the occlusal level where it is keratinized; at the junction there is often a whitish horizontal line called the **linear alba**. The cheeks have numerous minor salivary glands and in the region of the maxillary second permanent molar the parotid duct (**Stensen's duct**) can be seen marked by the parotid papilla.

Floor of the mouth

The floor of the mouth is made up of the mylohyoid, genioglossus, geniohyoid and the digastric (anterior belly) muscles. The floor of the mouth is covered by non-keratinised mucosa.

The lingual fraenum connects the under surface of the tongue to the floor of the mouth. On either side on this fraenum can be found the submandibular salivary ducts (**Wharton's ducts**). The ducts of the sublingual glands are numerous and can be found along the sublingual folds or **plica sublingualis**.

The tongue

The tongue is a muscular organ that plays an important part in mastication, taste, cleansing, speech, deglutition, suckling and exploring.

The **inferior surface of the tongue** is covered by a thin non-keratinised mucosa which is continuous with the floor of the mouth. On either side of the lingual fraenum lie the fimbriated folds ('frilly' folds) of tissue. The deep lingual vein is also visible.

The **dorsum of the tongue** is divided into the anterior two-thirds that lie within the oral cavity and the posterior third that faces the pharynx (Figure 1.18). A 'V'-shaped groove termed the **sulcus terminalis** separates the anterior part from the posterior part. At the apex of the 'V' is a small pit called the **foramen caecum**. A median fibrous septum runs from the tip of the tongue dividing the tongue into two halves.

The anterior two thirds of the tongue are covered by specialised keratinised mucosa. Four types of papillae can be found on the surface:

- **Circumvallate papillae**: these vary from 10–14 and can be found immediately in front of the sulcus terminalis. They are the most conspicuous papillae being large mushroom shaped, 1–2 mm in diameter and surrounded by a trough. Within these troughs can be

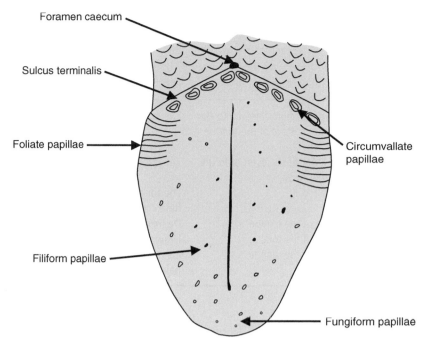

Figure 1.18 Diagram of the upper surface of the tongue.

Table 1.4 Intrinsic muscles of the tongue.

Intrinsic muscles of the tongue		
Muscle	Location	Function
Longitudinal fibres are grouped into superior and interior fibres	**Superior fibres**: found below the mucosa of the dorsum of the tongue, they run in an anterior–posterior direction from the tip of the tongue **Inferior fibres**: found at the base of the tongue they also run anterior–posterior direction	Contraction of the superior fibres causes the tip of the tongue to curl upwards and backwards Contraction of the inferior fibres pulls the tip of the tongue downwards When the inferior and superior fibres contract the tongue shortens in length
Transverse fibres	These fibres run horizontally from the fibrous septum to the borders of the tongue	Contraction narrows and increase the height of the tongue
Vertical fibres	These fibres run from the dorsum of the tongue to the under surface of the tongue	Contraction flattens and broadens the tongue

found taste buds and a special group of serous glands known as **Von Ebner's glands** which wash out these troughs.

- **Filiform papillae**: these are very numerous, conical elevations which create the rough texture of the tongue.
- **Fungiform papillae**: these are mushroom shaped, less numerous and can be seen as visible red dots at the tip and sides of tongue. They contain taste buds.
- **Foliate papillae**: found posteriorly along the lateral borders of the tongue, in parallel folds containing taste buds.

The posterior third of the tongue consists of lymphoid tissue covered by non-keratinized mucosa which has a nodular appearance.

Muscles of the tongue

The tongue consists of intrinsic muscles that alter the shape of the tongue and extrinsic muscles which move it to facilitate eating, swallowing and communication and originate from remote structures and insert into the tongue (Table.1.4).

A median fibrous septum divides the tongue into two halves, thus all the muscles are paired.

Table 1.5 Extrinsic muscles of the tongue.

Extrinsic muscles of the tongue			
Muscle	Point of origin	Point of insertion	Function
Genioglossus	Superior genial tubercle on the inner aspect of the mandible	Superior fibres insert into the under surface of the tongue	The superior fibres retract the tongue
		Inferior fibres insert onto the hyoid bone	The inferior fibres protrude the tongue when they contract
			The tongue is depressed when the superior and inferior fibres contract together
Hyoglossus	Hyoid bone	Side of the tongue	Depresses the dorsum of the tongue
Styloglossus	Styloid process	Side of the tongue	Draws the tongue upwards and backwards
Palatoglossus	Soft palate runs down the palatoglossal folds	Side of the tongue	Elevates the tongue to the palate and depresses the soft palate towards the tongue

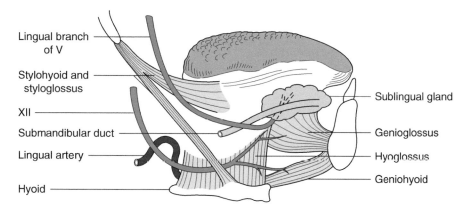

Figure 1.19 Diagram of the extrinsic muscles of the tongue. Reproduced with permission from Fiaz, O. and Moffat, D. Anatomy at a Glance, 2nd edn. Blackwell Publishing.

Extrinsic muscles

The extrinsic muscles of the tongue all have names ending in -*glossus* (Table 1.5 and Figure 1.19). Most of the muscles are innervated by the hypoglossal nerve (XIIth cranial nerve).

The palate

The palate separates the oral cavity from the nasal cavity. It is divided into the hard and soft palates.

Hard palate

The hard palate is lined with thick keratinised mucosa, which is tightly bound to the underlaying bone. Immediately behind the central incisors can be found the **incisive papilla**, an oval prominence overlaying the incisive foramen. Posterior to the incisive papilla is a midline ridge that extends vertically along the entire palate; this ridge is known as the **median palatine raphe**. Transverse ridges, the **palatine rugae**, radiate from the incisive papilla and the median palatine raphe.

At the junction where the hard palate meets the soft palate lie two small indentations in the midline; these are two small salivary ducts known as **palatine foveae**.

Soft palate

The soft palate extends backwards and downwards from the posterior aspect of the hard palate. It closes off the nasopharynx from the oropharynx during swallowing. The soft palate consists of a sheet of fibrous tissue covered by non-keratinised mucosa: in the midline a small conical projection called the **uvula** extends from the free edge of the soft palate. Laterally to the soft palate on each side can be found the **palatopharyngeal** and **palatoglossal arches**. Between these arches lies the **palatine tonsil**.

The gingivae

The gingivae are the part of the oral mucosa that surrounds the teeth and covers the adjacent alveolar bone and the oral mucosa. The detailed structure of the gingival tissues is described in Chapter 5.

Table 1.6 Functions of saliva.

Action	Function
Lubrication and protection	Keeps oral mucosa moist, prevents dehydration of oral mucosa, protects teeth and mucosa, acts as a barrier to irritants, aids speech, mastication and swallowing
Cleansing action	Assists in the self cleansing of oral cavity, clears loose particles of food
Taste	Dissolves substances into solution facilitating taste
Digestion	Contains enzyme amylase which converts starch into maltose
Buffering action	Helps neutralize plaque acids by increasing the pH of plaque
Maintaining water balance	Dehydration causes a reduction of saliva giving rise to dry mouth, encouraging individuals to drink
Antimicrobial action	specific immunoglobulins and antibacterial and antifungal mechanisms help to control oral microflora
Providing an ion reservoir	Saliva is saturated with inorganic ions preventing or reducing tooth dissolution. The ions also enhance remineralisation of enamel

The alveolar mucosa

The alveolar mucosa is loosely attached to the underlying bone, is non-keratinised and appears dark red. The **mucogingival junction**, or health line demarcates the attached gingiva from the alveolar mucosa.

The salivary glands

Salivary glands are compound **exocrine glands** (glands that discharge secretions, usually through a tube or a duct, onto a surface). They have special epithelial secretory cells that produce saliva. Saliva is produced by both major and minor salivary glands. The major glands are the parotid, submandibular and sublingual glands; the minor salivary glands are found throughout the oral cavity.

The functions of saliva are listed in Table 1.6.

- **Parotid gland**: this is the largest of the major salivary glands. It is located below and in front of each ear and lies on the surface of the masseter muscle. The parotid gland produces a pure serous secretion that enters the oral cavity through the parotid duct opposite the upper second molar tooth. The parotid gland is enclosed in a strong fibrous capsule. Several important structures pass through the parotid gland; namely the facial nerve, facial vein, external carotid and temporal vein. The parotid gland is supplied by the glossopharyngeal nerve.

- **Submandibular gland**: this lies in the submandibular fossa below the mylohyoid line on the inner aspect of the mandible. Part of the gland extends posteriorly around the free boarder of the mylohyoid muscle to lie above the mylohyoid muscle. The submandibular gland produces a mixture of serous and mucous secretions that enter the oral cavity though a small lingual papilla (**lingual caruncle**) on either side of the lingual fraenum. The submandibular gland is contained in a loose capsule through which passes the facial artery. Innervation is by the chorda tympani branch of the facial nerve and the lingual nerve.

- **Sublingual gland**: this is the smallest of the major salivary glands. It lies within the sublingual fossa on the inner aspect of the mandible above the mylohyoid muscle and below the sublingual folds. The sublingual gland produces a mixed secretion that is predominantly mucous, which enters the oral cavity through 8–20 small ducts (**plica sublingualis**) along the sublingual folds. The sublingual gland is not capsulated. The nerve supply is the same as for the submandibular gland.

The parotid glands receive their parasympathetic innervation from the glossopharyngeal nerve via the auriculotemporal nerve. The submandibular and sublingual glands receive their parasympathetic innervation from the chordae tympani, (branch of the facial nerve) via the lingual nerve and submandibular ganglion. The sympathetic nerve fibres are derived from superior cervical ganglion and follow the external carotid artery to reach the salivary glands.

Salivary flow

Both parasympathetic and sympathetic nerve fibres innervate the acini controlling the flow of saliva. The parasympathetic nerves fibres stimulate saliva production and the sympathetic nerve fibres increase the salivary composition and to some extent the salivary flow, however to a much lesser extent than the parasympathetic stimulation.

The salivary glands are capable of secreting approximately 0.5–0.6 litres of saliva per day. The normal adult unstimulated flow of saliva is between 0.3–0.4 ml per minute, of which approximately 25% comes from the parotid glands, 60% from the submandibular glands, 7–8% from the sublingual glands and 7–8% from the minor salivary glands. When stimulated, the flow can range from 1.5–2.0 ml per minute. A number of factors influence the flow rate (Table 1.7).

Table 1.7 Factors that influence saliva flow.

Decrease flow	Increase flow
Dehydration, loss of body fluids	Smoking
Position of body – lying down, sleep	Sight & smell of food
Exposure to light – saliva decreases in darkness	Vomiting
Side effects of drugs	Mastication
Fright/flight response	Taste
Sjögren's syndrome	
Radiotherapy to head and neck	

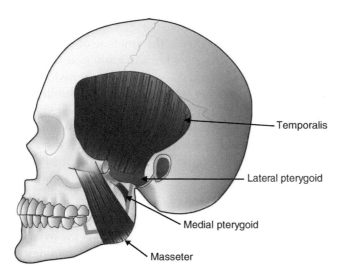

Figure 1.20 Diagram of the muscles of mastication.

Muscles of mastication

All of the muscles of mastication work together to perform a smooth co-ordinated series of movements of the mandible, they are innervated by the mandibular branch of the trigeminal nerve. The muscles of mastication can be seen in Figure 1.20; they are:

- **Temporalis**: an extensive fan-shaped muscle that covers the temporal region.
  Origin: superior and inferior temporal line of the parietal bone.
  Insertion: coronoid process and anterior border of the ramus of the mandible.
  Function: elevates and retracts the mandible. Mandibular condyles lead back to the glenoid fossa. This muscle is less powerful than the masseter.
- **Masseter**: a quadrangular muscle which has two heads deep and superficial.
  Origin: deep head is at the lower border of the zygomatic arch and the superficial head is at the zygoma.
  Insertion: lateral aspect of the ramus and the coronoid process of the mandible

Function: elevates and retracts the mandibular condyles back to the glenoid fossa. This combination is important in closing of the mandible
- **Medial pterygoid**: a thick, quadrilateral muscle that has two heads, deep and superficial
  Origin: deep head is at the medial surface of the lateral pterygoid plate and its superficial head is from the tuberosity of the maxilla.
  Insertion: the inner surface of the ramus and angle of the mandible.
  Function: It elevates, protrudes; and when only one (e.g. right) medial pterygoid contracts, it results in the mandible moving towards the opposite side (left).
- **Lateral pterygoid**: a conical muscle with its apex pointing posteriorly.
  Origin: It has two areas of origin the infratemporal surface of the greater wing of the sphenoid bone and the lateral surface of lateral pterygoid plate.
  Insertion: is into the articular disc and capsule of the temporomandibular joint and neck of the condyle.
  Function: Protrudes mandible important in opening mouth. Acts with medial pterygoid of same side (e.g. right) to move mandible to opposite side (left).
- **Digastric**: has an anterior and posterior part connected by a strong tendon.
  Origin: the posterior part originates from the mastoid notch medial to the mastoid process; it passes forward and downwards to the hyoid bone where it joins the anterior part via the tendon. The tendon passes through a fibrous sling attaching it to the hyoid bone.
  Insertion: the anterior part passes upwards and forwards to insert into the digastric fossa of the mandible.
  Function: Aids the opening movement.

The muscles of mastication move the mandible at the temporomandibular joint. This is not a simple hinge movement but a complex movement involving a combination of several different muscles.

The **buccinator**, although a muscle of facial expression, aids in maintaining the position of food within the oral cavity during chewing.

The temporomandibular joint

The temporomandibular joint (TMJ) is a double **synovial joint** consisting of the condylar process of the mandible articulating with the squamous portion of the temporal bone (Figure 1.21). A synovial joint is a joint made up of bone ends covered with cartilage, ligaments, a cavity filled with synovial fluid (joint fluid) and an outside fibrous capsule.

The articular joint surface of the temporal bone consists of a concave articular fossa and a convex articular eminence anterior to it. There is a fibrocartilaginous disc known as the **articular disc**; this disc is saddle-shaped and lies between the glenoid fossa and the condyle. The disc varies in thickness; the middle portion of the disc is thinner than the anteriorly and posteriorly portions. Posteriorly the disc is fused with the TMJ capsule and anteriorly it is attached to the lateral pterygoid muscle, dividing the joint into two distinctive compartments the upper and lower spaces. The upper joint space is bounded on the top by the articular fossa and the articular eminence. The lower joint space is bounded at the bottom by the condyle. The entire TMJ is enclosed in a fibrous capsule, the inner aspect of this capsule is lined with synovial membrane; this produces synovial fluid, which provides lubrication and nutrients to the TMJ.

The fibrous capsule is strengthened by the temporomandibular ligament, which runs from the articular eminence to the neck of the condyle. The sphenomandibular and stylomandibular ligaments limit excessive movements of the TMJ during mastication. The sphenomandibular ligament runs from the spine of the sphenoid to the mandibular lingula and the stylomandibular ligament runs from the styloid process of the temporal bone to the angle of the mandible.

The two movements that occur at this joint are forward gliding and a hinge-like rotation. When the jaw opens, the head of the mandible and articular disc move forwards on the articular surface. As this forward gliding movement occurs, the head of the mandible rotates on the lower surface of the articular disc. The disc serves to cushion and distribute the loading on the joint and provide stability during chewing. Tooth clenching (parafunction) or an alteration to the occlusal surfaces of the teeth such as due to an incorrectly contoured restoration, can initiate stresses in the joint which may lead to pain or dysfunction.

Muscles of facial expression

The muscles of the face are collectively known as the muscles of facial expression. (Figure 1.22) They are responsible for facial expressions and also they aid speech and chewing and are of importance to musicians. They are a large group of superficial muscles, which have their insertion into the skin and not the bone; they are innervated by the facial nerve.

The **orbicularis oris** muscle controls the opening of the mouth and other muscles radiate outwards from the orbicularis oris to move the lips or the angles of the mouth, these are:

- **Risorius** – draws the angles of the mouth sideways as in a grin.
- **Zygomaticus** – pulls the upper lip upwards and laterally.

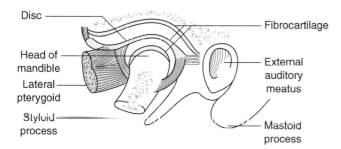

Figure 1.21 Diagram of the temporomandibular joint. Reproduced with permission from Fiaz, O. and Moffat, D. Anatomy at a Glance, 2nd edn. Blackwell Publishing.

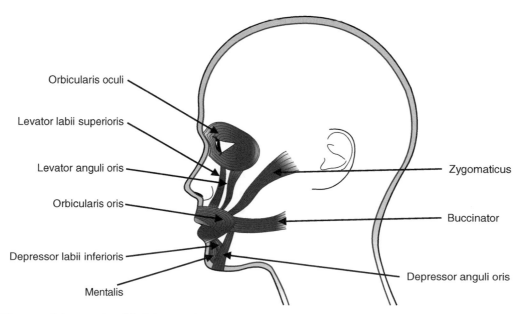

Figure 1.22 Diagram of the muscles of facial expression.

- **Levator anguli oris** – raises the angles of the mouth as in a smile.
- **Levator labii superioris** – raises the upper lip.
- **Mentalis** – turns the lower lip outwards as in pouting, wrinkles the skin of chin.
- **Depressor labii inferioris** – depresses and inverts the lower lip.
- **Depressor anguli oris** – depresses the angles of the mouth giving a sad appearance.

During chewing, the **buccinator** muscle works in conjunction with the masticatory muscles, by keeping the bolus of food on the occlusal surfaces of teeth. In infants, the buccinator provides suction for suckling at the breast.

Tooth morphology

During our life time we develop two dentitions: a primary dentition (deciduous) and a permanent dentition. The primary dentition consists of 20 teeth and the permanent dentition consists of 32 teeth. Teeth are arranged in maxillary (upper) and mandibular (lower) dental arches each arch is divided into left and right. There are four types of teeth: incisors, canines, premolars and molar teeth. Each primary tooth is recorded as a letter A, B, C, D and E and each permanent tooth is numbered from 1–8. (See Tables 1.1 and 1.2.)

Differences between primary and permanent teeth can be found in Chapter 12 Paediatric Dentistry.

Tooth identification

The main factors to look for when identifying teeth is size, shape, roots and colour.

A good understanding of the following terminology is essential (Table 1.8).

The permanent teeth (Figure 1.23a)
Permanent incisors
Identifying features of the maxillary permanent central incisor
Crown
This is the largest of all permanent incisors.

Labial surface
- Labial surface is convex with two faint grooves running vertically onto incisal edge to produce three small protuberances called **mamelons** (only seen in newly erupted teeth).
- Mesial surface straight and the mesial incisal edge is almost a right angle.
- Distal incisal edge is more rounded.

Table 1.8 Tooth identification terminology.

	Terminology
Mesial surface	Surfaces of teeth facing the midline
Distal surface	Surfaces of teeth faces away from midline
Lingual surface	Surfaces of teeth adjacent to the tongue
Palatal surface	Surfaces of teeth adjacent to the palate
Buccal surface	Surfaces of posterior teeth adjacent to the cheek (premolars and molars)
Labial surface	Surfaces of anterior teeth adjacent to the lip (incisors and canines)
Occlusal surface	Biting surface of posterior teeth
Incisal edge	Cutting edge of anterior teeth
Apex	Tip of the root
Bifurcation	Where a root divides into two
Cervical margin	The junction where the anatomical crown and anatomical root meet
Cingulum	Bulbous convex area found in the cervical third on palatal and lingual surfaces of anterior teeth.
Concave	Curved inwards making a depression
Contact area	An area where the crown of two adjacent teeth meet.
Convex	Curved outwards.
Fissure	A shallow groove found on the occlusal surfaces between the cusps
Fossa	A shallow rounded depression in a surface of a tooth
Marginal ridge	A ridge of enamel at the mesial and distal edges of a tooth.
Oblique ridge	A ridge of enamel running obliquely a cross the occlusal surface
Pit	Small pin point depression found in enamel
Transverse ridge	A ridge of enamel crossing the occlusal surface

Palatal surface
- Triangular in shape, concave in all directions producing the palatal fossa.
- Pronounced marginal ridges mesial and distal, which meet at a prominence called the **cingulum.**

Root
- Single root about 1½ times length of crown.
- The apex of the root frequently curves distally

Identifying features of the maxillary permanent lateral incisor
Crown
- Similar in form to the central incisors except it is much smaller. The crown can vary in shape.

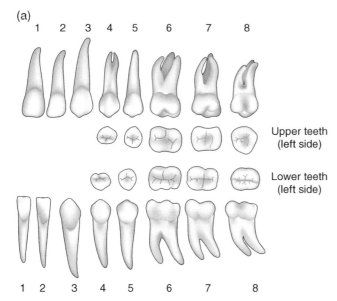

Figure 1.23a Upper and lower permanent teeth.

Labial surface

- More convex than the central incisors, mamelons and vertical grooves less prominent.
- Mesial incisal angle is sharper and distal incisal corner is more rounded than the central incisor.

Palatal surface

- Is triangular in form with rounded edges.
- Pronounced palatal fossa
- Often has a small pit where the marginal ridge meets the cingulum (**foramen caecum incisivum**).

Root

Single root, mesial and distal surfaces are flattened and grooved.

The apex of the root frequently curves distally.

Identifying features of the mandibular permanent central incisor
Crown

- Smallest tooth in the permanent dentition.

Labial surface

- Convex in cervical third and flattens out towards the incisal third.
- Mesial and distal incisal edge at right angles.
- Incisal edge has mamelons on newly erupted.

Lingual surface

- Is smooth and featureless, marginal ridges and cingulum being less developed.
- The crown is narrower on the lingual surface than the labial.

Root

- Single root, mesial and distal surface grooved, the distal groove being more marked.
- The apex of the root frequently curves distally.

Identifying features of the mandibular lateral permanent incisor
Crown

- Very similar to the lower central incisor. Crown appears fan shaped.

Labial surface

- The incisal edge mesiodistally is wider than the lower central and it follows the curve of the lower arch.
- Mesial side of crown is slightly longer than the distal.
- Distal incisal angle is rounded than the sharp mesial incisal angle.

Lingual surface

- Cingulum is off-centre to the distal, faint mesial and distal marginal ridges.

Root

- Single root.
- Crown of the lateral incisor tends to tilt distally on root, crown appears slightly askew.
- Mesial and distal surface grooved, the distal groove being more marked.
- The apex of the root frequently curves distally

Permanent canines
Identifying feature of the maxillary permanent canine
Crown
Labial surface

- Crown irregular diamond shape, convex in all directions.
- Incisal edge has a large pointed cusp. The distal slope of the cusp is longer than the mesial slope.
- Distal profile of crown more rounded than the mesial.
- The tip of the cusp is placed centrally in line with the long axis of the tooth.

Palatal surface

- Concave apart from a prominent convex cingulum.
- A vertical ridge runs from the cingulum to the tip of the cusp, on each side of this ridge is a depression (mesial and distal palatal fossae).
- The marginal ridges are also very prominent.

Root

- Single root, twice the length of the crown and the longest root of the permanent dentition.

- Mesial and distal surface is flattened and grooved. The distal groove may be more distinctive.

Identifying features of the mandibular permanent canine
Crown

- Resembles the upper canine; however, the crown of the lower canine is longer and narrower in the mesial distal direction.
- The single cusp is less pointed than the upper canine.

Labial surface

- Crown is convex.
- Mesial outline is straight and continuous with the mesial surface of the root.
- Distal outline is concave cervically but becomes convex at distal slope.
- Distal slope longer than the mesial slope.

Lingual surface

- Lingual surface concave.
- Cingulum is absent or very small.
- Marginal ridges not well defined.
- Faint ridge runs from the tip of the cusp to the cingulum, on each side are two shallow depressions (mesial and distal lingual fossae).

Root

- Single root.
- Mesial and distal surface is flattened and grooved.
- The apex of the root frequently curves distally.

Permanent premolars
Identifying features of the maxillary first permanent premolar
Crown

- Crown quadrilateral, two cusps buccal and palatal. Palatal cusp smaller in area and in height.
- Mesial slope of the buccal cusp is longer than the distal. (This is the reverse in the canine.)
- The cusps are separated by a fissure, which runs mesiodistal. The mesial fissure crosses the mesial marginal ridge and extends onto the mesial surface.
- The mesial surface has a marked depression called the **canine fossa**.

Roots

- Two roots, one buccal and palatal.
- Sometime has a single root which is grooved mesially and distally and may be bifurcated at the apex.

Identifying features of the maxillary second permanent premolar
Crown

- Crown appears smaller, less angular and oval in shape.
- Buccal and palatal cusps are almost equal in height and size.
- Distal slope of the buccal cusp is longer than the mesial.
- The tip of palatal cusp is always positioned off centre towards the mesial.
- A short fissure runs mesiodistally and confined to the occlusal surface.
- Mesial and distal surfaces are convex and the mesial surface does not have a canine fossa.

Root

- Single root, flattened mesially and distally.
- Roots are longer than the first premolar.

Identifying features of the mandibular first permanent premolar
Crown

- Crown appears circular in outline, except mesiolingually, where it is flattened.
- Two cusps one buccal and one lingual. Buccal cusp is much larger than the lingual cusp, it dominates the occlusal surface. The lingual cusp appears like a cingulum.
- The two cusps are connected by a central ridge of enamel – transverse ridge. On each side of this ridge is a mesial and distal fossa. The distal fossa is the larger.
- Mesial fissure runs from the mesial fossa and extends onto the lingual surface.
- Mesial and distal marginal ridges are well defined.

Root

- Single root, which is flattened on the mesial and distal surfaces, the mesial groove being more marked.
- The root may be bifurcated and curved distally.

Identifying features of the mandibular second permanent premolar
Crown

- Is larger than the lower first premolar.
- May either have two or three cusps, the three cusped type being more common.
- Mesial marginal ridge is higher than the distal.
- **Two cusped second premolar** – two cusps situated buccal and lingual.
- The cusps are connected by a faint ridge of enamel. On either side of this ridge lie the mesial and distal fossae, the distal fossa being the larger.

- A fissure runs from the mesial fossa to the distal fossa presenting either 'H' or 'C' fissure pattern.
- **Three-cusped second premolar** – more common. One buccal and two lingual cusps. Buccal cusp is the largest and the distolingual cusp is the smallest.
- The two lingual cusps are separated by a fissure which extends onto the lingual surface, presenting a 'Y'-shaped fissure pattern

Roots

- Single root. Grooves are not usually present.

Permanent molars

Identifying features of the maxillary first permanent molar
Crown

- Largest tooth in the upper arch.
- Rhomboid in outline with two acute and two obtuse angles.
- Four cusps: mesiopalatal, mesiobuccal, distopalatal and distobuccal.
- A fifth cusp may be present on the palatal side of the mesiopalatal cusp (**Cusp of Carabelli**).
- Mesiopalatal cusp is the largest, distopalatal cusp is the smallest.
- Buccal cusps are generally more pointed.
- Mesiopalatal cusp is joined to the distobuccal cusp by the oblique ridge. This divides the occlusal surface into two areas.
- Distal fissure runs parallel to the oblique ridge and extends onto the palatal surface.
- The mesial fissure runs from the mesial marginal ridge and extends buccally, between the two buccal cusps and extends onto the buccal surface.
- Occasionally the distal fissure may run across the oblique ridge joining the mesial fissure forming 'H'-shaped fissure pattern

Roots

- Three roots, two buccally and one palatally placed.
- Palatal root is the longest and most divergent. The buccal roots tend to curve distally.

Identifying features of the maxillary second permanent molar
Crown

- Is very similar to the upper first molar, rhomboid in outline.
- The crown is generally smaller.
- Distopalatal cusp is reduced in size and sometimes absent. If absent the occlusal outline is more triangular.
- Both distal cusps are smaller than the upper first molar.
- The cusp of Carabelli is never present.

Roots

- Three roots, similar to those of the upper first molar.
- Palatal root less divergent.
- Both buccal roots are same length, closer together with slight distal inclination.

Identifying features of the maxillary third permanent molar
Crown

- Similar to the upper first and second molars, but subject to considerable variations.
- Smaller than the upper first and second molars.
- Triangular in outline, distopalatal cusp is reduced in size.
- The distopalatal cusp is absent 50%, when this cusp is absent there is no oblique ridge.
- Largest cusp mesiopalatal.
- Occlusal surface usually has a wrinkled appearance due to additional fissures.
- Distal surface is more convex than the first and second molars, mainly because the distal surface is not in contact with a tooth.

Roots

- The roots are short, underdeveloped and rarely divergent.
- Roots often fused together with a distinct distal curve near the apex.

Identifying features of the mandibular first permanent molar
Crown

- This is the largest lower tooth.
- Rectangular in outline. Being longer mesial–distally than buccal–lingually.
- It has five cusps, three placed buccally (mesiobuccal, distobuccal, distal corner) and two cusps placed lingually (mesiolingual, distolingual).
- Lingual cusps more pointed.
- Occlusal surface has a central fossa where four fissures originate (mesial, distal, buccal and lingual).
- The mesial fissure runs mesially and bifurcates near the mesial marginal ridge.
- The distal fissure runs distally and bifurcates near the distal marginal ridge.
- A buccal fissure passes between the mesiobuccal and the distobuccal cusps and terminates on the buccal surface (buccal pit – **foramen caecum molarum**). Another buccal fissure runs between the distal and distal-buccal cusps and terminates on the buccal surface.
- The lingual fissure passes between the mesiolingual and distolingual cusp and extends slightly onto the lingual surface.

Roots

- Two roots, mesial and distal.
- Distal root is straight and shorter than the mesial root.
- Mesial root has a marked groove on the mesial surface and usually curves distally.

Identifying features of the mandibular second permanent molar
Crown

- Occlusal outline resembles a square with rounded corners.
- It has four cusps, two buccal (mesiobuccal and distobuccal) and two lingual (mesiolingual and distolingual).
- Lingual cusps are higher and slightly more pointed than the buccal cusps.
- Mesial cusps are larger than the distal cusps.
- The buccal surface is markedly convex while the lingual surface is flat.
- Distal surface slightly more convex than the mesial surface.
- Fissure pattern is similar to a 'hot cross bun'.
- The buccal fissure passes between the mesiobuccal and the distobuccal and terminates on the buccal surface.
- The lingual fissure passes between the mesiolingual and distolingual cusps and terminates on the lingual surface.

Roots

- Two roots, mesial and distal.
- Roots are closer together; occasionally the roots may be partially fused.
- Mesial root is larger than the distal.
- The roots curve distally.

Identifying features of the mandibular third permanent molar
Crown

- May be subject to considerable variations.
- A classic lower third molar has a crown form similar to the lower second molar, with four cusps.
- It is smaller and has many supplemental fissures.
- The occlusal outline may be similar to the other mandibular molars, some lower third molars a circular occlusal outline.
- The buccal surface is markedly convex while the lingual surface is flat.

Roots

- Two roots, mesial and distal.

- Similar to other lower molars, except that they are shorter and less developed and often fused together as one conical mass.
- The roots curve distally

Primary dentition
Incisors

- These teeth are smaller in size but similar in morphology to their permanent successors.
- The crowns are more bulbous.

Canines

- The crowns are much more bulbous than the permanent canines.
- When newly erupted the tip of the cusp is pointed, particularly in the upper canines.
- The mesial slope is longer than the distal slope in the maxillary and mandibular primary canine.

Primary molars (Figure 1.23b)
Identifying features of the maxillary first primary molar
Crown

- Outline of the crown trapezoid, the buccal surface is longer than the palatal surface and the mesiopalatal angle obtuse.
- Two cusps, buccal and palatal. Buccal cusp more like a ridge and is sometimes divided into two or three lobes.
- A fissure runs mesially–distally between the cusps is a fissure which bifurcates at each end.
- There is a pronounced bulge of enamel at the mesiobuccal corner of the crown near the cervical margin – Tubercle of Zuckerkandl.

Roots

- Three roots, two buccal and one palatal.
- The roots are widely divergent to accommodate the developing maxillary first permanent premolar.

Identifying features of the mandibular first primary molar
Crown

- The occlusal surface is elongated in the mesiodistal direction.
- It has four cusps, two lingual (mesiolingual, distolingual) and two buccal (mesiobuccal, distobuccal). The mesiolingual cusp is the largest.
- The mesiobuccal and the mesiolingual cusps are joined by a transverse ridge across the occlusal surface.
- On either side of this ridge is a fossa (mesial and distal fossae). The distal fossa is the largest.

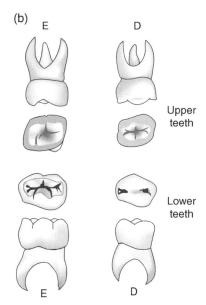

Figure 1.23b Upper and lower Primary Molars.

- Like the upper first primary molar, there is a pronounced bulge of enamel at the mesiolingual corner.

Roots

- Two roots, mesially and distally.
- Roots diverge to accommodate the developing lower first permanent premolar.

Identifying features of the maxillary second primary molar
Crown

- This tooth closely resembles the maxillary first permanent molar.

- There are four main cusps.
- Cusp of Carabelli may be present mesiopalatally.
- The oblique ridge is present, joining the mesiopalatal and distobuccal cusps.

Roots

- The roots resemble those of the maxillary first primary molars.
- They are larger and sometimes resemble the grab of a crane.
- They accommodate the developing maxillary second permanent premolar.

Identifying features of the mandibular second primary molar
Crown

- This tooth resembles the mandibular first permanent molar.
- It is smaller in size and has shallow fissures.

Roots

- Two roots, mesially and distally.
- Roots diverge to accommodate the developing mandibular second permanent premolar.

Further reading

Avery, J.K. (1999) *Essentials of Oral Histology and Embryology, a Clinical Approach*, 2nd edition, Mosby Publications, St Louis.

Bercoviz, B.K.S., Holland, G.R. and Moxham, B.J. (2009) *A Colour Atlas and Text of Oral Anatomy, Histology and Embryology*, 4th edition, Mosby Publication, St Louis.

Edgar, M., Dawes, C. and O'Mullane, D. (2004) *Saliva and Oral Health*, 3rd edition, British Dental Association, London.

Van Beek, G.C. (1983) *Dental Morphology: an illustrated guide*, 2nd edition, John Wright, Bristol.

2

General pathology

Henk S. Brand and Arjan Vissink

Summary

This chapter covers:

- The inflammatory response to tissue damage
- The functioning of the immune system
- The causes of cancer and different therapies to treat cancer
- The coagulation of blood and disorders which interfere with this process
- Atherosclerosis and other cardiovascular diseases

Introduction

The aim of this chapter is to introduce the reader to a broad overview and explanation of important and fundamental aspects of general pathology relevant to both dental hygienists and dental therapists. However, it is impossible to include all pathological conditions that can occur and may at some time influence clinical practice in a single chapter. A selection of texts is therefore included at the end of the chapter under 'Further reading', which are considered useful in directing the reader to explore additional areas of general pathology.

Inflammation and immunity

The integrity of the human body is continuously challenged by external and internal attacks. A few examples of these include:

- In the environment that surrounds us, microorganisms are the main menace.
- Physical injury can affect (oral) tissues.

- Internally we are threatened by the risk of tumour growth.

To protect our body against such injury, we possess an ingenious defence system, composed of a large number of components:

- The skin and mucosa form the **first barrier** of defence against intruders.
- If this barrier is passed, the intruders will be opposed by a **second barrier** of defence, consisting of inflammatory cells and soluble factors. Together, these two systems form the non-specific immune system, which is present at birth (**innate immunity**). Although this system is capable of immediately attacking the intruder, it has no specificity against it.
- When the intruder is not rapidly eliminated by the non-specific immune system, a **third barrier**, the specific immune system, will be mobilised. This specific immune system needs time to deploy its full effect, but has the utmost advantage in that it raises a defensive reaction specifically aimed against that intruder. In addition, after the first contact with a particular intruder, this specific defensive reaction is recorded in memory cells. As a result, a much faster and more potent reaction will result from a future confrontation with that intruder (**acquired immunity**). Both systems, the non-specific and the specific system, co-operate closely.

The non-specific immune system

Skin and mucosa

When intact, the skin and mucosal membranes provide the first barrier of defence. If this line is impaired, for example in a patient with severe burns, there is great risk

Clinical Textbook of Dental Hygiene and Therapy, Second Edition. Edited by Suzanne L. Noble.
© 2012 John Wiley & Sons, Ltd. Published 2012 by John Wiley & Sons, Ltd.

of invasive infections with microorganisms. Often these microorganisms originate from the so-called **commensal organisms**. Under normal conditions, these organisms live on the skin or mucosa without causing injury. Secretory products of glands located beneath the skin and mucosa also play an important role in the defence. Examples of local defence mechanisms against potential invaders are:

- The continuous flow of saliva through the oral cavity resulting in mechanical cleansing of the oral surfaces; e.g. in the case of a dry mouth the risk of development of dental caries and oral infections is considerably increased (Figure 2.1).
- The presence of antimicrobial components, such as **lysozyme** and **histatins**, in saliva.
- Fatty acids secreted by the skin.
- The production of tears (containing lysozyme).
- The low pH in the stomach due to secretion of hydrochloric acid.

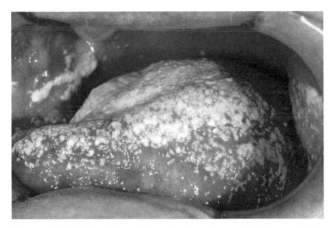

Figure 2.1 Reduced secretion of saliva has resulted in a shift in the composition of the oral flora. These patients are prone to candidiasis.

The normal (commensal) bacterial flora of the body is also an important defence mechanism. It suppresses the growth of many (potentially) pathogenic bacteria by competition for essential nutrients or production of inhibitory substances. This so-called colonisation resistance may be disturbed by the use of antibiotics. The result may be an overgrowth of pathogenic bacteria as their natural competitors are not present in sufficient numbers any more. In the gut, for example, such a disturbance may lead to a clinical infection with diarrhoea.

Cells of the non-specific immune system

When an intruder has passed the skin and/or mucosal surfaces, it will first encounter **macrophages**. These cells of the non-specific immune system, differentiated from blood monocytes, are present everywhere in the body. Depending on the tissue or organ where they reside, they have a more or less specialised structure and function (Table 2.1).

The function of macrophages is twofold:

- To recognise and clear intruders.
- To degrade the intruder into small protein fragments.

First, the macrophage attaches itself to the foreign structure, often a microorganism. This structure is 'swallowed' due to invagination of the cellular membrane of the macrophage. In this way a **phagosome** is formed. This process of 'eating' by the cell is called **phagocytosis** and is significantly accelerated when the microorganism to be swallowed is covered with antibodies and/or complement. Subsequently, the phagosome fuses with **lysosomes**, which are membrane-surrounded cell organelles in the cytoplasm of the macrophage containing **lytic enzymes** and **myeloperoxidase**. The latter enzyme produces an oxygen-derived free radical with powerful antimicrobial activity. The combined activity of the lytic enzymes and oxygen radicals kills and destroys the foreign structure.

Table 2.1 Mononuclear cells.

Location	Name	Major function (phagocytosing cells are also capable of antigen presentation)
Blood	Monocyte	Phagocytosis
Lymph node	Follicular dendritic cell	Antigen presentation
Thymus	Interdigitating dendritic cell	Antigen presentation
Brain	Microglia cell	Phagocytosis
Lung	Alveolar macrophage	Phagocytosis
Liver	Kupffer cell	Phagocytosis
Kidney	Mesangial cell	Phagocytosis
Skin	Langerhans cell	Antigen presentation

Second, the foreign structures are degraded into small protein fragments. These fragments, peptides with a length of 8–15 amino acids, are presented to the specific immune system. This process is a good example of the close collaboration between the non-specific and specific immune system.

If the intruder has succeeded in passing the above mentioned defence barriers and enters a blood vessel, it will be confronted with circulating phagocytosing cells (**monocytes**), which are comparable to the macrophages in tissues. In addition, blood contains large numbers of **granulocytes**. The name of these white blood cells is derived from the presence of granules in their cytoplasm. These granules contain lytic enzymes. The majority of the granulocytes are **neutrophils**, capable of phagocytosing foreign structures. Under certain conditions, neutrophils can leave the bloodstream and enter tissues. The **eosinophils** and **basophils** play a role in the defence against parasites.

A final group of cells from the non-specific immune system, present in the blood, are the so-called natural killer cells (**NK cells**). The NK cells can recognise aberrant structures on tumour cells. They make contact with these tumour cells and release the contents of their granules. The granules contain **perforins**, enzymes that are capable of making a hole in the membrane of the tumour cell, resulting in its death.

Table 2.2 and Figure 2.2 provide an overview of the cell types of the non-specific immune system.

Humoral factors of the non-specific immune system

Tissues and blood plasma also contain several chemical substances, mostly proteins, which are involved in the non-specific immune response. An important system is the **complement system**, which consists of a series of plasma proteins. Under normal conditions, these proteins are present in blood in their inactive form (Figure 2.3). The complement system can be activated in three ways:

- The classical pathway is activated by immune complexes (an antibody bound to the specific structure it recognises, e.g. part of a microorganism).
- The alternative pathway is activated by bacterial cell wall structures.
- The lectin pathway is also activated by bacterial cell wall structures.

Table 2.2 Cells of the immune system.

Cell	Reference values (healthy individuals)	Major function
Non-specific immune system		
Neutrophil	$2–7 \times 10^9$/litre blood	Phagocytosis + release of biologically active substances + release of toxic substances
Active eosinophil	$0–0.4 \times 10^9$/litre blood	
Basophil	$0–0.2 \times 10^9$/litre blood	
Mast cell	Localised in tissues	Tissue pendant of basophils, involved in allergic reactions
Monocyte	$0.2–0.8 \times 10^9$/litre blood	Functions comparable with granulocyte + antigen presentation
Macrophage	Localised in tissues	Tissue pendant of monocyte
Dendritic cell	Localised in tissues, small percentage present in blood	Antigen presentation
'Natural killer' cell	$0.1–1.4 \times 10^9$/litre blood	Non-specific killing of cells + release of biologically active compounds
Specific immune system		
T-lymphocyte	$1–4 \times 10^9$/litre blood	Cellular immunity (help, suppression and cytotoxic)
B-lymphocyte	$0.1–1 \times 10^9$/litre blood	Humoral immunity (production of antibodies)

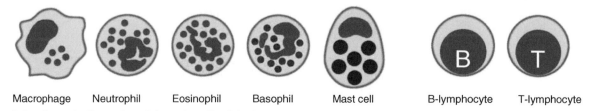

Macrophage   Neutrophil   Eosinophil   Basophil   Mast cell   B-lymphocyte   T-lymphocyte

Figure 2.2 Schematic illustration of the main cells of the immune system.

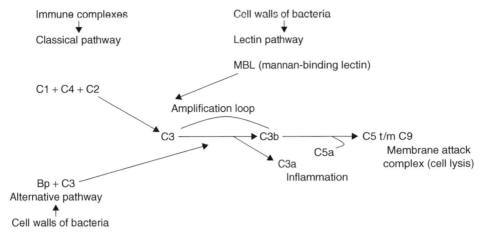

Figure 2.3 Simplified diagram of the complement system.

All three pathways lead to activation of the central part of the complement system, which is followed by self-amplification resulting in rapid activation of an enormous amount of complement proteins. This results in several biological effects. Some small complement fragments attract neutrophils. Other parts of the complement system form a cylinder-shaped structure in the membrane of bacteria resulting in cell lysis (destruction). Since macrophages and monocytes have receptors for complement C3b on their surface, they can phagocytose bacteria covered with this complement protein much faster.

A second important group of humoral factors is formed by the **cytokines**. These are low molecular weight compounds that are produced by many different cell types, including cells that are not part of the immune system. Cytokines can exert their activity on the producing cell itself (**autocrine activity**), on neighbouring cells (**paracrine activity**) or on cells far away (**endocrine activity**). Therefore, cytokines are the key mediators in the communication between cells.

The specific immune system

The specific immune system aims at a specific target and deploys a strong defensive reaction against that specific target. A structure that induces such a reaction is called an **antigen**. To be effective, this reaction needs time: approximately 7 days after the initial contact with the antigen. Simultaneously with this initial reaction an immunological memory is developed. Because of this memory, a much faster (about 2 days) and stronger reaction will occur on the next contact with the same antigen. This immunological memory forms the basis of **vaccinations**. First, a specific immune reaction is induced against a weakened or killed microorganism in order to raise a stronger and more rapid defensive reaction on subsequent infections with the same microorganism.

The defensive reaction itself can be exerted by antibodies and/or cells. Antibodies attach themselves to specific surface structures. This activates the classical pathway of the complement system. In addition, foreign structures covered with antibodies are phagocytosed much faster by monocytes and macrophages. Cells of tissues that have become infected with a virus or intracellular bacterium (e.g. *Mycobacterium tuberculosis*) will be rendered harmless by cells of the immune system.

The specific immune response consists of three phases:

- The initial phase is the so-called antigen presentation during which the antigen is presented to the specific immune system.
- During the second phase the system becomes activated and a memory against subsequent exposures with that antigen develops.
- The third phase is the **effector phase**. During this phase the ultimate defensive reaction takes place.

Antigen presentation

When an intruder passes the first barrier, it will be confronted with macrophages that are capable of phagocytosing the intruder and degrading it into small fragments, peptides of 8 to 15 amino acids. These peptides are admitted to the groove of **human leucocyte antigen molecules** (HLA molecules, see Figure 2.4). Next, the HLA molecules with peptide fragments in their groove move to the cell surface, where the peptide is presented to T-lymphocytes.

There are two classes of HLA molecules: HLA class I and HLA class II. HLA class I molecules can be subdivided into A, B and C antigens; HLA class II molecules are subdivided into DR-, DQ- and DP-antigens. HLA class I molecules are present on all cells with a nucleus; HLA class II molecules are restricted to antigen-presenting cells (macrophages, monocytes and B-lymphocytes).

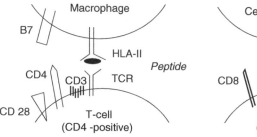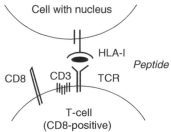

Figure 2.4 HLA class I and HLA class II mediated T-cell interactions.

Each individual has its own set of HLA molecules, which differ from those of other individuals. Only monozygotic (identical) twins possess exactly the same HLA molecules. Because of these individual differences in HLA molecules, tissues or organs from another person are recognised by the immune system of the acceptor as foreign. This may result in rejection of the graft, a major problem with transplantation.

Activation of the specific immune system and development of immunological memory

The specific immune system is composed of **lymphocytes**. Although each lymphocyte is only capable of recognising one specific antigen, together these lymphocytes can recognise an enormous variation in foreign structures. Lymphocytes are divided into B-lymphocytes and T-lymphocytes.

B-lymphocytes develop in the bone marrow. After activation, they can start forming antibodies. B-lymphocytes carry these antibodies on their surface and use them as receptors to recognise specific antigens. The variation in B-lymphocytes, each with their own antibody, is enormous.

After being created in the bone marrow, **T-lymphocytes** move to the **thymus** to mature. There are two kinds of T-lymphocytes: those with a CD4 molecule on their surface (which mainly function as **T-helper cells**) and those with a CD8 molecule on their surface (which mainly function as **cytotoxic cells**). T-cells also have a specific receptor on their surface, the T-cell receptor (TCR). The latter receptor enables them to recognise antigenic peptides. The TCR of CD4-positive T-cells can recognise peptides presented via HLA class II molecules; the TCR of CD8-positive T-cells can recognise peptides presented via HLA class I molecules (Figure 2.4). Each T-cell has one specific TCR. As a consequence, the total variation in T-cells is, like the variation in B-lymphocytes, enormous.

When a CD4-positive T-cell meets an antigen-presenting cell with a peptide in its HLA class II molecule that exactly fits in the TCR of this T-cell, that T-cell will be activated and start to produce the cytokine **interleukin 2**. This interleukin acts as an autocrine growth factor for this T-cell. Thereupon this cell starts to divide. As a result, activated T-cells become available to provide help to *specific* B-cells to form antibodies and/or to provide help to *specific* cytotoxic T-cells. The T-cell exerts this action mainly by producing cytokines. Some of the created T-cells remain in the body for a long time, circulating as memory cells. These cells are promptly available during future contacts with the antigen they are raised against, and will then provide a rapid and even stronger reaction.

The effector phase of the specific immune response

By producing interleukins 4 and 10, CD4-positive T-helper cells provide assistance to B-lymphocytes. For the activation of B-lymphocytes, two signals are necessary:

- A B-cell must recognise the antigen with the antibody on its surface.
- Assistance from a specific T-cell.

If both conditions are met, the activated B-cell (plasma cell) will start to produce antibodies. After the contact with an antigen, it takes quite some time before the first antibodies are produced (the so-called **primary immune response**); on average 7 days. These antibodies, of the immunoglobulin M (IgM) class, bind rather weakly to the antigen. Subsequently, IgG and IgA molecules are produced which can bind much more strongly with the antigen. After a second confrontation with the antigen this process is completed much faster due to the presence of memory T-cells with specificity for the antigen. This secondary immune response produces large numbers of IgG molecules, which bind strongly to the antigen (Figure 2.5). Bacteria-covered antibodies are rapidly and efficiently removed by phagocytosing cells. The production of antibodies is especially important for the defence against encapsulated bacteria like pneumococci and *Haemophilus influenzae*.

A large number of microorganisms (especially viruses, intracellular bacteria like *Mycobacterium tuberculosis* and certain fungi) conceal themselves from the immune system by entering the cells of the body. The infected cells, however, express on their surface HLA class I molecules containing microbial peptides. Subsequently CD8-positive T-cells are capable of recognising these strange peptides presented in an HLA class I molecule with their TCR. After recognition of the strange peptide, cytotoxic T-cells become activated and release substances like **perforins** that lyse the infected target cell. Specific T-helper cells provide assistance for the activation of cytotoxic T-cells by producing cytokines, mainly interleukin 2 and gamma-interferon. Cytotoxic T-cell reactions play

a special role in the defence against cells infected with a virus. A detailed diagram of the primary immune response is provided in Figure 2.6.

Inflammation

Acute inflammation

The development of an acute inflammatory response is well illustrated by the cascade of reactions that follows on penetration of the oral mucosa by a bacterium. In the tissue, the bacterium will be confronted with a macrophage that tries to phagocytose it. This process is facilitated by the complement system and, if immunity against that bacterium is present, specific antibodies. The macrophage becomes activated and starts to release cytokines, such as interleukin 1 and **tumour necrosis factor** (TNF). These cytokines exert an effect on the adjacent endothelium (epithelial lining) of capillaries. The endothelium becomes activated, resulting in a local expression of adhesion molecules on the endothelial surface. The blood vessels increase in diameter (**vasodilation**), which increases the blood flow through the vessels. Since the permeability of the endothelium increases simultaneously, the transport of fluid containing complement and antibodies to the tissue will increase.

Circulating neutrophils have structures on their surfaces that recognise the adhesion molecules that are expressed on the endothelium. As a result, the neutrophils adhere to the wall of the blood vessel and begin

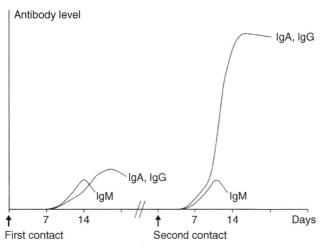

Figure 2.5 The primary and secondary immune response.

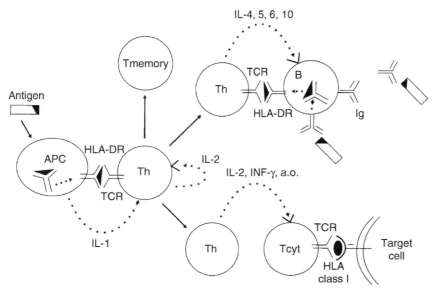

Figure 2.6 Diagram of the primary immune response. The antigen is phagocytosed by an antigen-presenting cell (APC), partially degraded and, in association with HLA class II (HLA-DR), presented to an antigen specific T-helper cell (Th) that recognises the relevant epitope with its T-cell receptor (TCR). The T-cell is activated and starts to proliferate, aided by interleukin 1 (IL-1 from the APC) and IL-2 (produced by the T-cell itself). T-memory cells and T-helper cells (Th) develop which, by direct interaction with B-cells and by production of cytokines (interleukins 4, 5 and 6), stimulate antigen specific B-cells to proliferate and to produce immunoglobulins (Ig). The T-helper cells also activate cytotoxic T-cells (Tcyt). Tcyt recognise antigen presented in association with HLA class I molecules on the target cell.

to move in the direction of the activated macrophage. This process is guided by substances released from the macrophage, the so-called **chemotactic factors**. In the area where bacteria have penetrated the mucosa, granulocytes are urgently needed because bacteria usually invade in large numbers. The granulocytes also begin to phagocytose bacteria, again helped by complement and specific antibodies. In doing so, the granulocytes become activated and release their lytic enzymes. This causes tissue damage and often the granulocytes have 'dug their own grave' as well. The disrupted granulocytes and necrotic tissue form pus.

This inflammatory reaction induces the five characteristic local clinical signs of acute inflammation, of which the first four were first described by the Greek doctor Celsus in the first century BCE:

- **Redness:** due to the local dilation of small blood vessels.
- **Heat:** vasodilation results in an increased delivery of warm blood to the area.
- **Swelling:** due to accumulation of fluid in the tissue.
- **Pain:** pus and swelling of the tissues press on nerve endings. Some chemical mediators of inflammatory response are also able to induce pain.

In the nineteenth century, the German **Rudolf Virchow** added a fifth sign:

- **Loss of function:** movements of an inflamed area are reflex inhibited by pain. In addition severe swelling may physically immobilise the tissues.

Inflammation of a specific tissue is denoted by the suffix '-itis' added to the name of the tissue. For example, an inflammatory response in the gingiva is called gingivitis, in the periodontium, periodontitis and in the mucosa, mucositis, etc.

In the case of a more extensive and/or longer-lasting local inflammatory reaction, a systemic reaction may occur that involves the other parts of the body. The cytokines interleukin 1 and 6, originating from the inflamed area, reach the brain where they reset the body's 'thermostat', inducing a higher body temperature (**fever**). In addition, these interleukins activate the liver to produce **acute phase proteins**. These proteins enhance host resistance and minimise tissue injury. Acute phase proteins are also responsible for the increase in the sedimentation rate of erythrocytes during inflammation, known as the **erythrocyte sedimentation rate** (ESR), which is often used as a clinical parameter of disease activity.

Chronic inflammation

When the inflammatory agent persists, the character of the inflammatory response changes. This can, for example, be due to extremely virulent bacteria that are resistant to breakdown by the acute inflammatory response, or

through the inability of a deficient immune system to clear microbes. In chronic inflammation, neutrophils become replaced by macrophages. Since the infectious agent persists, the immune response also plays a more prominent role. Therefore, a chronic infiltrate is composed of macrophages, lymphocytes and plasma cells.

A specific form of chronic inflammation is **granulomatous inflammation**. This type of chronic inflammation is characterised by the development of **granulomas**: large accumulations of macrophages and lymphocytes with a diameter of several millimetres. Granulomas also contain modified macrophages, which are called **epithelioid cells** because they resemble epithelial cells. Fusion of several epithelioid cells may result in multinucleated giant cells (**Langerhans' cells**), which possess some phagocytic activity. This type of chronic inflammation is especially observed in the reaction to infection with intracellular living pathogens, such as *M. tuberculosis*, which is resistant to digestion after phagocytosis. It can also be observed in the reaction to tissue damage by foreign non-digestible substances, such as silica particles and suture materials, or infections with *Actinomyces* species. The latter microorganisms are commensals of the oral cavity and only cause an inflammatory reaction in special cases, often related to trauma or a surgical procedure (e.g. local anaesthesia or the extraction of teeth).

Chronic inflammation is characterized by a sustained inflammatory process whose duration may vary from several months to years. In many cases chronic inflammation does not induce complaints and patients are often unaware of the chronic inflammation. For a definitive treatment, the cause of the chronic inflammation should be removed. This phenomenon is nicely illustrated by treatment of periodontitis as removal of accumulated plaque is an important element in the treatment of chronic periodontitis.

During the last decades, several studies showed a relation between periodontitis and systemic diseases, such as cardiovascular diseases, pulmonary diseases, diabetes mellitus and rheumatoid arthritis. This relationship will be described in more detail in Chapter 5, p. 99.

Wound healing

Primary intention

When the noxious agent is killed and removed, the body will start to repair the damage. An injury with little loss of tissue, for example a surgical incision, will be healed by **primary intention** (the healing together of clean, closely opposed wound edges). Since blood vessels are cut, some bleeding occurs, followed by aggregation of blood platelets and the production of fibrin. Together with clumped red blood cells, they form a clot that covers the wound and prevents infection. In fact, an acute inflammatory

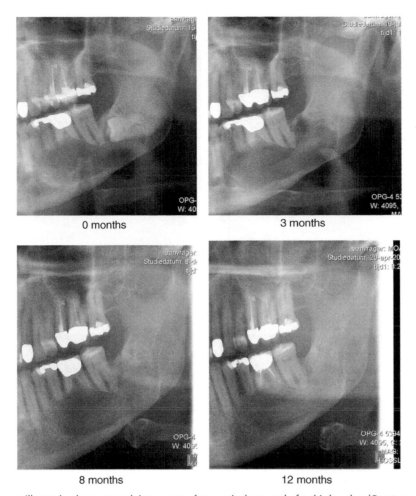

0 months

3 months

8 months

12 months

Figure 2.7 A series of X-rays illustrating bone growth into a cyst after surgical removal of a third molar. (Courtesy of Dr Baucke van Minnen.)

reaction is observed in the area of repair. Macrophages release cytokines that activate fibroblasts, myofibroblasts and endothelial cells residing in the wound margins. Guided by the meshwork of fibrin, these cells begin to grow into the clot, forming **granulation tissue**. This tissue is gradually replaced by collagen fibrils. The final result is a thin white line of collagen visible under the transparent layer of regenerated epithelium: a **scar**.

Secondary intention

When an injury results in a substantial loss of tissue, the edges of the injury cannot always be joined during healing. A larger clot will develop to fill this gap and more granulation tissue must be formed from the wound margins. In addition, contraction by myofibroblasts and shortening of collagen fibres induce wound contraction, which reduces the original size of the wound. However, this healing by **secondary intention** may lead to irregular mutilating scars.

Socket healing following extraction is a complex example of wound healing by secondary intention. Socket healing involves healing of both mucosa and bone. The regeneration of the mucosa starts at the mucosal wound margins. Although mucosal healing is in fact wound healing by secondary intention, mucosal healing usually does not result in irregular mutilating scars. The same applies to bone healing. Healing of bone also starts from the bone margins but it is a much slower process than mucosal healing. Therefore healing of the mucosa is already completed while bone healing is still in its initial phase. This is obvious when taking a radiograph of an extraction site just after completion of the mucosal healing. At that time, the contour of a root that has been removed is still clearly visible. It will take many months before the bone at the extraction site is regenerated and remodelled, and as a result is not visible on dental radiographs any more (Figure 2.7).

Hyperplasia, hypertrophy and atrophy

In most tissues in adults there is a very accurate balance between cell loss and cell production. With the continuous presence of an injurious agent or chronic irritation, tissues may, however, undergo an adaptive response. The general response of a cell to increased functional demand is to increase the tissue volume accordingly by

(a)

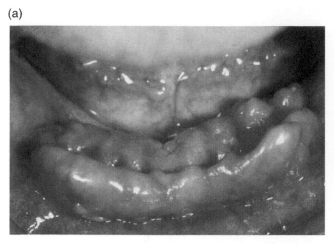

(b)

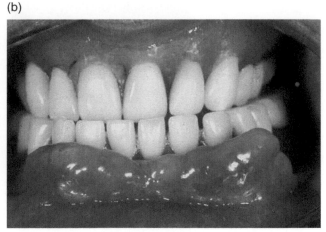

Figure 2.8 (a & b) Fibrous hyperplasia due to an ill-fitting lower denture. (a) Without lower denture. (b) Lower denture in place. The overextended border can be considered as a chronic irritating factor resulting in proliferation of fibrous tissue. (Courtesy of Dr G.M. Raghoebar.)

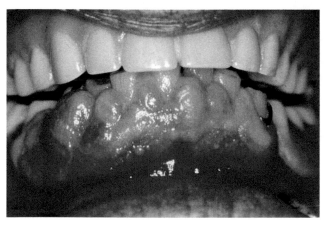

Figure 2.9 Gingival hyperplasia in a patient treated with immunosuppressive medication (ciclosporin A).

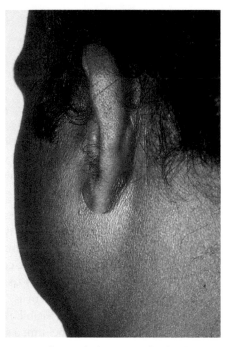

Figure 2.10 Swelling of the parotid gland is occasionally observed in metabolic disorders like anorexia nervosa and type 1 diabetes.

either increasing the volume without cell division (larger cells: **hypertrophy**) or by increasing the volume by cell division (more cells: **hyperplasia**). Since the stimuli for hypertrophy and hyperplasia are rather similar, these processes commonly co-exist. An example is the increase in oral epithelium in response to chronic irritation, for example by an ill fitting denture (Figure 2.8). When the irritation subsides, the tissue usually returns to normal. Some medication may also induce hyperplasia, specifically of the gingiva (Figure 2.9). Also, certain disease conditions may result in hypertrophy of tissues, such as a persisting, painless swelling of the parotid glands related to metabolic disorders such as anorexia nervosa or diabetes mellitus (Figure 2.10).

In contrast, **atrophy** is a decrease in volume and function of a tissue due to a reduction in cell size. A typical example is the muscle atrophy observed in a leg in plas-

ter. When the requirement of the organ is normalised, the atrophied cells are capable of restoring their original size. A well-known exception is the loss of alveolar bone related to the loss of teeth. The resulting atrophic mandible or maxilla is, however, not merely the result of shrinkage of cells, but the result of resorption of bone with loss of cells. Restoration of the original height with bone transplants will again result in a loss of bone as only the bone and not the teeth are replaced and thus the original function is not restored. Only if, for example, dental implants are placed and thus the (reconstructed) bone is functionally loaded, will the resorption process be greatly reduced.

Neoplasia

Characteristics of neoplasia

When the balance between cell loss and cell proliferation is disturbed for a long time, either by increased proliferation or decreased cell loss, the number of cells in a tissue increases gradually and a tumour develops. According to their behaviour, tumours are classified as benign or malignant. Cancer is a word used more by the general public to refer to malignant tumours. The term neoplasm is synonymous with the word tumour and is preferred in conversations with patients because it is usually not so alarming.

A **benign tumour** consists of cells that histologically resemble the normal cells of the tissue where the tumour develops. A benign tumour usually grows rather slowly and is often surrounded by a (fibrous) capsule. Benign tumours do not invade the adjacent normal tissues, but can push these tissues aside. This expansive growth of the tumour induces pressure on the adjacent tissues, which occasionally may even result in a fatal course of the disease, e.g. by inducing airway obstruction.

A **malignant tumour** consists of cells that histologically resemble the parent cell or tissue much less than do benign tumours (Table 2.3). The malignant tumour is less structured and rarely surrounded by a capsule. **Necrosis** (cell death) is common in malignant tumours, since the blood supply is not able to keep up with the rapid cell growth. A major characteristic of malignant tumours is their capacity to invade the adjacent normal tissues (e.g. connective tissue, bone, blood vessels, nerves, etc.) and the development of 'daughter tumours' or **metastases** in other organs.

In general, the name of a specific tumour describes the cell type from which it originates and whether the tumour is benign or malignant. The name of benign tumours ends in the suffix '-oma'; in tumours of mesenchymal origin they are preceded by the name of the cell of origin (Table 2.4). When malignant tumours consist of epithelial cells they are called **carcinomas** and if they consist of mesenchymal cells, **sarcomas**. These two categories can be further subdivided according to cell type. For example, malignant epithelial tumours with glandular tissue are called **adenocarcinomas** and malignant tumours from squamous epithelium are called **squamous cell carcinomas**. However, the names of a few tumours do not follow these general rules of nomenclature. For example, malignant tumours of lymphoid tissue are called malignant **lymphomas**. **Leukaemia** is the malignant growth of white blood cells and a **melanoma** is a skin tumour that develops from pigment-containing melanocytes.

Carcinogenesis

Carcinogenesis is the process by which normal cells are transformed into cancer cells. Tumours develop as a result of changes in cells, which enable cells to escape the control mechanisms that normally regulate cell growth. These changes are called **transformation** and are the result of genetic alterations in the cell (**mutations**). Several mutations are necessary to transform a cell. Subsequently, the transformed cell will develop into a tumour. This means that all cells of a tumour arise from one single transformed cell.

Environmental factors

Harmful environmental factors, and changes in the function of genes induced by these factors, play a role in the formation of tumours:

- **Chemical carcinogens** are compounds that can react with DNA. Some agents act directly; others require

Table 2.3 Characteristics of benign and malignant tumours.

Feature	Benign	Malignant
Type of growth	Expansive	Infiltrative
Metastases	Absent	Frequent
Growth rate	Slow	High
Necrosis	Rare	Frequent
Border	Regular	Irregular
Resemblance to original tissue	High	Variable, often poor
Structure of tumour	Regular	Irregular
Mitosis rate	Low	High

Table 2.4 Examples of tumour nomenclature.

Tissue type	Benign	Malignant
Epithelial		
Glandular	Adenoma	Adenocarcinoma
Squamous cell	Squamous cell papilloma	Squamous cell carcinoma
Mesenchymal		
Fat	Lipoma	Liposarcoma
Connective tissue	Fibroma	Fibrosarcoma
Striated muscle	Rhabdomyoma	Rhabdomyosarcoma
Blood vessels	Haemangioma	Haemangiosarcoma
Blood-forming tissue		Leukaemia
Lymphatic tissue		Malignant lymphoma
Pigmented cells		Melanoma
Nerve cells	Neuroma	Neuroblastoma

metabolic conversion to become an active carcinogen. The smoke of cigarettes and alcohol seem to be the most important carcinogens in oral health. Heavy smoking and alcohol abuse are associated with an increased risk of head and neck cancer and premalignant conditions, such as **leukoplakia.**

- **Ionising radiation** can also induce mutation in the DNA, causing cells to transform. A substantial amount of the radiation received by the body is background radiation, produced by inescapable natural sources. The radiation used for diagnostic and therapeutic purposes also has the potential to transform cells. However, this potential risk for patients and staff is minimised to an acceptable level by adequate safety regulations. Long and intense exposure to **ultraviolet light** is also capable of transforming healthy cells into tumour cells. A well-known example is the increased risk of skin cancer in people of the Caucasian race living in Australia related to 'overexposure' to the sun.

- Several **microorganisms** seem to play a role in carcinogenesis. The parasite *Schistosoma haematobium* causes bladder carcinomas. The bacterium *Helicobacter pylori* is thought to be involved in the development of stomach carcinomas. Carcinomas of the liver are frequent in those areas of the world where infection with hepatitis-B virus is endemic. The **Epstein–Barr virus** is frequently found in patients with nasopharyngeal carcinomas. The human immunodeficiency virus (HIV) is associated with the development of **Kaposi sarcomas.**

Genetic aspects

Around 1910, Rous observed that injection of cell-free homogenate of a chicken sarcoma developed the same type of sarcoma in the receiving animal. Later it was found that a virus that contained genes with a transforming capacity caused this. Afterwards, genes were observed in normal (non-transformed) human cells that strongly resembled these viral **oncogenes**. These normal human genes, called **proto-oncogenes**, are involved in the regulation of normal cell growth and cell differentiation. However, derangement of a proto-oncogene leads to a cellular **oncogen** which may result in aberrant cell growth. Derangement of proto-oncogenes can be induced by a point mutation, a chromosomal translocation (where part of one chromosome is moved to another chromosome) or infection with an oncogenic virus.

Fortunately, in healthy cells there are also genes present that suppress the development of tumours. However, when these tumour **suppressor genes** are not expressed or produce an aberrant inactive protein, a tumour may develop. An example of such a tumour suppressor gene is the p53 gene. The normal form of this protein inspects the DNA of the cell for possible damage. When injuries are observed, the p53 protein either delays the cell cycle, enabling repair of the damaged part of the DNA, or induces programmed cell death (**apoptosis**). The protein produced by the mutated p53 gene lacks these activities.

Metastasis

The most important characteristic of malignant tumours is their capacity to invade adjacent normal tissues. By invading blood vessels and lymphatic channels they can be spread to other organs to form secondary tumours (metastases). This process of metastasis consists of several consecutive steps:

- Aided by enzymes, the tumour first enters the wall of the blood or lymph vessel.
- Subsequently, a tumour cell is released which passively flows with the blood or lymph.
- Downstream, the drifting tumour cell gets stuck in a capillary blood vessel or a lymph node.
- There the tumour cell invades the extracellular matrix and, after several cell divisions, a metastasis has developed.

Sometimes, metastases are the presenting clinical feature of the disease. For example, bone pain due to skeletal metastases can be the clinical manifestation of a primary internal malignancy that is still without symptoms. Occasionally metastases are observed arising from an unknown primary tumour.

Staging of tumours

A widely used system for staging (measuring the progress) of tumours is the TNM classification (tumour, node, metastases). This classification includes:

- The size and spread of the primary tumour (T).
- The absence or presence of metastases in lymph nodes (N).
- The absence or presence of distant metastases (M).

The number behind these characters increases with the size of the tumour and the degree of metastasis. This is illustrated in Table 2.5, which provides the TNM classification for oral mucosal carcinomas. A tumour without any metastases is classified as M_0. The TNM system is only denoted once: at initial diagnosis and before any kind of treatment.

Treatment of neoplasia

Tumours can be treated by surgery, radiotherapy, chemotherapy, hormone therapy or a combination of these.

Table 2.5 TNM staging of tumours that develop in the oral cavity.

T stage (primary tumour)

T1	Tumour ≤ 2 cm
T2	Tumour > 2 cm and ≤ 4 cm
T3	Tumour > 4 cm
T4	Invasion of the tumour in local structures

N stage (regional lymph nodes)

N0	No metastases in lymph nodes
N1	One metastasis in ipsilateral (on the same side) lymph node ≤ 3 cm
N2a	One metastasis in ipsilateral lymph node > 3 cm and ≤ 6 cm
N2b	Several metastases in ipsilateral lymph nodes, all ≤ 6 cm
N2c	Several metastases in bilateral or contralateral lymph nodes, all ≤ 6 cm
N3	One or more metastases in lymph nodes > 6 cm

M stage (distant metastases)

MX	The presence of distant metastases cannot be assessed
M0	No distant metastases
M1	Distant metastases

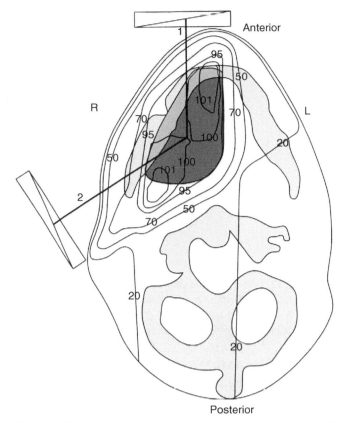

Figure 2.11 An example of radiation planning for a carcinoma of the tongue. Two beams are used to achieve a high dose within the tumour while sparing the surrounding tissue as much as possible.

Surgery

Surgical treatment is the primary treatment option for most solid tumours. During an operation, the blood vessels to and from the tumour are surgically closed as well as other vessels passing the target area. Next, the tumour is excised deep into the surrounding healthy tissue because the cut edges have to be completely free of tumour cells (particularly malignant tumours may invade the healthy tissue surrounding the tumour). When the tumour has a tendency for lymphatic metastasis, the local lymph nodes will also be removed surgically.

Radiotherapy

Radiotherapy uses ionising radiation, mostly produced by linear accelerators. These modern machines accelerate electrons almost to the speed of sound, resulting in a beam of high energy. Absorption of this energy by tissues results in the intracellular formation of radicals. electrons and radicals damage the DNA of the cell, ing in cell death during a subsequent cell division. he effect of radiation is predominantly observed that start to divide, radiotherapy will affect

rapidly dividing cells much faster than cells that divide at a much slower rate.

The radiation dose needed for the treatment of cancer is based on the location and type of malignancy, and whether or not radiotherapy will be used solely or in combination with other treatment options. In most patients with head and neck carcinomas treated with a curative intent, the total dose of radiation is given in small fractions (≈ 2 Gy) over a 5–7 week period, once a day, 5 days a week. This **fractionated radiation** is employed because there is a difference in the response of tumour tissue and normal tissue. In general, normal tissue repairs sublethal DNA damage, especially in the low dose range, better than tumour tissue. Giving radiation in small daily fractions magnifies the differences between tumour and normal tissues.

The radiation beam is given an optimal form, trying to spare the healthy tissues that surround the tumour as much as possible. In addition, usually multiple beams from several sides are used. This way, a high dose of radiation energy is achieved in the tumour, while the dose received by the normal tissues is divided over several areas, thus limiting damage to these normal (i.e. healthy), tissues (Figure 2.11). In **intensity modulated**

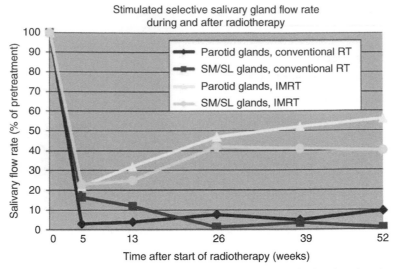

Figure 2.12 Loss of parotid and submandibular function following radiation therapy for head and neck cancer. Intensity modulated radiotherapy (IMRT) induces less damage to the salivary glands than conventional radiotherapy (Reproduced with permission from Vissink, A., Mitchell, J.B., Baum, B.J. et al. (2010) Clinical management of salivary gland hypofunction and xerostomia in head-and-neck cancer patients: Successes and barriers. International Journal of Radiation Oncology Biology Physics, 78, 983–991.)

radiotherapy (IMRT) a computer-driven machine moves around the patient, delivering thousands of tiny radiation beamlets from different angles which intersect at the tumour. Since the intensity of each beamlet can be controlled indivually, the normal surrounding tissues, are optimally spared (e.g. the salivary glands).

Normal tissues show remarkable differences in sensitivity to radiotherapy. The oral mucosa is very sensitive to radiation (epithelial cells have a rather short cell cycle) and therefore most patients that receive radiotherapy for head and neck tumours will develop **mucositis**. Damage to the salivary glands, both to the parotid and submandibular glands, is also common. IMRT has a clear clinical advantage over conventional radiotherapy, as it induces considerable less damage to the salivary glands (Figure 2.12).

Due to the severely reduced salivary flow, most patients suffer from **xerostomia** (sensation of a dry mouth) and have problems swallowing. They have an increased risk of oral infections such as **candidiasis** and the development of dental caries (Figure 2.13) and need support in maintaining an optimal oral hygiene.

Chemotherapy

Chemotherapy is the treatment of tumours with **cytostatic medication**. Cytostatics inhibit cell growth by damaging DNA or preventing the actual cell division. In general, tumour cells grow faster than the normal cells of the tissue where the tumour developed and therefore tumour cells are more sensitive to cytostatics. Cytostatics are especially used for treatment of disseminated neoplasms, such as tumours with metastases and leukaemia.

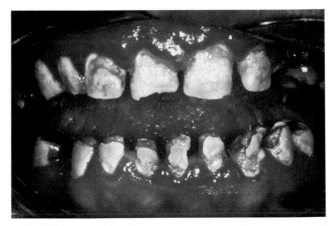

Figure 2.13 Example of radiation caries. Note the destruction of the smooth surfaces that are normally cleansed by the continuous secretion of saliva.

Unfortunately, like ionising radiation, cytostatics do not limit their action to tumour cells. Normal cells that divide at a high rate, such as the mucosa of the bowel and the oral cavity and stem cells in the bone marrow, are also sensitive to cytostatics. Therefore, potential acute side effects of chemotherapy are nausea, vomiting, diarrhoea and oral mucositis (Figure 2.14). The effects of cytostatics on the bone marrow result in decreased numbers of circulating leucocytes and thrombocytes in the blood. Another potential side effect of treatment with cytostatics is transient hair loss.

Patients with head and neck cancer are often treated with a combination of chemotherapy and radiotherapy (chemoradiotherapy). The cytostatics sensitize the tumors to radiation, thereby increasing survival of the patients.

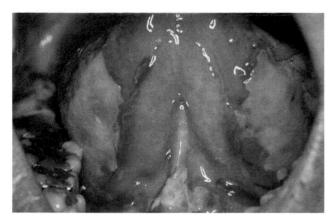

Figure 2.14 Example of chemotherapy-induced oral mucositis. (Courtesy of Dr. M. Stokman.)

Hormone therapy

Some tumours need specific human hormones for their growth. Examples of such tumours are breast cancer in women and prostate cancer in men. Hormone therapy tries to modify hormone concentrations in such a way that growth inhibition of the tumour occurs. Stimulating sex hormones can be withdrawn by surgical removal of the ovaries in women or the testes in men. Administration of **antihormones** is another possibility. Antihormones bind to the hormone receptors on the tumour cell, thereby blocking these receptors for normal hormones. An example of an antihormone is **tamoxifen**, used to treat breast cancer. Unfortunately, long-term clinical results of hormone therapy are limited.

Leukaemia

Blood cells develop from a relatively small number of stem cells in the bone marrow. These stem cells divide constantly, producing precursor cells that mature along several lines to produce the different types of cells in the blood. Since the lifetime of blood cells is rather short, blood cells must be produced in the bone marrow at a very high rate. On average, an adult individual produces 2×10^{11} erythrocytes, 2×10^{11} platelets and 10^{11} granulocytes per day!

In patients with leukaemia, the normal proliferation and maturation of the stem cells or precursor cells in the bone marrow are deranged. One malignant transformed stem cell results in an enormous offspring of identically altered cells. These deviant cells accumulate, disturbing the normal production of blood cells. This finally results in **anaemia** and a deficiency of platelets (**thrombocytopenia**) and granulocytes (**granulocytopenia**).

Leukaemias are divided into acute and chronic leukaemias. The classification according to the cell type that has overgrown the bone marrow is also important.

Acute leukaemia

In acute leukaemia there is an increase in the number of leucocytes in combination with a defect in the maturation of these leucocytes. The anaemia that develops may present as paleness, fatigue and shortness of breath. Infections of the throat and airway are the consequence of the granulocytopenia. Thrombocytopenia may cause spontaneous bleeding, for example from the oral mucosa and from the nose. The deviant leucocytes may accumulate in specific organs. This accumulation of leucocytes results in symptoms such as bone pain and lymph node enlargement, but gingival hyperplasia (due to leukaemic infiltrates) may also occur.

The first aim of the treatment is to normalise the production of blood cells. Cytostatic medication is administered to induce a complete remission: that is, leukaemic cells are no longer present when the bone marrow is microscopically investigated. The formation of blood cells in the bone marrow revives and the numbers of circulating blood cells normalise. When a remission is attained, additional treatment is necessary, consisting of intense chemotherapy or bone marrow transplantation.

Chronic leukaemia

In chronic leukaemia there is an increase in the number of white blood cells with different degrees of maturation (i.e. an increase in neutrophils, basophils and eosinophils). This indicates that in chronic leukaemia the capacity of the white blood cells to mature is maintained, in contrast to acute leukaemia.

In most patients with **chronic myeloid leukaemia** (CML) a translocation between a part of chromosome 9 and a part of chromosome 22 has occurred resulting in a characteristically small chromosome 22 (Philadelphia chromosome). Usually the symptoms of CML (anaemia, fatigue and loss of weight) develop slowly. A defect in the function of the platelets increases the bleeding tendency. The enlarged spleen may cause abdominal discomfort. Chemotherapy is given, in combination with alpha-interferon, in an attempt to normalise the blood count; for younger patients this is followed by bone marrow transplantation.

Chronic lymphocytic leukaemia (CLL) is characterised by increased numbers of B-lymphocytes in the blood. The B-lymphocytes infiltrate the normal lymphatic organs, such as bone marrow, spleen and lymph nodes. CLL is mostly observed in the elderly with a male predominance. A typical clinical feature of CLL is the swelling of several lymph nodes. During later stages, symptoms of bone marrow depression may develop (anaemia, granulocytopenia and thrombocytopenia), which are accompanied by an increased bleeding tendency and an increased risk of opportunistic infections.

Treatment of CLL consists of chemotherapy. Since the spleen plays an important role in the physiological removal of erythrocytes and thrombocytes, surgical removal of the spleen is sometimes performed in CLL patients with anaemia or thrombocytopenia.

The various types of leukaemia may cause oral complaints. Infiltration of peripheral nerves by leukaemic cells induces an oral prickling sensation or numbness. Infiltration of the gingiva occurs more frequently. The interdental gingiva especially may become oedematous, red and painful. In patients who have been treated with bone marrow transplantation, immune suppressive therapy is another potential cause of gingival hyperplasia. Periodontitis and multiple oral ulcers are also frequently observed in patients with leukaemia.

Haemostasis

For optimal circulation, the blood must remain fluid. Under conditions where blood unintentionally leaves the vessels, however, it is important that this fluid changes into a solid phase to minimise the loss of blood. The coagulation system maintains the delicate balance between keeping blood fluid inside the vessels and the capacity to coagulate outside the vessels. This implies that a defect in the coagulation system, resulting in a decreased capacity to coagulate, leads to (extensive) loss of blood. Such defects can be either congenital or acquired. On the other hand, defects of that part of the coagulation system that maintains blood in a fluid state will result in **thrombus** (blood clot) formation, causing vascular obstruction.

The coagulation process is composed of three parts: primary haemostasis, formation of a blood clot and finally, after some time, clot lysis.

Primary haemostasis

When a defect develops in the blood vessel wall, blood will come into contact with collagen from the underlying connective tissue. A protein present in blood, the **von Willebrand factor**, binds to this collagen. Next, the glycoprotein-Ib-receptor of the platelets binds to the von Willebrand factor. In this way, the platelets are tied to the vessel wall, the von Willebrand factor forming a kind of bridge. As a result of this adhesion, the platelets become activated and begin to express another receptor on their surface: glycoprotein-IIb/IIIa-receptor. Assisted by another protein in the blood, **fibrinogen**, the glycoprotein-IIb/IIIa-receptor makes contact with other platelets, resulting in an aggregation of these cells (Figure 2.15).

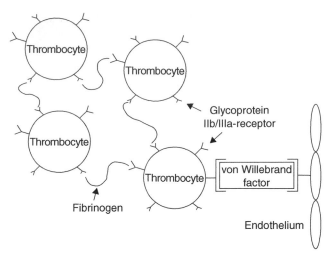

Figure 2.15 Diagram of platelet adhesion and aggregation. After adhesion of platelets to the wall of the vessel (by the glycoprotein-Ib-receptor and the von Willebrand factor) activation of the platelets occurs and the glycoprotein-IIb/IIIa-receptor is expressed on the surface. This receptor enables aggregation with other platelets via fibrinogen.

During activation of the platelets, several biochemical reactions occur. Substances are released from granules that further enhance the activation. In the platelet membrane, **arachidonic acid** is converted by the enzyme **cyclooxygenase** into **thromboxane A2**. Thromboxane A2 is capable of activating other platelets, which contributes to the formation of a platelet clot. Thromboxane A2 also has a strong vasoconstriction activity, which is important in reducing loss of blood. The enzyme cyclooxygenase is inhibited completely by acetylsalicylic acid, also known as aspirin. Therefore, in patients who use this analgesic, thromboxane A2 is no longer formed. As a consequence, the capacity of the platelets to aggregate is strongly reduced and the blood will not clot so readily.

Formation of the fibrin clot

The next step in the coagulation of blood is the formation of a fibrin clot. This is achieved through activation of **coagulation factors**. These factors are a group of proteins that are present in their inactive form in blood. Under the influence of an active factor, inactive factors become activated, in turn activating other factors. In this way, the coagulation system functions as a cascade resulting in large amounts of active factors. There are more than 10 different coagulation factors in blood, usually indicated by a Roman figure with a suffix 'a' for an activated factor (for example, factor VIIa is activated factor VII).

When the wall of a blood vessel is damaged, blood will leave the circulation and come into contact with the so-called tissue factor. The **factor VII** present in blood binds to this tissue factor and becomes converted into factor VIIa. In this way, a tissue factor/factor VIIa complex is created which can convert **factor X** into factor Xa. Subsequently, factor Xa (aided by **factor V**) can convert **prothrombin** (factor II) into **thrombin** (factor IIa). Under the influence of thrombin, **fibrinogen** is converted into **fibrin** which forms an insoluble network. In addition to this major route of the coagulation system, two amplification routes exist (Figure 2.16).

Inhibition of coagulation

Too much unintentional coagulation is undesirable since it may lead to **thrombosis** (a thrombus blocking a blood vessel). Therefore several inhibitors strictly regulate the coagulation system. These proteins can exert their activity at several levels of the coagulation system. The most important inhibitor is **antithrombin III**. This protein is capable of binding to thrombin (factor IIa) as well as to factor Xa, inhibiting both completely. Another inhibitor protein, **protein C**, can degrade the important cofactors **factor V** and **factor VIII**. For correct functioning, protein C itself also needs a cofactor, **protein S**.

Some people are deficient in one of these inhibitors. As a result, the activity of their coagulation system is increased leading to an increased risk of developing thrombosis. Some patients may have a congenital resistance to protein C because of a deviating factor V molecule (factor V Leiden), again leading to an increased risk of thrombosis.

Lysis of the clot (fibrinolysis)

Once the fibrin clot has developed, it forms a strong barrier against further loss of blood from the vessel. After a while, when the blood vessel wall and surrounding tissues have been repaired, the fibrin clot has to be removed to restore optimal circulation of the blood. The fibrinolytic system takes care of this. The final product of the fibrinolytic system is **plasmin**, a protein capable of degrading fibrin into small fragments. These degradation products are soluble, in contrast to fibrin, so the blood can remove them. Plasmin is the active form of **plasminogen**, another protein that circulates in the blood.

Coagulation disorders

A defect in the correct function of the coagulation system will result in spontaneous bleeding or in an abnormally large loss of blood, for example after a surgical procedure or the extraction of a tooth.

Disorders of primary haemostasis

Disorders of primary haemostasis can either be congenital or acquired during life. As described previously, platelets play a central role in achieving primary haemostasis. Therefore a shortage of platelets will result in an inadequate primary haemostasis. Under normal conditions blood contains $150–300 \times 10^9$ platelets per litre. A lack of platelets may be the consequence of an inadequate production, an increased degradation or an increased loss of platelets. Examples of diseases with deficient production of platelets are bone marrow diseases like leukaemia and chemotherapy-induced bone marrow suppression. Increased degradation may occur as the result of an autoimmune response against one's own platelets, while increased loss of platelets due to massive bleeding is rather rare, because the bone marrow can compensate rapidly for large losses of platelets by increasing the production rate.

A defect in primary haemostasis may also be due to a malfunction of platelets, although they are present in normal amounts. **Von Willebrand's disease** is caused by a deficiency in the von Willebrand factor, the protein that forms a 'bridge' between the platelet and the wall of the blood vessel. The disease has an autosomal dominant inheritance pattern.

Patients with von Willebrand's disease or a decreased number of platelets have an increased tendency of spontaneous gingival bleeding. Professional removal of plaque and calculus reduces this risk as it reduces the inflammatory burden to the gingiva, but such treatment should not be performed when the platelet number is lower than 50×10^9/l.

The use of medication is probably the most frequent cause of a defect in primary haemostasis. As described previously, acetylsalicylic acid (aspirin) irreversibly reduces the aggregation of platelets. A similar effect is induced by carbasalate calcium. Other non-steroidal

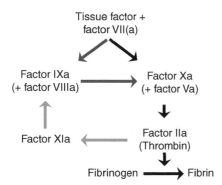

Figure 2.16 Diagram of the coagulation of blood. When blood is exposed to tissue factor, the tissue factor/factor VII complex can activate factor X, which in turn is capable of converting prothrombin to thrombin (black arrows). Amplification occurs because the tissue factor/factor VII complex also can activate factor IX leading to further activation of factor X (red arrows). Another amplification route consists of the activation of factor XI by thrombin, resulting in further activation of factor IX and subsequently factor X (green arrows).

anti-inflammatory drugs (NSAIDs), like ibuprofen, diclofenac and indomethacin, have a similar, but less prominent and mostly reversible effect on platelet aggregation. Obviously, these medications should not be used for pain relief in patients with lack of platelets or von Willebrand's disease.

Disorders of fibrin clot formation

Several diseases result in a deficient formation of a fibrin clot. Well known disorders are the hereditary deficiencies of factor VIII (**haemophilia A**) or factor IX (**haemophilia B**). In patients with such a deficiency, limited trauma may result in an extensive haematoma or prolonged bleeding. Spontaneous bleeding of the gingiva is not uncommon, and subgingival scaling and root surface debridement may cause extensive bleeding. In severe cases of haemophilia, factor VIII or factor IX is completely absent. From childhood, these patients suffer from spontaneous bleeding, especially into joints and muscles. Both haemophilia A and B are X-chromosome linked recessive disorders, almost exclusively affecting males. Treatment of haemophilia consists of the administration of the missing factor, purified from the blood of healthy subjects or produced by DNA-recombinant techniques.

Severe liver disease may also decrease formation of a fibrin clot. Most coagulation factors are synthesised in the liver, so an impaired function of the liver will result in decreased concentrations of these factors in the blood. Since **vitamin K** is an important factor for the production of factors II, VII, IX and X, a deficiency in vitamin K will also reduce fibrin clot formation. Treatment with vitamin K antagonists (acenocoumarol, phenprocoumarol) to prevent thrombosis also results in reduced concentrations of these four factors in the blood.

The effect of vitamin K antagonists is monitored using the **international normalised ratio** (**INR**), which compares the patient's prothrombin time with a normal control. In patients with an INR between 2 and 3.5, the risk of significant bleeding during dental hygiene treatment is small. The risk on bleeding can be reduced by using tranexamic acid which reduces the degradation of the bloodclot.

Atherosclerosis

Atherosclerosis is currently considered to be a continuous inflammatory response to a noxious stimulus, namely circulating low-density lipoprotein (**LDL-cholesterol**). Endothelial cells take up this LDL-cholesterol, but the LDL-cholesterol may also penetrate the wall of the vessel. In the blood vessel wall, LDL-cholesterol is oxidised to ox-LDL. Macrophages try to digest this ox-LDL, which is toxic for smooth muscle cells. If the amount of ox-LDL that enters the vessel wall exceeds the amount that can be processed by the macrophages, cells filled with lipid droplets begin to accumulate (**foam cells**). Smooth muscle cells also accumulate underneath the endothelium. Locations on the inner side of the blood vessel where foam cells and smooth muscle cells accumulate can be recognised as fatty streaks. These flat or slightly elevated linear lesions hardly obstruct the circulation of the blood. This early stage of atherosclerosis can be found in many people, even in young children.

Further accumulation of foam cells and smooth muscle leads to the formation of a thicker layer of fibrous connective tissue with a fatty mass in the middle. The fibrous cap, still covered with endothelial cells, may protrude into the lumen of the blood vessel and partially obstruct the circulation. Calcified atherosclerotic lesions of carotid arteries can occasionally be identified on dental orthopantomograms (Figure 2.17).

The term **atheroma** originally referred to the fatty deposit in the inner coat of the blood vessels, but is now

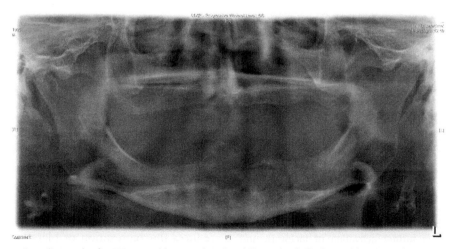

Figure 2.17 A panoramic radiograph of a 57-year-old man, showing bilateral calcified carotid artery atheromas.

used for the entire atherosclerotic lesion, also called **atherosclerotic plaque**. An atherosclerotic plaque also contains a large amount of tissue factor. When the plaque ruptures, collagen and tissue factor come in contact with blood. This will activate platelets and the coagulation system, resulting in the development of a blood clot (thrombus) with the concomitant risk of an acute total obstruction of the blood vessel. This illustrates that thrombosis is usually the terminal step of a long process in a vessel already narrowed by atherosclerosis. Arterial thrombosis has the additional risk of **embolisation**. For example, a thrombus may dislodge from the atherosclerotic plaque in the carotid arteries and be transported to the brain, where the sudden obstruction of an artery will cause a **cerebrovascular accident** (CVA) or stroke.

Atherosclerosis is most prominent in the large and medium arteries, especially at bifurcations of blood vessels. General risk factors for developing atherosclerosis are smoking, excess cholesterol levels in the blood, hypertension and diabetes.

Cardiac disease

The heart is a two-sided muscular pump that circulates the blood by co-ordinated contractions. The right side of the heart provides blood to the lungs; the left side is responsible for the general circulation. Both sides of the heart consist of an atrium and a ventricle. Valves are present between atrium and ventricle which prevent backwards blood flow during the contraction of the ventricle; on the right side, this is the tricuspid valve, on the left side, it is the mitral valve. Valves are also present between the right ventricle and the pulmonary artery (pulmonary valve), and between the left ventricle and aorta (aortic valve).

The wall of the heart is composed of three layers: an inner endocardium, a middle myocardium and an outer epicardium. The heart is surrounded by the pericardium. The myocardium forms the major part of the heart and is composed of striated muscle fibres. Two coronary arteries provide blood to the myocardium. The endocardium is the inner lining of the heart, including the heart valves, and consists of a thin layer of endothelial cells.

Ischaemic heart disease

Under normal conditions, the blood flow in the coronary arteries closely follows the metabolic demands of the myocardium. When the oxygen supply becomes insufficient, ischaemic heart disease results. This frequent cause of cardiac failure is usually due to atherosclerosis of the coronary arteries. The clinical presentation of ischaemic heart disease varies enormously, from symptomless to an acute myocardial infarct (see below).

Angina pectoris

The term angina pectoris refers to the presence of intermittent chest pain that may radiate to the arm, throat or jaw. Angina pectoris develops when the oxygen supply to the myocardium fails to meet the current oxygen demand. If the blood flow through the coronary arteries is hampered by atherosclerosis, an oxygen deficiency will occur during periods of increased activity of the myocardium, resulting in pain. Therefore, angina pectoris typically presents during exertion or periods of stress. In severe cases, angina pectoris may even develop at rest. The pain is usually relieved by rest (reduced oxygen demand) or a vasodilator like **nitroglycerin**. Within minutes after application, this vasodilator increases the blood supply to the mycocardium by coronary vasodilatation and reduces the cardiac workload by venous dilatation.

Further treatment of patients with angina pectoris is aimed at the prevention of oxygen deficiency, reduction of risk factors of atherosclerosis and prevention of a myocardial infarction. Reducing the heart frequency and the blood pressure with beta-blockers or calcium antagonists decreases the oxygen demand of the myocardium. Complementary treatment consists of prescribing medication to prevent platelet aggregation, like acetylsalicylic acid (aspirin) or carbasalate calcium.

When this treatment fails to reduce the frequency of angina pectoris attacks, a catheter can be inserted via a femoral artery or an inguinal artery into the beginning of the coronary arteries. After injection of a radiological contrast medium, the specific location(s) of the occlusion(s) of the coronary arteries can be identified. If the patient has a limited number of (small) **stenoses** (constrictions), the luminal diameter of these can be increased by inflating a small balloon at the tip of the catheter, which resolves the obstruction (**coronary angioplasty**). To prevent the wall from retracting into the lumen of the blood vessel again, sometimes a small metal tube is placed, a so-called **stent**. In patients with multiple or larger stenoses, surgical bypasses of these obstructions can be created using one or more veins from the leg.

Myocardial infarction

An infarct is a localised area of dead or necrotic tissue resulting from an obstruction of circulation to the area. An acute myocardial infarction is caused by a sudden, complete obstruction of a coronary artery. Usually the obstruction is caused by a thrombus that gets stuck on top of a ruptured atherosclerotic lesion already reducing the luminal diameter. The occlusion induces an acute lack of blood supply to parts of the myocardium.

In most cases, the myocardial infarction presents as an acute chest pain that, like angina pectoris, may radiate to the arm, throat or jaw. However, the pain lasts much longer than angina and is resistant to treatment with nitroglycerin. Associated symptoms are sweating, nausea, vomiting, breathlessness and collapse.

The acute management of a myocardial infarct is to restore the passage of the obstructed blood vessel. An early restoration of the blood supply is important to limit the damage to the myocardium. Because the coronary artery is usually obstructed by a thrombus, the enzyme **streptokinase** can be administered in an attempt to dissolve this blood clot. The lumen of the blood vessel can also be opened with coronary angioplasty (see angina pectoris).

An acute myocardial infarction frequently results in a cardiac arrest. Patients with a cardiac arrest lose consciousness immediately, stop breathing and lack an arterial pulse. If the loss of circulation lasts more than a few minutes, lack of oxygen will cause brain damage. Without treatment, a cardiac arrest will be fatal. Medical emergency services should be called immediately. Meanwhile, a combination of rescue breathings and cardiac compressions must be given to provide basic life support (see Chapter 16, p. 342).

Cardiac arrhythmia

Cardiac arrhythmia refers to a group of conditions in which the heart's normal rhythm is disrupted. Many arrhythmias are harmless, but some are life-threatening conditions. They can be classified according to the abnormal frequency: too slow (**bradycardia**, < 50/min) or too fast (**tachycardia**, > 100/min). Another classification is based on the location where the rhythm disorder originates. The relatively common **atrial fibrillation** is an extremely fast electrical activity of the atria (400–600/min), resulting in an irregular ventricular rhythm. As the atria do not functionally contract, patients with atrial flutter have a high risk of developing thrombosis, for which they receive oral anticoagulant treatment. **Ventricular tachycardia** is a fast heart rhythm that originates in one of the ventricles of the heart. This tachycardia decreases the cardiac output, which may induce hypotension and angina pectoris. A very rapid ventricular tachycardia may also lead to **ventricular fibrillation**. Ventricular fibrillation also frequently occurs after a myocardial infarction. During ventricular fibrillation there are chaotic electrical impulses that results in rapid, uncoordinated contractions of the muscle fibres in the ventricles. In ventricular fibrillation, the ventricles can not pump blood from the heart. Without resuscitation, the patient will die within a few minutes.

Pacemakers

A **pacemaker** is an implanted medical device which delivers electrical impulses by electrodes to the heart muscles. Pacemakers are used to speed up slow heart rhythms, to control fast heart rhythms and to make sure the ventricles contract normally in patients with atrial fibrillation. An implantable cardioverter defibrillator (**ICD**) is used in patients with a high risk of risk of developing ventricular fibrillation or ventricular tachycardia. The ICD monitors the heart rate continuously and when ventricular fibrillation or ventricular tachycardia is detected, a precisely calibrated electrical shock is delivered to terminate the arrhythmia.

There is some concern that the electromagnetic field from dental hygiene equipment could potentially interfere with the correct function of ICDs. However, this risk seems limited when the general precaution is followed to keep electrical appliances at least 15 cm away from the ICD and its electrodes (Brand *et al.*, 2007).

Infective endocarditis

Infective endocarditis is an infection of the thin layer of endothelium that covers the inside of the heart and the heart valves. Usually, infective endocarditis develops in patients who suffer from cardiac abnormalities that increase the flow rate of blood along the endothelium (e.g. deformed mitral valves or aortic valves). The increased blood flow damages the endothelium (**jetstream lesion**). On this damaged endothelium, a mesh of fibrin and platelets develops (a **vegetation**). When microorganisms subsequently enter the circulation, they can adhere to the vegetation. The synthetic material of an implanted prosthetic heart valve is another risk factor for developing infective endocarditis.

Although virtually any type of microorganism is capable of causing endocarditis, bacteria that are normally present on the skin or mucosa of the body, and can be introduced into the bloodstream as result of a surgical procedure, cause most cases. The chances of developing endocarditis largely depend on the ability of a microorganism to bind to fibrin. Once inside the vegetation, microorganisms are almost inaccessible for the immune system. The presence of microorganisms in the vegetation is an additional stimulus for coagulation and fibrin formation, increasing the size of the vegetation. This inflammatory process may invade the heart valve. The local effects of endocarditis vary considerably in severity, from an infected vegetation without tissue damage to a total destruction of the valve and adjacent tissue resulting in a sudden failure (Figures 2.18 and 2.19). A piece may also dislodge from the vegetation. In 15–35% of patients with infective endocarditis, these emboli will

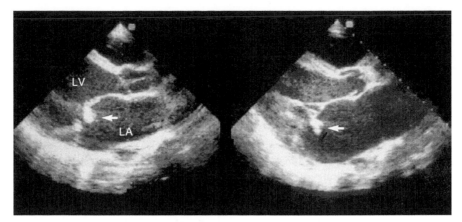

Figure 2.18 Echocardiogram of infective endocarditis of the mitral valve. The vegetation (arrow), present on the atrial side of the valve, is visible both during diastole (left) and systole (right). LA left atrium, LV left ventricle.

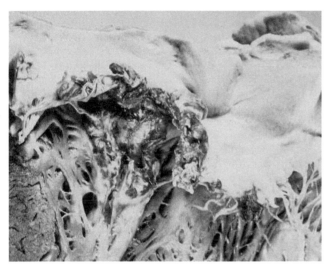

Figure 2.19 Infective endocarditis has resulted in total destruction of the mitral valve.

cause complications. The symptoms depend on the organ where the embolus obstructs the blood supply. The brain and lungs are involved most frequently.

The primary treatment of endocarditis is antimicrobial therapy against the (putative) microorganism for several weeks. About one third of the patients will ultimately need cardiac surgery to correct or replace damaged heart valves. Considering the severity of these complications, it is important that the chances of developing endocarditis are minimised after oral surgical or hygiene procedures that introduce microorganisms into the bloodstream, such as subgingival debridement or the extraction of teeth. Therefore antibiotics have been offered routinely as a preventive measure to patients with an increased risk of developing endocarditis prior to invasive treatment. However, there is little evidence that antibiotic prophylaxis is effective and any benefits

from prophylaxis need to be weighed against the risk of adverse effects for the patient and antibiotic resistance developing. As a result, the current UK guidelines recommend that antibiotic prophylaxis should not be offered to people undergoing dental procedures (www.nice.org.uk/CG064).

Hypertension

Throughout the cardiac cycle, blood pressure increases and decreases. The highest blood pressure (systolic blood pressure) occurs when the left heart ventricle contracts, pumping blood into the aorta. Then the heart muscles relax, allowing the heart to refill with blood and the lowest pressure is reached (diastolic blood pressure). **Hypertension** reflects a chronically elevated arterial blood pressure. Adults are classified as hypertensive if their systolic blood pressure is consistently at least 140 mmHg systolic and/or 90 mmHg diastolic.

Hypertension may develop secondary to, for example, endocrine disorders, kidney diseases or pregnancy. However, in 90–95% of the hypertensive patients no direct cause can be identified. Obesity, smoking, excessive use of alcohol and a sedentary profession are predisposing factors for hypertension. Hypertension is a major risk factor for developing atherosclerosis, myocardial infarction and a cerebrovascular accident. Treatment consists of a diet, lifestyle changes and antihypertensive medication. **Antihypertensives** are frequently accompanied by oral side effects such as gingival hyperplasia, xerostomia and taste alterations. Angioneurotic oedema may occur in patients that are using so-called angiotensin-converting enzyme inhibitors. Such a swelling may suddenly occur even after years of usage of this type of medication. When an angioneurotic oedema has

Table 2.6 Hypertension and dental (hygiene) treatment.

SBP	DBP	MRF	Guidelines
120–139	80–89	Yes/no	Routine treatment OK
140–159	90–99	Yes/no	Routine treatment OK, refer for medical consultation
160–179	100–109	No	Routine treatment OK, refer for medical consultation
160–179	100–109	Yes	Only urgent treatment, refer for medical consultation
180–209	110–119	No	No treatment without medical consultation. Refer for prompt medical consult
180–209	110–119	Yes	No treatment. Refer for emergency medical treatment
>210	>120	Yes/no	No treatment. Refer for emergency medical treatment

DBP: diastolic blood pressure; MRF: medical risk factor (such as prior medical infarction, angina pectoris, high coronary disease risk, stroke, diabetes, kidney disease); SBP: systolic blood pressure. (Modified from Merin, R.L. (2004) Hypertension guidelines. *Journal of the American Dental Association*, **135**, 1220–1222.)

occurred, further use of this type of antihypertensives is prohibited.

Guidelines for dental hygiene treatment in individuals with elevated blood pressure are provided in Table 2.6.

References

Brand, H.S., Entjes, M.L., Nieuw Amerongen, A.V. *et al.* (2007) Interference of electrical dental equipment with implantable cardioverter-defibrillators. *British Dental Journal*, **203**, 577–579.

Merin, R.L. (2004) Hypertension guidelines. *Journal of the American Dental Association*, **135**, 1220–1222.

Vissink, A., Mitchell, J.B., Baum, B.J. *et al.* (2010) Clinical management of salivary gland hypofunction and xerostomia in head-and-neck cancer patients: Successes and barriers. *International Journal of Radiation Oncology BiologyPhysics*, **78**, 983–991.

Further reading

Delves, P.J., Martin, S., Burton, S. and Roitt, I. (2006) *Roitt's Essential Immunology*, 11th edition. John Wiley & Sons, Chichester.

Faucci, A.S., Braunwald, E., Kasper, D.L., Hauser, S.L., Longo, D.L., Jameson, J.L. and Loscalzo, J. (2008) Harrison's principles of internal medicine. 17th edn. McGraw-Hill Professional, New York.

Kumar, V., Abbas, A.K., Fausto, N., and Mitchell, R. (eds) (2007) *Robbins Basic Pathology*, 8th edn. W.B. Saunders, London.

Roitt, I., Brostoff, J., Male, D. and Roth, D. (eds) (2006) *Immunology*, 7th edn. Mosby, St Louis.

Rubin, E., Gorstein F., Schwarting, R. and Strayer, D.S. (eds) (2004) *Rubin's Pathology: Clinico Pathologic Foundations of Medicine*, 4th edn. Lippincott, Williams & Wilkins, Baltimore.

Scully, C. (2010) *Medical Problems in Dentistry*, 6th edn. Churchill Livingstone, Edinburgh.

Underwood, J.C.E. and Cross, S.S. (eds) (2009) *General and Systemic Pathology*, 5th edn. Churchill Livingstone, Edinburgh.

3

Oral medicine and pathology

Paula Farthing

Summary

This chapter covers:

- Viral infections
- Oral ulceration
- White patches and premalignant lesion of the oral mucosa
- Oral cancer
- Soft tissue swellings of the oral mucosa
- Cysts of the jaws
- Conditions of the salivary glands
- Oral manifestations of systemic disease
- Common causes of facial pain
- Disorders of the temporomandibular joint
- Developmental tooth anomalies
- Tooth wear

Introduction

As dental care professionals (DCPs), hygienists and therapists will encounter the oral mucosa and the underlying supporting tissues as well as the teeth on a daily basis. They are therefore in a unique position to detect disease which may be either local or systemic in origin. In some cases detection may be life saving, in others recognition of the disease may affect the treatment plan, in yet others the patient may seek reassurance or an explanation of its implications. It is therefore important to have a thorough understanding of the causes and the clinical presentation of the common and important oral diseases and their effects upon both the treatment and the patient.

Viral infections

Unlike bacteria which are composed of single cells and capable of independent growth, viruses are composed of small nuclear fragments surrounded by a protein coat. They are unable to divide or replicate on their own and in order to survive must gain access to and live inside cells. Once inside they use the host cell's own synthetic processes to reproduce and, in the process, often destroy the host cell. In other cases the host will destroy the virally infected cell in order to eliminate the virus. It is this cellular destruction that is responsible for many of the clinical features of viral infections affecting the oral cavity.

The time taken for the virus to infect the host, replicate and for cellular damage and hence clinical symptoms to occur may be anything from 3 to 21 days and is known as the **incubation period**. Most severe viral infections last between 10 and 14 days, after which time the host has mounted an effective immune response and the infection resolves. Other less virulent infections may last only a few days. In general viral infections affect younger age groups, and viral infections occurring in older age groups raises the possibility of underlying immunosuppression.

The common viral infections affecting the oral cavity are:

- Herpes simplex: primary and secondary.
- Herpes zoster: primary and secondary.
- Hand, foot and mouth.
- Herpangina.

Clinical Textbook of Dental Hygiene and Therapy, Second Edition. Edited by Suzanne L. Noble.
© 2012 John Wiley & Sons, Ltd. Published 2012 by John Wiley & Sons, Ltd.

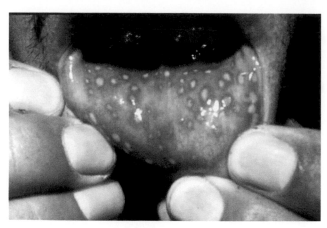

Figure 3.1 Young adult with primary herpes. Numerous small ulcers covered by a white slough and with erythematous margins are present on the labial mucosa.

Of these, infections caused by herpes simplex are the most common and important.

Primary herpes (primary gingivoherpetic stomatitis)

This is caused by herpes simplex virus type 1, which is transmitted in saliva, and it is usually children and young adults who are affected. The following features help in the diagnosis:

- The patient will complain of feeling unwell.
- They usually have a fever and enlarged lymph nodes in the neck (**cervical lymphadenopathy**).
- Painful blisters known as **vesicles** develop on the gingiva, palate, buccal mucosa and tongue and these are fragile and burst to form superficial ulcers covered in grey–white slough (Figure 3.1). The surrounding tissues are red (erythematous) and the lips may appear swollen and blood encrusted.
- In some cases the patients will be unable to eat or drink.

Patients are highly infectious and isolation and bed rest are advised. Most treatment is symptomatic and the disease is self-limiting, resolving in about 10–14 days. The diagnosis is made on clinical features. If antiviral agents are given early enough, they may shorten the course of the disease (see also Chapter 12, p. 261).

Although primary herpes may be very severe, in many instances the disease is subclinical and the patient will have no signs and symptoms.

Secondary herpes (cold sores)

In approximately a third of patients, the herpes virus remains dormant in the ganglion of the trigeminal nerve. It is reactivated by a number of agents including sunlight, stress and menstruation, and travels down the trigeminal nerve to form characteristic vesicles, which burst and crust over, on the lips. The lips may become swollen and the lesions are known as cold sores. They often recur in the same position and are preceded by a tingling or **prodromal phase**. Treatment with antiviral agents at this stage may significantly shorten the course of the disease which otherwise lasts 10–14 days. The patient is infectious during this time and dental treatment should be avoided.

Varicella zoster viral infection (chicken pox)

This is also caused by a herpes virus and is a common disease of children. It rarely affects the oral cavity but occasionally small ulcers may be seen in addition to the itchy, vesicular, crusting rash which occurs on the skin. The incubation period lasts up to 21 days and the disease 10–14 days. Like herpes simplex, the varicella zoster virus may also lie dormant in the trigeminal ganglion and upon reactivation forms a characteristic rash along the distribution of the nerve. This may occur on the face or rarely in the oral cavity. Such lesions are painful and may cause scarring.

Hand, foot and mouth and herpangina

These two infections are both caused by the **coxsackie A virus** and are relatively mild diseases usually affecting children. In both infections the lesions are characterised by vesicles, which break down to form shallow ulcers.

- In hand, foot and mouth disease almost any part of the oral mucosa may be affected together with the hands and the plantar surfaces of the feet.
- In herpangina the lesions may affect the soft palate, tonsils and pharynx and the patient usually complains of a sore throat.
- In both conditions lesions resolve within a few days.

Oral ulceration

The oral mucosa is composed of stratified squamous epithelium, which covers and protects the underlying connective tissues from the oral cavity. An ulcer is formed when there is a break or defect in the epithelial covering and the underlying connective tissue is exposed to saliva and microorganisms of the oral cavity. This results in an acute inflammatory response and the surrounding connective tissue becomes reddened and inflamed. The surface of the ulcer is covered by a white–grey slough.

There are many causes of oral ulceration but the two most common types are those caused by trauma and idiopathic aphthous ulceration. An important although rarer cause is malignancy and this is discussed in more detail in the section on oral cancer.

Traumatic ulceration

There are many causes of trauma in the oral cavity and these include mechanical, chemical and thermal.

Mechanical trauma may be caused by:

- Sharp cusps.
- Orthodontic appliances.
- Ill-fitting dentures.
- Teeth (biting lips or cheeks).

Diagnosis of this type of ulceration is usually not difficult and the position, shape and size of the ulceration should correspond to the suspected cause. Once this is removed the ulceration usually starts to heal within 10 days. If healing does not occur then other causes of ulceration should be suspected.

Chemical ulceration is relatively uncommon but may be caused by drugs and other oral preparations taken by the patient. Aspirin tablets placed in the oral cavity adjacent to a painful tooth may cause this type of ulceration.

Thermal injury is relatively common and is caused by the ingestion of very hot food or drinks. The oral cavity heals quickly and without scarring and thermal injury rarely causes a diagnostic problem.

Aphthous ulceration (recurrent aphthous stomatitis)

Aphthous ulcers are relatively common and affect younger rather than older individuals. Their characteristic feature is recurrence and typically they start in childhood and tend to decrease in frequency with age. The cause of aphthous ulceration is not known but there is a family history in about 45% of patients, indicating there may be a hereditary disposition. Other predisposing factors which have been implicated include stress, trauma and menstruation. In some cases aphthous ulceration is associated with iron-deficiency anaemia and treatment of the deficiency may result in resolution.

Three different clinical types have been identified: minor aphthae, major aphthae and herpetiform ulcers.

Minor aphthae

This is the most common type of ulceration and has the following characteristic features:

- Ulcers are typically small, about 2–5 mm across, oval and covered by a grey slough. The surrounding mucosa may be erythematous (Figure 3.2).
- In some patients the ulcers may be multiple.

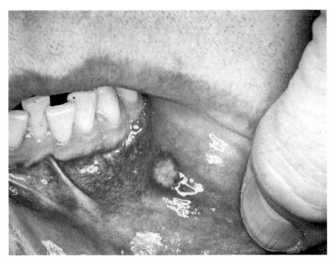

Figure 3.2 Minor aphthous ulcer on the labial mucosa.

- They affect the non-keratinised mucosa, i.e. the lateral border of tongue, floor of mouth, buccal mucosa and lips, and last about 10–14 days.
- The ulcers may be very painful and anecdotal evidence suggests that the pain increases towards the end of the 14-day period.
- The time interval for recurrence is variable.

Treatment is symptomatic if all possible underlying causes have been excluded.

Major aphthae

These ulcers are not as common as minor aphthae and differ in the following ways:

- They are larger and usually greater than 5–10 mm in diameter.
- They are often multiple and affect keratinised as well as non-keratinised mucosa; the lips, cheeks and soft palate are common areas.
- They last between 4 and 6 weeks and may be very painful.
- They may also heal with scarring.

Other causes of ulceration

A malignant ulcer caused by a squamous cell carcinoma is an important cause of oral ulceration. However, it has very characteristic features that help in the diagnosis and these are discussed below in detail. Ulceration following breakdown of vesicles is a feature of viral lesions affecting the oral cavity and also certain autoimmune blistering disorders, such as **pemphigus vulgaris**, but these latter conditions are rare.

The differential diagnosis and distinguishing features of oral ulceration are shown in Table 3.1.

Table 3.1 Differential diagnosis of ulceration of oral mucosa.

Type of ulcer	Clinical features
Traumatic: mechanical	Position of ulceration corresponds to suspected cause (dentures, teeth, orthodontic appliance) and disappears when cause removed
Idiopathic: minor aphthous ulceration	Recurrent, young individuals, painful, small lesions, lips, floor of mouth. Lasts 10–14 days
Neoplastic: squamous cell carcinoma	Long duration, non-healing ulcer, no obvious cause, raised rolled margins, firm/hard to touch. High-risk sites include floor of mouth, lateral tongue, retromolar area
Infective: herpes simplex	Preceded by vesicles, characteristic distribution on gingivae and palate, patients systemically unwell, lasts 10–14 days
Autoimmune conditions: pemphigus vulgaris, pemphigoid	Blisters which break down to give ulcers and erosions. Affects older individuals. Skin lesions with pemphigus vulgaris

Table 3.2 Differential diagnosis of white patches affecting the oral mucosa.

Type of white patch	Clinical features
Frictional keratosis	Position of lesion corresponds to cause (dentures, teeth, orthodontic appliance) and disappears when cause is removed. Common on cheeks, lateral border of tongue
Lichen planus	Bilateral reticular lesions affecting the cheeks, lateral tongue, gingivae. Skin lesions. Other clinical types. No obvious cause
Lichenoid reactions to drugs	Similar clinical appearance to lichen planus but associated with drugs
Lichenoid reactions to amalgam restorations	Unilateral on tongue or cheeks adjacent to large amalgam restoration. Resembles lichen planus
Leukoplakia – homogeneous	Smooth or undulating white patch, any site. Not associated with trauma or any other obvious cause
Leukoplakia – non-homogeneous	Irregular white patch. May have a raised, nodular or irregular surface and or show variations in colour with red areas. Highest risk of malignant change

White patches and premalignant lesions of the oral mucosa

In health the oral mucosa is pale pink, but pathological changes may result in white patches. In many instances this is brought about by changes in the keratinisation of the epithelium; for example, the cheeks are normally non-keratinised but if epithelium becomes keratinised they will appear white clinically. There are many causes of white patches on the oral mucosa and the most important are discussed below. The differential diagnosis and distinguishing features are shown in Table 3.2.

Frictional keratosis

White patches may occur in response to chronic trauma and are known as frictional keratosis. Such lesions are common on the buccal mucosa in a linear pattern adjacent to the teeth and this is known as an occlusal line. They may also be seen on the tongue or other intraoral sites and are often caused by:

- Chronic biting.
- A sharp cusp.
- An over-extended denture.
- An orthodontic appliance.

In order to make a diagnosis of frictional keratosis the source of the trauma must be identified and the position of the white patch should correspond to the trauma. If this is not the case then other causes of a white patch should be considered and these are discussed in more detail below.

Lichen planus

Lichen planus is a relatively common disorder, which may affect the skin as well as the oral mucosa. Middle-aged women are affected more than men and in most cases the disease is symptomless. However, some patients may complain of roughness or discomfort on eating spicy foods. Typically it is characterised by:

- Reticular, white, interlacing lines or striations which occur bilaterally on the buccal mucosa and tongue and occasionally the lips (Figure 3.3).
- Sometimes the free and attached gingivae may be affected and appear fiery red.
- Other patterns of disease may be seen: the white patches may be plaque-like rather than reticular or sometimes the mucosa appears erythematous and may show areas of erosion or ulceration. In these cases diagnosis may be more difficult.
- Skin lesions may be present on the wrists and shins and appear as violet papules.

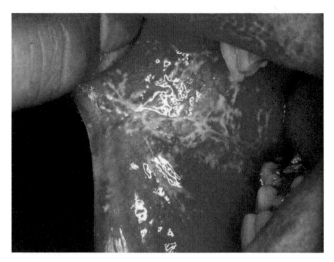

Figure 3.3 Lichen planus affecting the buccal mucosa. Note the lace-like white striations on the cheeks.

The histological changes in lichen planus show that the epithelium is keratinised, leading to the white striations seen clinically. In addition there is a band of lymphocytes beneath the epithelium which is associated with destruction of the lower epithelial layers. This and other observations have led to the belief that lichen planus is the result of a cell-mediated immune reaction. What precipitates this reaction is unknown.

Lichenoid reactions

Lesions that resemble lichen planus clinically may be caused by drugs and also dental materials. Lichenoid drug reactions are often caused by:

- Antihypertensive drugs taken for high blood pressure.
- Oral hypoglycaemic drugs taken for diabetes.

Lichenoid drug reactions start after commencement of drug therapy and resolve when the drug is withdrawn. Such lesions are usually bilateral and very difficult to distinguish from lichen planus unless a careful medical and drug history is taken.

Reactions to amalgam restorations are also common but in these cases lesions affect one side of the mouth only and are present on the mucosa in the contact area of amalgam. Quite often it is the buccal mucosa and lateral borders of the tongue that are affected. Removal of the restoration usually results in resolution of the lesion.

Leukoplakia

White patches that have no obvious cause and do not fall into any of the other diagnostic categories of white patches are known as leukoplakia. They are important lesions because a small proportion have a higher risk of turning malignant (i.e. developing into squamous cell

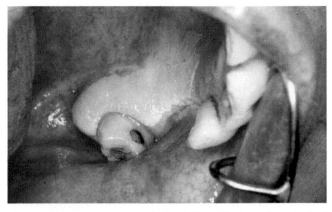

Figure 3.4 Homogeneous leukoplakia affecting the gingival margin and palate.

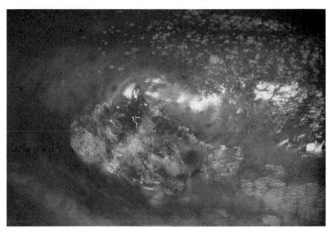

Figure 3.5 Non-homogeneous leukoplakia occurring on the lateral border of tongue. Note the variation in colour: red areas interspersed with white areas.

carcinoma) than does normal mucosa. Leukoplakia is therefore a **premalignant lesion** and identification of the 'high-risk' leukoplakias is important for the patient and dental care professional.

The clinical appearance of leukoplakia is very variable and they have been grouped into homogeneous and non-homogeneous types.

Homogeneous leukoplakia

- The lesions appear similar throughout and are usually flat, white patches, but some may have a regular undulating surface (Figure 3.4).
- This type of leukoplakia has a negligible risk of turning malignant.

Non-homogeneous leukoplakia

- The lesions may show variations in the surface contour; they may be nodular or spiky.
- They may show variations in colour with red areas interspersed with white areas (Figure 3.5).

- It is within this group that the highest risk of malignant transformation occurs (Axell *et al.*, 1996) and indeed some may be malignant from the onset.

The site of the leukoplakia is also important in determining the risk, as certain areas have a high risk of malignant change. These sites are the lateral border of the tongue, floor of the mouth and the retromolar area.

Aspects of the patient's social history are also important as the risk of malignancy increases in patients who smoke and drink. There is also an increased risk in patients who take **betel quid** and in these patients the leukoplakia is often found on the buccal mucosa.

Pathological changes in leukoplakia

It is often difficult, if not impossible, to determine the risk of malignant transformation in leukoplakia by clinical examination alone and for this reason biopsies are often performed on such lesions, i.e. a small piece is removed and sent for histopathological examination. From a histopathological point of view the risk of malignant transformation is related to how abnormal the individual epithelial cells appear (**atypia**) and the extent to which this is present throughout the thickness of the epithelium. These changes together are referred to as **dysplasia** which is graded as mild, moderate and severe. The highest risk of malignant transformation lies within lesions showing severe dysplasia and these are usually removed surgically. Patients with lesions showing mild or moderate dysplasia may be kept under review.

Oral cancer

Oral cancer refers to cancers which arise in the oral cavity including the lips, tongue, mouth, oropharynx and hypopharynx as well as other ill defined sites. Almost 90% are squamous cell carcinoma which is a **malignant neoplasm** that arises from the oral epithelium.

Epidemiology of oral cancer

Oral cancer is the sixth most common cancer worldwide with an estimated 405 000 new cases per year. Two thirds of these are in developing countries (Cancer Research UK). The highest incidence (i.e. rates of oral cancer per 100 000 population) is found in parts of South-East Asia, and in Bangladesh, Sri Lanka and Pakistan it is the most common cancer in men. In Europe the highest incidence in men is found in France and Hungary.

The following points are important in the epidemiology of oral cancer in the UK:

- There were 5410 new cases of oral cancer diagnosed in the UK in 2007 (Cancer Research UK) and the incidence has increased by 50% for both men and women since 1989.
- The highest incidence of oral cancer in the UK is found in Scotland and this correlates with higher rates of tobacco and alcohol consumption.
- The majority of new cases occur in individuals over the age of 40 years with a peak incidence between 60 and 70 years.
- Men are affected more than women but the incidence in women is rising.
- The incidence is rising in younger individuals particularly the 40–60-year-old age groups. It is thought this is due to changes in alcohol consumption rather than an increase in tobacco consumption (Hindle *et al.*, 2000) but one study has shown that a significant proportion of young patients have no risk factors (Llewellyn *et al.*, 2003).
- The percentage of people who survive 5 years after diagnosis of oral cancer (all sites) is in the region of 50%.
- The survival figures vary depending on the site of the cancer. Almost all patients with cancer of the lip survive 5 years but the percentage of people who survive 5 years with cancer of the posterior parts of the mouth is very low.

Aetiology of oral cancer

The causes or aetiology of oral cancer are complex. There is little evidence for a strong genetic predisposition to oral cancer and environmental factors appear to be important. The risk of developing oral cancer is increased in individuals who smoke, use smokeless tobacco in the form of snuff or betel quid and is further increased in those who drink and smoke together. There is some evidence that in a small subset of patients human papillomavirus infection may play a role.

The following points should be noted:

- The most commonly affected sites are the lateral border of the tongue, floor of mouth and the retromolar region and about 80% of cancers in the Western world occur in these sites. This is related to alcohol consumption and smoking, two important risk factors in the development of oral cancer. It is thought that the **carcinogens** (chemicals that cause cancer, which are present in tobacco), dissolve in saliva and pool in these regions of the mouth.
- Alcohol itself is not carcinogenic (i.e. it does not contain carcinogens) but it potentiates the effects of carcinogens by increasing the permeability of the oral mucosa.
- In South-East Asia many cases of oral cancer are caused by betel quid chewing and occur on the cheeks

adjacent to where the quid is placed. Studies have shown that immigrant populations from South-East Asia in the UK continue this habit and have a higher risk of developing oral cancer (Farrand *et al.*, 2001; Warnakulasuriya, 2002).

- Cancer on the lower lip is caused by sunlight and is prevalent in fair-skinned individuals with outdoor occupations or lifestyles.
- A diet low in fresh fruit and vegetables is a risk factor for the development of oral cancer.

Pathology of oral cancer

In health the oral epithelium forms a continuous layer on the surface of the mucosa but in oral cancer the epithelium proliferates excessively due to genetic changes and eventually the epithelial cells grow down into the underlying connective tissue. This is known as invasion and is a characteristic feature of malignancy (Figure 3.6). The tumour cells continue to divide and invade and will spread into and destroy the underlying tissues which will then feel hard and not function properly. Tissues affected in this way may include skeletal muscle, salivary glands and bone. Tumour cells will also invade lymphatic vessels and spread to the cervical lymph nodes in the neck. This process is called **metastasis**.

Once in the node, the tumour cells continue to proliferate and they destroy the node and sometimes spread out into the tissues of the neck. Nodes that contain tumour feel very hard and are usually painless. If the tumour has spread into the neck, the node will not be mobile, as is usual, but will be attached (fixed) to the surrounding tissues. In a small proportion of cases the cancer spreads beyond the lymph nodes, enters the blood stream and grows in other organs, but this is rare.

Clinical features of oral cancer

Recognition of oral cancer is important and early detection, particularly before the cancer has spread to the lymph nodes in the neck, may save lives. The following features are important:

- Some oral cancers arise in pre-existing leukoplakia; non-homogeneous lesions that have a raised nodular surface and show variations in colour with speckled red–white areas are particularly suspicious.
- Some cancers present as **erythroplakia**. These are velvety red patches which may be raised above the surrounding tissues (Figure 3.7). These lesions are very suspicious and nearly half are oral cancer on biopsy and the remainder show severe dysplasia which means they have a high risk of turning malignant.
- Long-standing ulceration is also a common presentation and typically the ulcers have raised, rolled margins (Figure 3.8).
- Some cancers fungate (grow out) into the oral cavity as well as invade into the underlying tissues.
- The site of the lesion is important; high-risk sites are the lateral border of tongue, the floor of mouth and the retromolar area.
- Tissues affected by oral cancer are firm or hard to touch and there may be destruction leading to loss of function.
- Lesions are usually painless in the early stages and many patients are unaware of the lesions until they are quite large.
- If the cancer has spread to the cervical lymph nodes these will feel rock hard and painless and may be enlarged.
- In advanced stage disease the patient may appear very thin and pale (**cachetic**).

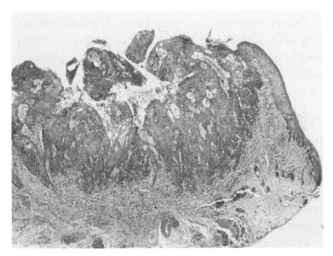

Figure 3.6 Histological changes in oral cancer. There is normal-appearing epithelium to the right of the picture. In the centre and towards the left, the surface is disrupted and islands of squamous cell carcinoma have invaded into the underlying connective tissue.

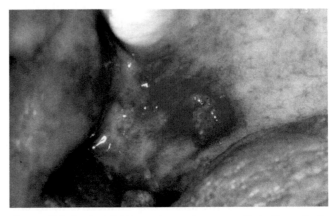

Figure 3.7 Erythroplakia on the oral mucosa. Note the velvety red appearance.

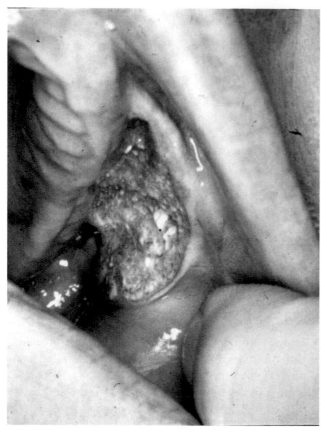

Figure 3.8 Oral cancer: long-standing ulcer in the buccal sulcus. Note the raised, rolled margins. The ulcer surface has a speckled red–white appearance.

Treatment

The diagnosis of oral cancer is made by biopsy and histopathological examination. Once the diagnosis is made it is important for the clinician to determine the extent of the disease and whether it has spread to the lymph nodes in the neck. Oral cancer is treated by surgery and/or radiotherapy, and the decision as to which is appropriate is taken at multidisciplinary team meetings attended by all who are involved in patient care.

Soft tissue swellings of the oral mucosa

Swellings may occur anywhere on the oral mucosa and are relatively common in the oral cavity. The overwhelming majority are benign, reactive or inflammatory lesions, that is they form in response to some injury or insult. A few are benign neoplasms or developmental lesions and only very rarely are swellings malignant neoplasms. Swellings may arise from the mucosa, the overlying epithelium or the underlying connective tissue and its component parts, or they may be related to the teeth, bone or salivary glands.

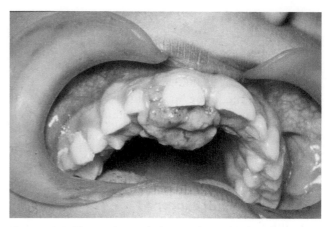

Figure 3.9 Fibrous hyperplasia on the palatal mucosa. It is caused by trauma from the lower incisor teeth which occlude onto the palate in a patient with an excessive overjet.

Swellings on the gingivae

A swelling on the gingivae is called an **epulis** and the three most common types are:

- Fibrous hyperplasia.
- Pyogenic granuloma.
- Giant cell granuloma.

Fibrous hyperplasia

These swellings are caused by an overgrowth of fibrous connective tissue in response to chronic trauma. This may be from:

- Plaque or calculus.
- Orthodontic appliances.
- Dentures.
- Malocclusion.

Often the hyperplasia is nodular and is known clinically as a **fibroepithelial polyp**. Fibrous hyperplasias are covered by oral epithelium and appear pale and the same colour as surrounding mucosa (Figure 3.9). They are treated by removing the cause of the trauma and by excision.

Pyogenic granuloma

Pyogenic granulomas are also formed in response to trauma and are the result of overgrowth of immature, vascular connective tissue (granulation tissue). They grow rapidly and as a result are ulcerated and not covered by epithelium. They are very vascular and therefore clinically appear red or red–blue and may bleed easily (Figure 3.10).

Pyogenic granulomas often form in response to calculus and plaque and are particularly common in pregnancy and during puberty when there is an exaggerated vascular response due to hormonal changes. They are sometimes referred as a **pregnancy epulis**. Treatment is to remove the cause, that is to improve oral hygiene.

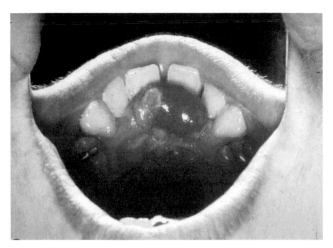

Figure 3.10 Pyogenic granuloma on the palatal gingivae behind the upper anterior teeth.

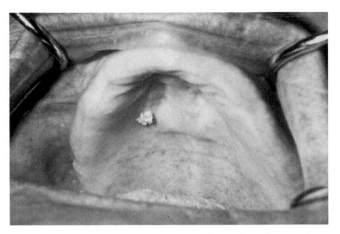

Figure 3.11 Papilloma on the palate of an edentulous patient. Note the spiky, cauliflower-like appearance.

Table 3.3 Differential diagnosis of localised gingival swellings.

Type of swelling	Clinical features
Fibrous hyperplasia (fibroepithelial polyp)	Smooth, mucosal coloured, related to trauma from teeth, orthodontic appliance or denture
Pyogenic granuloma	Red/red–blue, vascular, bleeds easily, related to poor oral hygiene. Patient may be pregnant or at puberty
Giant cell granuloma	Red/red–blue, vascular, anterior parts of mouth. Not related to poor oral hygiene
Dental abscess	Red–yellow, soft/fluctuant, associated with non-vital tooth

Some lesions may regress but more often it is necessary to excise them. In pregnant patients this may be delayed until after the baby is born.

Giant cell granuloma

Giant cell granulomas occur exclusively on the gingivae, usually in the anterior parts of the mouth. They may become quite large and extend over the labial aspect of the teeth. They are red–blue in colour and clinically difficult to distinguish from pyogenic granulomas. Their cause is unknown and treatment is excision.

The differential diagnosis of gingival swellings is shown in Table 3.3.

Swellings in other oral sites

Fibrous hyperplasia and pyogenic granulomas may occur at any intraoral site and show the same clinical characteristics as on the gingivae. A common cause of fibrous hyperplasia is overextended or ill-fitting dentures and large amounts of hyperplastic tissue may form under the denture on the palate or at the denture margins. This may also be associated with ulceration. Treatment is to improve the fit of the dentures and surgically remove the excess tissue. Other causes of swellings are described below.

Squamous cell papilloma

Squamous cell papillomas are formed as a result of overgrowth of the epithelium which becomes keratinised and thrown into folds or fronds. This results in lesions which have a white spiky or cauliflower-like appearance clinically. Common sites are the lips and palate (Figure 3.11) but any site in the oral mucosa may be affected. Some papillomas are the result of infection by the human papillomavirus. Treatment is simple excision.

Haemangioma

Haemangiomas are developmental malformations of blood vessels, which are increased in number and show an abnormal arrangement. As a result, haemangiomas appear red or blue–red clinically. Although they may present as a localised swelling it is important to realise that they may extend widely into the surrounding tissues. Because of the increased number of blood vessels, trauma to a haemangioma can result in excessive bleeding. In general practice it is therefore not advisable to perform any kind of surgical intervention in the region of a haemangioma.

Lipoma

These are benign tumours of fat and are common on the buccal mucosa. They may appear yellow but are often mucosal coloured. They are difficult to distinguish from

(a)

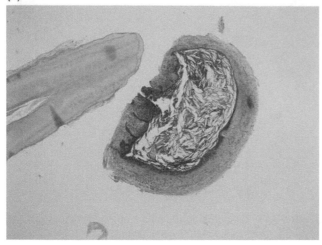

(b)

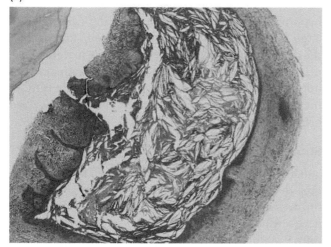

Figure 3.12 (a) Radicular cyst. Note the arrangement of the cyst wall, epithelial lining and lumen. (b) Enlarged view of (a).

fibrous hyperplasia but it should be noted that they are not associated with trauma.

Salivary gland swellings

Mucoceles are important causes of mucosal swelling and are common on the lower lip where they should be considered in the differential diagnosis. They are discussed in more detail in the section on salivary gland disease.

Cysts of the jaws

A cyst is a fluid-filled pathological cavity, which is usually lined by epithelium. The components of a cyst are:

- A lumen, which is filled with fluid.
- A lining, which is usually composed of epithelium.
- A wall, which is usually composed of fibrous tissue.

Their arrangement is shown in Figure 3.12.

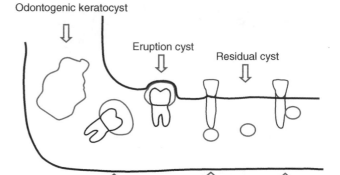

Figure 3.13 Position of odontogenic cysts relative to teeth and surrounding bone.

Cysts are relatively common in the jaws and many arise from the odontogenic epithelium that forms the teeth. The stimulus for cyst formation may be inflammatory or developmental and these two causes have been used as a basis for cyst classification.

The following are classified as inflammatory dental cysts:

- Radicular cyst.
- Residual cyst.

The following are classified as developmental odontogenic cysts:

- Dentigerous cyst.
- Eruption cyst.
- Odontogenic keratocyst.

Radicular cyst

Radicular cysts form at the apex of a non-vital tooth (Figure 3.13) and are the consequence of a spread of infection to the periapical tissues. The sequence of events leading to cyst formation can be summarised as follows:

- The necrotic pulp of the non-vital tooth causes an inflammatory reaction in the periapical tissues which results in destruction of bone and sometimes part of the root apex.
- The resulting space is filled with healing granulation tissue, i.e. fibroblasts and endothelial cells, but because the cause of the inflammation is still present, healing does not occur. At this stage the lesion is known as an **apical granuloma** and chronic inflammatory cells are present.
- Continued inflammation causes the epithelial rests present in the periodontal ligament (**cell rests of Malassez**) to proliferate.

- Eventually, the epithelial cells at the centre of these proliferations break down and a cyst is formed. The lumen becomes filled with fluid and the cyst grows by hydrostatic (fluid) pressure.
- This causes further resorption of bone and the cyst continues to enlarge.

Clinical features

Radicular cysts show the following features:

- They only occur in association with a non-vital tooth.
- They occur most commonly on upper anterior teeth but any tooth can be affected.
- They appear as an apical radiolucent area on a radiograph. The radiolucent area is usually centred on the non-vital tooth and is in continuity with the lamina dura. The margins may be well or ill defined.
- If there is a lateral root canal the radiolucency may appear lateral to the tooth.
- Many radicular cysts are symptomless but some patients complain of pain on biting or tenderness in the bone above the tooth root.
- If a radicular cyst becomes very large it may resorb the cortical plate which becomes thinned. If this area is palpated it may fracture and make a cracking sound which is sometimes described as **egg shell crackling**.

Management

Radicular cysts may resolve following root canal therapy or by replacing an existing root treatment if this is inadequate. After such a procedure the tooth should be monitored to check there is bony healing. Sometimes this does not occur but the tooth may be symptomless and, as long as the radiolucency does not get any bigger, it is permissible to monitor the tooth at regular intervals. If the tooth remains symptomatic then an **apicectomy** may be performed. During this procedure the cortical bone over the root apex is removed together with the cyst. Part of the root apex may also be removed and a retrograde root filling placed. If all these treatment options fail it may be necessary to extract the tooth.

Residual cyst

Occasionally a radicular cyst may remain in the bone after the non-vital tooth causing it has been extracted. Such cysts are known as residual cysts (Figure 3.13). They are treated by excision.

Dentigerous cyst

Dentigerous cysts form around unerupted or impacted teeth (Figure 3.13) and are most commonly associated with the lower third molars and upper canines. They are the result of fluid accumulation between the crown of the unerupted tooth and the surrounding follicle and reduced enamel epithelium. This fluid exerts hydrostatic pressure, which causes bone resorption and the cyst starts to grow.

Clinical features

- Dentigerous cysts are often symptomless and are discovered as an incidental finding on a radiograph.
- They appear as a radiolucent area surrounding the crown of an unerupted tooth and may grow to quite a large size before they cause symptoms.

Management

Dentigerous cysts are treated by removing the cyst, usually together with the unerupted tooth.

Eruption cyst

Eruption cysts are similar to dentigerous cysts in that they are formed by the accumulation of fluid between the crown and the follicle of the tooth. However, they differ because they form around teeth as they erupt through the mucosa and into the oral cavity (Figure 3.13). Clinically they appear as a tense, bluish swelling on the alveolar ridge and it is usually first permanent molars and primary (deciduous) teeth that are affected. They are treated by incision which relieves the pressure and allows the tooth to erupt.

Odontogenic keratocyst

Odontogenic keratocysts are relatively uncommon compared with radicular or dentigerous cysts. They form as a result of the proliferation of the epithelium forming the dental lamina rests, although what causes this is not known. Numerous dental lamina rests are found at the angle of the mandible and it is here that the odontogenic keratocyst is most common (Figure 3.13).

Odontogenic keratocysts differ from radicular and dentigerous cysts in several ways:

- They are lined by epithelium, which is keratinised – hence their name.
- They enlarge because of proliferation of the epithelial lining rather than due to hydrostatic pressure of fluid within the lumen.
- They recur if they are not completely removed.
- They extend through the bone rather than causing expansion and may reach quite large sizes.

Clinical features

Odontogenic keratocysts are often asymptomatic and are an incidental discovery on a routine radiograph. Typically they appear as a radiolucency at the angle of the

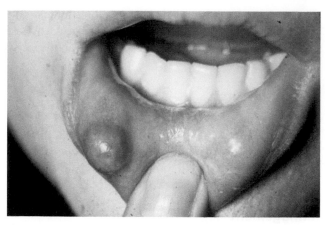

Figure 3.14 Mucocele on the lower lip. Note the blue colour.

mandible and this may have a multilocular appearance (i.e. the cyst appears to be divided by septae).

Management

Odontogenic keratocysts are treated by removal and curettage of the bone. Patients should be kept under a period of postoperative review.

Conditions of the salivary glands

Saliva is produced by three paired major salivary glands, the parotid, submandibular and sublingual glands, and numerous minor salivary glands which are present throughout the oral mucosa. Any of these salivary glands may be affected by disease. The most important disorders of the salivary glands are discussed below.

Mucocele

Mucocele is the clinical term given to a cystic swelling usually caused by trauma affecting the minor salivary glands. Their clinical features are as follows:

- They are common and usually occur on the lower lip and cheeks of young individuals.
- They appear as sessile (broad-based) blue swellings, which may be fluctuant (Figure 3.14).
- Patients often give a history of a rapid increase in size following trauma.

Two histological types are recognised: mucous retention cysts and mucous extravasation cysts.

Mucous extravasation cysts

These are the most common type and are the result of trauma to the minor salivary gland duct, which transmits saliva from the gland to the oral cavity. Trauma causes the duct to rupture and the saliva spills into the tissues rather than the oral cavity. The body mounts an inflammatory response and walls off the saliva with granulation tissue. Healing cannot take place, however, as the minor salivary gland continues to produce saliva.

Mucous retention cysts

Mucous retention cysts are relatively rare compared with mucous extravasation cysts. They are also caused by trauma but the duct becomes blocked usually by scar tissue. The saliva is unable to enter the oral cavity and the duct swells up rather like a balloon filled with water.

Management

The treatment of both lesions is excision including the underlying minor salivary gland.

Sialoadenitis

Inflammation affecting the salivary glands is known as sialoadenitis. It may be caused by infections such as mumps or by obstruction of the ducts. A **salivary stone** or **calculus** is a common cause of obstruction and the submandibular gland is most often affected. Obstruction to the duct causes the submandibular gland to become inflamed and the gland becomes infiltrated by chronic inflammatory cells.

Clinical features

The patient will complain of pain and swelling of the submandibular gland particularly just before or at meal times because the increased outflow of saliva is blocked.

Management

The stone is removed if it is accessible but sometimes it is necessary to remove the gland as well.

Sjögren's syndrome

Sjögren's syndrome is an autoimmune disease which may affect the salivary glands, lacrimal glands and many other organs in the body. Typically patients are middle aged and female. Two types of Sjögren's syndrome are recognised:

- Primary Sjögren's syndrome, in which patients have dry eyes and a dry mouth.
- Secondary Sjögren's syndrome, in which patients have another autoimmune disorder, such as rheumatoid arthritis, in addition to dry eyes and a dry mouth.

The aetiology of Sjögren's syndrome is not known. Patients have circulating autoantibodies in their blood and their salivary glands are destroyed by numerous lymphocytes which infiltrate into the glands. This leads to a lack of saliva and a dry mouth (xerostomia), one of the most distressing aspects of Sjögren's syndrome.

Clinical features of xerostomia

- Patients have trouble in eating and swallowing and cannot taste their food.
- They have an increased incidence of cervical and smooth surface caries. This is partly due to lack of saliva but some patients eat a high-sugar diet because of their lack of taste.
- They have a greater incidence of periodontal disease.
- Their mucosa appears smooth and red and they may suffer from fungal infections.
- Ulceration is also common.

Clinical importance

Dietary advice and good oral hygiene instruction together with topical fluoride can reduce caries and periodontal disease. Dryness may be treated by saliva substitutes.

Salivary gland neoplasms

A neoplasm may arise in any of the major and minor salivary glands and these may be benign or malignant. The overwhelming majority of salivary gland neoplasms are benign and the most common type is the **pleomorphic adenoma**. Malignant neoplasms are rare but **mucoepidermoid carcinomas** and **adenoid cystic carcinomas** are the most common. From a clinical point of view it is not necessary to know the details of each of these types of neoplasm but an appreciation of the differences in clinical presentation between a benign and malignant neoplasm is important.

Clinical features of benign neoplasms

Most benign neoplasms are slow-growing lesions with well-defined margins, which are easy to feel. They do not usually cause pain but may grow to a large size. If they arise from the minor glands in the oral cavity they do not usually ulcerate through the oral mucosa.

Clinical features of malignant neoplasms

Malignant neoplasms are characterised by rapid growth and, because they infiltrate into surrounding tissues, their margins are indistinct and difficult to feel. If they arise from minor glands in the oral cavity they often ulcerate through the mucosa. Malignant neoplasms arising in the major glands may affect nerve function and cause paraesthesia.

Oral manifestations of systemic disease

Many patients suffering from diseases which affect the whole body may show specific oral signs and symptoms. Those with important oral signs are listed below:

- Haematological disorders: iron-deficiency anaemia.
- Endocrine disturbances: type 1 diabetes.

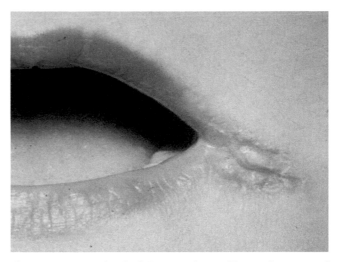

Figure 3.15 Angular cheilitis. Note the cracking at the corner of the mouth.

- Viral infections: infection with human immuno-deficiency virus (HIV).
- Malignant disease: advanced malignant disease, leukaemia.

Haematological disorders

Patients who suffer from iron-deficiency anaemia have a predisposition to certain oral mucosal diseases. These include:

- Aphthous ulceration.
- Angular cheilitis: soreness and cracking at the angles of the mouth caused by the fungus *Candida albicans* and/ or by the bacterium *Staphylococcus aureus* (Figure 3.15).
- Mucosal atrophy: the mucosa appears reddened and smooth.

It is important to rule out the presence of iron-deficiency anaemia in patients with aphthous ulceration and angular cheilitis. If iron-deficiency anaemia is detected then the underlying cause should be investigated.

Endocrine disturbances

Patients with type 1 diabetes have insufficient insulin and this may be controlled by diet, drugs or insulin injections. They may show the following:

- Symptoms of a dry mouth.
- Fungal infection by *Candida albicans*.
- Increased predisposition to periodontal disease.
- Poor wound healing.

Viral infections

Infection with HIV may cause marked immunosuppression and patients suffer from specific conditions in the oral cavity. These are:

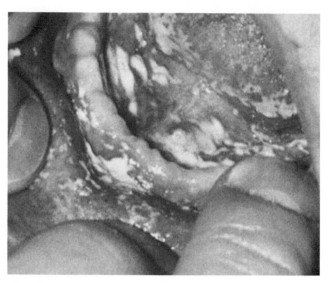

Figure 3.16 Thrush (pseudomembranous candidosis). Creamy white plaques are present on the floor of mouth and alveolar ridge.

- Fungal infections.
- Hairy leukoplakia – a white patch present on the lateral borders of the tongue on both sides. Unlike other leukoplakia, it is *not* premalignant and is associated with Epstein–Barr virus.
- **Kaposi's sarcoma**. These are red–purple patches, which are raised and granular and are commonly found on the gingivae and hard palate. They too are associated with a specific virus.
- Severe periodontal disease.
- Other severe viral infections, particularly those caused by herpes simplex and zoster and papillomatous lesions.

Malignant disease

Patients who have malignant disease arising in other parts of the body may suffer from oral symptoms, especially in the later stages of the disease. In particular they may suffer from **thrush** (acute pseudomembranous candidosis) caused by the fungus *Candida albicans*. This is characterised by thick, creamy white patches which may occur on any part of the oral mucosa and may be wiped off, leaving a raw reddened surface (Figure 3.16). Thrush may also occur in patients who are immunosuppressed, for example renal transplant patients who are taking immunosuppressant therapy and patients with HIV infection.

Leukaemia

Specific oral signs and symptoms may occur in patients with leukaemia. These are:

- Swollen (hypertrophied), ulcerated gingivae, which may exude pus. The degree of swelling is greatly in excess of the amount of plaque accumulation.

- Small haemorrhages (ecchymoses) or petechiae (pinpoint, flat red areas of haemorrhage) under the skin and mucosa.
- Patients will feel tired and lethargic and appear pale.

Common causes of facial pain

Dental healthcare professionals encounter many patients who complain of pain in the facial region. The vast majority of these patients suffer from tooth-related disorders, such as pulpitis, periapical infection, including abscesses, and dentine sensitivity. However, for some patients the pain is not tooth related and they experience what is broadly termed 'facial pain'. The non-dental causes of facial pain are listed below:

- Neuralgia – trigeminal, post-herpetic.
- Temporomandibular joint pain.
- Atypical facial pain.

Trigeminal neuralgia

Clinical features

This type of facial pain affects women more than men and usually occurs during middle age. It has very characteristic features, which are important in establishing the diagnosis. These are:

- A sharp, severe, episodic, stabbing or lancinating pain, which only lasts a few seconds.
- The pain is precipitated by touching a particular area of the skin or oral mucosa which is known as the trigger zone.
- The pain radiates along one of the three branches of the trigeminal nerve, usually the second and third branches, and does not cross the midline.

Trigeminal neuralgia can be very debilitating and patients will avoid touching the trigger zone. It is important to remember this when treating a patient with trigeminal neuralgia but it is highly likely they will remind you themselves. The episodes of pain come at varying intervals and in an unlucky few may seem almost continuous. The treatment of choice is the antiepileptic drug, **carbamazepine**. If this fails it is possible to ablate the nerve surgically but this procedure results in permanent anaesthesia.

Post-herpetic neuralgia

Pain which follows infection with recurrent herpes zoster (**shingles**) is termed post-herpetic neuralgia. It can be very debilitating and has the following characteristics:

- An intense aching and unpleasant pain, which may be continuous.
- Occurs in the distribution of the trigeminal nerve that was affected by herpes zoster.

This pain may affect up to 10% of patients but only in very few does it become chronic. Treatment is very difficult as the pain is often refractory (i.e. does not respond well to treatment).

Atypical facial pain
Clinical features

Atypical facial pain also affects middle-aged women more than men and is more difficult to diagnose than trigeminal neuralgia. The following features are seen in many patients:

- The pain is continuous and has usually been present for months or even years. It may show episodes of increased severity.
- It is described as gripping or vice-like.
- It affects the maxilla more than the mandible and may cross the midline and other anatomical boundaries.
- There are no clear precipitating factors.

It is important to exclude other causes of facial pain in these patients before the diagnosis is made. Many patients are depressed and it is important to take a thorough medical and social history. Antidepressant therapy helps in some patients.

Burning mouth syndrome

Burning mouth syndrome is relatively common and affects middle-aged women more than men. It shows the following features:

- A burning sensation which may affect the tongue, lips or hard palate.
- The sensation may be present on waking and remain the same or get more severe during the day.
- The mucosa appears normal.
- There are no precipitating factors.

It is important to exclude other causes of a burning sensation before a diagnosis of burning mouth syndrome is made. Blood tests to screen for iron-deficiency anaemia, folate or B12 deficiency should be carried out and it is wise to exclude candidal infection and systemic disease such as diabetes. Many patients are reassured if underlying systemic disease is eliminated but antidepressants may help in some cases.

Disorders of the temporomandibular joint

Temporomandibular joint disorder (myofascial pain–dysfunction syndrome)

Pain or dysfunction associated with the temporomandibular joint is very common and usually affects young individuals. It has the following characteristics:

- Pain associated with the joint or the attached muscles.
- Limitation of opening (**trismus**) or deviation of the jaw on opening.
- Clicking of the joint but this is not necessarily diagnostic.
- It may be associated with a headache and be misdiagnosed as migraine.

The pain is often worse in the morning but may vary in intensity. In most cases it is caused by spasm of the muscles of mastication although what causes this is not clear. There is an association with stress and bruxism (grinding of the teeth) and many patients have a night-time tooth grinding habit. It is possible that this is precipitated by premature occlusal contacts and some treatments aim to reduce these by providing soft splints which cover the teeth. In such patients it is important to ensure that any new restorations are fully contoured to the existing occlusion and do not initiate a grinding habit. There may also be an association with emotional stress.

Patients are managed by explanation of the condition and reassurance. A soft diet and jaw rest may be of value and in severe cases analgesics and anti-inflammatory drugs may be prescribed. The overwhelming majority of cases resolve but may require long-term management.

Developmental tooth anomalies

Developmental disturbances of the teeth may be inherited or they may be acquired and the result of environmental disturbances. In all cases the disturbances occur during the period of tooth formation which may be either before and/or after birth. Developmental disturbances which occur early in tooth development affect the shape (form) of teeth, their number or size. Those which occur later during the formation of the dental hard tissues result in disturbances of tooth structure.

Disturbances in the number of teeth

Hypodontia

Hypodontia is a decrease in the number of teeth compared with normal and is relatively common in the permanent dentition (although rare in the primary dentition). The most common missing teeth are:

- Lower third molars.
- Upper lateral incisors.
- Lower second premolars.

In some cases there is a hereditary trait but many cases appear sporadically.

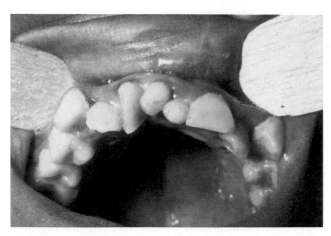

Figure 3.17 Two mesiodens: supernumerary teeth in the midline between the upper central incisors. Note the marked crowding.

Anodontia

Anodontia is a total absence of teeth and is very unusual. It usually occurs in association with a hereditary genetic condition, **hypohidrotic ectodermal dysplasia**. The condition is caused by a gene defect in which patients have very few or no teeth, and absence of hair and sweat glands.

Supernumerary teeth

An additional tooth in the arch is known as a supernumerary tooth. They are more common in the permanent than the primary dentition and affect females more than males. Supernumerary teeth may occur at any site but are more common in the anterior maxilla and the premolar region of the mandible. Different types of supernumerary teeth are recognised. These are:

- Mesiodens – a supernumerary tooth that develops between the upper central incisors. This is the most common type of supernumerary tooth (Figure 3.17).
- Paramolar – an additional molar tooth.
- Supplemental teeth – additional teeth that resemble normal teeth.

Clinical importance

Supernumerary teeth may prevent the eruption of a permanent tooth and should always be considered if a tooth fails to erupt. Similarly, a supernumerary tooth may cause displacement or malposition of teeth and, if unerupted, may resorb teeth.

Disturbances of tooth size

Tooth size is determined by genetic factors and abnormally large or small teeth may occur. Usually the entire dentition is affected but sometimes only a few teeth may be excessively large or small. Small teeth may occur in association with missing teeth; for example, one missing upper lateral incisor may be associated with a small peg-shaped lateral incisor on the other side.

Disturbances in tooth form

Variations in the form of crowns or roots of teeth are relatively common and may present as dilacerated teeth, double teeth, dens invaginatus and enamel pearls. These are fully described in Chapter 12, p. 246–247.

Disturbances in the structure of teeth

Disturbances in the structure of teeth may affect the enamel or dentine or sometimes both. Those which affect the enamel are more obvious clinically.

Disturbances of enamel

Developmental disturbances of enamel are relatively common and are usually the result of a localised or generalised environmental disturbance occurring during tooth development. Only a few are the result of a genetic defect. The causes are summarised below:

- Genetic disturbances
  - Amelogenesis imperfecta.
- Local disturbances:
  - Infection.
  - Trauma.
  - Idiopathic.
- Generalised disturbances:
  - Infections.
  - Fluorosis.
  - Neonatal events, e.g. premature birth, rhesus incompatibility.

Amelogenesis imperfecta

This is the name given to a group of inherited disorders which result in defective enamel formation. Most are the result of defects in genes which code for either enamel matrix production or the mineralisation of enamel.

The clinical features are variable and depend on which gene is defective:

- In some forms the teeth appear normal on eruption but, because the enamel is poorly mineralised, it is soft and soon wears away. The remaining enamel becomes stained and the teeth appear yellow–brown.
- In other forms the enamel is reduced in amount and the teeth are pitted and appear yellow–brown in colour.
- Some forms are carried on the X chromosome and boys are affected more severely than girls.
- The teeth are often sensitive, especially where the enamel is thin or has chipped away.

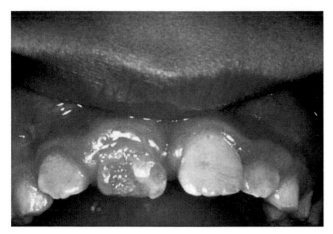

Figure 3.18 Turner tooth. The upper central incisor is markedly hypoplastic and brown in colour.

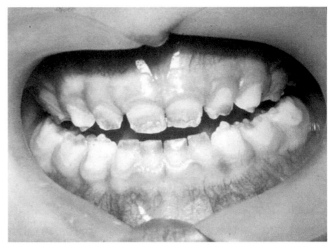

Figure 3.19 Chronological hypoplasia. Note the hypoplasia predominantly affecting the incisor teeth but present on the tips of the cusps of the more posterior teeth. The lower canine teeth are spared.

Acquired disturbances of enamel formation

Most acquired enamel defects result in areas of **hypoplasia**, which may be due to either a defect in matrix production or a defect in mineralisation. If only a single tooth is affected these are classified as localised disturbances, but if several teeth are affected then they are referred to as generalised.

Localised defects most commonly affect the upper incisor teeth and usually form as a result of infection or trauma to the deciduous predecessor. This affects the ameloblasts of the developing tooth, resulting in the production of enamel which may be yellow–brown, pitted or irregular. These teeth are sometimes referred to as Turner teeth (Figure 3.18).

Enamel opacities are opaque white spots sometimes seen particularly on the upper central incisors. They may become stained with time. The cause of these opacities is not known but they are relatively common.

Generalised defects are sometimes referred to as **chronological hypoplasias** and most are the result of a generalised or systemic infection or disturbance occurring during tooth development. The disturbance affects enamel formation and results in a linear horizontal band of hypoplasia. This may be characterised by ridging or grooving or pitting on the enamel surface and the teeth that are affected are those that were forming at the time of the disturbance (Figure 3.19). Thus with a knowledge of the times of crown formation it is possible to predict at what age a patient was systemically unwell.

The overwhelming majority of chronological hypoplasias are the result of disturbances in the first 10 months of life and the teeth affected are:

- The first permanent molars.
- Upper central incisors.
- Lower lateral incisors and canines.

However, disturbances may occur before birth or during the neonatal period. Common causes of disturbances are viral infections, such as measles and mumps, and excess fluoride ions. In the prenatal period, diseases affecting the mother may be important.

Fluorosis is the term given to changes in the enamel that are associated with excess ingestion of fluoride. These vary from localised white opacities to more severe brown–yellow mottling on the teeth. The precise effect depends on the dose of fluoride (from all sources), the duration for which it was taken and the age of the patient at the time of ingestion. Fluorosis when very severe (concentrations in the water supply greater than 6 parts per million) may result in extensive hypoplasia with brown staining (see Chapter 11, p. 226).

Disturbances of dentine

Like defects of enamel, the dentine may be affected by acquired and by genetic defects. However, acquired dentinal defects cause very few problems and only genetic defects are of clinical significance.

Dentinogenesis imperfecta

This genetic disorder is characterised by defective dentine matrix production and two types have been described. **Dentinogenesis imperfecta type 1** occurs in association with osteogenesis imperfecta, in which there is defective bone formation. It is very uncommon.

Dentinogenesis imperfecta type 2 is the commonest form. It has the following features:

- Both the permanent and primary dentition are affected.
- The teeth have a normal shape on eruption but appear amber–brown or purple–blue in colour.

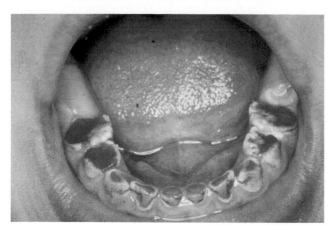

Figure 3.20 Dentinogenesis imperfecta. Note the brown colour of the dentine and the marked attrition.

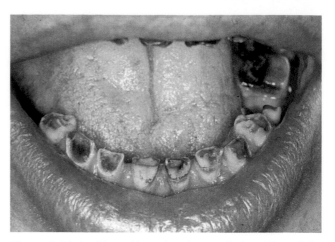

Figure 3.21 Attrition. This patient has marked attrition of the occlusal surfaces of most of his teeth.

- The enamel shears away from the poorly formed dentine, which quickly wears away (Figure 3.20).
- The pulps become obliterated with abnormal dentine.

Patients suffer marked attrition and this can cause severe problems. The aim of treatment is to prevent attrition with the restoration of lost tooth substance and the provision of crowns if necessary.

Tooth wear

Tooth wear is defined as loss of tooth tissue due to causes other than caries. Some tooth wear is normal and occurs with age. This is termed physiological tooth wear. However, excessive tooth wear is pathological. Three types have been described: attrition, abrasion and erosion. Although these may occur separately, in many instances they occur together.

Attrition

Attrition is tooth wear caused by tooth-to-tooth contact. It occurs as a normal part of ageing and it is usually the incisal edges which wear away first, followed by the occlusal surfaces of the molar teeth. There may also be loss of interproximal tooth tissue leading to mesial migration of the teeth. Excessive occlusal wear may occur in the following situations:

- Patients with bruxism. These patients grind their teeth excessively and in some cases this is triggered by occlusal irregularities (Figure 3.21).
- Patients who have lost several posterior teeth may show excessive attrition of the anterior teeth, especially if these are used for chewing.
- Patients who suffer from developmental disturbances of tooth structure, such as amelogenesis and dentinogenesis imperfecta, may suffer exceptional tooth wear.

Abrasion

Abrasion is frictional tooth loss caused by extrinsic agents. It is always pathological and may be caused by tooth brushing and habits such as biting on a pipe or a pencil. Toothbrush abrasion is characteristic and is caused by poor toothbrushing technique (i.e. patients brushing horizontally with excessive force). It has the following characteristics:

- It particularly affects the labial and buccal surfaces of the upper incisor, canine and premolar teeth.
- The resulting cavity is wedge-shaped with a sharp angle towards the occlusal surface and an obtuse angle towards the apical surface.
- The problem is often compounded by the use of hard toothbrushes and abrasive toothpaste.

Erosion

Erosion is the loss of tooth substance caused by chemical agents and is non-bacterial and therefore does not include loss by caries. Most erosion is caused by acids and is seen in the following groups:

- Those with gastric reflux and with **bulimia** and **anorexia**. Regurgitation of acid from the stomach particularly affects the palatal surfaces of the upper maxillary teeth.
- As an occupational hazard. Those who work in an acidic environment, e.g. in factories making batteries, and also in wine tasters. Erosion in these groups is relatively rare but because the acid is in the environment the erosion is particularly seen on the labial surfaces of both the upper and lower incisor teeth.
- Those who consume excessive amounts of carbonated soft drinks or fruit juices. This group is by far the largest and in the Western world it is particularly children,

adolescents and young adults who are affected. It has been estimated to affect up to 50% of 5-year-old and 30% of 14-year-old children in the UK. The teeth which are most commonly affected are the palatal surfaces of the upper anterior teeth. The teeth may appear yellow due to the reduction in the thickness of the enamel and typically the cavities are shallow and broad.

Patients with erosion may be unaware that they have a problem but others may complain of sensitivity, particularly on eating hot and cold foods.

Clinical significance

It is important to recognise that excessive tooth wear is taking place and to diagnose the most likely cause. In many cases the causes may be multiple. Abrasion caused by tooth brushing may be reduced by improving brushing technique. A careful history and detailed notes on the position of the erosion are important in order to determine the precise cause. Dietary analysis and advice are essential for those suffering from erosion due to dietary causes.

References

Axell, T., Pinborg, J.J., Smith, C.J. and van der Waal, I. (1996) Oral white lesions with special reference to pre-cancerous and tobacco related lesions: conclusions of an international symposium held in Uppsala, Sweden, May 18–21. 1994. International Collaborative Group on Oral White Lesions. *Journal of Oral Pathology and Medicine*, **25**, 49–54.

Cancer Research UK Information Resource Centre: http://info.cancerresearchuk.org/cancerstats/types/oral/ (accessed 22 September 2011).

Farrand, P., Rowe, R.M., Johnston, A. and Murdoch, H. (2001) Prevalence, age of onset and demographic relationships of different areca nut habits amongst children in Tower Hamlets, London. *British Dental Journal*, **190**(3), 150–154.

Hindle, I., Downer, M.C. and Speight, P.M. (2000) The association between intra-oral cancer and surrogate markers of smoking and alcohol consumption. *Community Dental Health*, **17**(2), 107–113.

Llewellyn, C.D., Linklater, K., Bell, J., Johnson, N.W. and Warnakulasuriya, K.A. (2003) Squamous cell carcinoma of the oral cavity in patients aged 45 years and under: a descriptive analysis of 116 cases diagnosed in the South East of England from 1990 to 1997. *Oral Oncology*, **39**(2), 106–114.

Warnakulasuriya, S. (2002) Areca nut use following migration and its consequences. *Addiction Biology*, **7**(1), 127–132.

Further reading

Bell, G.W., Large, D.M. and Barclay, S.C. (1999) Oral health care in diabetes mellitus. *Dental Update*, **26**(8), 322–330.

Cousin, G.C. (1997) Oral manifestations of leukaemia. *Dental Update*, **24**(2), 67–70.

Lamey, P.J. (1998) Burning mouth syndrome: approach to successful management. *Dental Update*, **25**(7), 298–300.

McIntyre, G.T. (2001) Viral infections of the oral mucosa and perioral region. *Dental Update*, **28**(4), 181–188.

Milosevic, A. (1998) Toothwear: aetiology and presentation. *Dental Update*, **25**(1), 6–11.

Rees, J.S. (2004) The role of drinks in tooth surface loss. *Dental Update*, **31**(6), 318–326.

Scully, C. and Boyle, P. (2005) The role of the dental team in preventing and diagnosing cancer: 1. Cancer in general practice *Dental Update*, **32**(4), 204–212.

Scully, C. and Porter, S. (1998) Orofacial disease: update for the dental clinical team: 2. Ulcers, erosions and other causes of sore mouth. Part I. *Dental Update*, **25**(10), 478–484.

Scully, C. and Porter, S. (1999) Orofacial disease: update for the dental clinical team: 2. Ulcers, erosions and other causes of sore mouth. Part II. *Dental Update*, **26**(1), 31–39.

Scully, C. and Porter, S. (1999) Orofacial disease: update for the dental clinical team: 2. Ulcers and erosions and other causes of sore mouth. Part III. *Dental Update*, **26**(2), 73–80.

Scully, C. and Warnakulasuriya, S. (2005) The role of the dental team in preventing and diagnosing cancer: 4. Risk factor reduction: tobacco cessation. *Dental Update*, **32**(7), 394–401.

Scully, C., Newman, L. and Bagan, J.V. (2005) The role of the dental team in preventing and diagnosing cancer: 2. Oral cancer risk factors. *Dental Update*, **32**(5), 261–270.

Scully, C., Newman, L. and Bagan, J.V. (2005) The role of the dental team in preventing and diagnosing cancer: 3. Oral cancer diagnosis and screening. *Dental Update*, **32**(6), 326–327.

Watson, M.L. and Burke, F.J. (2000) Investigation and treatment of patients with teeth affected by tooth substance loss: a review. *Dental Update*, **27**(4), 175–183.

Zakrzewska, J.M. and Atkin, P.A. (2003) Oral mucosal lesions in a UK HIV/AIDS oral medicine clinic. A nine year, cross-sectional, prospective study. *Oral Health and Preventive Dentistry*, **1**(1), 73–79.

4

Dental caries and pulpitis

Avijit Banerjee and Naveen Karir

Summary

This chapter covers:

- The aetiology, epidemiology, microbiology and development of the carious process
- The carious lesion and some of the important management rationales
- The operative techniques and technologies used to treat dental caries

Introduction

Dental caries is the major cause for loss of teeth in children and adults. It affects the enamel surfaces of teeth in children and adults and the exposed root surfaces of the teeth of the elderly. Dental caries is the result of the interaction of the bacteria on the tooth surface, the dental plaque or oral biofilm, the diet and specifically fermentable carbohydrate components of the diet, which are fermented by the plaque microflora to organic acids (primarily lactic and acetic acids), and the teeth acting together over time (Figure 4.1). Dental caries will occur only when the three factors are present together and when they act together over a sufficient period of time.

If the different factors are considered individually, it is possible to obtain a better understanding of the nature of their interactions and how these interactions may manifest as a carious lesion and, eventually, if not treated either preventatively or with a restoration, as pain and ultimately in the loss of the tooth.

Aetiology and microbiology of dental caries in relation to dental plaque

Dental plaque is a natural biofilm (Figure 4.2). The number of different bacterial species in dental plaque is not known, but sophisticated molecular biology studies have shown that over 700 different species may be identified; many more have yet to be characterised. The majority of these species have not been cultured in the laboratory using the current methods for bacterial isolation. It is also worthwhile noting that these molecular approaches have demonstrated that, for example, *Streptococcus mutans*, previously reported only to be isolated from the oral cavity after the eruption of the lateral incisors, is actually present in the mouth, colonising the tongue, within a few months of birth.

A **biofilm** is a community of microorganisms attached to a solid surface, with the bacteria encapsulated in polymers derived from the bacteria and exhibiting specific biofilm characteristics, including increased resistance to antimicrobials and biocides (chemicals used to kill bacteria) and the production of novel proteins. An appreciation of this type of growth has led to attempts to develop novel antiplaque strategies, which target the inhibition of function of novel biofilm-specific proteins.

Dental plaque biofilm is present on virtually all tooth surfaces and has a general structure whereby salivary and some bacterial proteins are initially deposited on the enamel surface to form the **pellicle** and the pellicle then absorbs further bacteria. The first bacteria to bind to the tooth surface, the pioneer organisms, include *Streptococcus oralis*, *Streptococcus sanguinius*, *Neisseria* and *Haemophilus* species and *Actinomyces naeslundii*.

Clinical Textbook of Dental Hygiene and Therapy, Second Edition. Edited by Suzanne L. Noble.
© 2012 John Wiley & Sons, Ltd. Published 2012 by John Wiley & Sons, Ltd.

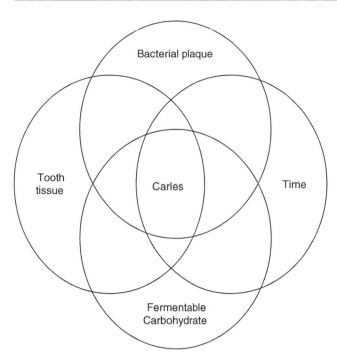

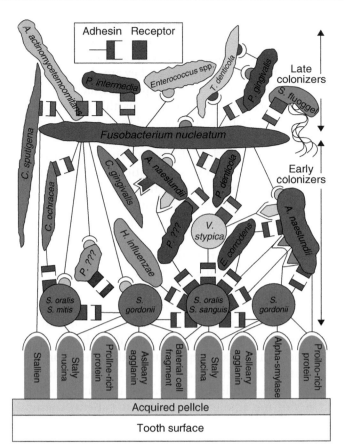

Figure 4.1 Schematic diagram to demonstrate the requirement for diet, bacteria and dentition to interact together over time to initiate caries.

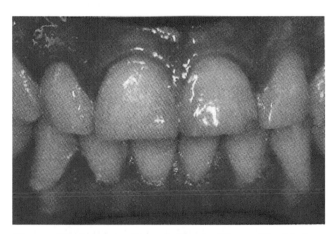

Figure 4.2 Anterior view of the dentition with 36 hour accumulation of plaque. (Reproduced with permission of Oxford University Press, Banerjee A. Watson TF (2011) *Pickard's Manual of Operative Dentistry*, 9th edition.)

These bacteria are isolated from cleaned tooth surfaces within 60 minutes of cleaning. Following the binding of these bacteria, other organisms bind and eventually plaque of full thickness develops, partly because of bacterial binding but primarily because of bacterial growth. The binding of bacteria to the pellicle and to other bacteria is mediated by specific interactions in which only certain bacteria bind to components of the pellicle and only certain bacteria interact. One of the major and most interactive of all the bacteria in dental plaque is *Fusobacterium nucleatum* which binds to many

Figure 4.3 Arrangements of bacteria within dental plaque showing potential attachments between bacteria and components of the pellicle (Reproduced from Kolenbrander, P.E., Andersen, R.N., Blehert, D.S., Egland, P.G., Foster, J.S. and Palmer, R.J. Jr. (2002) Communication among oral bacteria. Microbiology and Molecular Biology Reviews, 66(3), 486–505, with permission from ASM Press.)

other bacteria; it acts almost as a nucleus for plaque formation, cross-linking otherwise non-interacting bacterial species (Figure 4.3).

The composition of dental plaque varies over time. In supragingival plaque the flora becomes more anaerobic, with pigmented anaerobic rods such as *Prevotella* and *Fusobacterium* species becoming increasingly abundant as the plaque accumulates and ages, as it becomes a climax community. However, in sites where caries is initiated, in the stagnation sites (pits and fissures on the occlusal surfaces and at approximal sites on the enamel and at the gingival margin on exposed root surfaces) the composition of the plaque biofilm reflects the local acidic environment. Organisms most likely to be isolated from these stagnation sites are *Streptococcus mutans* and *Streptococcus sobrinus* (mutans streptococci), other streptococci (*S. oralis*, *S. intermedius* and *S. anginosus*), lactobacilli, *Actinomyces* and *Bifidobacterium* species. These organisms are Gram-positive, **acidogenic** (producing acid from sugars) and each includes strains which are **aciduric** (able to survive in acidic environments). At these stagnation sites yeasts, such as *Candida albicans*, may also be present as they are also both acidogenic and aciduric. *Veillonella* species, which are Gram-negative cocci, are also isolated, as this genus has the ability to use lactic acid produced from these other species to generate energy for growth.

Although it has long been known that bacteria are present on the teeth it was not until the 1950s that it was proven that without bacteria there was no tooth decay. Only in recent years has it become clear that the identification of the causative microbiological agents of tooth decay remains elusive.

Lactobacilli were regarded as the main microbiological agent of dental caries for many years until the 1940s, as they were, and still are, isolated in great numbers from active carious lesions. However, a definitive longitudinal study clearly demonstrated that lactobacilli colonised lesions after their formation and that they were not prevalent in dental plaque during the period of lesion formation (Hemmens *et al.*, 1946). Since lactobacilli proliferate in acidic environments, they are good indicators of the amount of sugar that patients consume. Monitoring the levels of these bacteria in saliva is a good way of establishing whether patients are following dietary advice and using adequate oral hygiene measures.

The studies which established once and for all that bacteria were essential for the initiation of tooth decay were carried out in the early 1950s using germ-free (**gnotobiotic**) rats. In these studies, rats were inoculated orally with single strains of bacteria isolated from the faeces of rats fed sucrose-rich diets and with tooth decay. Only rats inoculated with bacteria and fed sucrose in the diets developed caries. However, not all bacterial isolates were capable of forming carious lesions. In addition, bacteria, including *Streptococcus salivarius* and *Enterococcus* spp., which are not normally isolated in large numbers from dental plaque, also caused caries in rats. From these studies, *Streptococcus mutans*, isolated many years previously, appeared to be the most cariogenic of all the species tested, while other commensal bacteria (e.g. streptococci and *Actinomyces*), were less so. Some strains of *Streptococcus oralis* and milleri-group streptococci produced levels of caries that approached those found with *Streptococcus mutans* and *Streptococcus sobrinus*. However, all strains of mutans streptococci produced high levels of caries while only a few of the many other species, especially other species of streptococci, did so. It is now apparent that these non-mutans streptococci are heterogeneous (different) with respect to their ability to cause caries and that this is reflected in the range of acidogenic and aciduric properties of these organisms compared to the relatively homogeneous (similar) properties of the mutans streptococci.

It was for these reasons that for many years, mutans streptococci were regarded as the bacteria associated with the initiation of dental caries and the levels of these organisms were used to assess caries risk. Consequently, considerable research was undertaken to establish whether *Streptococcus mutans* was the cause of caries in humans. Despite definitive evidence that this was the case, a number of investigations were undertaken attempting to develop novel treatments to eradicate *S. mutans* from the oral cavity as a means of inhibiting caries formation. The methods which have been investigated include:

- Vaccine development.
- Passive immunisation with the direct application of anti-*S. mutans* antibodies directly on the tooth surface.
- Replacement therapies in which less cariogenic bacteria are introduced into the mouth to eradicate the more cariogenic *S. mutans* strains.

Some of these approaches work in laboratory animal models, and some eradicate *S. mutans* for short periods from the human oral cavity, but none has yet been shown to be effective at reducing the incidence of dental caries in humans. The reasons for the lack of success are still being determined. It is, however, well established that there is a clear association between the numbers and concentrations of *S. mutans* in plaque and/or saliva and the dental caries status of populations, and to a lesser extent to the caries status of an individual. It is also known that dental caries occurs in the absence of *S. mutans* and individuals with high levels of *S. mutans* do not necessarily have to have caries.

Caries-associated characteristics of caries-associated microorganisms

Laboratory investigations into the characteristics of bacteria, which might explain their involvement in the caries process, have focused on those related to interactions with sucrose, as it is the most cariogenic sugar and many bacteria make sticky polymers from it which may facilitate the adhesion of bacteria to the tooth surface and facilitate the caries process. As caries is mediated by acids formed by bacteria, the ability to produce large amounts of acid (**acidogenicity**) rapidly, to tolerate exposure to low pH environments (**aciduricity**) and to produce acid in an already acidic environment were considered features that bacteria initiating dental caries should exhibit. It was soon established that, in comparison with other bacteria, mutans streptococci are generally able to produce acid more rapidly, to produce the most acid in a low pH environment (pH 5.5 or less) and to survive exposure to acidic conditions. The mechanisms underlying the aciduricity of *S. mutans* have been investigated using modern molecular and protein analysis methods, but to date no precise mechanism has been identified. It is unlikely that the expression of any single gene is responsible solely for the aciduricity of mutans streptococci.

Mutans streptococci also possess a number of extracellular enzymes (glucosyltransferases and fructosyltransferase), which form a range of distinct polymers from sucrose. Uniquely, mutans streptococci produce a highly branched, water-insoluble glucan called **mutan**, which may facilitate its establishment in dental plaque. These polymers are necessary for the adherence of *S. mutans* to enamel; in rat studies, mutants with these genes inactivated and unable to produce these polymers are less able to colonise the dentition of rats and consequently are less able to initiate carious lesion formation. These characteristics have been extensively studied in mutans streptococci, but evidence has recently emerged that bacteria other than mutans streptococci also have these same acidogenic and aciduric properties and produce extracellular polymers promoting plaque formation.

It is difficult to find relevant information on the cariogenic characteristics of other oral bacteria other than the mutans streptococci since so much emphasis has been placed on enumerating mutans streptococci in dental plaque and analysing their physiological properties. However, a study of elderly Chinese subjects related the sucrose-induced pH response of dental plaque on sound exposed root surfaces to the microbial composition of the overlying plaque (Aamdal-Scheie *et al.*, 1996). The prevalence of a range of bacteria, including mutans streptococci, was determined and the pH of the plaque measured before and after the application of a sucrose mouth rinse. The plaque pH response on sound and carious root surfaces to sucrose was the same regardless of the presence or absence of mutans streptococci (Figure 4.4). Clearly, the rate of acid production from dental plaque was not determined by the presence of mutans streptococci nor was the final pH recorded following the sucrose rinse determined by the presence of mutans streptococci in the oral biofilm.

These *in-vivo* observations are different to those derived from *in-vitro* laboratory studies using single strains of planktonic organisms (organisms growing in liquid culture). The bacteria on the teeth grow in a biofilm and they grow as part of a very complex interacting microbial community. None of these features are present in many of the *in-vitro* studies, which found the acidogenicity of mutans streptococci to be significantly greater than that of other bacteria isolated from dental plaque. The results from the Chinese subjects clearly show that the magnitude of the cariogenic challenge was not determined by the presence of mutans streptococci and that other bacteria present in the dental plaque were responsible for caries initiation and progression. This idea that

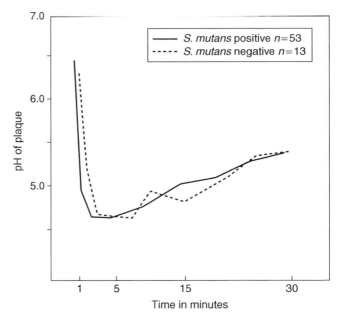

Figure 4.4 Stephan curves showing pH change in plaque of subjects with and without *Streptococcus mutans* (Reproduced with permission from Beighton, D. (2005) The complex oral microflora of high-risk individuals and groups and its role in the caries process. Community Dentistry and Oral Epidemiology, 33, 248–255. John Wiley & Sons, Ltd.)

bacteria other than mutans streptococci are associated with the initiation and progression of dental caries is now well accepted and new data have suggested roles for many other bacterial species in the caries process.

The acidogenicity and aciduricity of plaque bacteria and evidence for a multispecies aetiology of dental caries

The acidogenic composition of dental plaque reflects the dietary habits and caries status of an individual. A high acidogenic bacterial level was associated with active lesions or recent restorations, while individuals who were caries-free had a lower level of acidogenic bacteria. The acidogenic bacterial population also increased as the frequency exposure to dietary sugars increased. Streptococci, *Actinomyces* and *S. mutans* are also isolated amongst the acidogenic flora from dental plaque but no consistent relationship was found between either their isolation frequency or proportions and caries status, suggesting that the acidogenic population in plaque was heterogeneous. It was also apparent that bacteria other than mutans streptococci increased in plaque in response to an increased frequency of consumption of sugars.

It has been the studies of van Houte and colleagues (van Houte *et al.*, 1996) into the acidogenicity of bacteria isolated from a variety of sound and carious tooth sites that has shed most light on the role of bacteria other than

Table 4.1 Comparison of the percentage distribution of lactobacilli, mutans streptococci, *Bifidobacterium* and non-mutans streptococci, isolated from root caries lesions ($n = 84$) and sound tooth surfaces ($n = 223$) on the basis of their terminal pH in glucose broth. (Reproduced with permission from van Houte, J., Lopman, J. and Kent, R. (1996) The final pH of bacteria comprising the predominant flora on sound and carious human root and enamel surfaces. Journal of Dental Research, 75(4), 1008–1014.)

Organism	Terminal pH in 1% glucose broth					
	Advanced root caries lesions			Sound root surfaces		
	<4.2	4.2–4.4	>4.4	<4.2	4.2–4.4	>4.4
Lactobacillus	100	0	0	0	0	0
Mutans streptococci	100	0	0	100	0	0
Bifidobacterium	68	11	21	0	0	0
Non-mutans streptococci	78	18	4	16	51	33

mutans streptococci in the caries process. They found that other bacteria in dental plaque, presumably including *S. gordonii*, *S. oralis*, *S. mitis* and *S. anginosus*, outnumber the mutans streptococci in virtually all plaque samples. It was a logical extension of these observations to conclude that these bacteria may play a significant role in the caries process. There was clearly a selection for more acidogenic strains of non-mutans streptococci within carious lesions compared to those isolated from plaque on sound tooth surfaces (Table 4.1). It can be seen that lactobacilli and mutans streptococci all produced a terminal pH that was <4.2 while the other bacteria were heterogeneous. Of 100 isolates from root lesions, 78 produced a final pH of <4.2 but only 16 of 100 isolates from sound root surfaces produced the same low pH. van Houte and colleagues (1996) have reported that the emergence of mutans streptococci in plaque was usually preceded by an increase in the numbers of other types of acidogenic bacteria, including non-mutans streptococci. It was suggested that the initiation of caries, in the absence or presence of mutans streptococci, could be explained by the dynamic and positive relationship among the following factors:

- Carbohydrate consumption.
- Plaque flora composition.
- Plaque acidogenic potential.
- Caries activity.

The studies by van Houte reveal a little of the as yet poorly understood relationships between diet, microflora and caries initiation. However, they clearly demonstrate the heterogeneity of oral bacteria which may be exacerbated by exposure to fermentable dietary carbohydrates, and the consequent increase in acid production, by in turn exhibiting increased acidogenicity.

The aciduric flora of dental plaque has not been extensively studied in relation to dental caries initiation or progress. The variability observed by van Houte (1996) in respect to acidogenicity has also been observed for the aciduricity of dental plaque bacteria using molecular biology techniques (Figure 4.5). Here *S. oralis* strains were isolated from different people on media at pH 5.2 (acidic) and pH 7.0, and they were DNA fingerprinted using a method called **repetitive extragenic palindromic polymerase chain reaction** (REPPCR). These studies showed that this species was heterogeneous and that there exist distinct aciduric populations of *S. oralis*. Using the same methods the aciduric bacteria associated with root caries in the elderly were investigated by culturing plaque from different root surfaces on media at acid pH values. Plaque was taken from sound exposed root surfaces in subjects with no root caries activity, from sound root surfaces in subjects with root caries and from root carious lesions. It was found that the proportion of the flora that was isolated at pH 4.8 was significantly less from the sound surfaces in subjects with no root caries (0.008%) compared to the levels in the other groups, which were not significantly different. At pH 5.2 the recovery from the lesions was significantly greater than from the other two sites. From none of these samples were mutans streptococci recovered amongst the predominant aciduric bacteria. This study shows that the most diseased sites and those most at risk harboured the largest populations of aciduric bacteria, while the sites in subjects at least risk harboured the smallest populations of aciduric bacteria and that very few of the acidogenic bacteria isolated from these sites were mutans streptococci.

Together, these studies, derived using essentially conventional culture techniques supplemented with an assessment of genotypic and physiological characteristics, provide evidence that the microflora is heterogeneous. Individual species may be heterogeneous with respect to acidogenicity and aciduricity, features of

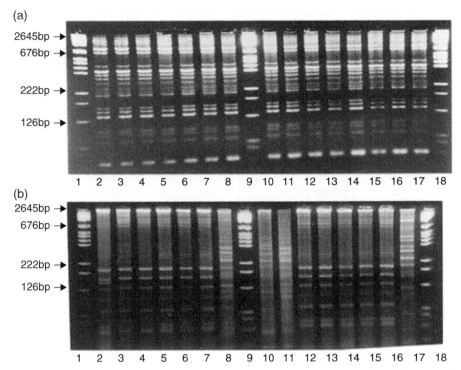

Figure 4.5 DNA fingerprint patterns of *Streptococcus oralis*. Strains grown at pH 7.0 or pH 5.2 from the same plaque sample. Evidence of heterogeneity within a species related to strain aciduricity. (Reproduced from Alam, S., Brailsford, S., Adams, R.S., Allison, C., Sheehy, E., Zoitopoulos, L., Kidd, E.A. and Beighton, D. (2000) Genotypic heterogeneity of Streptococcus oralis and distinct aciduric subpopulations in human dental plaque. Applied and Environmental Microbiology, 66, 3330–3336, with permission from ASM Press.)

mutans streptococci used to implicate these species in the caries process. While the associations between caries and the proportions of bacteria with acidogenic or aciduric traits were demonstrated, these studies provide only a basis for designing better investigations to enable a deeper understanding of the involvement of bacteria in the process of lesion formation. The changes in the flora from sound surface to white spot lesion through to cavitated lesion are not at all understood. The cross-sectional studies described clearly suggest microbial succession between these stages, but a definitive description of these flora and their physiological characteristics needs to be determined.

When it comes to considering the whole of the microflora of the dental plaque associated with dental caries, the newer techniques for studying bacterial populations provide a completely different insight into the causative bacterial species than has been previously understood from studies designed to associate mutans streptococci with caries. The modern studies use non-cultural methods and involve extracting DNA from whole plaque and analysing this to determine the number of species present or looking for the presence of a wide range of different, pre-determined bacteria.

From a study by Becker and colleagues (Becker *et al.*, 2002), the 16s rRNA genes, which are different in each bacterial species, were identified from dental plaque associated with sound and carious coronal sites in children. They analysed a total of 294 genes and found that these belonged to 68 species or phylotypes, of which 18 were uncultivated taxa and 10 were not previously identified; so 28 of 68 had not been previously encountered. The most complex flora was associated with plaque from sound intact tooth surfaces. Similar observations were made by Wade and Banerjee (Munson *et al.*, 2004) who investigated the microflora of five carious teeth and identified 95 different bacterial species amongst their samples, of which 44 were detected by the molecular method alone; 31 had never been previously described. All these studies demonstrate the great diversity of the microflora associated with dental plaque in both health and disease.

Using a more targeted approach, investigators at Harvard University used a semiquantitative method to determine the relationships between the presence and numbers of 23 well characterised species and the health or dental caries experience in children. They found the often-reported strong relationship between the numbers of *S. mutans* and caries but not between *S. sobrinus* and caries. However, other relationships were also demonstrated and these were that *Actinomyces gerensceriae*, *Bifidobacterium*, *Veillonella*, *S. salivarius*, *S. constellatus*, *S. parasanguis* and *Lactobacillus fermentum* were also associated with caries. *A. gerensceriae* and other *Actinomyces* spp. appeared to be associated with caries

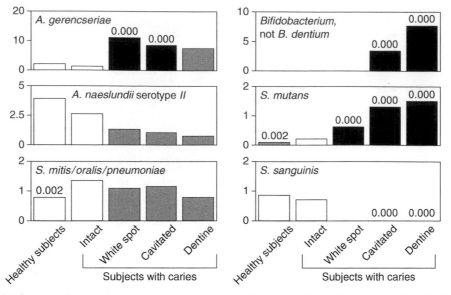

Figure 4.6 Relationship between bacterial numbers and caries status of teeth in children. (Reproduced from Becker, M.R., Paster, B.J., Leys, E.J., Moeschberger, M.L., Kenyon, S.G., Galvin, J.L., Boches, S.K., Dewhirst, F.E. and Griffen, A.L. (2002) Molecular analysis of bacterial species associated with childhood caries. Journal of Clinical Microbiology, 40(3), 1001–1009, with permission from ASM Press.)

initiation and a new *Bifidobacterium* species was associated with deep caries lesions (Figure 4.6).

These studies only serve to underline the complexity of the flora associated with caries and with caries initiation. They demonstrate that the proposed relationship between the presence of mutans streptococci and the aetiology of dental caries may be facile and simplistic. No matter how useful the relationship between the salivary or plaque levels of mutans streptococci and caries is in clinical practice, it must be regarded as an association and not a cause and effect relationship (see below). Caries occurs due to a complex interaction between dental plaque, whose physiological characteristics may be modified by carbohydrates in the diet, the diet itself and oral hygiene practices. These interactions are difficult to unpick and understand, especially as our knowledge of the microflora associated with health, disease and the transition from health to disease is minimal. It must also be recognised that the microflora associated with the transition state between health and disease may be different on different enamel surfaces (occlusal and approximal) and on exposed dentinal root surfaces.

Association and cause and effect

It is important to appreciate the difference between an association and cause and effect. For example, a study might show that a sample of the population which had a high incidence of skin cancer also consumed a greater than average quantity of ice cream. This does not mean that eating ice cream causes skin cancer; it merely shows an association, probably because people who expose their skin to sun radiation on the beach may also tend to eat more ice creams. A further example is that in the early part of the twentieth century, it was noticed that, when viewed over a measured period of time, the number of crimes increased with membership in the Church of England. This had nothing to do with criminals discovering religion. Rather, it was because both crimes and Church membership increased at the same time as the population increased. These two examples illustrate associations which are coincidental.

To establish a cause and effect, it is necessary to undertake a study which eliminates all other variables (**confounding factors**) which might influence the outcome other than the variable selected to be studied. This is usually achieved by dividing the study sample into two groups, a study group and a control group, and treating both groups identically except for the study group being exposed to the variable under consideration. It will be apparent how difficult this is to achieve with respect to the oral flora. Study design and the complexities of statistical analysis are outside the remit of this chapter and beyond the scope of this book and the interested reader is directed to more specialised texts in 'Further reading'.

The ecological plaque hypothesis

The microflora associated with health and disease are difficult to characterise accurately except in terms of the properties they possess, either individually or as a cariogenic biofilm. It also appears that the bacteria found in health are very similar to those found in disease. This realisation led Marsh (1994) to develop the ecological hypothesis for the aetiology of dental caries. Here the idea is that an external stimulus (dietary sugars) is converted to a localised stress (organic acids), which leads to ecological changes in the microflora at the site of acid production with only those species or genotypes of individual species able to survive and proliferate. These changes are dynamic and no particular bacterial species is implicated in the caries process; rather, any species may be present if it exhibits the appropriate level of aciduricity and acidogenicity.

The epidemiology of caries

It cannot be stated too often that dental caries has a multifactorial aetiology and the factors that have been identified as important in the development of caries are the consumption of fermentable sugars, the microflora of the dental plaque and the tooth surface. The prevalence and incidence of dental caries in a given population and in an individual are dependent upon the outcome of the interactions of these factors. These individual factors are, in turn, determined by a number of apparently unrelated factors which necessarily impact on them. The frequency of use of fluoride-containing toothpastes, which modify the tooth surface and may influence the acidogenicity of dental plaque, and the frequency of consumption of fermentable sugars by children may both, for example, be determined by the educational level and income of a parent, while the availability of fluoride-containing toothpastes may be determined by the commercial policy of the toothpaste producer. At a public health level, the factors that determine the level of tooth decay can be quite complicated. It is well established that in the UK caries levels are highest amongst poorer socioeconomic members of society; conversely, in developing countries the poorer people have the lowest levels of tooth decay since they are unable to afford the refined carbohydrates, which are an essential factor for caries development.

Historical studies

In 1883 Miller showed that carbohydrates when incubated with saliva caused demineralisation of extracted teeth. This showed for the first time that there was some scientific basis for dental caries being caused by diet. In 1940 studies by Stephan showed that dental plaque had a resting pH of 6.5–7; when exposed to fermentable sugars, such as sucrose, glucose or fructose, the pH fell rapidly to a pH well below 5, followed by a slow recovery to the original level over the next 30–60 minutes. The plot of plaque pH against time became known as the **Stephan curve** (see Figure 4.4). This is described more fully in Chapter 7, p. 148.

The relationship between sugar and caries

Epidemiological investigations

Interventional/epidemiological studies

Interventional studies or clinical trials are often seen as the best form of evidence. One of the earliest and most famous was the Vipeholm study, which is fully described in Chapter 7, p. 148–149.

Other epidemiological studies showed that caries prevalence was highest amongst children who ingested a high-sugar diet. Several studies showed that children living through the sugar restrictions of World War II had a reduction in caries prevalence. At the end of the war caries prevalence returned to prewar levels.

Observational studies

A classic observational study was undertaken on the inhabitants of the South Atlantic island of Tristan da Cunha. A volcanic eruption forced the occupants to move to England in 1962 where they were dentally examined and examined again on their return to the island in 1966. Before emigration, the islanders lived on a simple diet and their incidence of dental caries was low. The caries incidence of first permanent molars of 6–19-year-olds was zero in 1932 and 1937, increasing to 50% in 1962 (Holloway *et al.*, 1962) and to 80% in 1966 (Fisher, 1968a, b). The change of diet resulted in the development of caries to levels equal to those in England at the time. The change in sugar consumption in this study is described in Chapter 7, p. 149.

Animal studies

In the 1950s investigations on rats showed that those fed sugar via the mouth developed caries whilst those fed directly into the stomach did not (Kite *et al.*, 1950). Later, Konig, also using rats, showed a direct correlation between the severity of caries and the frequency of a cariogenic diet (Konig *et al.*, 1968). Rats were chosen for animal experimental work as the pathogenesis of caries in humans and rats is similar.

Enamel slab experiments

The effect of sugars and bacteria on sections of enamel placed on removable splints held in the mouth of volunteers is known as the demineralisation/remineralisation or **intraoral caries method** (ICT). At the end of the study period the amount of demineralisation is measured (Koulourides *et al.*, 1974; Brudevold *et al.*, 1984). Using this method, various forms of sugar and frequency of provocation can be assessed.

Acidogenicity studies

This method investigates the effects of food, meals and components of food on the pH of dental plaque. There are three methods of measuring the pH of plaque:

- **Plaque sampling**: plaque is sampled or collected from a number of sites at specific time intervals after eating or drinking sugars.
- **Touch electrode: Beetrode** pH electrodes or microelectrodes are used to measure the pH every few minutes for at least 30 minutes. A tip of a typical beetrode microelectrode is 0.1 mm diameter which is small enough to measure the pH of interproximal plaque.
- **Telemetry**: other electrodes connected to radio-transmitters (telemetry) are placed into intraoral splints and plaque pH change is measured over longer periods. They have been used extensively in the assessment of the cariogenicity of foods.

Incubational studies

Incubation laboratory studies are simple to perform but are generally considered to have the weakest relevance. The rate of acid production is recorded from foods mixed with plaque or saliva and the pH rise measured with electrodes. Another method is to mix whole enamel, powdered enamel or calcium phosphate with saliva and record the rate of the dissolution of the mineral. A measure of cariogenic potential is taken as the time for the process to cause demineralisation of the enamel (Clarkson *et al.*, 1984).

Fluoride

The introduction of fluoride into toothpaste and in the water in some UK cities (notably Birmingham and more recently, Southampton – see Chapter 11, p. 227) has reduced the average caries experience of most children. However, caries is still prevalent in poor socioeconomic areas, particularly in large cities. This reduction in caries experience has occurred in most developed countries. Although the addition of around 1 ppm of fluoride to the water supply has been shown to be effective, there are socially emotive reasons for stopping this being widespread. However, where water fluoridation has been undertaken, the reduction in caries experience is also seen in the poorer communities. In the more wealthy areas fluoride in toothpaste has an important role in caries prevention.

Effect of sugars

Caries develops on susceptible tooth surfaces which are normally covered by plaque. Sugars present within the diets provide the substrate for oral commensal bacteria to metabolise and produce lactic acid. The acid demineralises the enamel surface causing calcium ions to pass into the surrounding plaque. Mutans streptococci are the bacteria associated commonly with enamel caries. Provided sufficient time occurs between sugar intakes, the calcium ions present in the plaque start to

pass back into the tooth. This see-saw action will favour remineralisation if the frequency of sugar intake is more than 2–3 hourly. More frequent sugar intakes result in the calcium ions passing from the plaque into the saliva which is swallowed. If this continues the enamel surface becomes porous and a white spot lesion develops.

Features of enamel, dentine and root caries

It is the acidic pH that demineralises enamel and dentine. The **critical pH** for enamel is around 5.2–5.5 while for dentine it is around pH 6.0. The critical pH is defined as the pH at which the tooth tissue loses mineral to the saliva or plaque. The differences in pH are important in determining the rate of progression of enamel and root caries; root caries occurring on the exposed dentinal root surfaces of teeth. The root surfaces demineralise at a more neutral pH since the organic content of the dentine is considerably higher than that of the enamel. The tooth tissue does not dissolve when in contact with saliva, as saliva is supersaturated with calcium and phosphate ions and these are in equilibrium with the dentition. However, in acidic conditions, the saliva is able to sustain a higher concentration of these ions and so the teeth demineralise at specific sites (i.e. the stagnation sites where acid is produced by the dental plaque bacteria).

The following equation links these processes:

$$Ca_5(PO_4)OH \leftrightarrows 5Ca^{2+} + 3PO_4^{3+} + OH^-$$

The processes are reversible so that loss of mineral from the tooth surface may be replaced from the saliva when the pH of the site returns to the baseline pH value. Caries is a reversible process but if the process of loss of mineral in the acidic environment occurs too frequently, then the process cannot be reversed and it will progress to cause a clinically detectable carious lesion. In the acidic environment following consumption of dietary sugars and acid formation by the dental plaque, the hard tooth substance (hydroxyapatite) becomes more soluble. This is because the concentration of hydrogen ions (H^+) increases and these react with the $PO_4^{3+} + OH^-$ ions, so driving the equilibrium towards dissolution of the tooth substance.

The appearance of enamel caries
Macroscopic

Early enamel lesions appear as white or demineralised areas of increased porosity (**white spot lesions**) over an intact enamel surface (Figure 4.7). This increase in enamel porosity represents a reduction in its mineral content with an associated change in refractive index of the component parts. If the plaque remains undisturbed,

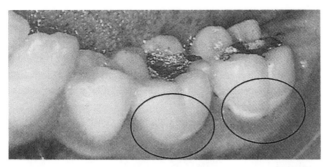

Figure 4.7 Early white spot enamel lesions on the cervical-gingival margins of both the mandibular left molars (circled). (Reproduced with permission of Oxford University Press, Banerjee A. Watson TF (2011) *Pickard's Manual of Operative Dentistry*, 9th edition.)

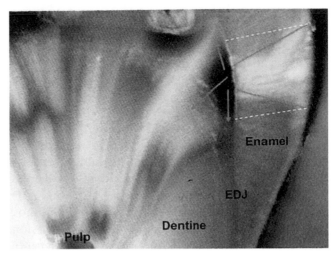

Figure 4.8 A mesiodistal section through a carious tooth highlighting an approximal lesion. The red lines outline the inverted cone cross-sectional histological shape of the enamel lesion and the blue lines the direction of spread of the lesion having crossed the enamel–dentine junction (EDJ) into dentine. The white dotted lines show how the extent of the spread of the dentine lesions subjacent to the EDJ is associated with the same lateral extent of the enamel lesion on the tooth surface, both governed by the presence of the plaque biofilm on the tooth surface. (Reproduced with permission of Oxford University Press, Banerjee A. Watson TF (2011) *Pickard's Manual of Operative Dentistry*, 9th edition.)

the lesion progresses and the size of the pores increases as the mineral ions are lost. As the lesion progresses the surface begins to break down and the lesion starts to spread laterally. At this point there is no alteration in the dentine. As caries progresses discrete periods of demineralisation and remineralisation occur which are seen as colour changes on the surface of the enamel. The remineralisation periods usually produce brown or yellow discoloration on the enamel surface. The progression of the lesion depends on the enamel and the continuation of the supply of nutrient.

As the lesion progresses into dentine, collapse of the enamel occurs, leaving voids in the surface. Proximally, a lesion starts just below the contact area. On the buccal and lingual surfaces, the early (incipient) enamel lesion starts just above the gingival margin. On the occlusal surfaces the lesion starts along opposite walls of a fissure. Although the appearance differs at each site, the basic mechanism remains the same. For example, in an occlusal fissure two smooth surface lesions develop on the adjacent walls of the enamel fissure.

Root surface lesions are quite different in appearance as the carious attack is into a tissue with a lower mineral content than enamel lesions. The root surface lesions tend to initiate at the gingival margin and are first apparent clinically as softened areas of dentine, which are identified using a blunt dental explorer. The soft lesions are active and undergoing demineralisation. If plaque control is instituted these lesions undergo repair as a result of remineralisation and pass through stages described as leathery and eventually hard.

Microscopic

An initial enamel lesion starts as a wedge shape with the point towards the dentine. There appears to be an outer intact layer, 20–50 µm thick, and a deeper body of the lesion where the pore volume is increased. Two other zones are visible on ground sections viewed under transmitted light (Figure 4.8). The dark and translucent zones represent the gradual loss of mineral from the tissues. The deeper **translucent zone** has slight loss of mineral whilst the outer and narrower **dark zone** represents an area of previous remineralisation. However, the distribution of the various zones varies greatly.

The appearance of dentine caries

Macroscopic

The progression from enamel to dentine caries is a continuum representing a change from a hard to a softer substrate. The concept that the enamel is undermined by the advancing lesion in dentine is untrue. Despite the fact that dentine is softer than enamel, the lateral progression of the advancing lesion is the same in both tissues. The changes in pore size and increase in permeability of the spreading lesion in enamel are mimicked below with the lateral spread into dentine.

The progression of caries changes the surface features of the tooth and results in a breakdown of the integrity of the crown. It starts with a localised collapse of enamel to expose dentine to plaque formation/stagnation, so promoting the progression of the lesion.

Eventually collapse of cusps and fractures of the crown can occur, exposing the pulp. As the destruction continues, the tooth becomes extensively carious, approaches the gingival tissues or invades the pulp and becomes increasingly more difficult to restore and eventually may require extraction.

The most important predictor for the activity of caries in dentine is the surface texture of the lesion. Bacterial destruction causes a reduction in hardness of dentine (due to demineralisation), which is detected by probing with a sharp instrument. In the dentine lesion adjacent to the enamel–dentine junction (EDJ), the **caries-infected dentine** is very soft, and almost wet. It comprises the carious biomass of the lesion, is easily separated and the surface can be peeled away with an excavator. The deeper **caries-affected dentine** zone is less infected and gradually becomes harder and more resistant to probing. There is a strong correlation between the bacterial infection and the softness of the dentine. There is also a change in colour from yellow to browner shades. Although colour changes are common they should not be interpreted as active caries. Hard stained dentine has a low level of infection by bacteria, whereas soft stained dentine has a high infiltration of bacteria.

Microscopic

The first sign of change in dentine is the formation of tubular infill ('sclerosis'), part of the dentine–pulp complex defence reaction to the carious process. This mineral infill along the dentinal tubules can form as a result of the progression of the enamel lesion. Tubular sclerosis starts before the advancing enamel lesion has penetrated the dentine. Once the lesion spreads into dentine, bacterial invasion occurs with plaque accumulation. The action of acids on the surface causes superficial tissue destruction. This area is called the **zone of destruction** and coincides with the zone of caries-infected dentine described above. With a rapidly advancing lesion, **dead tracts** can be seen within the dentine structure where the odontoblasts have died and not laid down further mineral within the tubules. These resulting empty tubules allow bacterial infiltration leading to further tissue destruction. As these areas combine they form **liquefaction foci**.

The appearance of root caries
Macroscopic

Root caries begins along the gingival or cervical margins of teeth. It can occur on the buccal, lingual or interproximal surfaces and, like enamel caries, starts with tissue decalcification (Figure 4.9). As the lesion progresses it spreads into the dentine and undermines the

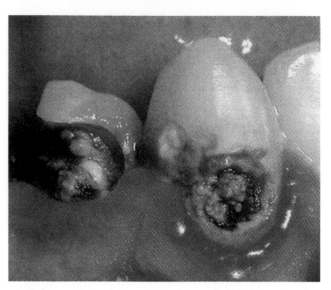

Figure 4.9 Grossly cavitated buccal carious lesions on LR3 and LR4 with quantities of stagnant dense plaque deposited on the exposed dentine – MICDAS 4. (Reproduced with permission Oxford University Press, Banerjee A. Watson TF (eds) (2011) *Pickard's Manual of Operative Dentistry*, 9th edition.)

surrounding enamel, causing further tissue breakdown. Like dentine caries, the most important determinant of activity is the texture. Soft carious dentine is heavily infected with bacteria and needs removing, whereas harder surfaces may indicate that the process has become inactive. Remineralisation of root caries produces light and dark brown areas, which are hard to probe and may be aesthetically displeasing, but do not represent active lesions.

Microscopic

Early root lesions normally start in dentine and follow a similar pathological process.. Like enamel caries there is an outer surface zone which varies widely in thickness and represents surface remineralisation. Unlike enamel caries, however, the surface may become softer at an earlier stage as the bacteria invade the dentine. Therefore, surface disruption with probing can cause more damage earlier in the process than that found with occlusal caries. At the same time scaling and polishing should be avoided as this causes more breakdown of the surface layer. Before scaling is undertaken the lesion should be arrested with improved oral hygiene and patient maintenance.

Root caries lesions have distinct microscopic appearances for each of their diagnostic stages:

- The **soft lesions** have extensive breakdown of the organic material, primarily collagen, and extensive demineralisation of the hydroxyapatite crystals with the residue of the structures embedded in an actively metabolising bacterial mass.

- Once the lesions start to heal the **leathery lesions** start to mineralise and bacterial metabolism is reduced; often a surface layer of mineral may be observed above the lesion.
- In the **hard lesions** the new mineral has no specific structure, the crystals are amorphous and bacterial cell wall ghosts may be seen within the mineral.

The driving force behind the reversal of these lesions is control of the plaque biofilm overlying the lesion surface and the presence of saliva to drive the remineralisation of the tissues.

Diagnostic methods for dental caries

Clinical methods

Caries can occur on the occlusal, proximal and buccal/lingual surfaces of teeth. On smooth surfaces the lesions normally develop close to the gingival margin and are covered in plaque biofilm. Lesions developing in fissures and on proximal surfaces are more difficult to detect and diagnosis usually involves indirect methods. Diagnostic tests have been developed to maximise the accuracy of caries detection on each surface. On the buccal and lingual surfaces the optimal assessment is the visual appearance of the surface. A white spot lesion can be seen when enamel has been cleaned and dried. The area is often covered in plaque. On those surfaces hidden from direct visual examination, radiographic examination is the most commonly used diagnostic technique.

Visual

The **modified International Caries Detection and Assessment System (mICDAS)** (Table 4.2) uses the link between visual appearance of the lesion surface to its underlying progressing histopathology. As the carious process advances into dentine there is a suggestion that the enamel can become undermined. Ekstrand et al. (1998) showed in microbiological studies that there is

Table 4.2 mICDAS criteria used to assess the depth and activity of occlusal caries (column 1) and criteria to measure the depth, the activity and the level of infection histologically. (Modified with permission from Ekstrand, K.R. (2004) Improving clinical visual detection –potential for caries clinical trials. Journal of Dental Research, 83(Spec Iss C), C67–C71.)

Column 1	2	3[a]	4	5[b]
Original criteria used in the visual examination (Ekstrand et al., 1998)	Original criteria used in the histological examination	Criteria used for assessment of activity (Ekstrand et al., 1998)	Methyl red (pH-indicator) indicates pH ≤5.5, no color or yellow > 5.5	Level of infection at the enamel-dentine junction (Ricketts et al., 2002)
0 = No or slight changes in enamel translucency after prolonged air-drying (>5 s)	0 = No enamel demineralization or a narrow surface zone of opacity (edge phenomenon)	As in column 1	No colour or yellow	0
1 = Opacity or discoloration hardly visible on the wet surface, but distinctly visible after air-drying	1 = Enamel demineralization limited to the outer 50% of the enamel layer	1 = Opacity (white) hardly visible; 1a = Opacity (brown) hardly visible.	Red. No colour or yellow	0
2 = Opacity or discoloration distinctly visible without air-drying	2 = Demineralization involving between 50% of the enamel and 1/3 of dentine	2 = Opacity (white) distinctly visible . 2a = Opacity (brown) distinctly visible .	Red. No colour or yellow	+
3 = Localized enamel breakdown in opaque or discoloured enamel and/or greyish discoloration from the underlying dentine	3 = Demineralization involving the middle 1/3 of the dentine	As in column 1	Red	++
4 = Cavitation in opaque or discolored enamel exposing the dentine beneath	4 = Demineralisation involving the inner 1/3 of the dentine	As in column 1	Red	+++

[a](The criteria 1, 2, 3, and 4 indicate active lesions, while 1a and 2a are indications of arrested lesions. Score 0 denotes sound surfaces.
[b]Level of infection: 0, no infection; +, lightly infected; ++, moderately infected; +++, heavily infected.

an equivalent demineralisation front occurring in the overlying enamel. This progression can be examined using a simple process. A clean and well-dried enamel surface is assessed for surface integrity and enamel demineralisation and whitening (equivalent to increase in surface porosity). The enamel surface must be thoroughly cleaned and dried. An intact surface without demineralisation indicates a non-advancing lesion. White demineralisation and a break in the enamel surface show that dentine is involved. If the surface is completely dry it is possible to see that the spread of the enamel decalcification matches that of the spread of caries in dentine.

Probably the most difficult lesion to assess is recurrent caries occurring around existing restorations. Marginal gaps and ditching are common around most amalgam and tooth-coloured adhesive restorations. The distinction between caries and localised material collapse is difficult, with many clinicians interpreting the same appearance in different ways. Marginal gaps which are sticky to probing and are wider than the width of a periodontal probe would encourage plaque biofilm stagnation and generally mean that caries is present and there is a need for operative intervention. However, pure ditching (which is a breakdown of the amalgam at the tooth surface) does not require restoration if the surface can be maintained plaque-free. Shadowing and a blue–brown discoloration within the tooth and surrounding the restoration can indicate an active lesion, although this can be misleading as the appearance of metallic restorative materials under disease-free enamel can have a similar appearance.

Radiography

Bitewing radiographs are relatively reliable for detecting proximal lesions but less so for occlusal lesions. Radiolucencies developing below the contact areas usually appear like horizontal V-shaped notches in enamel-only lesions (Figure 4.10). As the lesion progresses into dentine, a mushroom formation occurs as the enamel appears to be undermined along the EDJ. The situation is more difficult to assess on the occlusal surfaces as the more mineralised and thicker enamel together with the superimposition of enamel from adjacent cusps partly obscures the lesion progression. The advancing lesion is therefore relatively underdiagnosed by radiographs. A rough guide suggests that a lesion clinically is 25% more advanced than when estimated from a radiograph. It is important to remember that a clinician must not decide to intervene operatively on the radiographic appearance alone but must take into account numerous other factors when making this important decision. A bitewing radiograph needs to be taken correctly to have the optimal diagnostic yield. Film holders yield the most accurate results and ensure that the X-rays pass perpendicularly through the crown of the tooth. This reduces the amount of overlap proximally. A clear outline should be visible of the enamel overlying the dentine and allows good distinction between the two tissues. A change in the radiolucency of the tooth can then be seen. Caries appears as diffuse radiolucent shadowing and occurs at susceptible sites. Approximally, this will occur below the contact area and above the alveolar bone. Beneath the occlusal surfaces the faint outline of caries can be detected. The radiolucent zone appears as a diffuse zone beneath the enamel. The extent of the lesion spread is more difficult to visualise as the bulk of

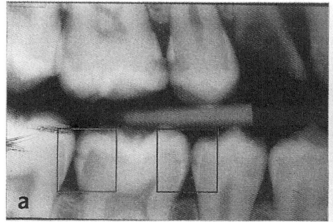 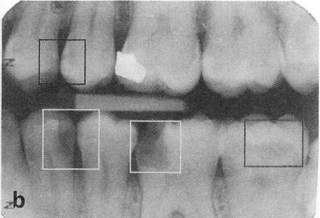

Figure 4.10 (a)Left (b) Right bitewing radiographs from two different patients both with high caries experience; showing caries lesions within enamel and outer third of dentine (E2–D1 blue squares), approaching middle third dentine (D2, red square) and very close to the pulp (D3, yellow square). Note other lesions can be detected on these films. (Reproduced with permission of Oxford University Press, Banerjee A. Watson TF (eds) (2011) *Pickard's Manual of Operative Dentistry*, 9th edition.)

the enamel and dentine partly obscures the X-rays; this results in a less accurate assessment of occlusal caries compared to that occurring proximally. Care is needed to interpret the cause of the radiolucency within the crown – a well-defined shadow beneath an existing restoration may be caused by the presence of a relatively radiolucent restorative material (e.g. lining or bonding agent).

The frequency of bitewing radiographs should be assessed for each individual. A high caries risk individual (one with recent caries – see Chapter 11, p. 224) might require radiographs taken at six monthly intervals whereas someone with no caries experience for a number of years would need them less frequently (e.g. every 2 years).

Transillumination

This is a technique used rarely to assess caries on molars and premolars but used more commonly on anterior teeth. Direct light reflected by dental mirrors on to the teeth can highlight darkened shadows present between the approximal surfaces of upper anterior teeth. A carious lesion appears as a darkened shadow in dentine surrounded by a normal coloured zone. Visual blue light curing lamps can be used to examine the surfaces as white intraoral lights are not common. These lights need to be directed between the contacts of teeth and have sufficient intensity to show the caries. Generally, ambient light sources need to be reduced to improve the reliability of the diagnosis.

Tooth separators

Orthodontic separators have been reported to be useful for examining directly the approximal areas between contacting teeth. Orthodontic elastic bands are placed between teeth and over a few days gradually separate the teeth so that direct visual inspection of the surfaces can be undertaken. Once the contacts are broken, the lesion is inspected and, if sufficient access is available, operative management commenced if necessary. This procedure is, however, rarely used in clinical practice due to the need for extra appointments. Proprietary interdental wedges can be used to separate teeth more rapidly within the same appointment. After infiltrating some local analgesia, the wedge can be pushed through the contact area from the buccal aspect. After a few minutes, it can be further advanced through towards the lingual/palatal aspect, eventually permitting direct inspection of the proximal surfaces.

Other techniques
Electronic caries meters

Research has suggested that changes to the electrical impedance of enamel can indicate an active lesion. Small d.c. voltages have less resistance in carious enamel than

that through an intact surface. The instrument needs a clean and dry surface to work efficiently and is generally used on the occlusal surfaces of molars and premolars. The advantage of using this technique is that it is the occlusal surfaces of molar and premolar teeth where radiographic assessment of caries is less accurate than the proximal surface. The tip of the probe is less than 1 mm in diameter and can detect changes in the impedance of enamel over very small areas. This means that over small areas the instrument might be very accurate at detecting early carious lesions, but the reliability over larger areas has been questioned. This technique has the potential to overdiagnose caries by giving false-positive results and thus its clinical application is limited.

Laser fluorescence

This technique, available commercially as an instrument called the DIAGNOdent (KaVo), is meant to detect the fluorescence characteristics changes of the carious lesion when compared to its sound counterpart. However, the light reflectivity from a carious and non-carious surface is different and can easily overpower the changes in fluorescent signal from the carious lesion. The instrument is calibrated in an attempt to detect this difference and informs the operator through a numerical read out (Figure 4.11), but like the electronic caries meters, these instruments can overdiagnose caries (false positive readings) and potentially confuse stained surfaces with

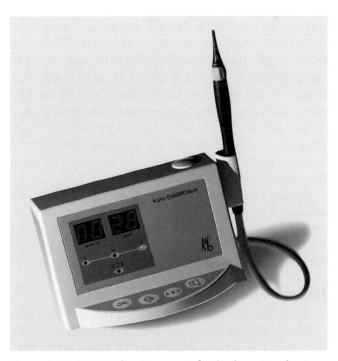

Figure 4.11 DIAGNOdent instrument for the detection of carious lesions. (Reproduced with permission from Kavo.)

carious ones. In addition, some restorative materials have shown similar fluorescent/reflective values to those of carious dentine and its application for the detection of secondary caries seems questionable. A systematic review of the performance of laser fluorescence device for detecting caries found that despite its high sensitivity for detecting caries, its likelihood for false positive readings limits its use as a clinically viable diagnostic technique.

Non-surgical management of dental caries

It is important to distinguish the difference between prevention and control of caries. The biochemical carious process cannot be prevented at the tooth surface, but by regulating the factors alluded to earlier in this chapter, can be controlled. The manifestation of the disease process, that is the hard tissue lesions in enamel and dentine, can be prevented with suitable tailored-made interventions for both the patient and from the dental team.

Prevention

The most important preventive roles are improving plaque biofilm removal and modification of the patient's diet to reduce the frequency of sugar consumption (see Chapter 7, p. 151).

Oral hygiene instructions should aim to improve biofilm removal and produce a reduction in the bacterial load in the mouth. Careful flossing techniques, although difficult to learn, are efficient at removing cariogenic bacteria from interdental areas. More recently, the introduction of interdental brushes has largely superseded dental floss in terms of interdental plaque removal except in very tight interproximal spaces. Although much of the emphasis in the UK is aimed at dietary reduction of refined carbohydrates, other parts of Europe consider efficient tooth cleaning as important if not more so than dietary advice. Whichever is more important, efficient plaque removal reduces the bacterial load but, without changes to the diet by reducing the frequency of sugar intake, neither will be effective.

Dietary changes are notably difficult to achieve, but smaller less intrusive modifications can be effective. Dietary analysis utilising tools such as diet diaries (see chapters 7, p. 156 and 12, p. 251) are an effective method for educating patients into dietary sources of sugars.

Fissure sealants

The concept of separating the lesion from the oral bacteria has also been utilised with fissure sealants. This technique is described in Chapter 12. Provided the sealant remains intact and the oral hygiene procedures as well as the diet of the individual improve, sealants have been shown to be effective in arresting caries activity. However, continuation of a cariogenic diet along with plaque biofilm stagnation can result in caries developing in adjacent sites next to the fissure-sealed areas. The unfilled or partially filled resin-based materials are not resistant to occlusal wear and will be worn away over time and so will need regular inspection and replacement. However, the materials should be sufficiently flowable to pass into the occlusal fissures. Even though the occlusal surfaces may be worn away over time, residual parts within the deep occlusal fissures remain to protect the tooth. Fissure sealants are generally not indicated for all young patients and are usually targeted at those with a higher caries risk (see Chapter 12).

Surgical management of dental caries

Removal of carious dentine

Access is the term used to describe the procedure for gaining clearance to visualise and remove caries surgically. This generally involves cutting sufficient enamel away with burs (or hand instruments if the enamel is weak) to provide sufficient access to the carious dentine. Burs coupled to high-speed handpieces can be used to remove weakened undermined or unsupported enamel to expose the softer dentine which is then excavated using hand instruments (spoon excavators) and/ or burs, ideally coupled to a slow-speed handpiece. The most important clinical parameter to judge the extent of dentine caries removal is its texture and hardness. The amount of caries removed should be gauged by analysis of the following factors: the pulp status and proximity, the amount of supragingival coronal tooth structure retained, the caries risk of the patient and the clinical factors involved in placement of the restoration (operator access, moisture control, etc.). The biological depth aspect (that is caries-infected vs. caries-affected vs. sound dentine) and the lateral extent of the lesion (that is the extent from the EDJ to the pulp) must be also evaluated. With the increased use of adhesive materials and minimally invasive principles/techniques to restore cavities, the achievement of a seal between the tooth substrate and the restorative material is paramount in preventing lesion progression. This seal is best achieved at the EDJ, the peripheral margin of the overall restoration. Currently, the best seal is obtained when the restoration is coupled to sound enamel, followed by sound dentine, followed by caries-affected dentine. Therefore consideration must be given to the histological quality of the tissue retained at the cavity walls and floor. Histologically sound enamel and dentine would be ideal at the EDJ whereas overlying the pulp, affected dentine (and in some cases, even infected dentine remnants) may be retained, termed **residual caries**. The clinical differences in carious dentine layers can be difficult to judge objectively without experience but the texture and hardness differs through the zones. Caries-infected dentine is soft, wet and mushy; affected dentine is intermediate with a simultaneous scratchiness and tackiness elicited with a sharp dental explorer drawn across the dentine surface whereas sound dentine is completely hard and scratchy. A balance needs to be achieved between removing sufficient carious tissue to prevent disease progression and yet conserve the pulp's vitality and tooth structure allowing the tooth to be restored successfully. Provided the soft dentine that appears wet is removed, the vitality of the pulp should be protected. Depending on the restorative material, the pulp itself can be protected physically and chemically from further bacterial onslaught with the use of **indirect or direct pulp capping techniques**. The term 'lining' should be considered obsolete in modern dentistry. The techniques and treatment options in operative dentistry for children are described in Chapter 12 and for adults in Chapter 13.

'Stepwise excavation' – biological caries management

The knowledge that caries progression is dependent upon a continual supply of substrate has been utilised in the concept of stepwise excavation. If the supply of sugar is stopped, the bacteria are no longer able to metabolise a substrate; therefore their numbers reduce and the lesion activity slows. Originally, this method involved sealing the carious lesion from the oral cavity with a, provisional restorative material. After excavating the caries-infected soft and wet dentine layer, the residual caries was covered with the restorative material and left for a few months. Thereafter, the restoration was removed, the arrested carious dentine excavated further and the final cavity restored with a definitive material, such as composite or amalgam. The isolation of the bacteria from the oral cavity results in the lesion arresting, the remaining dentine hardening and a reduction in the number of bacteria to levels which do not maintain lesion progression. With the improvement in adhesive dental materials along with their ability to seal to carious dentine, the hardening of the residual arrested dentine means that operative re-entry is not indicated and it is no longer necessary to remove the caries-affected dentine overlying the pulp. This helps to preserve the pulp integrity and prolongs the life of the tooth. This original technique was first suggested in the 1960s but has gained favour following more recent research (Bjorndal and Thylstrup, 1998) and innovations in dental materials science. The principles of minimally invasive (MI) dentistry with the concomitant biological approach

to excavating dentine caries has now made the term stepwise excavation unnecessary.

Chemomechanical caries removal

Sodium hypochlorite dissolves organic material. This property is used in the formulation called Carisolv (Orasolv, Goteburg, Sweden). The material is presented in a gel formulation and applied on to the surface of a carious dentine lesion. The hypochlorite, given sufficient time, partially breaks down the organic material and kills the bacteria, rendering the lesion caries free. The gel is placed over the carious lesion (Figure 4.12). The dentine caries is then abraded with specially designed hand instruments and the caries-infected dentine emulsifies into the gel turning it cloudy. Several applications of the gel may be required to achieve adequate caries removal and after the final cavity wash can be restored with an adhesive material. It has the advantage of being a painless procedure (does not require local anaesthesia), and although a bur is not needed to remove carious dentine, one may still be needed to access the lesion. A bur is used to remove enamel to gain access to the body of the lesion.

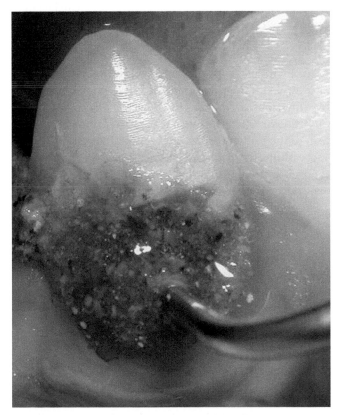

Figure 4.12 Buccal cavitated carious lesion (MICDAS 4) on the LR3. Gel and carious dentine agitated with a mace tip hand instrument using toothbrush force. (Reproduced with permissions of Oxford University Press, Banerjee A. Watson TF (eds) (2011) *Pickard's Manual of Operative Dentistry*, 9th edition.)

Studies have shown that the technique is successful in removing caries but it has not become a common clinical procedure in general practice. It has perhaps a greater application for **atraumatic restorative treatment** (ART) in underdeveloped healthcare systems often in developing countries because of the minimal requirement of rotary instrumentation. With the philosophy of minimally invasive operative treatment of caries, these techniques will be used more commonly.

The histopathology of pulpitis

Acute pulpitis

Early changes within the pulp instigated by the advancing carious lesion lead to the production of **tertiary dentine** by the odontoblasts. Tertiary dentine, also known as irregular secondary dentine, contains fewer tubules than primary or secondary dentine. Tertiary dentine may be **reactionary**, laid down by primary odontoblasts in response to a mild stimulus, or **reparative dentine**, laid down by secondary odontoblasts differentiated from other pulp cells if the primary odontoblasts are irreversibly damaged by the initial rapid stimulus. This attempt at creating a barrier to the advancing lesion can be effective if the lesion progresses slowly and particularly so if it arrests. However, with the advancing lesion, bacteria invade the odontoblasts and destroy the surrounding tissues. Clinically it is characterised by the patient feeling pain in response to temperature change which lasts for the duration of the stimulus. There is normally no pain on biting or when the tooth is percussed. The inflammation of the pulp is reversible and the cause can be treated successfully, for example by the removal of the caries. As the pulpal inflammation becomes more severe, the pain experienced as a result of temperature change becomes greater and persists after the removal of the stimulus usually for several minutes or longer.

As the lesion approaches the pulp, inflammatory responses are detected ahead of the advancing lesion. Once the bacteria have penetrated the pulpal complex, the inflammatory process becomes more profound resulting in an increase in the number of inflammatory cells together with an accumulation of inflammatory exudate within the confines of the pulpal dentinal walls. The inability of the pulp chamber to expand to alleviate the build up of pressure results in the clinical symptoms of acute pulpitis. These are:

- A constant, throbbing pain in the affected tooth that is often made worse by reclining or lying down.
- A lack of pain on biting unless the inflammation has spread beyond the confines of the pulp.
- The inability to obtain relief from the pain.

Other processes which can lead to bacteria penetrating the pulp are trauma (e.g. a fractured tooth or traumatic exposure during cavity preparation; iatrogenic), tooth wear, via the periodontal membrane or, rarely, via a bacteraemia (e.g. induced by a tooth extraction from another site; **anachoresis**).

Chronic pulpitis

Chronic pulpitis may be the result of persistent mild to moderate irritation of the pulp or it may follow a period of acute pulpitis. The symptoms are:

- A mild intermittent pain over an extended period of time.
- Pain of varying intensity.
- Pain which is often difficult to localise.
- Pain usually induced by thermal change or sweet liquids or solids.

Symptoms may be relieved by taking analgesics which act on the central nervous system (see Chapter 10). Patients have been known to try to alleviate the symptoms by placing an analgesic tablet, (e.g. aspirin), adjacent to the suspected tooth. Aspirin has no analgesic affect locally and is likely to compound the discomfort by inducing a mucosal burn because of the high local concentration of acetylsalicylic acid.

The result of bacterial invasion is an influx of anti-inflammatory cells (macrophages) into the pulp and an increase in lymphocytes and plasma cells. This produces dead bacteria, other necrotic debris and sometimes discrete areas of calcification including pulp stones. The ratio of dead to living cells increases and can lead eventually to death of the pulp.

Abscess formation

Acute abscess

Once the pulp dies the pulpal space is invaded by bacteria which progress to the apical tissues. Early changes involve localised tissue response to bacteria and their by-products. Unless the carious lesion is large and associated with extensive tissue breakdown, the only exit pathway for necrotic tissue in the pulp is through the apical foramen and into the supporting bone. The leaching of bacteria and inflammatory factors released from dead inflammatory cells causes an inflammatory response in the apical tissues which is experienced clinically as pain on biting or tenderness to percussion and is termed **apical periodontitis**. The potential exists for this to increase to produce an area that contains predominantly dead cells from the bacteria, bone and inflammatory cells. Accumulation of these cells in an enclosed space produces greater tissue destruction and the formation of **pus**, a liquid containing large numbers of polymorphonuclear cells, necrotic tissue and bacterial toxins. The pus increases in amount until tissue expansion results in a breakout, usually along the line of least resistance into the soft tissues, either via the periodontal ligament or directly into the mouth. It may also spread into the soft tissues to create a **cellulitis**. Such spread can be dictated by the related anatomical structures. Infection via fascial planes can be rapid and extend some distance from the original abscess site, resulting occasionally in occlusion of the airway by oedema (e.g. **Ludwig's angina**). Rarely it may also spread into the deeper medullary space of the alveolar bone producing a spreading **osteomyelitis**. There can also be an indirect spread of infection, either via the **lymphatic system** to the regional lymph nodes in the head and neck (the submental, submandibular, deep cervical, parotid or occipital), which can become enlarged and tender, or more rarely, via the blood vessels to other organs such as the heart or brain.

The onset of an abscess is usually characterised by a severe throbbing pain, often easily localised by the patient, with or without an obvious clinical swelling intra-or extraorally depending on the site of infection. The tooth is normally very sensitive to biting and percussion because of the inflammation of the supporting structures. Due to the increase in pressure in the periapical region with a periapical abscess, the tooth is usually elevated in the socket which results in increased mobility and causes the patient to experience additional pain due to a premature contact on occlusion. The initial treatment for an apical abscess is to establish drainage via the tooth (endodontic access) or via an incision into the affected tissues which can be intraoral or extraoral.

Chronic abscess

When the abscess bursts through the bone into the adjacent soft tissues, there is usually an immediate reduction in the symptoms and, providing the abscess can continue to maintain drainage, it will tend to go into a chronic phase which is frequently asymptomatic. In the chronic phase, a **sinus** links the main abscess cavity with the skin or mucosal surface and allows further drainage to take place. This process can be associated with both primary and permanent teeth. In both cases the progression from a carious lesion to a chronic abscess may be completely asymptomatic and visual examination will reveal a discharging sinus usually adjacent to the carious tooth. The sinus drainage pathway may become blocked, resulting in an elevated lesion or **gum boil** at the gingival margin. As the pressure increases this will intermittently burst and discharge into the oral cavity.

A dentoalveolar abscess is usually polymicrobial consisting of predominantly anaerobic organisms which include *Streptococcus sanguis*, milleri-group streptococci, *Actinomyces* spp., *Porphyromonas gingivalis* and *Fusobacterium nucleatum*.

References

Aamdal-Scheie, A., Luan, W.M., Dahlen, G. and Fejerskov, O. (1996) Plaque pH and microflora of dental plaque on sound and carious root surfaces. *Journal of Dental Research*, **75**(11), 1901–1908.

Alam, S., Brailsford, S., Adams, R.S., Allison, C., Sheehy, E., Zoitopoulos, L., Kidd, E.A. and Beighton, D. (2000) Genotypic heterogeneity of *Streptococcus oralis* and distinct aciduric subpopulations in human dental plaque. *Applied and Environmental Microbiology*, **66**, 3330–3336.

Becker, M.R., Paster, B.J., Leys, E.J., Moeschberger, M.L., Kenyon, S.G., Galvin, J.L., Boches, S.K., Dewhirst, F.E. and Griffen, A.L. (2002) Molecular analysis of bacterial species associated with childhood caries. *Journal of Clinical Microbiology*, **40**(3), 1001–1009.

Beighton, D. (2005) The complex oral microflora of high-risk individuals and groups and its role in the caries process. *Community Dentistry and Oral Epidemiology*, **33**, 248–255.

Bjorndal, L. and Thylstrup, A. (1998) A practice-based study on stepwise excavation of deep carious lesions in permanent teeth: a 1-year follow-up study. *Community Dentistry and Oral Epidemiology*, **26**(2), 122–128.

Brudevold, F., Attarzadeh, F., Tehrani, A., van Houte, J. and Russo, J. (1984) Development of a new intraoral demineralization test. *Caries Research*, **18**, 421–429.

Clarkson, B.H., Wefel, J.S. and Miller, I. (1984) A model for producing caries-like lesions in enamel and dentin using oral bacteria in vitro. *Journal of Dental Research*, **63**, 1186–1189.

Ekstrand, K.R. (2004) Improving clinical visual detection – potential for caries clinical trials. *Journal of Dental Research*, **83**(Spec Iss C), C67–C71.

Ekstrand, K.R., Ricketts, D.N., Kidd, E.A., Qvist, V. and Schou, S. (1998) Detection, diagnosing, monitoring and logical treatment of occlusal caries in relation to lesion activity and severity: an in vivo examination with histological validation. *Caries Research*, **32**, 247–254.

Fisher, F.J. (1968a) A field survey of dental caries, periodontal disease and enamel defects in Tristan Da Cunha. 1. The background. *British Dental Journal*, **124**, 398–400.

Fisher, F.J. (1968b) A field survey of dental caries, periodontal disease and enamel defects in Tristan da Cunha. *British Dental Journal*, **125**, 447–453.

Hemmens, E.S., Blaney, J.R., Bradel, S.F. and Harrison, R.W. (1946) The microbic flora of the dental plaque in relation to the beginning of caries. *Journal of Dental Research*, **25**, 195–205.

Holloway, P.J., James, P.M. and Slack, G.L. (1962) Dental caries among the inhabitants of Tristan da Cunha. (d). The last count. *Royal Society of Health Journal*, **82**, 139.

Kite, O.W., Shaw, J.H. and Sognnaes, R.F. (1950) The prevention of experimental tooth decay by tube-feeding. *Journal of Nutrition*, **42**, 89–105.

Kolenbrander, P.E., Andersen, R.N., Blehert, D.S., Egland, P.G., Foster, J.S. and Palmer, R.J. (2002) Communication among oral bacteria. *Microbiology and Molecular Biology Reviews*, **66**, 486–505.

Konig, K.G., Schmid, P. and Schmid, R. (1968) An apparatus for frequency-controlled feeding of small rodents and its use in dental caries experiments. *Archives of Oral Biology*, **13**, 13–26.

Koulourides, T., Phantumvanit, P., Munksgaard, E.C. and Housch, T. (1974) An intraoral model used for studies of fluoride incorporation in enamel. *Journal of Oral Pathology*, **3**, 185–196.

Marsh, P.D. (1994) Microbial ecology of dental plaque and its significance in health and disease. *Advances in Dental Research*, **8(2)**, 263–271.

Munson, M.A., Banerjee, A., Watson, T.F. and Wade, W.G. (2004) Molecular analysis of the microflora associated with dental caries. *Journal of Clinical Microbiology*, **42(7)**, 3023–3029.

Ricketts, D.N., Ekstrand, K.R., Kidd, E.A. and Larsen, T. (2002) Relating visual and radiographic ranked scoring systems for occlusal caries detection to histological and microbiological evidence. *Operative Dentistry*, 27(3), 231–237.

Stephan, R.M. (1940) Changes in hydrogen concentration on tooth surfaces and in carious lesions. *Journal of the American Dental Association*, **27**, 718–723.

van Houte, J., Lopman, J. and Kent, R. (1996) The final pH of bacteria comprising the predominant flora on sound and carious human root and enamel surfaces. *Journal of Dental Research*, **75(4)**, 1008–1014.

Further reading

Banerjee, A. Watson, T.F. (2011) *Pickard's Manual of Operative Dentistry*, 9th edition. Oxford University Press, Oxford.

Beighton, D., Lynch, E. and Heath, M.R. (1993) A microbiological study of primary root-caries lesions with different treatment needs. *Journal of Dental Research*, **72**(3), 623–629.

Bulman, J.S. and Osborn, J.F. (1989) *Statistics in Dentistry*. BDJ Books, London.

Fisher, F.J. (1981) The treatment of carious dentine. *British Dental Journal*, **150**, 159–162.

Kidd, E.A.M. and Joyston-Bechal, S. (2005) *Essentials of Dental Caries: The Disease and its Management*. Oxford University Press, Oxford.

Marsh, P.D. and Martin, M.V. (2005) *Oral Microbiology*, 5th edition. Elsevier Limited, Oxford.

Section 2
Clinical

5

The periodontium, tooth deposits and periodontal diseases

Philip R. Greene and Maggie Jackson

Summary

This chapter covers:

- Periodontal health as the key to maintaining lifelong tooth support
- Dental plaque as the principal cause of inflammatory diseases leading to destruction of tooth-supporting bone
- Cigarette smoking, diabetes and increasing age as the main risk factors in destructive periodontitis
- Effective treatment protocols
- Antibiotics in periodontal therapy
- The control of periodontal diseases in the long term

Introduction

Periodontics is the fundamental dental science. All restorative dentistry relies on healthy periodontal support for its longevity so it is therefore essential that all practitioners of dentistry understand the structure of the periodontal tissues, know how problems develop and are adept at managing periodontal problems.

The normal periodontium

The periodontium (periodontal tissues) hold the teeth in the mouth. The normal periodontium consists of:

- The gingiva.
- Bone.
- Cementum.
- The periodontal ligament.

The appearance of healthy tissue varies between patients, and 'normal' healthy tissue can look quite different in different individuals (Figure 5.1a, b, c).

The gingiva

There are two components to the gingival tissues:

- The attached gingiva.
- The alveolar mucosa.

Attached gingiva

The normal attached gingiva frames the crowns of the teeth on the buccal and lingual aspects and forms a strong protective cuff at the necks of the teeth, keeping food away from the delicate epithelial attachment. Covering the bony attachment to the teeth, it varies in colour, texture and architecture. Most Caucasians have a coral pink gingiva with a light stippling reminiscent of orange peel. This is because the tissue is a true mucoperiosteum and the stippling corresponds to a fibrous attachment of the epithelium to the periosteum. Therefore, the attached gingiva does not move (Figure 5.2).

Gingival tissue is normally 2–3 mm thick and 1–5 mm wide, increasing in width with age. It has a dull surface and a firm consistency. At its coronal aspect the gingiva terminates in the **free gingival margin**, which is scalloped in outline to follow the contour of the teeth. At the apical aspect of the attached gingiva is the **mucogingival junction**, which separates it from the looser, more flexible, alveolar mucosa.

The biologic width

The 'free' gingival margin is free because it is not attached to the tooth on its inner (crevicular) aspect. There is a **gingival crevice**, on the inner aspect of the free gingiva, anything from 1–3 mm deep, usually deeper interproximally than labially or lingually. At the base of the crevice the gingiva is attached to the tooth by means of a 1 mm

---

Clinical Textbook of Dental Hygiene and Therapy, Second Edition. Edited by Suzanne L. Noble.
© 2012 John Wiley & Sons, Ltd. Published 2012 by John Wiley & Sons, Ltd.

(a)

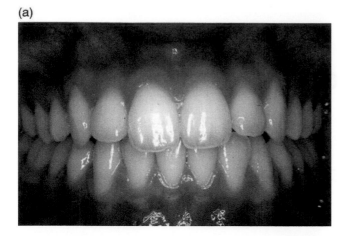

(b)

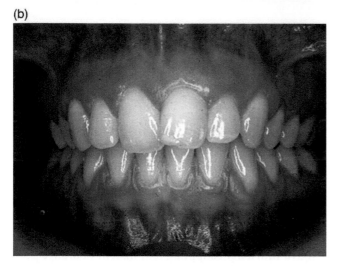

(c)

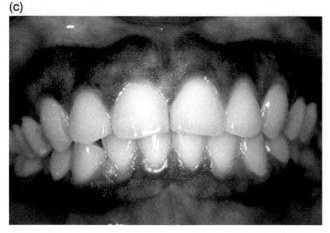

Figure 5.1 (a,b,c) Three very different, but all normal healthy gingival types.

wide layer of epithelial cells attached to the cementum surface in the same way as they are attached to each other. This band is known as **the junctional epithelium**. One millimetre beyond the gingival crevice, the junctional epithelium gives way to a band of connective

tissue, approximately 1mm wide, containing collagen fibres arranged in groups (Figure 5.3).

These three elements, the gingival crevice, junctional epithelium and connective tissue attachment, make up the **biologic width of the gingiva**. It will always re-establish itself after any damage to the gingiva and must not be violated beyond the gingival crevice by restorative dentistry. A restoration margin located beyond the crevice, in the area attached by junctional epithelium or connective tissue, will cause persistent inflammation and this may be both uncomfortable, due to pain and bleeding, and unsightly due to swollen and discoloured tissue. The restorative dentist or therapist, therefore, must respect the biologic width. Errors in tooth preparation can sometimes only be corrected by crown-lengthening surgery.

The gingival papilla

Between the teeth, the attached gingiva forms a triangular papilla on both buccal and lingual aspects. If it could be viewed transversely (i.e. from in between the teeth), the papillae would resemble two peaks and a valley and the contact areas between the teeth determine the shape of the valleys. Between the anterior teeth the papillae have the shape of a pyramid, and between the posterior teeth the papillae are more flattened. The valley between the two peaks of the papillae is known as the **interdental col**.

Microscopically, the attached gingiva has a layer of **keratin** (a tough fibrous insoluble protein) on the surface, covering a layer of connective tissue known as the lamina propria. The basal layer of the epithelium is in contact with the periosteum, which is in direct contact with the underlying bone. The **periosteum** is a richly vascular layer of dense connective tissue, containing osteoblasts in the deeper part and with fibres embedded in the bone surface making it very difficult to separate the periosteum from the bone. The gingiva derives much of its blood supply from the periosteum.

Gingival periodontal fibres

Although the gingival tissue contains randomly arranged collagen fibres everywhere, there are four groups of recognisable fibres closely associated with the attachment of the gingiva to the tooth: Dentogingival fibres, Dentoperiosteal fibres, circular fibres, and trans-septal fibres.

- **Dentogingival fibres** are embedded in the cementum in the connective tissue attachment area, and fan out in a coronal direction towards the free gingival margin.
- **Dentoperiosteal fibres** are embedded in the same area as dentogingival fibres, but turn in an apical direction towards the root of the tooth.

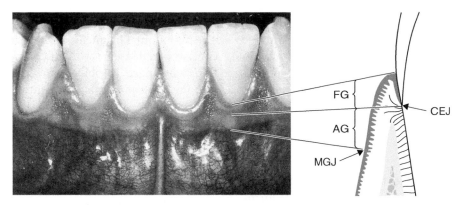

Figure 5.2 Gingival anatomy. (Reproduced with permission from *Clinical Periodontology and Implant Dentistry*, 4th edition (eds J. Lindhe, T. Karring, and N. Lang). Blackwell Munksgaard; p. 6, Figure 1.6.)

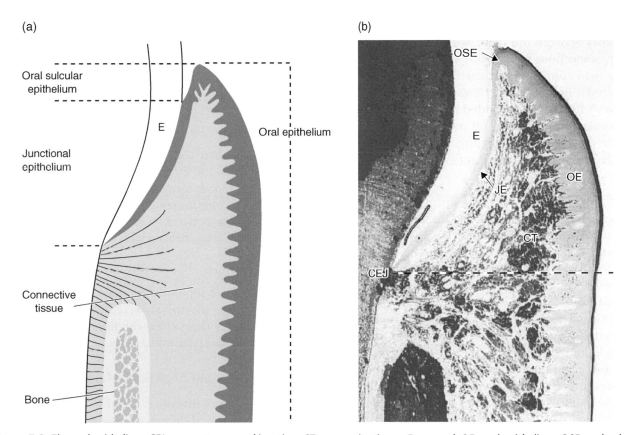

Figure 5.3 The oral epithelium. CEJ, cemento–enamel junction; CT, connective tissue; E, enamel; OE, oral epithelium; OSE, oral sulcular (crevicular) epithelium; JE, junctional epithelium. (Reproduced with permission from Clinical Periodontology and Implant Dentistry, 4th edition (eds J. Lindhe, T. Karring, and N. Lang). Blackwell Munksgaard; p. 8, Figure 1.14a & b.)

- **Circular fibres** encircle the tooth like a ring.
- **Transeptal fibres** are embedded in the cementum of adjacent teeth and run above the bone crest.

These gingival collagen fibres are responsible for the stippling seen in healthy gingival tissue, and for maintaining a tightly attached gingival cuff around the tooth. They are damaged or destroyed in gingivitis and periodontitis, and severed by the raising of a surgical flap. This explains why:

- The gingivae become glazed when the tissues are inflamed, changing the surface to a smooth texture.
- Teeth become looser due to gingivitis and periodontitis, and become tighter after successful treatment as the fibres regrow.
- Teeth become looser when a surgical flap is raised, severing the transeptal and circular fibres, and tighter after surgery when the tissues heal; healing takes approximately 3–4 months.

Alveolar mucosa

Alveolar mucosa is a softer and more flexible tissue than attached gingiva. It has a much thinner keratin layer on the surface and is continuous with the mucosa of the buccal and lingual sulci. It is therefore a darker red than the attached gingivae and has a smooth shiny surface.

Bone

The bone that supports the teeth, the **alveolar bone**, grows with the teeth as they erupt into the mouth forming the alveolus of both maxilla and mandible. The alveolar bone supports the teeth by absorbing and distributing occlusal forces. The wall of each tooth socket is formed from a thin layer of dense compact bone. The areas between the tooth sockets are composed of spongy **cancellous bone**, which contains many more spaces than compact (**cortical**) bone. The ends of the periodontal ligament fibres, which are also known as **Sharpey's fibres**, are embedded into the cementum and the alveolar bone of the socket walls.

Bone is a constantly changing dynamic tissue, always remodelling in response to functional change and needs.

Cementum

The cementum is the calcified surface tissue covering the dentine of the root of the tooth. It has a similar structure to bone, but it has no blood supply, no nerves, does not remodel and is more resistant to resorption than bone. This resistance to resorption is important in orthodontic treatment, allowing the tooth to move by alveolar bone resorption in response to controlled applied pressure, without root resorption. The cementum attaches the periodontal ligament (Sharpey's) fibres to the root of the tooth and contributes to the process of repair after the root surface has been damaged. The cementum protects the underlying dentine and compensates for occlusal attrition by increasing in thickness in the apical area (**cementosis**). Cementum therefore does not remodel in response to functional changes, but instead gradually increases in thickness with age by the deposition of new layers; where this increase is excessive it is known as **hypercementosis**.

Connective tissue

Connective tissue consists of a ground substance containing fibroblasts, macrophages and neutrophils (defence cells) and lymphocytes (active in the immune response process) and fibrous tissue. The fibrous tissue is made up of elastic **elastin** fibres and non-elastic **collagen** fibres.

Periodontal ligament

The periodontal ligament (PDL) surrounds the tooth. It consists of a dense network of collagen fibres (Sharpey's fibres) arranged in oblique rows, inserted at one end into the bone and at the other into the cementum. This is the means by which the tooth is attached to the bone. The fibres are elastic in nature, giving them the ability to extend in response to occlusal loading (biting pressure), and this extension acts as a cushion for the tooth, allowing it to absorb functional forces thus reducing the likelihood of damage to the supporting structures and making chewing more comfortable.

Connective tissue fills the spaces between the fibres, through which run the blood vessels that supply the tooth attachment apparatus with blood, and the small nerve fibres that make the PDL so sensitive. Whereas pain from a dental pulp is poorly localised – the patient usually cannot tell which tooth is hurting – pain from the PDL is very accurately localised. The patient can describe exactly which tooth is the source of pain.

Blood supply

Blood is brought to the gingival tissues by small branches of the superior and inferior dental arteries. The gingiva receives its blood mainly from blood vessels on the surface of the periosteum arising from various facial arteries. A fine network of small vessels traverses the tissue and can often be seen with the naked eye.

Nerve supply

The gingivae are supplied with nerves from the various branches of the trigeminal nerve, the same nerves that supply the teeth themselves with fibres carrying sensory input (sensation) back to the brain.

The classification of periodontal disease

A classification of diseases is useful so that we can make sense of the clinical information we collect and to help us to take a rational approach to planning treatment for our patients. The classification presented here is based on the American Academy of Periodontology (AAP) Classification of 1999. A simplified version of this is described in Table 5.1. It has been simplified for the purposes of this book, however the full classification can be obtained from the AAP website (www.perio.org/).

Chronic gingivitis

The term gingivitis means inflammation of the gingiva. The most common cause is the accumulation of dental bacterial plaque at the gingival margins if not effectively removed by the patient. Unlike periodontitis, gingivitis

Table 5.1 The classification of periodontal disease.

I	Gingival diseases	Plaque induced	Gingival diseases associated with or without other local contributing factors (see VIII)		
			Gingival diseases modified by systemic factors	Associated with blood dyscrasias	Hormonal (puberty, menstrual, pregnancy) Diabetes
				Associated with endocrine system	Leukaemia associated Non-leukaemia associated
			Gingival diseases modified by medications		
			Gingival diseases modified by malnutrition		
		Non-plaque induced	Bacterial origin		
			Viral origin		
			Fungal origin		
			Genetic origin		
			Manifestation of systemic conditions		
			e.g. mucocutaneous disorders, allergic reactions and reactions attributable to toothpastes, mouthrinses, foods and food additives		
			Trauma (chemical, physical or thermal)		
			Foreign body reactions		
			Not otherwise specified		
II	Chronic periodontitis	Localised Generalised			
III	Aggressive periodontitis (affecting adults under 35 with >50% attachment loss)	Localised Generalised			
IV	Periodontitis as a manifestation of systemic disease	Associated with haematological disorders Associated with genetic disorders Not otherwise specified (NOS)			
V	Necrotising periodontal diseases e.g. ANUG				
VI	Abscesses of the periodontium				
VII	Periodontitis associated with endodontic lesions				

results in *reversible* damage to the gingival tissues. The effect of the plaque on the tissue varies between different individuals and may be modified by various factors, as listed in the AAP classification (Table 5.1).

Clinical features

The signs of gingivitis are the same signs as can be found in any other inflammatory condition, and, in particular, erythema (redness), oedema (swelling), and pain or tenderness can be identified by close examination of the gingival tissues. The symptoms are that the patient may notice bleeding, and perhaps some tenderness of the gingivae when brushing, although pain is not normally a clinical feature of gingivitis. Inspection of the gingivae with a good white light may show a red line at the margin with swelling and redness of the papillae initially and later the margins, with a tendency to bleed on gentle probing with a blunt periodontal probe. The probing depth does not exceed 3 mm in gingivitis unless the tissue is so swollen that the gingival tissue is larger than normal. The level of the attachment of the gingivae to the tooth remains unchanged. Plaque can frequently be seen at the gingival margins corresponding to the signs of inflammation. It takes 2–3 days for unnoticed plaque to result in the development of gingivitis. Some patients brush vigorously just before attending for treatment and may have removed the plaque, but signs of the tissue having bled on brushing will then be seen. The examiner should not be deceived when looking closely! (Figure 5.4).

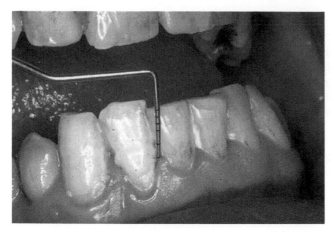

Figure 5.4 Chronic marginal gingivitis in a 72-year-old man; probing depth does not exceed 3 mm.

Chronic periodontitis

Susceptibility

For most patients with gingivitis, the inflammation does not progress beyond the gingival margins; however 10–15% of patients are susceptible to a more destructive process known as **chronic periodontitis**. In the most recent UK Adult Dental Health Survey (1998) it was found that 54% of dentate adults had some periodontal pocketing of 4 mm or more and 5% had deep pocketing (6 mm or more); 43% had some loss of attachment of 4 mm or more and 8% had loss of attachment of 6 mm or more. The prevalence of pocketing and loss of attachment increased with age. For example, the proportion of dentate adults with some loss of attachment increased from 14% among those aged 16–24 years to 85% of those aged 65 and over.

The initiation of periodontitis in an individual is thought to be due to a gene polymorphism, which causes a change in the behaviour of **cytokines**, substances that regulate the movement of immune system defending cells. This behaviour change leads to the destruction of bone and connective tissue, which usually takes place very slowly, and is mostly asymptomatic, so that affected teeth may lose their attachment to the bone over a period of 30–50 years. The genetic element explains why chronic periodontitis frequently affects several members of the same family.

The technology exists to identify the genetic abnormality (which in the future may well turn out to be one of many) that is thought to determine the susceptibility to destructive disease and this knowledge would be very helpful in deciding about the long-term prognosis of the affected teeth and therefore in treatment planning. There is no chair-side test currently available in the UK to assess genetic susceptibility or the presence of periodontal pathogens.

It follows that susceptibility cannot be 'treated'. Once susceptible, the patient will always be so because this characteristic is genetically determined. Treatment of periodontitis is directed towards elimination of the substance to which the patient is susceptible (i.e. the plaque). Susceptible patients, once treated, must therefore be monitored for the rest of their lives to ensure that periodontitis does not become re-established.

General risk factors

Cigarette smoking

The most important known risk factor for periodontitis is cigarette smoking. Smokers have more periodontal problems than non-smokers, and the results of treatment are poorer in smokers. This is thought to be due to:

- A reduction in gingival blood circulation (which results in a reduction in bleeding on both brushing and probing in smokers).
- Impaired white blood cell mobility and function.
- Impaired wound healing.
- An increased production of inflammatory substances (**cytokines**), particularly due to nicotine, which results in an increased production of **collagenase**.

Many studies (Palmer *et al.*, 2005; Preshaw *et al.*, 2005) have shown that treatment outcomes are not as good for smokers as for non-smokers, and recurrence of disease is more likely.

Diabetes

Diabetes increases the risk of periodontal diseases and because the way in which diabetic complications develop is a similar pathological process to periodontitis, it is not surprising that there may be a close relationship between the two diseases. It has even been reported that treatment of periodontitis may improve diabetic control (Grossi *et al.*, 1997). Wound healing is adversely affected by diabetes, especially if poorly controlled, and this can make treatment of diabetic patients more difficult.

Other systemic conditions

Hormonal changes can affect the response of the gingival tissues to plaque and to therapy. **Puberty**, pregnancy, and the **menopause** are all known to cause changes in gingival response. The increase in the severity of gingivitis during **pregnancy** has been attributed to the increased circulating levels of progesterone causing increased permeability of gingival vessels and a consequent increase in bleeding and swelling.

An enlargement of a gingival papilla, known as a **pregnancy epulis**, is frequently seen during pregnancy. These lesions can be up to 2 cm in diameter; removal is best deferred until after parturition if possible although they can be quite large and troublesome. Thorough plaque control is essential and the lesions tend to resolve spontaneously at the end of the pregnancy.

Leukaemias, resulting in altered leukocyte function, are likely to increase the incidence of periodontal disease.

Age

Older patients are more likely to have periodontitis than younger patients due to many years of exposure to plaque and to the various risk factors known to be associated with periodontitis.

Stress

Many clinicians believe that stress is a factor modifying the host response to plaque. The evidence is inconclusive, but it has been suggested that stress can have a direct effect on immune responses to plaque. Equally, stress may exert an influence by way of behavioural change, reducing the thoroughness and therefore the effectiveness of oral hygiene.

Periodontal diseases and general health

There is a growing body of evidence suggesting that there is an association between periodontitis and various systemic conditions, in particular the incidence of premature low birth weight babies and coronary heart disease. Various studies have been published suggesting that there appears to be a benefit in improving the periodontal health of expectant mothers expressed as a reduced incidence of adverse pregnancy outcomes.

The association between periodontitis and cardiovascular disease is thought to be mediated by inflammatory markers, in particular C-reactive protein. Periodontitis is also thought to be associated with raised levels of serum cholesterol and further research is in progress to elucidate this.

Local risk factors

Anything that makes it easier for plaque to accumulate at the gingival margins is a local risk factor for periodontitis. This includes:

- Calculus.
- Enamel pearls (a small, focal excessive mass of enamel on the surface of the tooth. They occur most frequently in the bifurcation or trifurcation of the tooth and are occasionally supported by dentine and very rarely contain pulp tissue).
- Root grooves and concavities.
- Malpositioned teeth (Figure 5.5).
- Overhanging, poorly fitting or contoured restorations.
- Removable partial dentures.

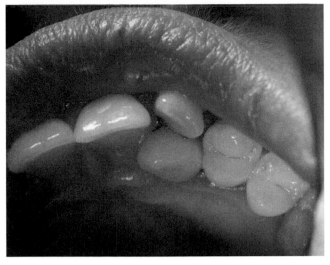

Figure 5.5 Palatally placed upper canine.

- Weak or malpositioned contact areas between the teeth.
- A deep overbite causing direct gingival trauma.

Clinical features

Gingivitis becomes periodontitis when the junctional epithelium is damaged and migrates apically. The clinical result of this is an increase in the depth of the gingival crevice beyond 3 mm. The gingival crevice now has become a **periodontal pocket**, and the implication of this is that the patient can no longer remove the plaque that is located at the base of the pocket, thereby allowing the condition to progress towards the apex of the tooth. Periodontal probing will now show depths deeper than 3 mm and it is well established that the inflammation quickly progresses to involve the connective tissue that is situated between the junctional epithelium and the periodontal ligament (PDL).

The same clinical features seen in gingivitis are also commonly seen in periodontitis i.e. oedematous (swollen), erythematous (red) and discoloured gingival margins and papillae, with bleeding on gentle probing with a blunt periodontal probe. The most important diagnostic information is obtained by the use of the periodontal probe. Inserted into the gingival crevice, aligned with the long axis of the tooth, the probe is moved apically until resistance is felt to gentle probing. In some cases this will be uncomfortable for the patient, and will always cause bleeding if the subgingival tissues are inflamed. There will be no bleeding to gentle probing if the tissues are not inflamed or if the blood supply to the gingivae has been reduced by cigarette smoking, disguising the true condition of the tissues.

Periodontal measurements are recorded on a chart and can then be used to assess the severity of the condition, and to compare measurements taken at previous visits. The progress of the condition can thereby be quantified. Other clinical features that may be observed are:

- Detachment of papillae.
- Swelling of papillae.
- Gingival sinuses.
- Hyperplasia of papillae or gingival margins.
- Exudation of pus on digital pressure or probing.
- Mobility.
- Gingival recession: this may be associated with destructive periodontitis because the gingiva derives much of its blood supply from the underlying periosteum. If bone is destroyed by periodontitis the gingiva will tend to follow the bone crest in an apical direction; the thinner the gingival tissue, the more likely this will be to happen (Figure 5.6).
- Clinical evidence of furcation involvement by means of probing into the inter-radicular space.

Measurement of tooth mobility

Tooth mobility is assessed using two handles of two hand instruments positioned buccally and lingually. The tooth is moved buccolingually with the instruments and the degree of movement recorded (Table 5.2).

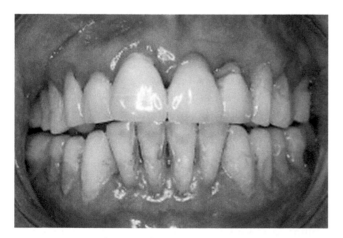

Figure 5.6 Atrophic periodontitis where gingival tissue is thin; pocketing is predominantly shallow.

Table 5.2 Measuring tooth mobility.

Grade	Mobility
1	Horizontal movement of the crown 0.2–1 mm
2	Horizontal movement of the crown >1 mm
3	Horizontal movement of the crown >1 mm and additional movability in a vertical direction

This crude system is very subjective but remains the only method in universal use. Recent research has resulted in the development of an electronic device for measuring tooth mobility, the **Periotest**, which uses an accelerometer to measure the resistance of the tooth to a force applied 16 times over a four second period by a small metal cylinder. This method employs a 60-point numerical scale ranging from −10 (ankylosed teeth or osseointegration e.g. implants) to +50 (extreme mobility) and has the advantage of providing results that are reproducible and comparable with previous readings. Increasing or decreasing trends in mobility of individual teeth can thereby be more accurately assessed (Figure 5.7).

Aggressive periodontitis

Among the relatively small proportion of the population who are susceptible to periodontitis, a small subgroup suffers more rapid bone destruction, so that by the age of approximately 35, they may have lost half of their total tooth attachment; this can be clearly seen on radiographs. This condition is known as aggressive periodontitis and it may affect all the teeth equally, only incisors and molars, or even just a small number of isolated teeth. It is essential to identify this group of patients as early as possible in the progress of the condition, because early treatment can be effective and long lasting, whereas delayed diagnosis can be disastrous for the survival of the teeth (Figure 5.8a and b).

This highly destructive form of periodontitis is characterised by rapid attachment loss with destruction of the periodontal ligament and supporting bone in an otherwise healthy young adult usually below the age of 35, but older patients may be affected. There is

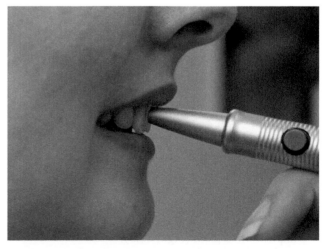

Figure 5.7 The Periotest, for assessment of tooth mobility using an accelerometer.

(a)

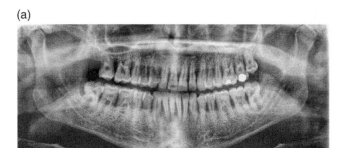

(b)

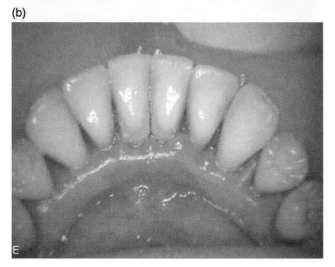

Figure 5.8 (a and b) Aggressive periodontitis in a man aged 22.

often a familial tendency (other members of the family have been affected) and this condition is thought to be associated with high levels of specific bacteria, notably *Aggregatibacter actinomycetemcomitans* and *Porphyromonas gingivalis*. There is some evidence of altered leucocyte function and also increased production of some immune system mediators.

Clinical features

Aggressive periodontitis, formerly known as **early onset periodontitis**, frequently presents with a lack of overt gingival inflammation, relatively good oral hygiene and low levels of visible plaque, which is inconsistent with the aggressive nature of the disease, and the diagnosis can therefore easily be missed. Clear signs of supporting bone loss are to be found on radiographs, however, and these should therefore be scrutinised in all cases. Vigilance is required on the part of the dentist, therapist and hygienist to ensure that aggressive cases are diagnosed as early as possible.

Aggressive periodontitis is rarely seen affecting children below the age of puberty. When it does occur at this age it is known as **prepubertal periodontitis**.

Localised and generalised forms of aggressive periodontitis are recognised corresponding to the older terms **rapidly progressive periodontitis** and **localised juvenile periodontitis. Localised aggressive periodontitis** (LAP) involves the incisors and molars, with onset around or soon after puberty, and is characterised by interproximal attachment loss on at least two permanent teeth, one of which is a first molar, and involving no more that two teeth other than first molars and incisors.

Generalised aggressive periodontitis (GAP) usually has a later onset, before the age of 30, and is characterised by generalised attachment loss involving at least three permanent teeth other than first molars and incisors. There is a more episodic nature to the progress of GAP.

Most studies put the prevalence of aggressive periodontitis among 13–20-year-olds at well below 1%; however, this still represents a large number of people who may be affected and the disease is so destructive that early detection, by means of periodontal screening for all teenagers, is essential in the protection of those individuals who may develop this condition.

Vigorous treatment, including mechanical plaque removal and systemic antibiotics, can be just as successful in controlling these conditions, as it is in controlling the more common forms of periodontitis

Histopathology of periodontal diseases

Five histopathological states are recognised in the gingiva (Lindhe *et al.*, 2003) namely:

- **Pristine gingiva** (only really found in experimental animals) has an intact layer of epithelium lining the gingival crevice, and no inflammatory cells in the connective tissue. There is a continuous sparse migration of neutrophil leucocytes into the coronal part of the junctional epithelium and gingival crevice.
- **Normal healthy gingiva** has a small number of inflammatory cells in the junctional epithelium and connective tissue. Even though gingivitis at this stage is not clinically detectable, inflammatory changes can be found microscopically.
- **Early gingivitis** is seen after 10–20 days of plaque accumulation. There are an increased number of inflammatory cells in the tissue and an increase in the number of neutrophils emigrating into the gingival crevice. The junctional epithelium becomes thicker. The gingival connective tissue becomes more heavily infiltrated with inflammatory cells and dilated blood vessels.
- **Established gingivitis** has a more dense infiltration of inflammatory cells in the connective tissue, with plasma cells becoming much more evident (10–30%). Collagen loss increases due to an outpouring of the

enzyme collagenase and the epithelium lining the gingival crevice continues to increase in thickness.

- **Periodontitis** is characterised by the apical migration of the junctional epithelium – the first stage of attachment loss. The same dense infiltration of inflammatory cells can be seen with plasma cells now dominant, (>50%). Bone loss now begins to occur.

Gingival recession

Gingival recession, which is a lack of complete coverage of the tooth root exposing the root surface, is very common, and is a cause of concern to many patients. The main causes are:

- Disproportion in sizes of teeth and alveolar bone – the tooth is too wide for the supporting alveolar bone; this situation may be exacerbated by abrasion from a toothbrush, especially if the patient is using an over-aggressive technique.
- Attachment loss due to chronic periodontitis.

Recession is often associated with a lack of keratinised mucosa and a highly placed muscle attachment is often found aggravating the situation. This can cause discomfort, and may lead to difficulty in maintaining plaque control, which results in inflammation, infection and a deterioration of the situation in relation to the tooth involved. Mostly, however, gingival health can be maintained in spite of recession, and with little or no attached gingiva. Where there is an adequate zone of keratinised mucosa associated with the defect, the problem is usually self-limiting and stops when the gingiva reaches a level at which it is in harmony with the underlying bone.

Recession may also cause aesthetic problems if it affects the anterior teeth, and may also result in sensitivity of the root surface to hot, cold or acidic foods and fluids. Where the patient experiences such problems, there are several predictable surgical techniques available to alleviate symptoms and sometimes achieve coverage of denuded root surfaces (Figure 5.9a and b).

Acute periodontal conditions

Necrotising periodontal diseases

The incidence of these conditions has declined in the UK over the last 30 years except for human immuno-deficiency virus (HIV)-positive patients. There are three types of necrotising periodontal diseases (NPD) defined according to the extent of tissue destruction:

- **Necrotising gingivitis**, which is confined to the gingivae.
- **Necrotising periodontitis**, where there is attachment loss.

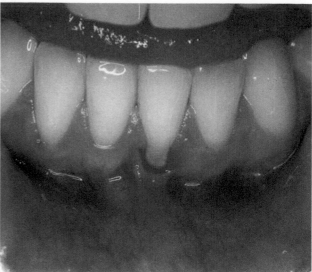

(a)

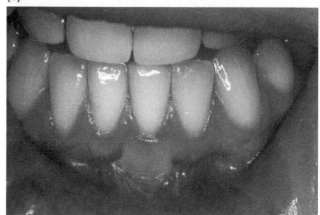

(b)

Figure 5.9 (a and b) Gingival recession corrected with a free gingival graft.

- **Necrotising stomatitis**, where the surrounding tissues are involved.

The predisposing factors are:

- Poor oral hygiene; associated with all the necrotising diseases.
- Cigarette smoking; commonly seen in all NPDs.
- Raised stress levels, e.g. students at exam time or soldiers in action.
- Malnutrition; associated with poor protein intake in developing countries.
- Fatigue.
- Immune dysfunction or suppression of the immune system.
- Pre-existing gingivitis.
- Systemic conditions such as leukaemia or HIV.

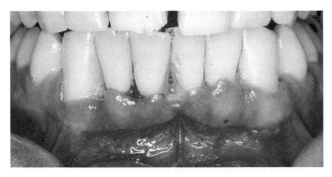

Figure 5.10 NUG. Note the loss of papillae and the grey pseudomembrane. (Reproduced with permission from *Clinical Periodontology and Implant Dentistry*, 4th edition (eds J. Lindhe, T. Karring, and N. Lang). Blackwell Munksgaard; p. 245, Figure 10.3.)

Clinical features

There is a visible change in gingival contour accompanied by bleeding, pain, and the loss of the apex of the papilla producing a punched out appearance. A grey slough, known as a **pseudomembrane** is frequently seen on the surface and there is tissue necrosis that causes an unpleasant but typically unforgettable odour (Figure 5.10). Patients may present with swollen lymph nodes (lymphadenopathy) or more rarely pyrexia. Destruction of tissue may progress to necrosis of the periodontal ligament and bone, which may be rapid and extend to the interproximal or facial bone, forming a fragment of dead bone known as a **sequestrum**.

Histopathology

Ulceration of the epithelium can be seen under the microscope, with necrosis (tissue death) and many inflammatory cells. Infecting organisms (spirochetes and fusiform bacilli) can be found in the tissues (not just on the surface) and in the necrotic slough.

Treatment of necrotising diseases

The most important therapeutic measure is **debridement**, (i.e. the removal of the soft and hard plaque, slough and calculus deposits), as soon as possible. This should be accomplished, or at least started, at the first visit as soon as the diagnosis has been made. The use of ultrasonic scalers makes this process much quicker, gentler and therefore more tolerable for the patient.

Hydrogen peroxide as a mouth rinse or applied directly to the ulcerated tissue is beneficial due to its mechanical cleansing properties and its ability to release oxygen into the area, damaging the environment for the predominantly anaerobic infecting organisms.

Chlorhexidine mouth rinse (0.2%) is an effective way of reducing plaque growth; it can be very helpful because the patient may not be able to brush thoroughly due to the pain of the infection.

Systemic antibiotics may be required if the patient shows signs of being generally ill, with fever, lassitude or severe lymph gland involvement. Metronidazole (200 mg, three times daily for 3–5 days) has been found to be very useful in NPD as well as penicillin and tetracyclines. Topical antibiotics have no place in the treatment of NPD because of the presence of bacteria within the tissues where there is no penetration of the antibiotic.

Patients with NPD should be seen frequently, perhaps daily, until the acute phase is over. Thereafter, completion of debridement and maintenance treatment as required should be arranged. In view of the association between NPD and other systemic conditions, consideration should be given to advising the patient's medical practitioner so that further investigations can be considered.

Acute herpetic gingivostomatitis

Patients with this condition can present with pyrexia, lymph gland involvement, flu-like symptoms, stomatitis, oral ulceration, gingivitis and pain. The causative organism is the herpes simplex virus. The condition, which has an incubation period of about 7 days, is highly contagious and is spread from the oral lesions. Treatment is by maintaining adequate fluid intake and by the use of antipyretics and topical antiseptics. Antiviral drugs such as **Aciclovir** are not normally prescribed except when the patient is immunocompromised. Subsequent reactivation of the virus can occur (e.g. following trauma or exposure to sunlight) when it manifests itself as **cold sores** (herpes labialis).

Abscesses of the periodontium

Abscesses of the periodontium are classified into three types:

- **Gingival abscess**: usually caused by trauma from a foreign body.
- **Periodontal abscess**: usually arising from an established periodontal pocket (Figure 5.11).
- **Pericoronal abscess**: usually related to an operculum (flap of gum) overlying a partially erupted third molar.

It is important to distinguish between periodontal and periapical abscesses and this may be difficult if both conditions are present at the same time. Sometimes the periodontal and periapical diseases meet half way along the root and coalesce, to form a combined lesion (Figure 5.12). All these abscesses can be acute (active, painful and destructive) or chronic (painless and slowly progressing). The difference may be due to occlusion

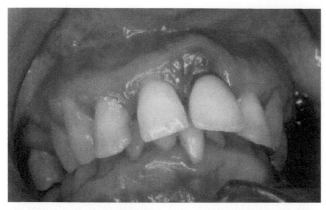

Figure 5.11 Periodontal abscess arising from a central incisor.

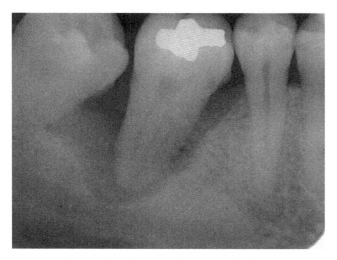

Figure 5.12 A combined endoperio communication lesion.

of the pocket entrance. If a chronic abscess cannot drain, the pressure increases in the pocket and an acute infection results. This may follow incomplete scaling and it is therefore very important to debride any pocket entered *completely* to avoid an embarrassing return by the patient for emergency treatment a day or two after scaling.

Microbiology

The bacteria in a periodontal abscess are the same as are found in a chronic periodontal pocket. The precise mechanism by which they become active and virulent enough to become an acute abscess is not yet known.

Aetiology

Trauma, the presence of a foreign body or the arrival of new, more virulent bacteria can all initiate the change from chronic periodontitis to an acute abscess. Incomplete scaling with the retention of calculus is another frequent cause of acute abscesses.

Treatment

Correct diagnosis is all-important. Once an abscess has been declared periodontal rather than periapical, treatment follows the same principles as for NPD. In the early stages, debridement is the best and quickest way to resolve the infection. Antibiotics are indicated if the patient has facial swelling, is medically compromised, or is showing signs of systemic illness. Follow-up is essential after the acute phase to consider long-term management and prevention of recurrence.

Microbiological aspects of periodontal disease

It has been observed that the human body is made up of more than one hundred billion cells, of which only 10% are mammalian! The rest are microorganisms or resident flora, of which 80% are indigenous (normal flora), and 10% are transient. This means that there are very many microorganisms present in the human body and the mouth is a moist, warm environment, with plentiful nutrients and an ideal environment for bacterial growth.

The development of dental plaque

The oral bacterial flora attaches itself to tooth surfaces in an organised and recognisable way. A film of glycoproteins known as the **tooth pellicle** covers the tooth surface within minutes of being cleaned. It is colonised by a layer of so-called pioneer species, forming first a thin layer, and later palisades (piles) of cells perpendicular to the tooth surface. By 24 hours a wide variety of bacteria (mainly Gram-positive facultative streptococci) can be identified and more new bacteria join the plaque over the next 24–36 hours until a fully mature plaque – known as a **climax community** has developed.

Further investigation has identified specific microorganisms that are associated with periodontal health and disease states. Socransky *et al.* (1988) have grouped them into colour complexes (Figure 5.13).

The red (particularly) and orange complexes of bacteria are thought to be the most influential in causing periodontitis. Complexes to the left of the diagram, green and yellow especially are thought to be compatible with gingival health.

The composition of plaque is influenced by diet. A high-protein diet produces a more alkaline plaque, associated with an increase in gram-negative organisms and the presence of peptides, which may have an offensive odour. A high carbohydrate diet will tend to be associated with a more acidic plaque favouring a reduction in Gram-negative organisms.

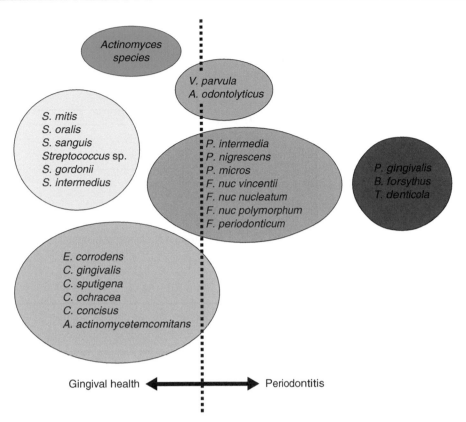

Figure 5.13 Bacterial complexes in dental plaque.

The bacteria, suspended in a matrix of water and various other substances, stick to the tooth surface to form a **biofilm**. This increases in thickness primarily due to bacterial cell division. The matrix fluids provide nutrients for the bacteria and enable the plaque to resist toxic substances, and this is why antibiotics have difficulty penetrating the biofilm to kill the organisms. In order for periodontal therapy to be successful, the plaque biofilm must be mechanically disrupted. Some form of root surface instrumentation is essential.

Calculus

Calculus is a hard deposit of calcium salts found on the surface of the teeth. Initially this consists of octocalcium phosphate (**brushite**) but after about 6 months this matures to **hydroxyapatite**. It tends to form more rapidly close to the parotid (buccal to the upper first and second molars) and sublingual salivary ducts (lingual to the lower anterior teeth) where saliva enters the mouth. Two main types of calculus are recognised based on its location.

- **Supragingival calculus** forms at and above the gingival margin. It is usually yellow in colour and clearly visible.
- **Subgingival calculus** forms below the gingival margin and is therefore invisible on superficial examination. It is frequently dark brown or green in colour due to the inclusion of haem, a blood breakdown product.

A highly alkaline saliva favours the production of calculus and when saliva flow rates are high, a high proportion of bicarbonate is found, raising the pH. It forms more readily within plaque and is often thought of as **mineralised plaque**.

Calculus is a local environmental factor for periodontal disease because:

- It has a rough surface always covered with pathogenic bacteria.
- It increases plaque retention.
- The contour changes produce overhangs and increase plaque retention.
- It is almost impossible to control periodontal disease in the presence of calculus.

Principles of periodontal examination

Every dental examination should include a periodontal examination because it is fundamental to the assessment and attainment of dental health. Six steps are required:

Step 1 – Get to know your patient

The Pankey Philosophy (www.pankey.org) of dental treatment includes the sensible axiom: *never treat a stranger*. The more we know about the patient, the more effective our therapy can be. The first step therefore includes asking open-ended questions, and most importantly *listening* to the answers (see Chapter 6).

If the patient does not volunteer the information, specific questions should be asked to identify the signs and symptoms of periodontal disease. In particular:

- Gingival bleeding on brushing, flossing, nocturnally or at any other time.
- Tooth mobility.
- Bad taste and halitosis.
- Pain, swelling or changes in shape of the gums.
- Difficulty in chewing effectively and comfortably.
- Smoking habits and history.

The use of simple language that is easily understood by the patient is much more effective than the use of jargon or technical terms.

Step 2 – External examination of the patient

Unusual external facial features should be recorded and also signs of disease or asymmetry. The height of the upper lip when smiling should also be noted as this may be an important factor in restorative treatment planning.

Next the submandibular and cervical **lymph glands**, located under the body and ramus of the mandible, and in front and behind the sternocleidomastoid muscle in the neck on each side should be palpated. This may give an early warning of inflammatory or other diseases in the head and neck area.

Step 3 – Examination of the mouth

Accurate periodontal probing is the essential step to avoid periodontal disaster.

Gingival recession is measured first because it is non-invasive, totally painless and allows the patient to relax, making later subgingival probing more acceptable.

The **probing depth** at any site dictates the patient's ability to maintain optimal plaque control. Probing depths in excess of 3 mm are considered to be too deep for plaque control with toothbrushes and floss. These sites should be considered for active periodontal therapy.

The periodontal probe provides the answer to two key questions:

- **Where is the base of the gingival crevice?** How far is it below the gingival margin and how far from the amelocemental junction? This is a measure of periodontal attachment loss, but it must be remembered that the recession is added to the probing depth to give the clinical attachment level. This is always the parameter used for long-term monitoring (Figure 5.14).

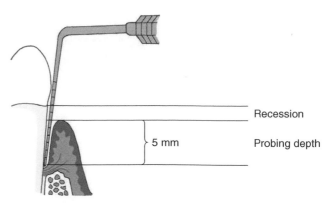

Recession + probing depth = clinical attachment level

Figure 5.14 Clinical attachment.

Table 5.3 The basic periodontal examination (BPE).

UR8–4	UR3–UL3	UL4–8
LR8–4	LR3–LL3	LL4–8

- **Does the tissue bleed when touched?** This is a measure of inflammation, not necessarily active tissue destruction. No bleeding on probing usually means no inflammation. Therefore, no inflammation means no breakdown of support at the time of examination. This is the only safe endpoint for periodontal therapy. Clinicians must remember, however, that in smokers the gingival circulation is impaired and this often results in reduced bleeding on probing, even in active periodontal pockets.

Four different types of probe are in common use:

The Basic Periodontal Examination (BPE) probe should be is used to screen every new and recall patient for periodontal diseases and enables the clinician to identify patients who have suffered some degree of attachment loss. The probe markings are at 3.5 and 5.5 mm.

For a BPE Examination the mouth is divided into six sextants as shown in Table 5.3.

Probing depth measurements are made from the free gingival margin to the base of the pocket. A score is given for the worst affected site in each sextant based on the criteria set out in Table 5.4.

The **standard 10 mm Williams Probe** is necessary for detailed data collection required to monitor the progress of specific sites. The probe is inserted into the gingival crevice with minimal force aligned with the long axis of the tooth, until the base of the crevice is felt and the depth at that point is measured and recorded, preferably by the dental nurse or by direct entry into a computer program. It should be remembered however that a probe would tend to penetrate further in inflamed tissue than in healthy tissue when using the same probing force;

Table 5.4 Bpe Scoring.

Code	Signs	Treatment
Code 0	Probing depth 0–3 mm No bleeding on probing No calculus or root roughness	Oral hygiene reinforcement
Code 1	Probing depth 0–3 mm Bleeding on probing No calculus or root roughness	Oral hygiene instruction
Code 2	Probing depth 0–3 mm Bleeding on probing Calculus or root roughness	Oral Hygiene instruction – Removal of plaque retentive factors including all sub and supragingival calculus
Code 3	Probing depth 3.5–5.5 mm Bleeding on probing Calculus or root roughness	Oral Hygiene instruction – root surface debridement, followed by detailed reassessment in affected sextants
Code 4	Probing depth >5.5 mm Bleeding on probing Calculus or root roughness	Oral Hygiene instruction – root surface debridement, assess the need for more complex treatment, referral to a specialist may be indicated
Code*	Furcation involvement	Oral Hygiene instruction – root surface debridement, assess the need for more complex treatment, referral to a specialist may be indicated

(a)

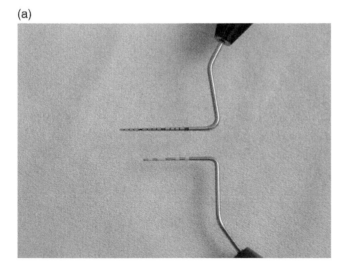

(b)

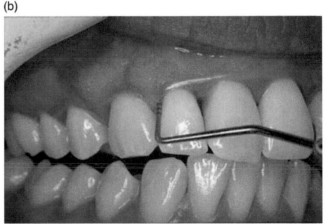

Figure 5.15 (a and b) Williams and Extended Williams periodontal probes; the probe is aligned with the long axis of the tooth.

this can influence the interpretation of results when the inflammation has been resolved. Various periodontal data charts are available for manual data entry.

The **15 mm Extended Williams Probe** is essential for difficult-to-reach areas on the lingual aspect of lower molars, and where there is recession in addition to deep pocketing (Figure 5.15a and b).

The **Nabers Furcation Probe** is very useful in assessing the prognosis of molars. It is a large curved instrument that can be easily manipulated into furcation areas (Figure 5.16).

Finally, **tooth mobility** is recorded (Table 5.2).

Step 4 – Record your findings

Periodontal data should be recorded on a pre-printed chart, computer, official General Dental Services (GDS) periodontal chart, or modified dental record card. The minimum standard (based on the British Society of Periodontology (BSP) parameters of care document www.bsperio.org.uk) includes:

- Probing depths.
- Gingival recession.
- Bleeding on probing.
- Mobility.

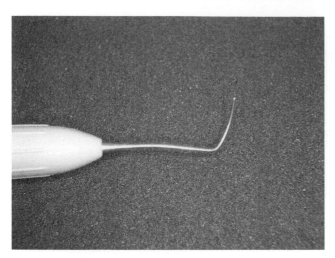

Figure 5.16 Nabers furcation probe.

The **plaque index** is optional in daily general dental practice, because bleeding on probing indicates the location of the plaque. This written record guides periodontal therapy for the affected sites, allows monitoring of treatment and shows the patient how well they have done. It could also be used to resist a patient's complaint of inadequate diagnosis and treatment. It is advisable to also note in the patient's clinical records the fact that the problem was fully explained to the patient and that, where the patient has declined all or part of the recommended treatment, appropriate treatment or referral for specialist advice was offered.

Periodontal indices

It is sometimes useful to express the patient's condition in numerical terms as a means of monitoring progress over a period of time. An expression such as this is known as an Index. A simple periodontal index would be the **bleeding index**, which is computed as follows:

1 Probe six sites on each tooth (i.e. mesial, mid and distal on both buccal and lingual surfaces).
2 Multiply the number of teeth by 6.
3 Score bleeding as present or absent.
4 Count the number of sites where bleeding is present.
5 Divide the number of sites where bleeding is present by the total number of sites in the mouth and multiply by 100 to express the bleeding index as a percentage.

Figures 5.17(a and b) show how this is recorded in a clinical situation.

The same method can be used for developing a plaque index, however a more sophisticated plaque index is that devised by Silness and Loe (1964), which is more qualitative in that absence of plaque deposits is scored as 0, plaque disclosed by running the probe around the gingival margin is scored as 1, visible plaque as 2, and abundant plaque as 3. The index is calculated by scoring the plaque present on mesial, distal, buccal and lingual surfaces on each of six teeth usually the upper right first molar and lateral incisor and left first premolar, and the lower left first molar and lateral incisor and the right first premolar. This gives a representative sample of the mouth without having to score every tooth (in WHO notation: 16, 12, 24, 36, 32, 44). The average scores for each tooth are added together and divided by 6 to give an average for the mouth. This is the plaque index. In clinical practice bleeding on probing, as an indicator of inflammation is the most useful and practical method of assessing changes that are relevant to the patient's periodontal prognosis.

Step 5 – Radiographs

Diagnostic radiographs enable the clinician to visualise the dental hard tissues, i.e. the teeth, jaws and related structures. A great deal of information relevant to the periodontal health of the patient can be derived from well-angulated, exposed and developed radiographs, in particular:

- The anatomy, shape and position of the teeth.
- The presence of related anatomical structures, pathology (such as granulomas. cysts and tumours) and foreign bodies.
- Interdental contacts and relationships.
- Root surface deposits.
- Root resorption.
- Root fractures.
- Interproximal caries.
- Deficient and overhanging restoration margins.
- Patterns of bone loss related to periodontally involved teeth, including furcation involvements.
- The relationships of the teeth to the maxilla and mandible, and an overview of the occlusion.

The **oral pantomograph** (OPG) panoramic radiograph gives a good overview and shows the position of major anatomical structures such as the inferior alveolar canal and maxillary sinuses. The distorted image produced by panoramic radiographs, however, compromises accuracy and intraoral views are required for a more detailed diagnosis and appropriate treatment planning. **Bitewings**, vertical or horizontal, are very useful in giving undistorted views of interdental areas, and **periapical** views are needed to show the entire teeth. Long-cone paralleling techniques are advisable to ensure a true representation on the film, and to allow more accurate comparisons to be made between radiographs taken at different times.

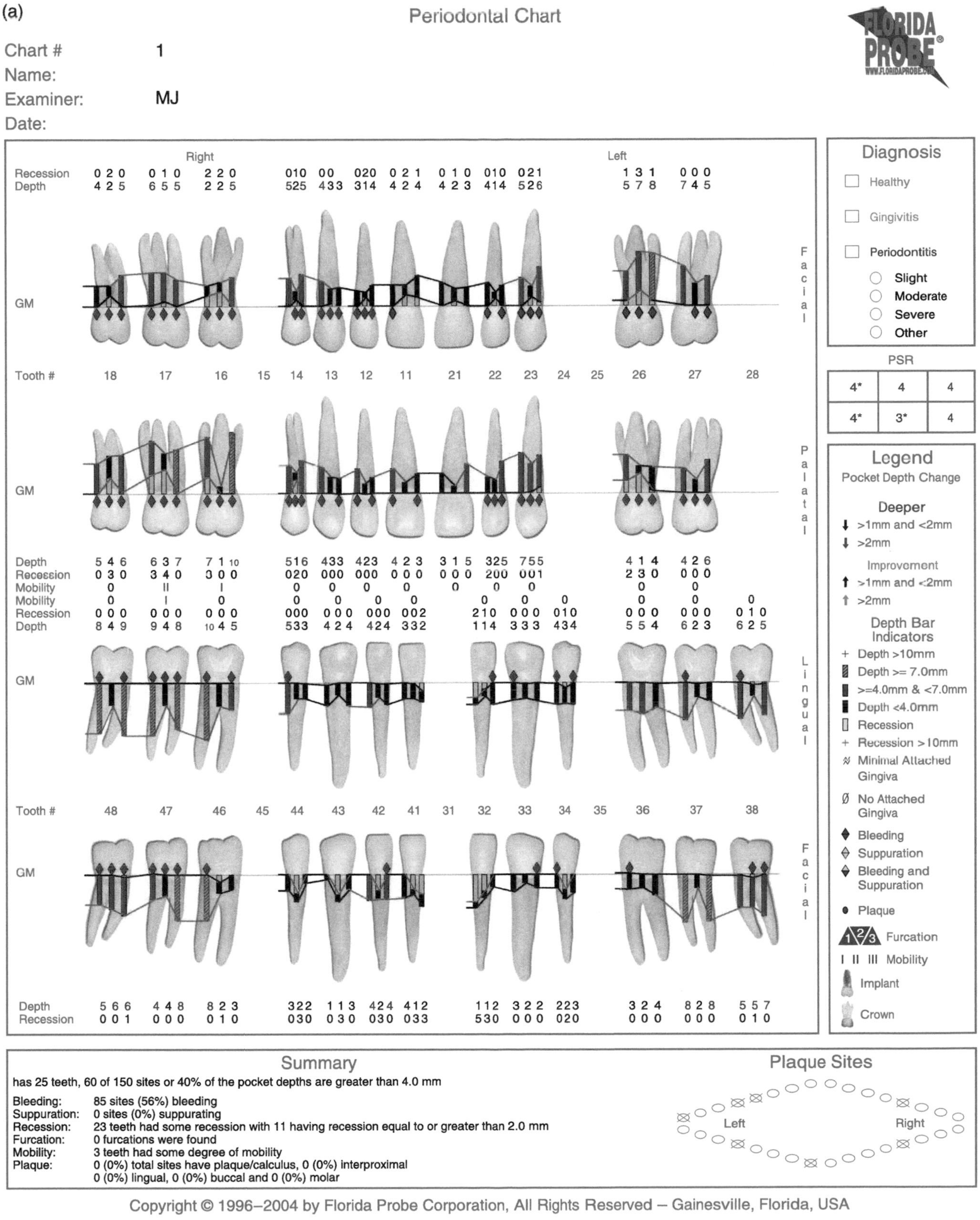

(a)

Periodontal Chart

FLORIDA PROBE®
WWW.FLORIDAPROBE.COM

Chart #   1
Name:
Examiner: MJ
Date:

	Right												Left	
Recession	0 2 0	0 1 0	2 2 0	010	00	020	0 2 1	0 1 0	010	021	1 3 1	0 0 0		
Depth	4 2 5	6 5 5	2 2 5	525	433	314	4 2 4	4 2 3	414	526	5 7 8	7 4 5		

Diagnosis

☐ Healthy

☐ Gingivitis

☐ Periodontitis
  ○ Slight
  ○ Moderate
  ○ Severe
  ○ Other

Facial

GM

| Tooth # | 18 | 17 | 16 | 15 | 14 | 13 | 12 | 11 | 21 | 22 | 23 | 24 | 25 | 26 | 27 | 28 |

PSR

4*	4	4
4*	3*	4

Palatal

GM

Depth	5 4 6	6 3 7	7 1 10	516	433	423	4 2 3	3 1 5	325	755	4 1 4	4 2 6		
Recession	0 3 0	3 4 0	3 0 0	020	000	000	0 0 0	0 0 0	200	001	2 3 0	0 0 0		
Mobility	0	II	I	0	0	0	0	0	0	0	0	0		
Mobility	0	I	I	0	0	0	0	0	0	0	0	0	0
Recession	0 0 0	0 0 0	0 0 0	000	000	000	002	210	000	010	0 0 0	0 0 0	0 1 0
Depth	8 4 9	9 4 8	10 4 5	533	4 2 4	4 2 4	332	114	3 3 3	434	5 5 4	6 2 3	6 2 5

Legend
Pocket Depth Change

Deeper
↓ >1mm and <2mm
↓ >2mm

Improvement
↑ >1mm and <2mm
↑ >2mm

Depth Bar Indicators
+ Depth >10mm
▨ Depth >= 7.0mm
▩ >=4.0mm & <7.0mm
▮ Depth <4.0mm
▢ Recession
+ Recession >10mm
⋈ Minimal Attached Gingiva

Ø No Attached Gingiva

♦ Bleeding
♦ Suppuration
♦ Bleeding and Suppuration

● Plaque

▲1 2 3 Furcation

I II III Mobility

Implant

Crown

Lingual

GM

| Tooth # | 48 | 47 | 46 | 45 | 44 | 43 | 42 | 41 | 31 | 32 | 33 | 34 | 35 | 36 | 37 | 38 |

Facial

GM

| Depth | 5 6 6 | 4 4 8 | 8 2 3 | 322 | 1 1 3 | 424 | 412 | 112 | 3 2 2 | 223 | 3 2 4 | 8 2 8 | 5 5 7 |
| Recession | 0 0 1 | 0 0 0 | 0 1 0 | 030 | 0 3 0 | 030 | 033 | 530 | 0 0 0 | 020 | 0 0 0 | 0 0 0 | 0 1 0 |

Summary

has 25 teeth, 60 of 150 sites or 40% of the pocket depths are greater than 4.0 mm

Bleeding: 85 sites (56%) bleeding
Suppuration: 0 sites (0%) suppurating
Recession: 23 teeth had some recession with 11 having recession equal to or greater than 2.0 mm
Furcation: 0 furcations were found
Mobility: 3 teeth had some degree of mobility
Plaque: 0 (0%) total sites have plaque/calculus, 0 (0%) interproximal
               0 (0%) lingual, 0 (0%) buccal and 0 (0%) molar

Plaque Sites

Left   Right

Figure 5.17 Recording of periodontal indices (a) Initial condition, (b) at re-evaluation.

(b)

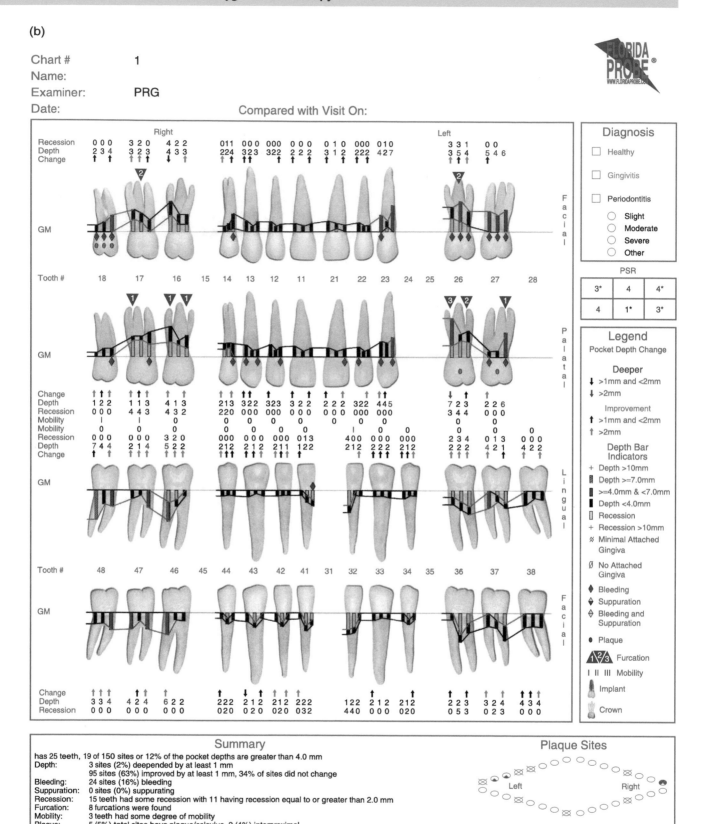

Chart #   1
Name:
Examiner: PRG
Date: Compared with Visit On:

Figure 5.17 (*Continued*)

Digital radiography

Modern digital radiographic techniques allow almost instantaneous viewing of radiographic images which can be enlarged, enhanced, included in correspondence, and transmitted around the world to enable interaction and co-operation between clinicians without the inconvenience, time delay and health hazards associated with chemical development. Digital radiography also eliminates the potential for processing errors, which can render the radiograph of limited or no diagnostic value. Because the radiograph can be viewed almost instantaneously, it provides the operator with the opportunity to retake an unsatisfactory film at the same patient visit thereby avoiding the temptation with conventional radiography to diagnose from a film of limited diagnostic value in order to avoid recalling the patient.

Step 6 – Explain your findings and recommendations

Every time a patient attends a dental practice it provides a window of opportunity for the dental professional to tell them something that will help to improve their dental health. It is important to use the right approach and appropriate language, which can be the key to unlocking the patient's co-operation and inducing a change in their behaviour. It is worth taking the time to explain the problem to the patient, in words they can understand (i.e. **speak their language** – see Chapter 6). The patient will not be impressed by a discussion about pocket depth reduction, bleeding indices or even more frighteningly 'bone-loss'. They are interested in issues that they understand and are important to them, such as absence of blood on the pillow on waking, no bad taste, sweeter breath, a stronger bite, keeping their teeth and not having to wear dentures. The questioning and listening process at the first meeting with the patient is designed to reveal what worries and motivates each particular person. If you can give them something personal to take home that reinforces your dental health message, such as a booklet or the diagram you may have drawn to help explain the problem, so much the better.

Treatment of chronic periodontitis

Treatment of all forms of periodontitis follows the basic principle of plaque control, which can be summarised as follows:

- A diagnosis is reached on the basis of clinical and radiographic examination identifying the type of periodontitis observed. Whilst dental hygienists and therapists may undertake the radiographs under the prescription of a dentist, it is the dentist's responsibility to write up the radiographic report.

- The patient is taught how to remove the accessible plaque deposits.
- The hygienist or therapist must remove plaque that is inaccessible to the patient and also must remove calculus.
- Where access for the therapist is not possible via the gingival margin, surgery may be required to provide access to the inaccessible areas.
- Antibiotics may be required *as an adjunct to mechanical therapy* (never alone) in order to eliminate tissue-invading bacteria in aggressive or resistant forms of periodontitis or in cases where there are recurrent or chronic abscesses likely to become acute if disturbed.
- The patient's condition should be re-evaluated after initial plaque control therapy.

Principles of plaque control therapy

The patient must remove deposits of plaque that are accessible to their oral hygiene equipment. The therapist is therefore responsible for the removal of all deposits of plaque that the patient has been unable to remove and calculus located supra and subgingivally beyond the reach of the patient.

Plaque removal by the patient

It has been said that there is nothing the clinician can do that will compensate for what the patient will *not* do. The clinician must rely on the patient to remove plaque thoroughly every day, and it is the clinician's responsibility, therefore, to ensure that the patient is sufficiently well motivated, educated and equipped for this task.

Motivation

Persuasion is getting the patient to do what **you** want him or her to do. Motivation is getting the patient to do what *he or she* wants to do. In order to achieve this, the therapist needs to take the patient through a five-step process.

1. The patient must understand that they have a **problem**.
2. The problem has potentially serious **effects** for the patient.
3. There is a **solution** to the problem
4. The patient must **participate** in the solution
5. Treatment will bring far-reaching **benefits** for the patient.

The problem and solution should be explained to the patient using simple language, avoiding technical terms and dental jargon. Drawing a personalised diagram may be helpful, especially for patients who like to receive information visually. A face mirror is an essential aid in demonstrating the problems (e.g. periodontal pockets, bleeding on probing, and loose teeth), to the patient.

Basic communication skills is covered in Chapter 6; however it is of considerable additional benefit to have a basic understanding of different personality types and learning styles so that the therapist can then tailor the language used to suit each individual patient.

Personality types

Personality typing began in ancient Greece; Hippocrates outlined four temperaments and, later the psychologist Carl Jung described four personality types, which have been developed with many different terms, and are used in many business and educational training programmes.

The four types are described as follows:

The ruler

Rulers are leaders, with management or officer positions. They frequently occupy positions of responsibility in business and industry. They are business-like and prefer to be in control. They are goal or task-oriented and their time is valuable. They are not particularly interested in detail or in relationships; the bottom line is all-important. Rulers make decisions quickly and confidently. They can be recognised by their confident walk and dress style, their strength of voice and their clear desire to make a decision and then see it through to a conclusion.

It is important to see these patients on time if possible, and to address the main issues quickly, stressing the benefits of treatment. Offer them options to choose from (allowing them control) and explain the pros and cons of the alternatives that are available to them.

The amiable

Amiables are pleasant, caring and people-orientated, making them likely to seek occupations such as nursing, teaching, and other caring professions. Making friends and maintaining relationships are important to them and they characteristically avoid conflict, preferring to walk away rather than cause trouble. They therefore make good team players and often soothe the anger of those around them. They make decisions slowly and prefer not to be rushed. They can be recognised by their gait and gentle voice, and as with all types, their language often betrays their personality style. They tend to make decisions slowly and thoughtfully and therefore tend to require more time.

When treating amiables, it is helpful to match your tone of voice and posture to theirs, to build a feeling of togetherness and friendship. Show sensitivity to their feelings and remember that they do not care how much you know until they know how much you care. Take time, do not rush the amiable patient, and be aware that, when used judiciously, a touch, such as a warm handshake or a supporting hand on their hand or shoulder may help the patient to feel more comfortable with you.

The analytical

Serious, scientific detail-lovers, the analytical people consider all the aspects of a problem and think through the consequences of action before making decisions. For this reason they make good lawyers, doctors, architects, and, yes, periodontologists!

Precise detail is important to them, so they will be very interested in the periodontal data chart and would appreciate a copy. They like to see proof of their condition, and of changes, and are more likely to be impressed by the data than by changes they can feel. Although slow to decide, they will be assiduous and thorough once convinced. They are recognised by their precision in describing their condition, lack of interest in feelings and fashions and their questions, designed to dig deeper for information.

When treating an analytical patient, it is helpful to show them the detail, explain logically and show how the proposed treatment will bring a benefit to them. Any numerical evidence, such as percentage success rates, will help them to feel more comfortable.

The entertainer

Often referred to as extrovert, entertainers are recognised by their bright approach and dress, interest in other people, and cheerful, positive disposition. They are a fountain of great ideas, but may not be good at seeing projects through to completion. Image is important and aesthetics will play an important part in their requirements. Decisions are made quickly and based more on emotion than on logic. Entertainers may be volatile and moody, and they relish approval and any personal touches that show their friendship is important to you.

When treating an entertainer, try to match their tone of voice and body language, and show them how your treatment will make them more comfortable and attractive in order to build and reinforce their self-esteem.

These four personality styles can be shown visually on a matrix as in Figure 5.18, based on assertiveness and emotionality. Individuals will not necessarily be typical of one particular personality type to the exclusion of all the others but every individual will have a place somewhere on this matrix and all will have a predominant place or 'home base' in one of the four quadrants. If you can discover where it is you will have a powerful key to unlock the co-operation you need for successful periodontal therapy.

It is important to understand that most people show characteristics of more than one personality type, and that people who are naturally of one type may develop the other aspects of their own personality. As an example,

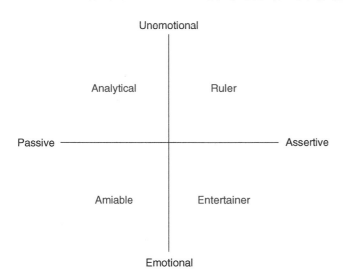

Figure 5.18 Personality matrix.

consider the principal of a periodontal practice: he needs leadership skills to build and direct his practice team, analytical skills to collect and interpret periodontal data, people skills to make working relationships with many different types of patients, co-workers, technicians, company representatives, and an amiable, caring approach to deal sensitively with his patients at times of concern and distress.

Learning styles

As well as personality typing, it is also very useful to know the preferred learning style of your patient. There are three styles:

- Visual learners:
  - prefer information they can see, such as a mirror, diagram, or key words
  - like to have a clear view of the teacher's facial expressions and body language
  - use colour to highlight important points in text
  - visualise information as mental pictures to help them remember.
- Auditory learners:
  - prefer information they can hear, such as a verbal description of their problem
  - participate in class and group discussions
  - read or repeat information out loud
  - use a tape recorder rather than take notes
  - use verbal analogies and stories to illustrate points.
- Kinaesthetic (tactile) learners:
  - like to touch, feel and sense the situation as much as possible; they may need to play with an object, such as a pen or pencil, during explanations
  - work at a standing position
  - tend to chew gum while learning

  - listen to music while learning
  - skim through reading material to get a rough idea of what it is about before reading it in detail.

Observation of the patient will often reveal their preferred style. Some people have a preference for more than one style. A presentation that incorporates all three styles is more likely to resonate with any individual patient than one that is only verbal or only visual. The clinician should try to develop an explanation of periodontal disease that combines the three styles, using visual, verbal and tactile methods for explanation.

The principles of mechanical plaque control by the patient

Key concepts

Once patients have understood that they have a problem, it is important to teach them their role in controlling their plaque. Plaque control by the patient is as important as plaque removal by the therapist. The options chosen for each patient must be achievable and effective. The features and benefits of each oral hygiene device should be explained to the patient. The patient needs to understand that thorough plaque control may take longer than they are used to and that one *thorough* plaque removal each day is better than more frequent but less efficient brushing.

- As has been stated, the development of plaque biofilm takes 2–3 days before signs of inflammation start to develop. Therefore, the thorough removal of plaque once daily is enough to control and prevent gingivitis and periodontitis.
- It is vital to remove plaque from interdental spaces daily with interdental brushes or dental floss. Excessive pressure or long scrubbing movements should be discouraged. New habits can be formed within a few days after which the routine will become easier.
- A methodical approach, always starting and finishing in the same place, is easiest for the patient to learn.
- Attention should be focussed on areas of difficulty. In some cases a disclosing solution may be helpful but it is important to first evaluate where plaque is being retained; it may not be visible to the patient in their bathroom mirror with normal domestic lighting. Facial surfaces are often almost plaque free and the patient's inability to see plaque in the buccal and posterior regions may give a false impression of how well they are performing. It can be more productive to explain where and why they need to prioritise their cleaning.
- The patient needs to understand that their gingivae will be likely to bleed at first when they practice a new method of plaque removal, and that persistence will

lead to a reduction in inflammation and therefore a reduction in bleeding. After selection of the best aids for each patient, a demonstration of both the interdental cleaning method and toothbrushing technique is important, initially taking between only 5 or 10 minutes in all, so the patient is not overloaded with information. This can be reinforced and developed at subsequent appointments.

Step 1: removal of interdental plaque

An efficient toothbrushing technique only cleans approximately 65% of the tooth surface, leaving the vulnerable interdental col area untouched. Some form of interdental plaque control is therefore essential for patients who are susceptible to periodontitis, and advisable for all patients who may be susceptible to gingivitis (i.e. everybody else) as a preventive measure.

Where there is no loss of interdental papillae, dental floss will be required to remove interdental plaque. However, floss is difficult for most people to learn and simpler methods are preferable. Where there has been loss of interdental tissue, including bone, or where natural spaces exist between the teeth, interdental brushes can provide a more effective answer. They are easier to use, and therefore more effective, than dental floss for patients with periodontitis. Wood sticks are easy to use but tend to break if used too vigorously and do not remove plaque as effectively as brushes or floss. Toothpicks are inappropriate because their circular shape prevents them from adapting to the interdental spaces, leaving them ineffective and likely to cause gingival trauma.

Interdental cleaning should be demonstrated to the patient in their mouth, regardless of whichever aid is chosen, sticks, floss or interdental spiral or 'bottle brush'. The interdental brush must be a snug fit between the teeth in order to remove plaque effectively. If it is too small it will not reach subgingivally, and will therefore not be as effective at controlling periodontitis. *Interdental spaces are not all the same size*, so the patient needs a range of sizes ensuring a snugly fitting brush for each interdental space to achieve efficient plaque removal. The patient who has already experienced interdental attachment loss will typically need three to four sizes of interdental brushes for the whole mouth (Figure 5.19a and b).

Correct and effective use of floss or interdental brushes takes time to learn so, for the first few days, patients may need to set aside about 10 or 15 minutes each day to practise the hygienist's or therapist's instructions.

Instructions on the use of floss

It helps for the patient to practise with the fingers first without the floss to assess their ability to reach all parts of the mouth. It is recommended that this is done 'by

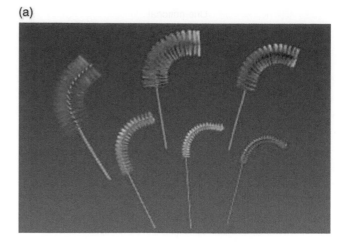

(a)

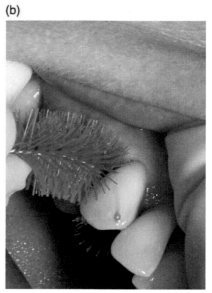

(b)

Figure 5.19 (a) Interdental brushes. (b) Interdental brush between canine and and premolar.

feel' rather than looking in a mirror, as this may be less confusing than a reversed mirror image, which can be obscured by the patient's hands. There is no need for more than two fingers in the mouth at any one time. It is best to keep the other fingers in a loose fist and out of the way.

It is important to emphasise that the floss takes up a C-shape round the mesial and distal surfaces of the teeth, a fact that many patients fail to appreciate (Figure 5.20).

A number of different types of floss aids (floss held between plastic fingers or prongs joined by a handle) are available for patients who need to use them and who, for a variety of reasons, find flossing difficult to manage (Figure 5.21).

There does not appear to be any significant difference between waxed or unwaxed dental floss, or between floss and the thicker dental tape; this choice can be left

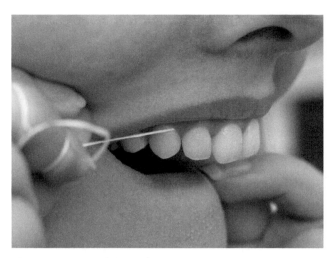

Figure 5.20 Use of dental floss.

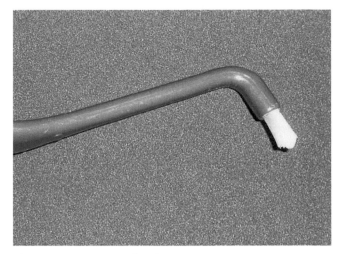

Figure 5.22 Interspace brush.

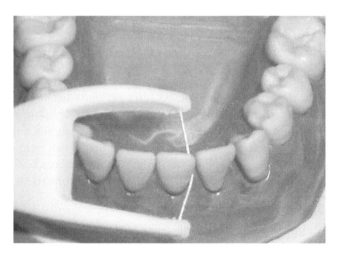

Figure 5.21 Flossing aid.

to personal preference. Whichever is chosen, the patient should understand that the floss is positioned gently in the gingival crevice and applied to the tooth as it is withdrawn in a coronal direction. A gentle sawing motion may be helpful in guiding the floss between a tight interdental contact; however, the force applied should be *just enough* to slip the floss between the teeth; any more than this may cause damage to the soft tissue. Persistent and patient practice is required until the technique is mastered and the patient should be encouraged to keep trying.

For patients new to the use of floss, it is helpful to work on the upper and lower six anterior teeth first, mastering these areas before graduating to the posterior teeth.

Interdental brushes

Where there has been interdental attachment loss, with loss of interdental papillae or the underlying bone (this can be identified from the radiographs or pocket depths),

a curved interdental brush works best to reach subgingivally and into the interdental col or pocket (Figure 5.22). The convexity of the curve is used against the papillae. Some brushes are supplied precurved; others can be curved round a finger before use. This not only helps to avoid catching or stabbing the papillae but also can gently compress the soft spongy papillae, removing subgingival plaque and debris.

Interdental brushes should be used once a day *before the toothbrush;* this is easier for the patient to remember and has the additional benefit of fluoride in the toothpaste penetrating between the teeth when used with the conventional toothbrush later.

No toothpaste should be used on interdental brushes because most pastes are abrasive. It is possible to remove plaque effectively without rubbing back and forth if the brush fits snugly and the head is 20–25 mm long. A long-headed brush encourages a 'once in once out' operation avoiding scrubbing habits and disrupts the plaque without leaving an accumulation of debris on the palatal or lingual surfaces, which can occur with a brush that is too short.

The use of chlorhexidine or stannous fluoride gels may be of some benefit in highly caries-susceptible patients.

Although many interdental brushes have a handle, compression of the gingiva to reach into the deepest part of the pocket (where the col may have deepened to become a crater beneath the contact point) is important to achieve subgingival plaque removal requires both direction and control; by holding the brush close to the tip it can be guided gently between the teeth.

Brushes with a strong fine wire that can resist thrust along their length should be selected. This will make them last longer. Brushes that collapse after a single use need constant replacement and this can de-motivate the patient and add unnecessary expense.

Step 2: conventional toothbrushing

There are many different designs of toothbrush and all can be effective (nylon are cheap and have a consistent bristle size – see Chapter 11) Choose the shape and texture of the brush for the individual patient, taking into consideration:

- the size of teeth and oral cavity
- the ease of accessibility
- the quality and anatomy of the gingivae
- any vulnerable or sensitive places.

Sensitive areas, such as those with minimal keratinised mucosa, or where surgery has just been completed, may need a very soft brush for a few weeks during the healing phase.

The Bass technique

Emphasis should be placed on the position of the toothbrush filaments at the gingival margin. A firm pressure should be applied towards the gingival margin, using a side-to-side vibration (known as the Bass technique) to 'jiggle' the bristles into the gingival crevice with the shortest possible movement. This emphasis focuses on a 'polish' rather than a 'scrub' movement, which is required to break up the plaque biofilm. By demonstrating the technique by brushing the patient's teeth for them, an important sense, of 'how it feels', during tooth cleaning is developed. The hand mirror should be used at the end of each demonstration for a brief glimpse to demonstrate the angle of the brush head at the gingival edge, the very short brush movement, and the subgingival reach of the interdental brush. A scrubbing technique tends not to be as effective at removing the plaque biofilm and also can significantly contribute to tooth abrasion.

The brush is kept dry to improve awareness of the filaments on the gingival margin. A shirt button sized smear of toothpaste on the dry brush is sufficient so that the feeling of the filaments of the brush is not reduced by the presence of the paste.

Manual versus electric toothbrushes

Many studies have been conducted into the relative efficiency of electric and manual toothbrushes. The consensus is that electric brushes are at least as effective as manual brushes. Some studies have shown greater efficiencies for electric brushes. Most conclude that further longitudinal investigation is needed to evaluate the clinical significance of these findings; however if they are at least as good, and easier to use, there is a strong argument for recommending electric brushes for all patients, especially those with any problems related to manual dexterity.

Other aids

There are many other oral hygiene aids that may be beneficial for certain situations or patients including:

- A tufted interdental brush for tight areas of overcrowding (Figure 5.22).
- Extra thick floss for plaque removal under bridge and implant superstructures.
- Chlorhexidine mouthwash: for short-term use (because it has an unpleasant taste and deposits a brown stain on the teeth) and to reduce the risk of bacterial resistance.
- Water jets and irrigators for subgingival delivery of water and medicaments: subgingival irrigation in specific deep sites may prevent further breakdown in an otherwise untreatable situation, but this requires a skilful and persistent patient.

Professional plaque removal

The objective of root surface instrumentation is to remove all the contaminants that cause inflammation of the periodontal tissues. A rough, contaminated surface retaining pathogenic bacteria prevents healing of the tissues surrounding the tooth. Current opinion is that thorough debridement need not include significant removal of root substance, the clinical endpoint being healing which is dependent on the balance between bacterial contamination and the natural defences of patient.

Scaling

Scaling is the removal of calculus deposits, both sub- and supragingival, from the root surfaces of the teeth. It may be necessary to discuss with the dentist the removal of overhanging margins of restorations in order to eliminate niches for retention of plaque.

Root debridement

Root debridement is the removal of the soft tooth surface deposits, mainly bacterial biofilm. A curette is used for root planing and root debridement.

Root planing

This is the establishment of smooth root surfaces by the removal of root surface material and contaminated cementum. This technique has been superseded in recent years by the less aggressive root debridement.

Hand instrumentation versus ultrasonic instrumentation

The advantages of hand instrumentation over ultrasonic instrumentation are:

- It can cause the patient less discomfort.
- The instruments are cheaper to buy and maintain.

- There are no aerosols.
- A chairside dental nurse is not essential.
- It can be easily undertaken in a domiciliary setting.
- Generally not as uncomfortable for the patient as ultrasonic scaling.

The advantages of ultrasonic instrumentation over hand instrumentation are:

- It is easier for the operator.
- Tactile sensitivity tends to increase over a 45 minute treatment period (Ryan *et al.*, 2005).
- There is generally a shorter instrumentation time.
- It requires minimal stroke pressure.
- There is less iatrogenic damage to the periodontium.
- There is minimal cementum removal.
- Generally quicker than hand scaling to acquire the necessary skills.
- It is not dependent on permanently sharp instruments.
- The fluid lavage flushes out debris, bacteria and unattached plaque.
- Precision-thin tips have been shown to penetrate deeper than hand instruments.

Hand instrumentation is hard work and requires time, strong fingers, a delicate touch, great patience and permanently sharp instruments to produce an effective end result. Local analgesia may be required for either procedure and failure to use it where the patient is finding the sensitivity intolerable may dissuade the hygienist from being as thorough as necessary. Research has shown however that the clinical outcome, if both methods are carried out thoroughly, remains the same (Hallmon and Rees, 2003).

Scaling technique

There are many different designs of scalers and unlike curettes, they have sharp tips. All have a triangular cross section (Figure 5.23) and are designed for removing supragingival calculus and plaque from the tooth surface around and above the gingival margin and in shallow pockets only.

Only the tip should be used in the gingival crevice because the shape of the instrument is not designed to conform to the subgingival root shape and it may therefore tear the gingival tissue. Both sides of the double edged working tip should be sharpened to maintain a keen edge, and taper to the tip forming a sharp toe in order to reach into narrow interdental spaces.

The scaler is inserted into the gingival crevice and carried beyond the edge of the calculus deposit. The tip is then engaged against the root surface and withdrawn from the crevice bringing the calculus with it (Figure 5.24). Many designs of scalers are available,

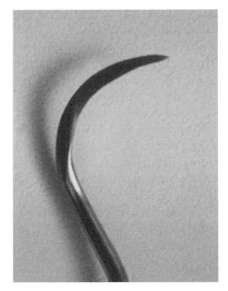

Figure 5.23 Scaler.

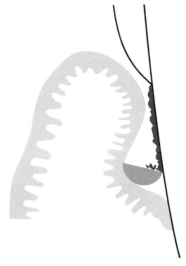

Figure 5.24 Scaler on tooth. (Reproduced with permission from *Clinical Periodontology and Implant Dentistry*, 4th edition (eds J. Lindhe, T. Karring, and N. Lang). Blackwell Munksgaard; p. 437, Figure 20.9d.)

with personal preference the main determining factor. The H6/H7 design can be used in most situations, with mini-versions and elongated patterns useful in difficult areas.

Curette technique

Good tactile skills are needed for the detection of deposits on the root surface. The sharpened curette (Figure 5.25) is gently inserted to the bottom of the pocket, past the calculus deposits to ensure that no deep calculus is left behind before applying the instrument to the tooth, beyond the deepest deposit. The edge of the instrument is drawn firmly along the tooth surface to remove the deposit. This movement is repeated in long overlapping strokes to render the root surface free of both plaque and calculus. The instrument should be firmly grasped with a pen grip, using the second or third finger on an adjacent tooth as a rest.

Many different designs of curette are available. **Gracey curettes** are popular in the USA. The Columbia 4L/4R is regarded as a universal curette, effective in virtually all sites (Figure 5.26). The Gracey series of 7 double ended curettes were designed in the 1930s by Dr Clayton

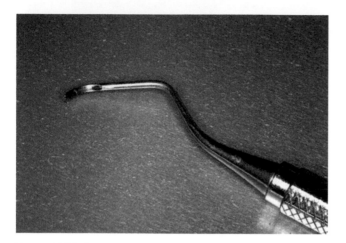

Figure 5.25 Curette.

Gracey at the University of Michigan. They have a tip angled at 70° to the shank and each tip, sharpened only at the lower edge, has a specific site of use.

The **Langer series** of four curettes, each double ended, with 90° tips and sharpened on both sides, are easier to use and have similar shapes, from straight to doubly curved. All sites can be reached with this series of instruments.

Curettes require regular sharpening. This, and pressure against the root surface being applied only on the 'up' stroke, will avoid burnishing of calculus on to the root surface The test of a sharp instrument is to listen as it is drawn up the tooth surface. A characteristic scraping sound will be heard if the instrument is engaging with the surface and removing the deposits effectively. When the surface is clean the tooth should feel smooth to the touch of the sharp edge of the curette. This may also be checked with a periodontal probe. The Old Dominion University (ODU) explorer is a useful instrument to explore root surfaces and detect subgingival calculus.

Periodontal hoes

Periodontal hoes are large and have a flat surface and therefore fail to conform to the curvature of the tooth surface, so they are used less frequently. Some authorities recommend their use during surgical open curettage procedures when access to the root surface is improved.

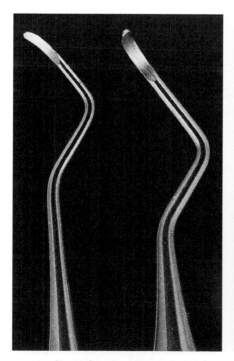
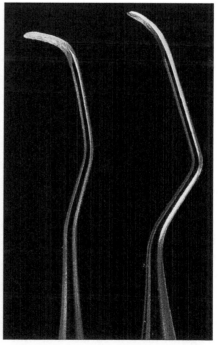

Figure 5.26 Gracey curette. (Reproduced with permission from *Clinical Periodontology and Implant Dentistry*, 4th edition (eds J. Lindhe, T. Karring, and N. Lang). Blackwell Munksgaard; p. 434, Figure 20.3.)

Power-driven instrumentation

Sonic and ultrasonic scalers are water-cooled mechanical devices that produce a fine vibratory movement of a metal tip, which causes fine droplets to form in the water coolant – a phenomenon known as **cavitation**. The streaming of water from the instrument (known as **microstreaming**) together with the small water droplets produces a flushing effect (lavage), which dislodges plaque and may disrupt the bacterial cell walls – even beyond the physical reach of the instrument tip. At the same time, the vibration of the tip dislodges calculus from the root surface with less effort than that required using a scaler or curette.

One disadvantage of this is that damage may be caused to the root surface cementum; this is undoubtedly more than with a hand instrument; however, clinical studies have shown that this does not have an adverse effect on the outcome of treatment.

Modern ultrasonic scaling units have fine, slim tips that are ideally suited to subgingival use, some straight, some curved like hand curettes and scalers. The instrument should be kept parallel to the tooth surface, constantly moving the tip, relying on the vibratory movement and cavitation at the tip to dislodge hard deposits from the tooth surface. There is no evidence that any one design of power-driven scaler is more effective than the others.

The instrument should not be applied to the tooth with any force or repeatedly in one line of action; a crisscross pattern is more effective, trying to cover the entire accessible tooth surface. The ultrasonic scaler is often the best choice for furcation areas where the furcation entrance is narrower than the tip of a curette restricting access to the tooth surface. There is good evidence that the ultrasonic tip can dislodge plaque deposits beyond the physical reach of the instrument and this is a great advantage in places where access is difficult (Figure 5.27).

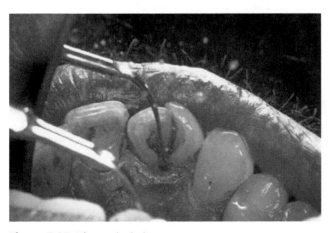

Figure 5.27 Ultrasonic tip in use.

Moore *et al.* (1986) showed that 99% of the bacterial endotoxin, in the form of lipopolysaccharide, can be removed from the root surface by rinsing and brushing, suggesting that almost complete elimination of the bacterial pathogens in periodontitis can be achieved with relatively simple and atraumatic measures.

The ultrasonic and cavitation effect produced by the vibration of the ultrasonic tip disrupts the biofilm and destroys bacteria and plaque microflora. There is also a washing effect on the root in addition to the direct physical contact effects of removing calculus, and flushing out of debris. In spite of the emphasis placed on the use of ultrasonic scalers, hygienists should develop their skills using both manual and mechanical scalers in treatment since it is not always possible to reach all areas adequately with mechanical devices. The preference, experience and skill of the operator remain important factors.

Chemical methods of plaque control

Since bacteria cause periodontal diseases, antibacterial agents and antiseptics have become part of the periodontal armamentarium.

Antiseptics

Antiseptics inhibit the growth of bacteria without actually killing them. There are several chemical types in common use:

- **Quaternary ammonium compounds** such as cetylpyridinium chloride are used in mouthrinses.
- **Phenols and essential oils** include triclosan and are used in toothpastes and mouthrinses.
- **Natural herbal products**, such as sanguinarine have been used in both mouthrinses and toothpastes.
- **Bisguanide antiseptics**. Chlorhexidine, the most well known member of this group, was developed by ICI in England as an antiseptic for skin wounds. A study by Loe and Schiott (1970) showed that rinsing for 1 minute with 10 ml of 0.2% chlorhexidine could inhibit plaque re-growth and the development of gingivitis. Since then it has become one of the most used and investigated materials in dentistry. Unfortunately it has a bitter taste and deposits a brown extrinsic stain on the teeth although the stain can be polished off albeit with some difficulty. Chlorhexidine is used as a mouthrinse in tooth gels and sprays, and can be applied as a varnish. It has also been incorporated into a gelatin chip (**Periochip**), which slowly biodegrades, releasing the active ingredient for 10 days.

Chlorhexidine mouthrinse has shown antibacterial activity lasting over 12 hours. It is important to realise that, because of their differing electrical charges, chlorhexidine is inhibited by the use of toothpaste, which should therefore precede the use of chlorhexidine by at least 30 minutes.

Chlorhexidine is the most effective mouthrinse in reducing the growth of plaque and it has therefore become the standard prescription for many oral diseases, including all forms of ulceration as well as its use in the reduction of gingivitis. It is also used after periodontal surgery and at any other time when the patient is unable to maintain good mechanical plaque control.

It is important to remember that mouthrinses do not penetrate subgingivally, and therefore they are only of value in supragingival plaque control.

Antibacterials in periodontal therapy

Antibiotics (as a means of combating infection) work either by killing bacteria (bactericidal) or by stopping them from multiplying (bacteriostatic). They can be applied in two ways: **systemically** (distributed round the body via the bloodstream) or **topically** (applied directly to the site of activity).

In order for an antibiotic to be effective it must be present in a high enough dose to overwhelm the bacteria that are present for a long enough period of time for the bacteria to be affected. Ideally, the clinician has identified the bacteria that are present so that an antibiotic known to be effective against those specific bacteria can be chosen. Until recently this has been impracticable in general dental practice because the bacteria known to be associated with periodontal diseases are anaerobic and difficult to grow in a laboratory. Recent technological advances have enabled known periodontal pathogens to be identified by comparing the DNA on the cell walls of bacteria in plaque samples taken from a patient with reference DNA in the laboratory. The test has become known as the **DNA probe test** and such testing is currently available in the USA and Europe. The relative load of the eleven most likely pathogens, including *Aggregatibacter actinomycetemcomitans* (Aa), can be identified and this helps in the choice of antibiotics.

Plaque samples are taken simply by placing a paper point in a periodontal pocket for 10 s. Single sites can be tested, or samples from several sites in the same mouth can be pooled together. This test is currently not available in the UK. Figure 5.28 illustrates a typical laboratory analysis.

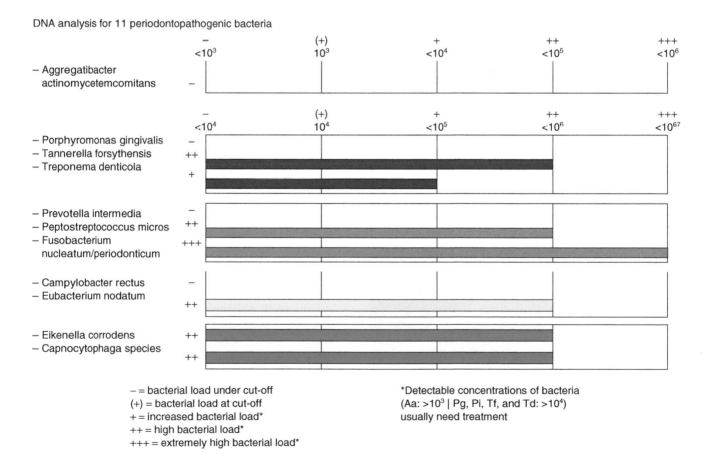

Figure 5.28 Typical bacteriological analysis.

Systemic administration, for example by swallowing a tablet, distributes the antibiotic around the body, thus diluting the concentration at any point and even though some antibiotics are concentrated in the gingival crevicular fluid, the dose available may not be high enough to overwhelm the bacteria present in the plaque biofilm. A large number of antibiotics are available for the systemic approach, and the cost, for most of them, is relatively inexpensive. On the other hand, we rely on the patient's compliance in taking the tablets exactly as instructed and this is not always guaranteed. Unwanted side effects of antibiotics are well known, and include the elimination of harmless but essential **commensal bacteria** and the development of bacterial resistance to antibiotics. This has led to a reduction in the use of antibiotics in recent years and a strong indication is therefore required for a prescription of systemic antibiotics.

Current opinion is that there is no place for systemic antibiotics in the management of slowly progressive chronic periodontitis because this can usually be controlled by mechanical therapy (i.e. plaque control and subgingival debridement) alone. Systemic antibiotics are useful for:

- Aggressive periodontitis.
- Chronic periodontitis resistant to mechanical therapy.
- Multiple periodontal abscesses as part of a full mouth disinfection approach.
- Acute infections in medically compromised patients in conjunction with root debridement of the affected area.
- Patients showing systemic symptoms such as pyrexia and glandular involvement.

Antibiotics in current use include amoxicillin, Augmentin, metronidazole, doxycycline and minocycline. Metronidazole, alone or in combination with amoxicillin, has been found to be very effective in cases that have proved resistant to non-surgical periodontal treatment.

Topical application of antimicrobials

Problems with the use of systemic antibiotics have led to the development of local (or topical) antibiotic delivery systems. These materials enable the dentist to administer a very high dose of antibiotic exactly where it is required, without the need for patient compliance and with no side effects. This implies that topical antibacterials are best suited to a situation where there are a relatively small number of isolated sites that have not responded to therapy, or to recurrently inflamed sites discovered at a recall visit.

Early topical delivery systems included a polyvinyl acetate fibre impregnated with tetracycline, (**Actisite**)

The fibres are packed in layers into the pocket and kept in place by means of a cyanoacrylate adhesive and removed after ten days of sustained release of tetracycline. Actisite is currently only available in the USA.

These were later followed by gels containing minocycline (**Dentomycin**) and metronidazole (**Elyzol**) supplied in simple syringes. Gels are easy to apply but do not remain in place for more than a few hours, so they must be re-applied several times in order to maintain a therapeutic dose for long enough to be effective.

The factors to be considered when choosing the mode of antibacterial to be used are listed in Table 5.5.

Other chemical devices

PerioChip (Figure 5.29) is a hydrolysed gelatine chip containing 2.5 mg of chlorhexidine in a biodegradable chip with controlled release and no risk of antibiotic resistance. PerioChip may be effective in sites that have not responded well to initial non-surgical therapy.

The local delivery of antimicrobials may be beneficial in the control of periodontitis but do not provide

Table 5.5 Antibiotic delivery in periodontitis.

Systemic application	Topical delivery
Low dose in gingival crevicular fluid (GCF)	High dose in GCF
Sustained activity	Short period of activity
Low cost	High cost (gels)
Relies on patient compliance	No compliance required
Wide choice of antimicrobials	Restricted choice of antimicrobials
Wide distribution in the body	Small area of activity
Risk of systemic side effects	No risk of side effects

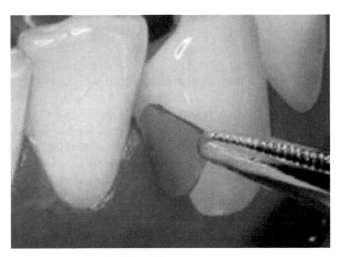

Figure 5.29 Chlorhexidine chip.

a superior result when compared to scaling and root surface debridement. They may, however, offer a greater potential for success when used together with conventional treatment in a small number of non-responding sites. Factors that must be considered in using local antibiotics include the risk of the development of antibiotic sensitivity and the time and cost of therapy.

Host modulation

Some systemic medications may modulate host response or periodontal pathogens. These include:

- Flurbiprofen (a non-steroidal anti-inflammatory drug used to treat pain caused by rheumatoid arthritis and osteoarthritis) may slow rates of bone loss.
- Hormone replacement therapy (HRT) may influence the activity of osteoclasts and osteoblasts in the periodontium.
- **Periostat®**, is a sub-antimicrobial dose of doxycycline that has been shown to inhibit the activity of collagenase, an enzyme capable of breaking down collagen. This therapy has been shown to be effective as an adjunct to subgingival scaling and root planing.

Full mouth disinfection – putting it all together

The notion of eliminating all pathogenic bacteria at once is an attractive proposition, not least for the patient who wants to get the mechanical removal of plaque and calculus over with as quickly as possible. It also avoids the possibility of reinfection of treated sites with periodontal pathogens from sites as yet untreated. The technique involves complete root surface debridement of the whole mouth within a 24-hour period, supplemented by a prescription of systemic antibiotics. This could be done at one or two sessions, under local analgesia. When two sessions are used, the right and left sides are usually treated separately; however the individual patient's condition dictates the best way of sequencing the treatment.

Ultrasonics are preferred for the reasons given above, and a methodical approach is needed, using the periodontal chart as a guide to sites to be treated, spending 30–40 seconds in each pocket, moving the tip of the instrument up, down and across the root surface, to cover all the surface if possible. It is important to feel the base of each pocket with the instrument tip to ensure that the entire tooth surface has been debrided.

The choice of antibiotics depends on the bacteria present and the tolerance of the patient. The pathogens present are not always known, although commercially available DNA probe tests are now available for use. A combination of amoxicillin (250 mg) and metronidazole (200 mg) given three times daily is used most often, particularly if *Aggregatibacter actinomycetemcomitans* (Aa) is present. Metronidazole can be used alone if the patient is allergic to penicillin, or if Aa is absent. Other antibiotics have also been used. Some clinicians advocate the use of chlorhexidine twice daily for 2 weeks after debridement.

Perhaps the greatest advantage of full mouth disinfection is the rapid improvement that can be achieved in comparison with the more conventional sessional treatment programme. This makes the patient more comfortable quickly, and the rapid improvement encourages the patient to work on their plaque control to ensure that the disease does not return.

Full mouth disinfection is most useful in the following conditions:

- All forms of aggressive periodontitis.
- Cases of multiple periodontal abscesses.
- Cases where the gingivae are uncomfortable, or where the patient is distressed about the condition for any reason.
- Situations where time is short.

Re-evaluation

After a programme of non-surgical therapy the patient should return to the clinician for re-evaluation. This is a crucial stage in the patient's treatment. When the patient has completed a course of initial treatment the relationship which has developed between the therapeutic team and the patient and the response to plaque control treatment, often referred to as **cause-related therapy,** can be assessed. This is the time for long-term decision making.

A full periodontal examination, exactly the same as at the outset of treatment, is repeated so that the data can be compared. Healthy sites should be maintained. Unhealthy sites are assessed for additional or revision therapy. Periodontal surgery can be considered at this stage to provide access to deeply placed plaque and calculus deposits, for regeneration of lost attachment, and for treatment of furcation involvement. The prognosis for individual teeth and the dentition as a whole can be reviewed with a view to long-term management.

The role of periodontal surgery

Even the most skilful hygienist is hampered by an inability to see the root surface.

Periodontal surgery provides access to root surfaces for investigation of residual periodontal pockets. The periodontal surgeon is able to complete the debridement and scaling of the root surfaces, and has access to furcation areas and osseous defects for therapy which may

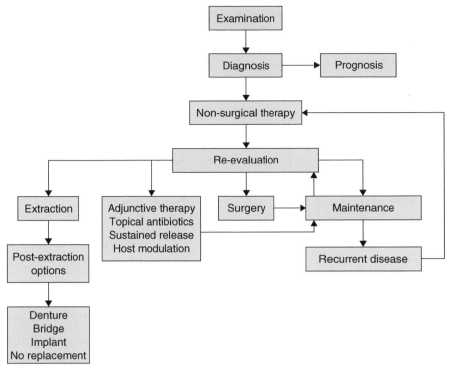

Figure 5.30 Decision making in periodontal therapy.

include amputation of a root or an attempt to regenerate periodontal attachment (i.e. cementum, bone and periodontal fibres) that have been destroyed by periodontitis. In addition, periodontal surgery may be able to improve mucogingival defects and enhance the outcome of implant-related treatment.

Surgery requires some form of anaesthesia, usually local, and perhaps intravenous sedation, so this form of treatment is more invasive, time consuming and costly for the patient. At the re-evaluation stage the clinician needs to decide whether any residual pockets would benefit from surgical intervention. Among the factors that influence this decision are:

- Access for surgical therapy.
- The strategic importance of the tooth or teeth to the dentition as a whole.
- The degree of mobility.
- The endodontic status of the tooth.
- The likelihood of regeneration occurring, e.g. how many bony walls does the defect have?
- The proximity of nearby anatomical structures, e.g. the mental or lingual nerves.
- The prospects for replacing the tooth or teeth with bridgework or implants.
- The prospects for improvement with other non-surgical methods such as topical antibiotics.
- The patient's wishes.

Supportive phase of therapy

Susceptibility to periodontal disease is immutable. It cannot be changed, but it can be successfully managed. When periodontal therapy has controlled the periodontitis the patient needs a long-term maintenance programme to prevent recurrence of the disease. Recalls at 3-month intervals are usually recommended. At each recall the patient should be examined for periodontal pockets, bleeding on probing, plaque deposits and mobility. Residually inflamed sites should be re-treated by subgingival root-surface debridement and the patient's plaque control refined and changed if necessary. Adjunctive methods, such as topical antibiotics can be considered at this stage. The decision-making process, used at each recall examination, is shown in Figure 5.30.

Conclusion

The treatment of periodontal diseases requires a thorough and detailed diagnosis, a knowledgeable, persistent and co-operative patient, an enthusiastic therapist, and meticulous long-term maintenance therapy. Every dental clinician needs to develop the skills required because all restorative dentistry depends on good periodontal health for long-term success. The ability to change inflamed, discoloured, swollen and bleeding gingivae into pink healthy tissue, to eliminate a bad taste and halitosis and to stop the loss of a patient's teeth, giving them the peace of mind of a healthy and maintainable mouth is one of the most satisfying and rewarding aspects of clinical dental practice.

References

Grossi, S.G., Skrepcinski, F.B., DeCaro, T. *et al.* (1997) Treatment of periodontal disease in diabetics reduces glycated hemoglobin. *Journal of Periodontology*, **68**, 713–719.

Hallmon, W.W. and Rees, T.D. (2003) Local anti-infective therapy: mechanical and physical approaches. A systematic review. *Annals of Periodontology*, **8**(1), 99–114.

Lindhe, J., Karring, T. and Lang, N. (eds) (2003) *Clinical Periodontology and Implant Dentistry*, 4th edn. Blackwell Munksgaard. www.idpride.net/learning styles. Learning Styles Internet site.

Löe, H. and Schiott, C.R. (1970) The effect of mouthrinses and topical application of chlorhexidine on the development of dental plaque and gingivitis in man. *Journal of Periodontal Research*, 5(2), 79–83.

Moore, J., Wilson, M. and Kieser, J.B. (1986) The distribution of bacterial lipopolysaccharide (endotoxin) in relation to periodontally involved root surfaces. *Journal of Clinical Periodontology*, **13**(8), 748–751.

Palmer, R.M., Wilson, R.F., Hasan, A.S. and Scott, D.A. (2005) Mechanisms of action of environmental factors – tobacco smoking. *Journal of Clinical Periodontology*, **32** Suppl 6, 180–195.

Preshaw, P.M., Heasman, L., Stacey, F., Steen, N., McCracken, G.I. and Heasman, P.A. (2005) The effect of quitting smoking on chronic periodontitis. *Journal of Clinical Periodontology*, **32**(8), 867–868.

Ryan, D.L., Darby, M., Bauman, D., Tolle, S.L. and Naik, D. (2005) Effects of ultrasonic scaling and hand-activated scaling on tactile sensitivity in dental hygiene students. *Journal of Dental Hygiene*, **79**(1), 9.

Silness, J. and Loe, H. (1964) Periodontal disease in pregnancy. II. Correlation between oral hygiene and periodontal condition. *Acta Odontologica Scandinavica*, **22**, 122–135.

Socransky, S.S., Haffajee, A.D., Cugini, M.A. *et al.* (1998) Microbial complexes in subgingival plaque. *Journal of Periodontology*, **25**(2), 134–144.

UK Adult Dental Health Survey (1998) http://www.statistics.gov.uk/downloads/theme_health/DHBulletinNew.pdf. (p. 5, Figure 6).

Further reading

American Academy of Periodontogy Position Paper (2000) Sonic and ultrasonic scalers in. *Journal of Periodontology*, **71**, 1972–1801.

American Academy of Periodontology (2005) *Implications of Genetic Technology for the Management of Periodontal Diseases.* American Academy of Periodontology, Chicago, IL.

Armitage, G. (1999) *Annals of Periodontology: Development of a Classification System for Periodontal Diseases and Conditions.* American Academy of Periodontology, Chicago, IL.

Bandler, R. and Grinder, J. (1981) *Frogs into Princes: Introduction to Neuro Linguistic Programming.* Real People Press, Boulder, CO.

Bollen, C.M., Mongardini, C., Papaioannou, W., Van Steenberghe, D. and Quirynen, M. (1998) The effect of a one-stage full mouth disinfection on different intra-oral niches. Clinical and microbiological observations. *Journal of Clinical Periodontology*, **25**(1), 55–66.

Grossi, S.G. (2001) Treatment of periodontal disease and control of diabetes: an assessment of the evidence and need for future research. *Annals of Periodontology*, **6**(1), 138–145.

Heanue, M., Deacon, S.A., Robinson, P.G. *et al.* (2005) Manual versus powered toothbrushing for oral health. The Cochrane Database of Systematic Reviews, 2005, Issue 2.

Leon, L.E. and Vogel, R.I. (1987) A comparison of the effectiveness of hand scaling and ultrasonic debridement in furcations as evaluated by differential dark-field microscopy. *Journal of Periodontology*, **58**(2), 86–94.

Oda, S., Nitta, H., Setoguchi, T., Izumi, Y. and Ishakawa, I. (2004) Current concepts and advances in manual and power driven instrumentation. *Periodontology 2000*, **36**, 45–58.

Preshaw, P., Hefti, A.F., Novak, M.J. *et al.* (2004) Subantimicrobial dose doxycycline enhances the efficacy of scaling and root planing in chronic periodontitis: a multicenter trial. *Journal of Periodontology*, **8**, 1068–1076.

Seymour, R.A. (2005) Does periodontal health improve general health? *Dental Update* 37(4), 206–212.

6

Oral health education and promotion

Jane M. Pratt

Summary

This chapter covers:

- The meaning of health
- Defining health education and health promotion
- Models of health promotion
- Considerations while planning health education and health promotion strategies
- Planning a teaching session
- Evaluating health promotion and education
- Oral health promotion and education samples
- Conclusion

Introduction

The purpose of this chapter is to define the meaning of health education (HE) and health promotion (HP). The two terms are sometimes interchangeable. Both health professionals and lay people promote and control health. For example, a dental hygienist/therapist may educate a patient on oral hygiene as they have been taught as an undergraduate, the link between dental plaque/bacteria and periodontal disease and dental caries. A lay parent, despite no dental training, may still promote twice daily toothbrushing to her/his child. On a wider scale HP is linked to government initiatives. HP can be delivered in various forms, such as via the media, health professionals or by national campaigning of certain groups and topics. Therefore, everyone is involved in HP and HE.

On a global level, oral disease has a high prevalence in populations that are disadvantaged, either by income and/or socially. Historically, HP and HE focused on individual behaviour that may contribute to ill-health. However, it has been recognised that achieving good oral health goes beyond risk-taking behaviour. Therefore, effective public health strategies and the collaboration of different organisations and health educators contribute to the reduction of poor oral health.

Many white papers have been released from the government to improve health. *Choosing Health; Making Healthier Choices Easier* (DoH, 2004) identified the need for patients to make informed choices. It outlined that choice may be influenced by a person's own health needs and expectations. Therefore, the health professional's role is to assist patients in making healthy choices, which may be facilitated by collaboration between different partnerships. A year later, there was a focus on oral health – *Choosing Better Oral Health; An Oral Health Plan for England* (DoH, 2005) identified contributions to poor oral health. It recognised that in order to improve oral health, education and different initiatives are essential in order to influence long-term behaviour and develop skills.

However, oral health advice may conflict with other health professionals' advice. An example may involve the intake of medication with a high sugar content on a regular basis. From an oral health promoter's point of view, this regular intake may increase the risk of dental caries. It is important that when promoting oral health, that evidence-based information is given. One such guidelines is the *Delivering Better Oral Health Evidence-Based Toolkit for Prevention* (DoH/BASCD, 2009). Hence, the

Clinical Textbook of Dental Hygiene and Therapy, Second Edition. Edited by Suzanne L. Noble.
© 2012 John Wiley & Sons, Ltd. Published 2012 by John Wiley & Sons, Ltd.

same messages are being given to patients from all health professionals.

A Dental Care Professional (DCP) will be involved in both HP and HE. Therefore, in order to teach and promote health to others, it is essential that the theoretical aspect of HP and HE are understood. Thus, this chapter will discuss various HP models, as well as the psychology of the interaction, such as communication styles, between the health educator and patient/client.

Meaning of health

It is important for health educators and promoters to be able to define what health means to them and to their patients/clients. Of course, the word 'health' has various meanings to different people. Some may relate their idea of health to their present day situation, while others may compare their health in relation to past ill-health or to that of an ill relative/spouse. The concept of health is also influenced by cultural, spiritual and ethnic factors. Whatever its meaning, one thing is clear is that health is essential for everyday living.

How would *you* define 'health'? A young person may report health as being able to run a certain distance, or having the right body image. In contrast, an elderly person may report being healthy, despite a complex medical history and regular medication.

The World Health Organization (WHO) defined health further as; 'Health is not merely the absence of disease, but a state of complete physical, mental and social well-being' (WHO, 1946).

This statement identifies that health is not only related to physical well-being, but also other factors. Furthermore, it appears that if certain resources are lacking, then this may affect health. Is it possible to attain 'complete health'? The WHO definition gives an impression of an Utopian-type view of health, whereby if we cannot have the 'completeness' of the factors that contribute to health, then we can never aspire to attain 'complete health'. Seedhouse (2001) also suggested that people will achieve their own realistic health potential. However, what has been highlighted for many years, is that ill health can be influenced by several factors. In 1974, The Lalonde Report (Lalonde, 1974) identified four areas that could be targeted in order to improve health. These were:

- Genetic/biological factors – may determine predisposition to a certain disease.
- Lifestyle – certain behaviours which may contribute to disease such as smoking.
- Environment – poor housing, overcrowding and pollution.
- Health services – some patients may not have access to dental care.

Thus, education on its own is not enough. The above factors need to be addressed by using different strategies and collaboration with different services.

Defining health education and health promotion

The term 'health promotion' and 'health education' are sometimes difficult to define separately. However, HP is a broad concept which also covers HE.

Health education

Generally in simple terms, HE is the active process of transferring information from an organisation/person to a client/patient. This can involve the explanation of cause and effect of disease and the influence of behaviour on health. The aim of HE is to encourage good health by using different strategies. It may include written/verbal information, as well as advising, supporting and developing people's skills. HE can be given one-to one or to a group. Traditionally, HE may have been delivered in 'health' settings, although in recent years HE now influence's social policies, community action and health of employees (Needs and Postans, 2006).

Health promotion

In 1986, a WHO international conference, The Ottawa Charter, put forward a definition of health promotion as: 'The process of enabling individuals and communities to increase control over the determinants of health and thereby improve their health'.

Hence, HP is a combination of health education and various support services that enable people to improve their health. It also focuses on groups and aims to prevent disease. Therefore, HP attempts to target the health of a population and incorporates a top-down approach, whereby policies and strategies are put forward to improve health. As already discussed, health is a global concern, as identified in *Health for All by the Year 2000* (WHO, 1977, 1985), which highlighted the need to reduce disease and to promote health. On a national and local level, health authorities and primary care trusts incorporate global strategies and targets. Furthermore, partnerships between different groups can promote health. Traditionally, oral health professionals have focused on preventing oral disease by giving advice on their lifestyle/behavioural aspects, such as smoking cessation. However, this is a reductionist point of view, as behaviour and lifestyle choices are influenced by social factors. Likewise, social behaviour is further influenced by economic, environmental and cultural factors. Thus, highlighting the negative effects on health as a result of the patient's behaviour, may have limited results (Watt, 2005).

The Ottawa Charter (WHO, 1986) put forward five main areas of health promotion strategies in order to improve health education/promotion and promote health and reduce inequalities:

- **Build public policies that support health**. For example, the government level may introduce labels on food, so that consumers are given the correct information and make a choice. Local level policies may concentrate on healthy eating within the nurseries and schools.
- **Supportive environments**. An example is supporting healthy diets at school.
- **Strengthen community action**. Involves empowerment of local people. Therefore, this may involve group activity. An example may include local mothers working together to manage sports activities for their children.
- **Develop personal skills**. This incorporates health education and assists people in developing skills that will contribute to good health. An example of this is the demonstration of interdental cleaning and a 'tell, show, do' within the dental setting.
- **Reorientate health services**. There has been a lot of this in recent years. Different services question why there is poor health and develop strategies in order to overcome this.

Later, the further development of services in order to improve both HE and HP delivery were put forward by The Jakarta Declaration on *Leading Health Promotion into the 21st Century* (WHO, 1997).

Thus, HP should involve a more collective responsibility in achieving health. Furthermore, in order to empower people to introduce changes to their lifestyle, public policies and community action need to facilitate these changes and ensure that healthy choices.

Promotion of oral health

Oral health can be described as being without disease and a state whereby the individual can carry out the normal physiological aspects such as eating and speaking. Watt (2005) further suggested that good oral health contributes to general health as it also satisfies psychological and social needs such as communication and appearance.

Oral health education (OHE) may relate to the transfer of information and teaching of new skills to an individual or small group, usually patients. (Needs and Postans, 2006) Oral health promotion (OHP) also includes OHE, but it also focuses on a wider scale; it incorporates different groups, plans different strategies and sometimes legislation.

The DCP needs to be aware of current oral health issues. In 2003, *The World Oral Health Report* was released (WHO, 2003). WHO determined areas that could contribute to improved oral health such as reduced tobacco use, healthy diet, use of fluoride, promotion of oral health in schools and to the elderly. It also suggested development of 'oral health systems' and the need for research to improve oral health. However, inequalities still exist with regards OHP programmes. One reason for this is that the groups that would benefit most from oral health promotion are not able to do so as resources may not be available or limited. Furthermore, it has been reported that dental caries and periodontal diseases have been recognised as the most important key areas for improvement in the status of oral health at a global level (Peterson, 2008). It has also been suggested that other negative influences exist, which may affect the person's ability to achieve improved oral health. These factors include lifestyle choices/issues, habits that have been established from childhood and therefore may be difficult to change and external pressures such as work and time (Needs and Postans, 2006).

Who is involved in oral health education/promotion?

Many people are involved in OHE and OHP. The previous sections have highlighted the need for collaboration between different services and health professionals. So who is involved in OHE and OHP? The first that come to mind are those that work within the dental settings, such as oral health promoters, dentists, DCPs (hygienists, therapists, dental nurses, lab technicians) and receptionists.

Dental companies and dental/health agencies may promote oral health via a variety of ways, such as the delivery of leaflets, posters, use of media and by advertising. Water companies have introduced public water fluoridation. Other health professionals include health visitors, dieticians, pharmacists and nurses. OHE may also be taught in nurseries and schools as part of the teaching curriculum. On a larger scale, WHO, organisations, governments, the NHS, primary care trusts also are involved. They are responsible for social change and public health policies, as well as forming partnerships between different organisations.

Models of health promotion

Many health promotion models have been introduced and the given examples in this chapter are just a few. Models should be seen to allow a framework in order to guide health promotion programmes.

Ewles and Simnett model (2003)

This model involves five different approaches to the delivery of health promotion. It includes;

- **The medical approach** aims to have freedom from disease. This approach may be incorporated during different levels of prevention. An example may include promoting the ill-effects of smoking to a smoker. The medical approach is evidence-based; therefore it has a more scientific background.
- **The behaviour change approach** focuses on individual behaviour. This could be included in smoking cessation advice to an established smoker. However, patients may feel that they are to 'blame' for their 'ill-health'.
- **The client-centred approach** focuses on the patient's own agenda. It involves empowering the patient; they 'lead' their own health promotion/ intervention activity. An example of this approach is a smoking cessation programme devised, only after the patient has identified smoking as a health concern and the strategy that they want to follow in order to improve their health.
- **The educational approach** imparts knowledge to groups and individuals. It allows the individual to make an informed choice about a particular behaviour or activity.
- **The societal change** promotes a healthier environment via social change. An example of this approach was the ban on smoking in public places.

The Ewles and Simnett model puts forward a clear framework in how to promote a certain health promotion subject. But not all approaches may be relevant to the DCP. For example the social change may refer more to organisations that can put forward policies and strategies. Nor does it examine why people make certain choices regard their behaviour, or why people want to improve their health.

'Stages of Change model' (Prochaska and DiClemente, 1984)

The Stages of Change model (Prochaska and DiClemente, 1984) is based on different types of theories that explain human behaviour. The model has been used to describe addictive behaviour such as smoking, as well as defining clear stages, as outlined in Figure 6.1.

These stages can be described as follows:

- **Precontemplation stage**. The patient may not be aware that they have a health problem or that it is necessary to change their behaviour. What can the DCP do at this stage? The problems with trying to persuade a smoker to give up smoking is that they may not

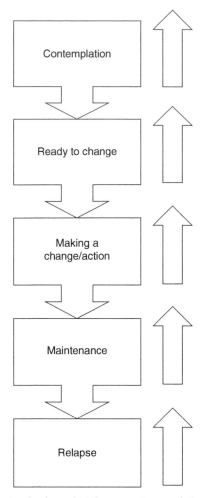

Figure 6.1 Prochaska and DiClemente 'Stages of Change Model'. (Adapted from Prochaska, J. O. and DiClemente, C. C. (1984) Self-change processes, self efficacy and decisional balance across five stages of smoking cessation. *Progress in Clinical and Biological Research*, **156**, 131–140.)

consider that they are smoking much. Or they may enjoy the social aspect of smoking or may be negative to any smoking cessation advice. Hence, the DCP must first require a willingness of the patient to change their habits before they can accept further help and support. However, education may alert the patient on the health issues associated with smoking.

- **The contemplation stage**. At this stage, the client may accept that smoking may have a negative effect on their health. They may not have actually sought an action plan yet, such as seeking pharmacological interventions. They are, however, ready to accept advice and guidance. The DCP needs to work through the factors that can contribute to smoking as well as actions to be taken in the smoking cessation programme.
- **Ready to change**. The patient has weighed up the costs and benefits of smoking. The associated

psychological, social and health factors may spur the patient on to make a change to their behaviour. The patient may actively seek advice and guidance from the DCP.

- **Making a change/action**. The patient may now demonstrate actual commitment to change behaviour, such as seeking out nicotine replacement therapy patches. This action process may be a short or long duration. It is important for the DCP to constantly support and encourage the client in their new regime. This can be achieved by setting goals and review smoking cessation progress. It helps to formulate an agreed plan with the client. Support may also be given by family and friends.
- **Maintenance**. Not everyone may reach this stage. The same encouragement and support should be given as in the action phase. Sometimes clients may enter this phase briefly before entering the action phase again.
- **Relapse**. An ex-smoker may move back into the cycle, as the change has not been maintained.

This model has been used many times during health promotion activities, although it does not explain why people may decide to move from one stage to another. It outlines the 'process' of behaviour change, yet not everyone moves through these stages in a synchronised fashion, nor does everyone move through all the stages. It also does not take into account social, ethnic and environmental factors that may contribute to a person's behaviour. However, it does give guidance to health professionals as to the stages of behaviour change and the support that can be given to the patient. The model does not view the relapse as an end point, but just another stage in the continuous cycle.

Health Belief model (Becker, 1974)

This model, explores the psychological aspect of 'risk' behaviour. Thus, a person's behaviour is influenced by factors such as beliefs, culture, class, religion and education. It also depends on the 'value' that people may place on their health. Behaviour is also shaped by affective attitudes such as emotions and preferences. Behaviour of course is the outward display of these influences. The Health Belief Model suggests that an individual may adopt a certain behaviour after assessing the pro's and con's of a particular action. Therefore a person's cognitive attitude (knowledge that they possess about a particular health subject) influences their behaviour (Needs and Postans, 2006).

Behaviour is also affected by socialisation, which is a process which enables the individual to participate in group life. By doing so, the individual acquires many human characteristics that may be unique to that group, such as health beliefs. Thus, 'primary socialisation' occurs within the family and 'secondary socialisation', refers to settings such as within schools or work (Needs and Postans, 2006).

This model explains why people may act in certain ways, but does not give guidance regards planning for a health promotion intervention. The model however, could serve as part of an ethical model and as guidance for oral education delivery.

Determining the type of need

In order to communicate with patients and to ensure that the appropriate health message is being delivered, the DCP needs to determine the level of need that is required by an individual or group. But how can the DCP determine need? This can be obtained from information gained from patients and parents via questionnaires or informal discussions. On a wider scale, demographic health surveys may determine need of a population both globally and nationally. This information can then influence government strategies to improve health.

Different types of need were originally defined by Bradshaw (1972).

- **Normative need**. This can be determined at global, national and local levels. We as DCPs may also determine this type of need and given our 'scientific' background may be influenced by the medical approach. Normative needs also reflect views and values that are held by health professionals. For example a child may have a high incidence of plaque and gingival inflammation. Because of the DCP's understanding of plaque induced inflammation, the DCP may give intense oral hygiene instruction. The problem with this type of need is that not all professionals may agree on the degree of need. This can lead to loss of confidence from patients.
- **Felt need or perceived need**. This is actually what the patient feels that they need in relation to their own assessment. This type of need can be identified by questioning the patient. Therefore, the patient with the high level of plaque may not feel that he/she needs oral hygiene instruction. Their own perceived need may be tooth whitening.
- **Expressed need**. Patients may actually 'express' or demand what they require. The expressed need is a request for treatment and therefore requires action. The expressed needs however, need co-operation with normative needs, although ideas may be opposed.
- **Comparative need**. This type of need is compared between groups or populations. For example, epidemiology studies may identify high decayed, missing and filled teeth (*dmf*) scores of certain groups in

specific areas. This type of need therefore requires some professional input. Health advice and support can be given to groups at 'risk' from oral disease.

By looking at the different levels of need, health promoters and organisations can attempt to incorporate all four levels. However, these needs are influenced by certain factors such as targets, finance and resources and so not all needs may be met.

Considerations while planning health education and health promotion

It is important for the DCP to consider certain factors which may influence both HE and HP sessions.

Environmental and social factors

Policies have outlined certain factors such as environmental and social issues that can affect health. Certain groups may require HP interventions more than more affluent groups. However, reaching these groups in need may be problematic due to barriers, such as lack of access to facilities, difficult to reach groups, such as travellers, the homeless, certain ethnic groups, limited resources and language barriers.

Top-down or bottom-up approach?

Health promotion involves different types of approaches – top-down and bottom-up.

The top-down refers to health education and health promotion initiatives that are led by health professionals. Example of this approach includes policies and strategies put in place by the government and primary care trusts. A bottom-up approach is led by people and communities. This approach focuses on the group's felt and expressed needs, although partnerships with health professionals and other organisations are also needed (Munday *et al.*, 1999).

Ethical issues

It is important to point out that health educators/promoters may influence other people's lives. By educating the patient/client, they are placing responsibility on that person to change their current behaviour. Hence, the DCP need's to ensure that patient's find themselves in supportive environments. It is also important to motivate patients/groups in a positive way, in order for them to develop skills and support them in modifying their behaviour. Other responsibilities include respecting people's autonomy, allowing patients/clients to make an informed choice and ensuring patients increase their self-esteem.

When should oral health messages be promoted? It is every DCP's duty to actively promote good oral health, without enforcing the patient into accepting their views. Instead, the DCP and patient should want to work together as a team. Of course, if the DCP has been invited to promote an aspect of oral health, as in a planned teaching session, there may be a willingness of the group to comply with the intended oral messages.

Teaching style

There are various methods that can be used to transfer information from the 'teacher' to the learner. It does of course depend on the location, the type of learners and situation. The traditional method of teaching, for example a didactic approach, involves the transfer of information to a passive learner. As this involves a more top-down approach, it offers little interaction between the teacher/educator and patient/client. Nor does it allow opportunity for feedback and opinions. It does however, guide the patient and some patients/clients may prefer this clear concise method. Another method may involve a more paternalistic approach; the educator takes on the role of highlighting the patient's current behaviour. Therefore the patient may feel anxious about their behaviour and may change their behaviour as a result. The patient may have little choice in discussing further options, although some patients may feel the need to be shown in order to change their behaviour.

Another approach may involve informing the patient/client regards a certain behaviour or health condition. The patient may therefore make an informed choice and as a result develop their own action plan without interference from the health educator. While this approach does not use 'victim blaming', the patient may not have developed the most cost-effective or easiest treatment. Some patients need to be guided with treatment.

An alternative approach may involve informing the patient, but allowing a two-way interaction between the educator and patient. Both listen to each other and an agreement is met.

Effective communication

The DCP has to be good communicator in order to get the health message across to the patient/group. It is not always the message that is important, but how the message has been communicated, that makes a difference to the patients' understanding. Communication is also a core skill which will enable the DCP to build a relationship with the patient/client. Of course, we may think we know how to communicate – after all it is an everyday activity. However, there is a variation of communication between health professionals and not all groups communicate at the same level. Some people may prefer first name use, while others may dislike the overfamiliarity (Needs and Postans, 2006). It is not enough to churn out a list of facts to the patients/ groups. It is how you actually engage with your group that will determine whether the health intervention is a success. Ask yourself, what are you trying to achieve? The DCPs aim should be to improve health by promotion and education. The required action of the patient, in order to achieve this is by perhaps behaviour change. They can only do this if they can listen effectively, interact with the educator and be empowered to change their behaviour. Communication is achieved via various methods, such as verbal, that is the actual use of words, para-linguistics – how we deliver the words and finally, non-verbal communication – the use of body language.

Use of language

The DCP should use simple language and short sentences whilst presenting the relevant and important message first. Furthermore, it is important to introduce medical language carefully. Explanations should be used with these 'scientific' words so as not to confuse the patient/group and to share knowledge between the educator and the target group. Likewise, consider the age and intellect of the patient and use appropriate words accordingly. For example, the word 'bugs' may be fine for children, while 'bacteria' will be more appropriate for adults. A way to build rapport with the patient/audience is to share a style of speech, although care should be taken so as not to patronise them. Health promoters should be aware of semantics. This is the meaning of words and may differ between groups of people, for example differences in age, experience, background/ culture and values. The DCP should also be aware that some ethnic groups may not share the Western view of health and interpretation of certain words is difficult.

Delivery

Needs and Postans (2006) suggested that the delivery of speech can determine whether the communication process is effective. Thus, factors need to be considered such as the pattern of speech, the speed, variation and level of voice and the use of pauses. Facilitation of the communication process by the DCP is important, as well as repeating the last sentence or paraphrasing, as this demonstrates understanding and allows clarification.

Questioning skills

Questioning has many purposes, such as helping develop a relationship between the DCP and the patient. The DCP can also determine baseline information, such as the oral hygiene regime of the patient or the level of understanding of a particular topic of a group, prior to a teaching session. Questions are also used in order to receive feedback in order to evaluate a health promotion session. Effective questioning allows both accurate and relevant information. The DCP should be aware of effective questioning techniques.

What type of questions?

Closed questions will result in short answers such as a yes, no. An example would be; 'Do you use floss?' These allow data to be collected quickly, but do not allow further information. **Open** questions may be more interactive and may begin with a when, how and what. An example would be; 'What toothbrush do you use?' While, a **focused** question may ask 'How did you get on with that toothbrush that I gave you last time?' This allows a more comprehensive answer, perhaps with the addition of opinions and emotions. This enables a clearer rapport and facilitates teamwork between the educator and patient. **Multiple** questions involve asking many questions at once. These questions are confusing and the patient cannot remember all that was asked. An example would be; 'How did you get on with that toothbrush that I gave you last time. What did you think of the bristles? Have you found the same make in the supermarket?' The patient will be unsure as what to answer first!

Also, be careful of asking **leading** questions whereby it may appear that the DCP wants to lead the patient in a particular direction, such as; 'So you are using the brush twice daily as I recommended you to?' The patient may feel that they have to agree even if they haven't! Thus, care must be taken with questioning in order to prevent negativity and opinions being conveyed across to the patient. Nor should **offensive** questions be used, so as not to offend the patient/group.

Non-verbal communication
Body contact and proximity

The amount of body contact depends on the relationship between people. There will be less contact between the health professional and the patient than the patient and spouse. However, there is more body contact between the clinician and patient than the receptionist or shop assistant. People follow certain rules regarding body space (proximity). Kay and Tinsley (2004) suggested that certain zones of body space exist; first (intimate), second and third zone, whereby we allow certain people, dependent on our relationship with them. During a OHE session, it is acceptable to be within the second zone, with a distance between 0.4–1.2 m. It is also important to consider different ethnic groups' perception on what is acceptable regards body contact and proximity.

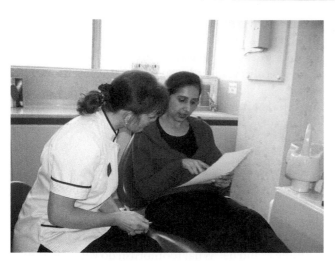

Figure 6.2 Sitting at the same level as the patient.

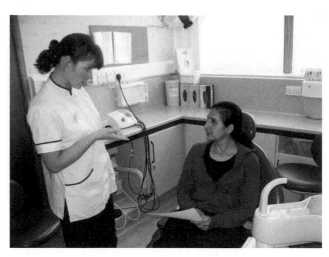

Figure 6.3 Standing above the patient while educating the patient can be confrontational.

Eye contact

The DCP need's to maintain eye contact in order to make the patient valued. This will also facilitate trust from the patient. However, too much eye contact may make a patient feel self-conscious, while maintaining eye-contact with a particular member of a group during a health promotion talk may make the listener feel uncomfortable. Therefore, the speaker should look away and gaze at several different people. During the clinical interaction, the DCP should avoid delivery of OHI while writing up notes, as the actual communication process and eye contact are lost.

Movements and posture

The delivery of OHE to a patient, while carrying out clinical work is not advisable, as this only allows a one-way conversation. Furthermore, talking to a patient while sitting behind them, does not allow effective communication. Therefore, the DCP should sit at the same level as the patient in a relaxed manner, at the same head height. Also, the DCP should incline their body to the patient, thus implying that they find their communication important. Sitting towards the patient at an angle, rather than directly in front, may be more non-confrontational (Figure 6.2). Likewise, it is not recommended that the DCP stands in front of a seated patient, while giving OHE (Figure 6.3). Folding arms and turning away from the patient/group acts as a barrier and suggests to the listeners that you are uncomfortable talking to them. Instead, unfold arms, which demonstrates a more open and friendly position to your audience. Also, be aware of flapping hands while talking. This is off-putting to the listener and they may become so distracted that they may miss out on key health messages!

An understanding 'open' face is more welcoming, rather than an angry or hostile facial expression.

Listening

This is an important, often under-rated skill. In order to develop a rapport with the patient/group, the DCP needs to be able to listen to them, just as they expect the patients to listen to them. However, listening is not a passive activity as it does involve assimilation of how the speaker is conveying their meaning. The listener also has to be aware of their own body language so that they suggest that they understand and are open to the speaker's opinions.

How can we ensure that we are good listeners? Think about the nervous withdrawn patient, perhaps by asking an opening question, we can engage the patient more and begin to build a rapport through verbal communication. An occasional nod of the head and use of non-words signify to the patient that you are following their dialogue and that they have your full attention.

Appearance

It is important, that as a health professional, that the DCP is a representative of the dental profession. Therefore, the patient may be making a judgement of the DCP, not only by their communication skills, but also by their appearance. Care needs to be taken with body odour, cleanliness and cosmetics. The DCP should be trying to portray a positive image of health! Of course, certain factors regarding the appearance can act as a barrier to learning. For example, in a medical environment, the uniform, may hinder learning, especially with children, whereby a more informal dress may be appropriate.

However, a uniform may also lend authority to the speaker, so that the patient will trust what they are instructed regards their oral care. Larger teaching sessions, outside the clinical area, allow the use of non-clinical dress, although it is important that the DCP still dresses smartly.

Barriers to effective communication

The DCP should consider barriers to effective communication:

- **Environment**. Clinical environments may not be conducive for learning for more nervous patients. The actual environment may also be noisy and distracting. It may be difficult for both the patient and the DCP to effectively listen and communicate.
- **Beliefs and attitudes**. People may have different values of oral health, sometimes based on family values, cultural beliefs, ethnicity, economics and oral health expectancy. The attitude of the educator may inhibit communication, such as patronising the patient or an accusation of 'risky' behaviour. There may also be conflict between the patient/group's interest or agenda and the educator.
- **Ineffective verbal/non-verbal communication**. Some groups may not share the same language as the DCP. Other patients may be visually and hearing impaired. Therefore, an interpreter may need to be organised and alternative methods used to communicate.

Planning a teaching session

Why is it important to plan an OHP activity? Generally, OHE given at the chairside within a clinical setting will be targeted to that particular patient's needs, it may be ad hoc, depending on the oral health status of that patient. It will be a shorter duration, than a planned oral health session to a group, outside the clinical setting. However, an OHP session to a group will not only be a longer duration, but also requires planning and thought in order to enable efficient use of resources. The DCP need's to determine the type of need, what messages will be delivered and the methods in which to do so.

Background information

A DCP may target certain groups of people, or they may be promoting particular subjects, such as smoking cessation or oral cancer awareness. It is helpful to draw on existing policies to determine the proposed strategies, epidemiology and evidence-based advice.

Ewles and Simnett (2003) suggested using a checklist to determine the health needs and education needs. What is the existing knowledge and is this the first time that this group will be involved in a health intervention, or have they been involved in previous OHP/OHE sessions? What type of group is at risk? Is this OHP programme feasible?

In order to find out this information, the DCP may want to find out existing knowledge of the group and previous interventions so that an appropriate OHP session can be delivered. This can be found out by the use of questionnaires or surveys.

Audience

This is the target group and may be one to one or a group. A one-to-one session is more specific and personalised. It may involve more questions, of a shorter duration and may involve a closer sitting proximity between the patient and the DCP. A group in comparison may require a longer teaching session. The DCP needs to be aware of the group dynamics and the need to engage all members of the group, as some members of the group may become more distracted. Hence, the session may require more visual aids and activities to prevent this. Factors that apply to both groups are considerations of age of the audience, the understanding, culture and language. Thus, the delivery may have to be modified accordingly. It is important to remember that some people may be well-informed regards health issues. They are also exposed to different forms and sources of media regarding the topic of health. Therefore, the audience may have existing opinions regard a subject.

Environment

The DCP needs to consider where the teaching session will take place. If it is within the dental setting, most of the resources are to hand. However, some people may find this environment threatening due to existing dental fears, while others may find it a novel environment in which to learn.

An external environment may need a pre-visit in order to determine the available resources, such as tables, seating and electronic equipment. Is the laptop compatible with the media systems within the teaching environment? The DCP will have to decide whether to hand out lecture notes or whether the audience will be required to make their own notes. Is the room noisy and therefore likely to distract the group? This has previously been outlined, as possible barriers to learning. Space is also important; there needs to be a balance between a crowded room and a small enough group to allow some interaction between the speaker and the audience, as well as between the group itself. Comfortable chairs are a must, although this may be out of the control of the speaker.

Aims and objectives

An aim is a general statement of what the health promotion intervention is trying to achieve or its intention. The session should also have set objectives so that this aim can be achieved. Put simply, an objective is what the health educator will hope to achieve in more detail, in order to satisfy the aim of the session (Needs and Postans, 2006). The aims and objectives should be stated at the beginning of the session, so that the audience can follow and understand the sequence of the teaching session. However, try and link these statements personally to the target group and they should also relate to all members of the audience.

Objectives should commence with words such as 'describe, define, identify, name, label, list, match and select'. (Needs and Postans, 2006) The objectives should also fit the **SMART** acronym:

Specific – the message should relate to the oral health aim and should be clearly defined. Do not attempt too many objectives!

Measurable – Can the DCP ensure that at the end of the teaching session, that the aims and objectives have been achieved? If so, how can the DCP determine this? Is it quantifiable?

Achievable – does the teaching session relate to the audience? Is the language relevant to the group? Does the aim relate to the learners ability? For example educating the use of interdental aids is inappropriate for preschool children!

Realistic – Will the teaching session achieve the set aim and objectives? Is the DCP attempting too much in a short space of time? In order to determine and plan an appropriate teaching session, a questionnaire could find out the needs of the group.

Time – there should be a recognised time in which to deliver the oral health messages. This may be pre-set as in national campaigns, or determined by the DCP, organisation or the group. Sometimes, there may only be one day in which to deliver the message, or even one session. Will there be a follow-up?

An example of setting an aim and its objectives may be;
Aim; To educate the use of interdental cleaning.

Objectives: At the end of the session, the patient will be able to:

- Describe the relationship between plaque, bacteria and periodontal disease.
- Demonstrate an effective interdental cleaning regime.
- List the interdental cleaning aids in order to achieve efficient interdental plaque removal.

Delivery

Now that the background information and the aims and objectives have been set, the DCP needs to plan the actual delivery of the OHP/OHE session. Let us consider different learning styles:

- **Cognitive learning** – involves learning facts.
- **Affective learning** – involves learning of emotions, behaviour and attitudes.
- **Psychomotor learning** – involves learning of practical skills (Needs and Postans, 2006).

The DCP needs to determine how these learning styles can be adapted to different activities. For example, cognitive learning will involve the intake of factual information, such as the reasoning for regular flossing, Learning to floss is modifying behaviour so involves affective learning, while the actual physical act and learning of the new skill involves psychomotor learning. Hence, a good OHP session will consist of combination of all learning styles. It has also been suggested that people like to be involved in practical demonstrations and activities and this reinforces their learnt theoretical knowledge (Needs and Postans, 2006).

Other methods used in OHP sessions include group work and brainstorming. These are more engaging for learners, as they allow discussions, active learning, dialogue and enquiry. However, too much 'free' discussion may result in loss of control of the session. Therefore, the DCP must consider the target group and the time of the session. It is therefore important to be flexible.

So how can the session begin? The start of the session could include an icebreaker, a statement, question or quiz. A story works well with younger children. It may be helpful to wear name badges, both for the educator and the group. A written lesson plan is useful as it guides the educator regards the topic and the timing. However, make sure that the lesson plan is not too intense, as it will be difficult to follow, especially when nervous. Perhaps the DCP could practise the teaching session with a trusted colleague. Also be prepared for the lesson plan to be modified, due to certain factors, such as the mood of the group and time constraints.

Consider the various methods of communication and how the group may be perceiving the speaker. Ensure eye-contact as this will help with the interaction with the audience, although it is important to attend to each member of the group evenly (Needs and Postans, 2006). Speak clearly and at a reasonable pace. Reading from notes puts a barrier between the educator and the group. The DCP should allow questions from the group, although guidelines should be outlined as to when they should ask questions, so as not to interrupt the flow of the lesson.

Be aware of the content of the OHP. Is it relevant and appropriate? Is it non-judgemental? Is it racist or sexist? Is the information evidence-based?

Conclude key points. The oral health promoter could ask questions in order to evaluate the teaching session.

Include goody bags for the audience. Ask the audience to fill in a feedback sheet regarding the teaching session.

Activities/participation

The teaching session should appear seamless to the audience. Different activities may be included, although care must be taken to ensure that these do not overrun. Examples include group work/discussions, brainstorming, experiments, videos, games, quizzes, questionnaires, interviews and role-play. However, don't forget that learner activities can also include listening, looking/watching and writing.

If the session involves the teaching of practical skills, approach with a demonstration, rehearse and practise (Needs and Postans, 2006). Build up the patient's/group's skills. For example, start with a mouth model and then finish and transfer the new skill within the patient's own mouth. The DCP should build up the participant's confidence, encourages, motivates and reinforces the oral health messages and skills.

Resources

Visual aids can reinforce the OHE session, both within the clinical and informal setting. However, the DCP has to consider whether the visual aids may really be appropriate for achieving the aims of the lesson. For example, written information such as leaflets are not effective on their own. An actual practical demonstration of toothbrushing may be better. Could other types of resources be used that are more economical? Sometimes a PowerPoint presentation may not be available, but photographs may be just as good (Needs and Postans, 2006).

The health education resources should be ethical, relevant and use appropriate language. They should not be judgemental and should avoid the use of 'victim-blaming' Written information should avoid too much medical 'jargon', although they should be evidence-based and relevant to the target group. Shorter sentences work well. Be aware of the literacy and knowledge level of the target group. Are the resources reproduced in other languages? Are the resources available in other formats, such as Braille or large type?

The resources should avoid being racist (stereotyping people into certain racial groups or roles that are based on particular ethnic groups), information should be sound and evidence-based (Needs and Postans, 2006). Resources should also be non-sexist (stereotyping men and women into certain roles or characters based on their gender). Furthermore, resources should not make references about sexual orientations of people (Needs and Postans, 2006).

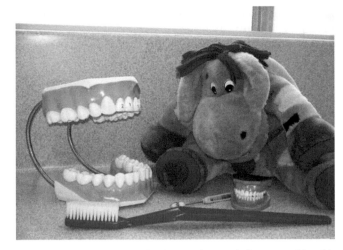

Figure 6.4 Various visual aids can be used during oral health promotion and education sessions.

Different resources include posters, leaflets, handouts, videos, films, tapes, blackboards, white boards and flipcharts. Exhibitions and displays may include oral health resources, such as mouth models and brushes (Figure 6.4). These can be obtained from dental companies, hospitals, dental surgeries and health promotion organisations. However, care must be taken whilst using material from dental companies, as they will contain advertising; target groups may be given the impression that the DCP are endorsing the dental companies' products.

Resources can also be made. Whatever the type and source, the educator needs to ensure that the resources are effective in order to engage to learner. Hence, important factors include the use of colour, writing, font and text. This should be bold so that they can be viewed from a distance.

Contrasting colours work well. The educator also needs to consider language, use of space, lighting and so on. These points are particularly important when setting up exhibitions and displays.

Evaluation

The DCP needs to ensure that the patient/group will change their behaviour in order to achieve good health, as a result of the OHP/OHE session. In order to determine that our teaching has been effective, the session needs to be evaluated. Of course as well as behaviour changes, the DCP can also assess whether the groups' attitude, knowledge, skills and behaviour have changed (Needs and Postans, 2006).

So what does evaluation actually mean? It means testing the effectiveness and the outcomes of a particular activity and whether they have actually worked. Why should the DCP evaluate oral health promotion interventions? Reasons include:

- Assess whether aims and objectives have been met.
- Determine whether OHP/OHE and health intervention has worked.
- Need to determine benefits of intervention.
- Improve health services.
- Demonstrate cost-effectiveness of interventions and determine future funding.
- Feedback to all involved staff.
- Determine process and delivery of OHP.
- Identify problems with any aspects of the OHP project.
- Inform policies.

The type of evaluation depends on the OHP activity. For example, a one-to-one oral hygiene session to a patient, can be evaluated by assessing their skills at the end of the session, along with their knowledge. The behaviour and attitude can be evaluated by quantitative measures, such as the recording of indices in the patient's notes, which can reflect improved gingival health and oral hygiene. Qualitative evaluation can include verbal discussion (Ewles and Simnett, 2003).

A health promotion session that is delivered to a group however, may require a more formal written evaluation at the end of a session. It could also involve a quiz, which can then determine the new acquired knowledge of the patient/group. OHP sessions/programmes on a larger scale, such as policies and legislation which facilitates social change, may require evaluation of the population. This takes time, even years and the evaluation has to be quite sophisticated.

A poster/exhibition may require written feedback with either open or closed questions, with a section for comments. It may be possible for some verbal feedback, which can be very valuable, although it should be done soon after the event. It does not however, allow the verbal feedback to be anonymous, if given to the actual OH promoters.

So, what specific methods can be used to determine the outcomes? The DCP could test people's knowledge as a result of the OHP by asking questions in a verbal or written form. The patients/clients could be formally or informally interviewed. They could be observed to see if they can demonstrate their new knowledge/skills. While designing the evaluation questionnaire, the DCP has to consider the proposed time required for the participant to complete it. Closed questions, which provide quantitative data and which give a yes, no, or don't know can quickly be filled in.

While qualitative questions are more time consuming to complete, they can give additional valuable feedback.

Whatever the design, the disadvantage's of obtaining feedback from questionnaires are that they require honesty from the participants, they rarely provide a 100% response rate and they are particularly time-consuming to design well. However, the DCP could encourage participants to complete the evaluation forms soon after the OHP, to ensure a high response. However, evaluation should not be narrow-minded and just focus on the end-result. Interventions need to be assessed for the actual process too. In other words, how were the outcomes achieved? Was it easy for people to achieve the outcomes? Was it expensive and were there any barriers to learning? The factors that may hinder health promotion have been considered, such as negative communication techniques and the psychology of the interaction between the educator and learner. From a learner's point of view, consider some scenarios whereby you thought it was a good session and why. Have you experienced a bad teaching session, if so, what could have been improved? The environment may hinder the OHP, such as poor seating, lighting, equipment, internal and/or external distractions and crowding. What was the relationship to the teacher? Was the speech delivery at the right pitch and pace? Were there pauses at the right times and was there a rapport between the teacher and learners or was the teacher dispassionate and disinterested? Also consider the actual presentation, sequence of information, learners' participation and use of resources.

Finally, it is a good idea to reflect/evaluate one's own practice as an educator, to determine what went well and/or what could be improved. This of course should be a continuous process, which may take weeks, months or even years, depending on the HP programme. It is also beneficial for the educator to be peer-reviewed, so that further recommendations can be put forward within a supportive framework.

Oral health promotion/education examples

In the dental surgery

- Given at the chairside, whilst treating patients. One-to-one session.
- Does not involve written aims and objectives and is therefore spontaneous.
- The information given is specific to that particular patient.
- OHE can involve oral hygiene demonstration within the patient's own mouth.
- The patient's own needs can be easily identified.
- Evaluation is more informal. The DCP can follow up changes in the patient's behaviour, attitude, knowledge and skills at the next appointment.

- Advice given to the patient should be written in the patient's notes. This should also include recommendations for specific oral hygiene aids, techniques and whether a practical demonstration was given.
- Evaluation can be followed up at the next patient visit. It may be helpful to repeat the key messages. Motivating the patient and continuing support is important.
- Use appropriate language for specific patients. Consider different approaches for different groups of patients, for example the use of a interpreter.
- A wide range of visual aids and written material may support the oral health messages. Ensure advice given is evidence-based.

Nurseries

- Preschool children aged 0–5 years. Therefore there is a variation of oral health messages, due to the age and parental control.
- Involves aims and objectives.
- More detailed advice is given to parents/carers of the children while simple delivery of OHP/OHE is given to the preschool children.
- The session is interactive for children. They enjoy stories and dressing up.
- The DCP needs to educate parents/carers on diet, such as the reduction of sugars, sugary/erosive drinks and the reduction of pacifiers. The DCP has to be aware that some children may not like milk, pacifiers may be needed to manage behaviour of a child, and bottles may be seen less messy than cups.
- Hence, the DCP can influence the parent/carer by educating on the side effects of these habits, such an increased risk of caries, affected speech and appearance.
- Avoid using too much medical jargon, keep the information straightforward and be aware of ethnic differences.
- Evaluation can be carried out by nursery staff and/or parents/carers.

School-age children/adolescents

- Age group ranges from 5–16 years old. Therefore, different approaches are needed for the wide age range.
- Consider influences on oral health and diet choices. There is a move from parental control to a more independent child, who has particular choices. As the child becomes older, he/she may conform to peer pressure. This does not always comply with the advice given to them from parents/carers and authority figures.
- Involves aims and objectives.

- The younger age group is still receptive to advice and particularly enjoy interactive activities such as games, simple quizzes and dressing up. They will have some simple knowledge of teeth. This knowledge increases as the child gets older.
- Activities for the older groups include simple experiments such as the effect of dietary acid on teeth, oral hygiene techniques, the structure and function of teeth using 3D models and using actual food samples to demonstrate healthy options versus food containing sugar. Other examples may involve worksheets and word search.
- Therefore, the DCP should check the educational syllabus to determine existing knowledge. The supervising teacher could also be approached to determine what activities the children have carried out regards oral health.
- Preplanning the teaching session is paramount.
- Evaluation can be carried out by the target group using various methods.

Nursing/residential homes

- The target group may have a different range of capabilities, understanding and oral health needs.
- Some residents may be either completely edentulous, partially or fully dentate.
- Some residents may not have control over their oral hygiene or diet. They may have to rely on nursing support for oral hygiene, while regular medication may also contain sugar.
- Oral hygiene habits may not have changed from childhood. Therefore behaviour is firmly established.
- Older people may have lower expectations regarding their oral health. Therefore this and other physical factors such as poor manual dexterity, poor co-ordination and poor eyesight may contribute to declining oral health.
- Aims and objectives may be written to target residents or to the staff.
- Topics include oral hygiene, denture care, diet and caries and periodontal disease.
- Teaching activities could include demonstrations on models, cleaning dentures and videos/DVD's to demonstrate oral hygiene methods. Adaptation of toothbrushes could be highlighted to enable the older person to grasp the brush in order to facilitate toothbrushing.

Exhibitions

- Range from a simple poster to a more interactive team-approach.
- Exhibitions are a very good approach to promote public awareness of oral health. Such examples in the

UK include 'Smile Month', 'Oral Cancer Awareness' and 'National No Smoking Day'.

- Topics include smoking cessation, oral hygiene advice, use of fluoride, oral cancer awareness, periodontal disease, diet and dental caries. Different aspects of dentistry and associated oral hygiene care can be highlighted, such as orthodontics, prosthetics and implants.
- Target groups could include mothers, pregnant women, children, elderly, groups with specific health problems and ethnic groups.
- The display should be bold and catch the audience's attention. Colours should be contrasting, ensure a striking heading and a large font. The material should be organised in order of importance.
- Resources include leaflets, posters, table displays and videos.
- Activities could include drawing competitions, guessing the number of toothpastes or toothbrushes in a container, practical demonstrations of oral hygiene and experiments to demonstrate amount of sugar in food.

The above examples highlight the variance of needs, type and amount of dental education and activities. It is paramount that the educator delivers evidence-based information. *The Scientific Basis of Oral Health Education* (Levine and Stillman-Lowe, 2009) delivers four long-standing key messages:

1 Diet – to reduce the consumption and frequency of drinks, confectionary and foods with sugars.
2 Toothbrushing – thoroughly twice every day with a fluoride toothpaste.
3 Fluoride – includes water fluoridation to enable a safe and effective public health measure.
4 Dental attendance – an oral examination to be carried out every year, although patients who are at risk from dental disease may be required to attend more frequently.

Conclusion

The main points of OHE are:-

- To plan the teaching sessions accordingly.
- The information given should be evidence-based and up to date.
- The educator should be aware of his/her communication techniques and how this may influence the patients.
- It is also important to constantly encourage, empower and support patients in the acquisition of their new skills.

- Teaching sessions should be evaluated so that teaching practices are constantly updated and improved.

References

Becker, M.H. (ed) (1974) *The Health Belief Model and Personal Health Behaviour*. Charles B. Slack, New Jersey.

Bradshaw, J. (1972) The concept of social need. *New Society*, **30 March**, 640–643.

Department of Health (2004) *Choosing Health; Making Healthier Choices Easier*. Department of Health, London.

Department of Health/British Association for the Study of Community Dentistry. (2009) *Delivering Better Oral Health; An Evidence-Based Toolkit*, 2nd edition. Department of Health, London.

Department of Health/Dental and Ophthalmic Services Division (2005) *Choosing Better Oral Health; An Oral Health Plan for England*. Department of Health, London.

Ewles, L. and Simnett, I. (2003) *Promoting Health; A practical guide*, 5th edition. Baillière Tindall, Edinburgh.

Kay, E.J. and Tinsley, S.R. (2004) *Communication and the Dental Team*. Stephen Hancocks Ltd, London.

Lalonde, M. (1974) *A New Perspective on the Health of Canadians*. Ministry of Supply and Services, Ottawa.

Levine, R.S. and Stillman-Lowe, C.R. (2009) *The Scientific Basis of Oral Health Education. A Policy Document* , 6th edition. British Dental Journal Books, London.

Munday, P., Plimley, W. and Stillman-Lowe, C. (1999) A guide to policy development within pre-school settings. In Watt, R.A (ed.) *A guide to Effective Working in Pre-School Settings*. Health Education Authority, London, pp. 30–31.

Needs, K. and Postans, J. (2006) Oral health education and promotion. In Ireland. R. (ed.) *Clinical Textbook of Dental Hygiene and Therapy*. Blackwell Munksgaard, Oxford.

Peterson, P.E. (2008) World Health Organization Global Policy for Improvement of Oral Health – World Health Assembly 2007. *International Dental Journal* **58**, 115–121.

Prochaska, J.O. and DiClemente, C.C. (1984) Self-change processes, self efficacy and decisional balance across five stages of smoking cessation. *Progress in Clinical and Biological Research*, **156**, 131–140.

Seedhouse, D. (2001) *Health; The Foundations for Achievement*, 2nd edition. John Wiley & Sons, Ltd, Chichester.

Watt, R.G. (2005) Strategies and approaches in oral disease prevention and health promotion. *Bulletin of the World Health Organization* **83**(9).

World Health Organization (1946) Preamble to the Constitution of the World Health Organization as adopted by the International Health Conference, New York, 19 June–22 July 1946.

World Health Organization (WHO) (1977, 1985) *Health for All by the Year 2000*, WHO, Geneva.

World Health Organization (WHO) (1986) *Ottawa Charter for Health Promotion*. WHO, Geneva.

World Health Organization (WHO) (1997) *The Jakarta Declaration on Health Promotion into the 21st Century*. WHO, Geneva.

World Health Organization (WHO) (2003) *The World Oral Health Report; continuous improvement of oral health in the 21st century – the approach of the WHO Global Oral Health Programme*. WHO, Geneva.

7

Diet and nutrition

Suzanne L. Noble

Summary

This chapter covers:

- The components of a balanced diet
- The dietary requirements of groups of people with special needs
- The relationship between diet and dental caries
- The relationship between diet and dental erosion
- Antioxidants and periodontal diseases
- The role of the dental hygienist and therapist in dietary advice and counselling

Introduction

Diet

In general, the term diet refers to food and drink consumption (*diaita* (Greek) 'way of life'). The type of food and the amount eaten is an environmental factor in the aetiology of several diseases and variations in the morbidity and mortality between the world's populations. More specifically the term diet is used to refer to a prescribed course of eating and drinking for therapeutic benefit. This involves regulation of the quantity, timing and category of food and drink, either under professional guidance or self regulated.

Nutrition

Nutrition refers to a process by which living organisms physiologically absorb and metabolise food to ensure growth, energy production, repair of tissue and ultimately reproduction of the species (*nutritio* (Latin) 'to nourish') (Macpherson, 1995). The intake of the appropriate requirements is essential for survival. According to **Maslow's hierarchy of needs** (cited in Naidoo and Wills, 1998), basic physiological needs, such as hunger or thirst, must be satisfied first before an individual can find self-fulfilment. The science of nutrition includes the study of diets and dietary diseases.

The relationship between diet and disease

A **'balanced'** diet refers to the minimum consumption of nutrients to provide the essential requirements of the body. Deficiency states, whilst no longer an overt problem in developed countries, continue to cause disease states in underdeveloped countries, due to famine or war. Where one or more of the essential nutrients are absent in the diet or there is inadequate absorption from the gastrointestinal tract, this is referred to as **malnutrition**.

Conversely, the majority of diet-related health problems in developed countries relate to excessive intake of essential and non-essential food and drink. Excessive consumption of refined carbohydrates, saturated fats, salt and alcohol have been linked to obesity, cardiovascular disease, high blood pressure, type 2 diabetes, dental caries and certain cancers. Obesity and malnutrition may occur in the same individual. Health promotion in affluent nations, in which these dietary components are freely available, is aimed at awareness and empowerment of the individual to eat a 'healthy' diet, i.e. one in which the essential nutrients are present but not consumed to excess. Education concerning obesity should be focused on awareness that food consumption must match physical activity. Current trends indicate that a third of the adult population will be obese by 2020. The dietary requirements of an individual throughout life are dependent upon the energy and growth requirements, for example during pregnancy, lactation and childhood. In addition the degree of physical activity and concomitant disease status must be considered. The 'balance' in the diet must take into account the dynamics of the human being.

Consumption of energy – basal metabolic rate

When the body is at rest a minimum amount of energy is needed to regulate involuntary life processes, such as:

- Respiration.
- Circulation.
- Digestion.

The basal metabolic rate (BMR) is measured by the amount of oxygen inhaled compared to the amount of carbon dioxide excreted. It is usually higher in women than in men.

Total energy output is made up of:

- BMR (70%).
- Physical activity.
- Thermogenesis.

Thermogenesis is the increase in energy output in response to food intake, cold exposure and psychological influences.

In general obese people have a higher BMR and total energy output than lean people. Obesity is graded according to a person's weight in kilograms, divided by their height in metres squared, and is known as the body mass index (Table 7.1). Obese people do not appear to have a reduced capacity for thermogenesis.

Energy is measured in calories:

- **Gram calorie** (cal): the amount of heat required to raise 1 g of water 1 °C in temperature.
- **Kilocalorie** (kcal): the amount of heat required to raise 1 kg of water 1 °C in temperature.

In the moderately active woman, the BMR accounts for 1500 kcal a day out of a total daily energy expenditure of about 2300 kcal. For an average man the

Table 7.1 Classification of obesity.

Grade of obesity	Ratio of weight in kilograms (w) to height in metres (h), squared (w/h²)
III	>40
II	30–40
I	25–29.9
Not obese	<25

BMR accounts for 1600 kcal out of a total energy expenditure of 2500 kcal. Hence the proportion of energy expenditure by the BMR is approximately two thirds of the total.

The process whereby the energy derived from food products is made available to the various forms of work required by the body is known as **metabolism**. This can be subdivided into two separate processes:

- **Anabolism**: the constructive chemical and physical processes by which food materials are adapted for use by our body, e.g. amino acids to build proteins.
- **Catabolism**: the destructive process by which energy is produced with the breaking down of tissue into waste products.

Sources of energy are fat (9 kcal/g), alcohol (7 kcal/g), protein (4 kcal/g) and carbohydrates (3.75 kcal/g).

The current national dietary recommendations

A 'balanced' diet should include the following nutritional groups:

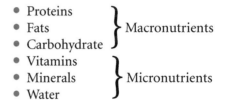

- Proteins
- Fats   } Macronutrients
- Carbohydrate
- Vitamins
- Minerals   } Micronutrients
- Water

Dietary standards have been used in Britain since the 19th century and are published to improve the health of the nation. The recommended daily amount (RDA) dates back to 1979 and was meant to be applied to groups of people to minimise the risk of undernutrition and was set high compared with the average requirement. The Committee on Medical Aspects of Food Policy's (COMA) Panel on Dietary Reference Values published their report in 1991. **Dietary reference values** apply to healthy people rather than those with diseases. The reader is recommended to review *Scientific Basis of Nutritional Education: a Synopsis of Dietary Values* (Health Education Authority, 1992), for specific detail, but dietary reference values are an estimate of the range of requirements of nutrients for a population or group and are intended for guidance. Such guidance is required for a scientific basis for food counselling, meal provision and food labelling. In this chapter the dietary reference values are given for the macronutrients. For the micronutrients the **reference nutrient intake** (RNI) is used, which represents the amount of nutrient which is sufficient for almost all individuals.

Macronutrients

Carbohydrates

Carbohydrates contain carbon, hydrogen and oxygen with the formula $C_n(H_2O)_n$. The term is applied because the hydrogen and oxygen are in the proportion to form water (hydrates). They should be the major source of energy in the diet (55%). They are broken down by enzymes to form simple sugars. Carbohydrates are stored in liver and muscle as glycogen, but excess is converted into fat for storage.

Carbohydrates can be classified as follows:

- Sugars: should make up no more than 15% of the carbohydrate intake and can be subdivided into monosaccharides and disaccharides.
- Polysaccharides: do not have the crystalline form of sugar, and are used in the human diet as a source of starch and roughage.

Consumption of sugars (**refined carbohydrates**) is a major aetiological feature in dental caries and is discussed later. A classification of carbohydrates and dietary sources is given in Table 7.2.

The glycaemic index (GI)

The glycaemic index measures the rate at which glucose is absorbed through the intestine and its subsequent level in the blood. It runs from 0 to 100. The rate at which pure glucose is absorbed and raises the blood glucose level is given a score of 100. All other carbohydrate products are measured against this:

- High-GI foods: 70+.
- Medium-GI foods: 56–69.
- Low-GI foods: <55.

High-GI foods trigger the release of insulin for the removal of excess glucose from the blood for storage as glycogen or fat. Excess insulin is produced in response to a diet high in high-GI foods. Insulin excess creates hunger pangs and the desire to overeat. Low-GI foods are digested slowly and raise glucose level in the blood by a small amount, and hence only low levels of insulin are produced and the body feels satisfied for longer. Table 7.3 gives examples of high-, medium- and low-GI foods.

Fats (lipids)

Fats in the diet should be called lipids. They are a more concentrated source of energy than carbohydrates. They should make up no more than 30% of the diet of which a maximum 10% should be saturated fats.

Animal fat is a mixture of triglycerides:

- Stearic acid + glycerol.
- Plasmatic acid.
- Oleic acid.

Animal fats and dairy products are saturated fats. They are solid at room temperature. Vegetable oils are unsaturated fats, are liquid at room temperature and include soya bean, maize and sunflower. Fish oils are also unsaturated (e.g. cod liver oil).

The functions of fat are as follows:

- Energy source.
- Cushion to protect vital organs.
- Insulates the body by forming a layer under the skin.
- Carrier of fat-soluble vitamins A, D, E and K and carotene.
- Maintenance of cell membranes.
- Production of hormones, e.g. oestrogen.

Table 7.2 Classification of carbohydrates and dietary sources.

Type	Example	Dietary source
Monosaccharide	Glucose	Honey
	Fructose	Fruit
Disaccharide	Sucrose	Cane sugar, beet sugar, molasses, confectionery
	Maltose	Beer, cereal, barley
	Lactose	Milk
Polysaccharide	Starch	Rice, potatoes, pasta, bread cereals
	Cellulose	Skins of fruit and vegetables (indigestible but provide roughage)

Table 7.3 High, medium, and low glycaemic index foods.

High	Medium	Low
Cornflakes	Granary bread	Bran
Biscuits	Pitta bread	Oats
Baguettes	Basmati rice	All beans except
Cakes	Fruit yoghurt	broad beans
White bread	Low-fat ice cream	Barley
Rice	Bananas	Cottage cheese
Butter	Eggs	Milk
Cheese		Herbal tea
Cream		Unsweetened juices
Alcohol		Decaffeinated coffee
Soft fizzy drinks		Most fruits
Sausages		Lean meat
Bacon		Vegetables
Confectionery		
Potatoes		

Cholesterol

Cholesterol is a sterol, a waxy material derived from animal and vegetable tissues. It is essential in the body to the production of sex hormones and for repair of membranes. It is found in the brain, nervous tissue, adrenal glands and skin. Dietary sources are red meat, egg yolks and butter.

A high blood cholesterol level (i.e. >6 mmol/l), is correlated with **atheroma**, which is associated with coronary thrombosis, high blood pressure and strokes. The liver can produce all the bodily requirements for cholesterol, but a high consumption of saturated fats leads to high blood levels of circulatory cholesterol.

Proteins

Proteins consist of chains of **amino acids**, linked together. Proteins constitute an essential part of the diet as a source of energy and for replacement and repair of tissues. Proteins contain nitrogen, which is an essential constituent of the body.

Proteins should make up about 12% of the diet. To be digested, proteins have to be broken down into the constituent amino acids. The adult human requires eight amino acids which it cannot produce or store and these are known as essential amino acids (Table 7.4). The body can produce non-essential amino acids, but a diet of mixed proteins is recommended for health. Protein for vegetarians is available as nuts, Quorn (yeast) and pulses. Examples of pulses are peas, beans and lentils. The soya bean is high in protein, and is available as tofu (soybean curd) and miso (fermented bean paste).

The functions of proteins are:

- Growth, repair and maintenance.
- Energy source (after carbohydrates).
- Production of hormones and enzymes.

Micronutrients

Vitamins

Vitamin is a term that applies to a group of substances which are required in small amounts and are essential for growth and development. They exist in natural foods but most have been produced synthetically. The absence of vitamins leads to certain dietary diseases and growth retardation (Figures 7.1, 7.2 and 7.3). Many vitamins are coenzymes, which have an essential function in a chemical reaction catalysed by a specific enzyme. Vitamins are

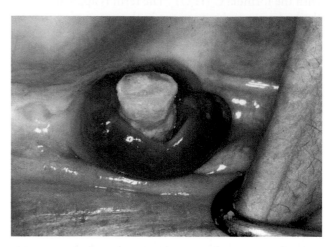

Figure 7.1 Oral scurvy: a manifestation of vitamin C deficiency.

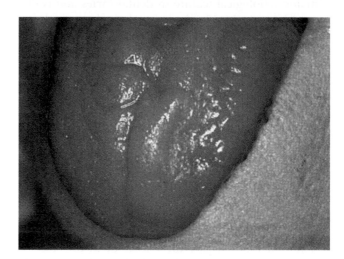

Figure 7.2 Lobulated tongue in folate deficiency.

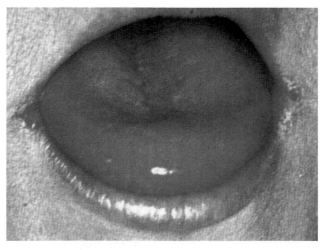

Figure 7.3 Angular cheilitis, a sign of deficiency of the B vitamins, iron and folate.

Table 7.4 Sources of essential amino acids.

Sources of all eight amino acids	Sources of some of the essential amino acids
Beef	Nuts
Eggs	Vegetables
Soya	Grains
Cows' milk	Barley
Fish	Wheat
	Oats

classified into fat-soluble A, D, E, K and water-soluble B complex and C. Table 7.5 outlines sources of vitamins, their function and deficiency states, including those of oral relevance.

Vitamins and antioxidant activity

Carotenes, including beta-carotene, vitamin C and vitamin E, are among the many substances in food that have antioxidant properties. This attribute can help to counter the effects of reactive oxygen species (free radicals) which are produced by the body's normal metabolic processes. If they accumulate they can damage key cellular molecules, such as DNA and proteins. Cells with damaged DNA may be more prone to developing cancer. Free radicals readily oxidise polyunsaturated fatty acids in food and in cell membranes in the body to give lipid peroxides which can also damage cells. Peroxides, for example those formed by the oxidation of low-density lipoprotein (LDL) cholesterol, may play a part in the formation of the 'plaque' which can build up on the walls of the arteries and eventually cause heart disease.

People who consume large amounts of yellow fruits and dark green or orange vegetables seem to be less prone to some forms of cancer. Beta-carotene (but not

Table 7.5 Sources of vitamins, their functions and deficiency states including those of oral relevance.

Vitamin	RNI/day	Source	Function	Deficiency	Oral relevance
A Retinol	700 µg	Liver, kidney, fish liver oils, eggs, cheese and added to margarine. In precursor form in carrots and dark green and yellow vegetables	Epithelial differentiation	Night blindness Xerophthalmia	Keratosis of mucous membrane, impaired salivary flow, enamel hypoplasia
B1 Thiamine	1.0 mg	Yeast extract, cereals, fortified flour, eggs	Coenzyme in energy metabolism	Beri-beri	Burning mouth, reduced taste perception
B2 Riboflavin	1.3 mg	Yeast extract, dairy products, whole grains	Coenzyme in energy metabolism		Angular cheilitis, glossitis, aphthous ulcers
B3 Niacin	17 mg	Yeast extract, eggs, liver	Coenzyme in energy metabolism	Pellagra	Glossitis, angular cheilitis, mucosal atrophy
B6 Pyridoxine	1.4 mg	Liver, meat, grains, milk, peanuts	Coenzyme in amino acid metabolism	Peripheral neuropathy, depression	Glossitis, ulceration, burning mouth, lip inflammation
B12 Cobalamin	1.5 mg	Liver, kidney, eggs, milk	Coenzyme, needed for haemoglobin and essential for cellular function	Pernicious anaemia	Atrophy, glossitis, aphthous ulcers, angular cheilitis
B Complex Folic Acid	200 µg	Yeast, kidney, liver, green leafy vegetables	As B12	Megaloblastic anaemia	Aphthous ulceration, papillae atrophy of tongue
Biotin		Egg yolk, kidney, liver, yeast, nuts	Coenzyme	Fatigue, nausea, muscle pains/scaly skin	Glossitis, mucosal soreness, swollen and sore tongue
Pantothenic Acid		As other B vitamins	Coenzyme	Rare	
C Ascorbic Acid	40 mg	Green vegetables/citrus fruits, blackcurrants, tomatoes	Antioxidant, collagen production	Scurvy	Gingivitis/periodontitis, aphthous ulcers, impaired wound healing
D Calciferol	10 µg	Fish oils, margarine, eggs, sunlight on skin	Controls calcium and phosphorus in blood	Rickets and osteomalacia	Enamel and dentine hypoplasia
E Tocopherols		Vegetable oil/seeds/grains	Antioxidant	Malfunction of reproduction	None
K Coagulation		Spinach, cabbage, liver, gut bacteria	Production of clotting factors	Rare	Gingival bleeding

From Health Education Authority in: *Scientific Basis of Nutritional Education: A Synopsis of Dietary Reference Values* (1996), pp. 14–31. Reproduced with permission. © Crown Copyright.

preformed vitamin A) may play a role in the body's natural defence mechanism against cancer by helping to destroy reactive oxygen species, but more research is needed to clarify this.

Vitamin C may also form part of the body's defence against the harmful effects of reactive oxygen species. It may work directly by destroying free radicals, indirectly by helping to reactivate vitamin E, or in both of these ways. Research is continuing into the possible role of vitamin C in the prevention of heart disease and cancer.

Alpha-tocopherol (and to a lesser extent other tocopherols) can help prevent the oxidation of LDL and the formation of free radicals that may damage cells and cause heart disease.

People at risk of vitamin deficiency

These include:

- Anorexics and bulimics.
- People suffering from Crohn's disease and other intestinal diseases affecting absorption of nutrients.
- Vegans and vegetarians.
- Low socioeconomic groups.
- The elderly.
- People with liver disease, including alcoholics.

Vitamin supplements – are they necessary?

Most people should be able to obtain their vitamin requirements by eating a healthy balanced diet. Vitamins are only needed by the body in small amounts and high doses can be harmful. Taking vitamin supplements is not a substitute for an unhealthy diet. Fruit and vegetables are a good source of water-soluble vitamins but they also contain fibre and antioxidants, which are not provided by a vitamin tablet. There is currently no evidence that vitamins prevent colds and, until such time as the evidence proves that vitamin supplements are beneficial to the healthy person, they are best avoided. Some groups, such as pregnant women, vegans, etc., may benefit after consultation with a physician.

Minerals

Minerals are inorganic substances, which are required in the structural composition of the hard and soft body tissues. They also participate in the contraction of muscles, nerve conduction and blood clotting. They are classified into major and minor (or trace) elements. Table 7.6 gives sources of minerals, their function and deficiency states, including those of oral relevance.

Water

Water is not formally a nutrient but additional sources of water are essential in the diet. As 65% of body weight is water, a 10% loss can cause metabolic problems or even death. The recommended daily intake is 1–2 litres and the body can only survive a few days without water. There is increased demand in hot climates, following strenuous exercise, in times of fever and in diarrhoea and vomiting. It has become fashionable to drink bottled water which may be carbonated at source or by the

Table 7.6 Sources of minerals, their function and deficiency states, including those of oral relevance. Minor elements include copper, zinc, fluorine, chromium, molybdenum and selenium, which are components of many enzymes and are essential in trace amounts.

Mineral	RNI/day	Source	Function	Deficiency	Oral relevance
Sodium	1600 mg	Table salt, excessive amounts in processed food, bread	Fluid balance	Muscle cramps	
Calcium	700 mg	Milk, cabbage, figs, wholemeal bread	Formation of bones and teeth. Stored in skeleton	Osteoporosis, tetany	Hypoplasia, and deficiency during tooth development
Phosphorus	625 mg	Milk and wide distribution	As for calcium, energy metabolism	Rare	
Magnesium	270 mg	Vegetables	Nerve and muscle activity	Tremors and convulsions	
Iron	14 mg	Meat, fish, dark green vegetables, pulses	Haemoglobin and myoglobin formation	Anaemia	Glossitis, angular cheilitis, candidiasis
Iodine	140 µg	Water, added to table salt	Thyroxin synthesis	Thyroid goitre, hypothyroidism in infants	
Potassium	3500 mg	Widely found	Nerve and muscle activity	?excessive use of diuretics	

From Health Education Authority in: *Scientific Basis of Nutritional Education: A Synopsis of Dietary Reference Values* (1996), pp. 14–31. Reproduced with permission. © Crown Copyright.

manufacturer before bottling. Mineral waters contain calcium, hydrogen sulphide and sodium. People with oedema, high blood pressure or heart diseases should check the sodium levels of bottled water. Excessive intake of carbonated water may lead to enamel erosion.

The functions of water in the body are:

- A carrier of nutrients and waste products to and from cells.
- Helps regulate body temperature.
- Essential to digestion and metabolism.
- Lubricates the joints, nervous system and eyes and aids respiration.

Summary

In summary, the **Food Standards Agency** (FSA) states that the key to a healthy diet is to eat a variety of foods, which for most people means eating:

- More fruit and vegetables.
- More bread, cereals and potatoes.
- Less fat, sugar and salt.
- A third of their diet made up from bread and cereals, choosing wholegrain, wholemeal, brown or 'high-fibre' varieties whenever possible.
- At least five portions of fruit and vegetables every day, including fresh, frozen, tinned, dried or juiced. Fruit and vegetables should make up about a third of food eaten each day.
- A moderate amount of meat, fish and alternatives such as pulses, eggs, nuts and beans, choosing lower-fat versions when possible. At least two portions of fish per week should be eaten, one of which should be oily fish.
- Less fatty and sugary foods and drinks, such as margarine, butter, cream, chocolate and biscuits, soft drinks, sweets, jam, cakes and ice cream.
- Milk, cheese, yoghurt, fromage frais and other dairy products in moderate amounts, choosing lower-fat varieties whenever possible.
- Less salty foods. Most adults are eating too much (on average 9 g of salt per day (two teaspoonfuls) which should be reduced to less than 6 g). Most (about 75%) of the salt in our diets comes from processed foods.

Alcohol

Alcohol has no nutritional value and is a drug. If it is drunk to excess it may be a contributory factor in systemic and oral diseases. The reader is directed to Chapter 11, p. 236 for further details.

Figure 7.4 is a pictorial representation of a balanced diet, published by the **Health Education Authority**.

Dietary requirements of groups with special needs

Pregnancy and lactation

A woman's nutritional needs increase during pregnancy and lactation. This is necessary to provide for the development of the child and to meet the physiological changes of the mother's body. These need to be provided by an increased intake of essential carbohydrates, proteins, iron, calcium and folates and vitamins C and D. In the final 3 months of pregnancy, an additional 200 kcal are required daily, and in lactation 500 kcal extra a day. There is some evidence that vitamin D deficiency in pregnancy can cause enamel hypoplasia and thus predispose to caries in the deciduous dentition (Rugg-Gunn, 1993). In the case of calcium deficiency in the mother, calcium cannot be removed from the calcified tissues of her teeth, and any increase in caries is due to a high-sucrose diet. Vomiting in early pregnancy is a frequent symptom and the dental hygienist/therapist has a role to play in giving advice about the avoidance of dental erosion.

Weaning

Good nutrition is essential to the development of the primary and secondary dentitions. Solid food is usually introduced at 3 months and before 6 months of age. Breast-fed babies tend to have a lower dental caries experience than bottle-fed babies. Milk has a low cariogenicity factor but if mothers add sugar to the bottle or supplement the bottle with reservoir feeders containing fruit syrup, there is a strong relationship between their use and the incidence of dental caries (Rugg-Gunn, 1993). Comforters must not be dipped in sugary foods (Figure 7.5). If the child uses either of these methods as a comforter before bedtime the risk of caries will increase because the secretion of the salivary buffers will decrease during sleep.

Diet and nutrition do not influence teething but the child may benefit from biting on hard sugar-free foods to gain some relief from symptoms. It is important to develop good dietary habits during the weaning period, to reduce the frequency of sucrose-containing drinks and snacks and hence establish patterns of eating behaviour which will benefit both general and dental health.

Food intolerances

Certain foods may lead to **hypersensitivity** in some people, and such reactions may be acute, leading to **anaphylactic shock**. These reactions to substances such as peanuts, eggs and shellfish may be sudden and total, following contact with a mere trace of the substance.

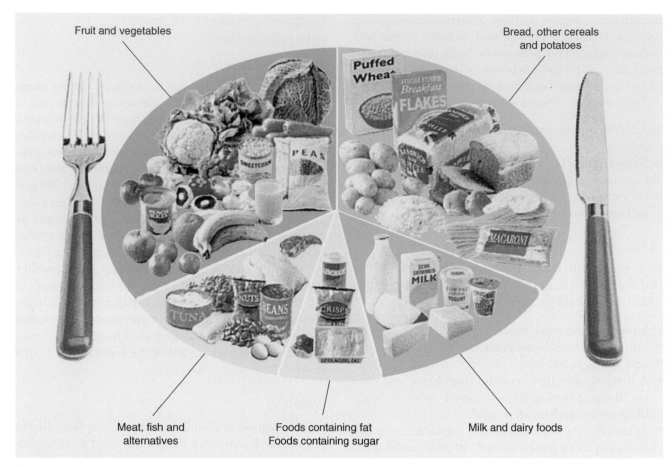

Fruit and vegetables

Bread, other cereals and potatoes

Meat, fish and alternatives

Foods containing fat
Foods containing sugar

Milk and dairy foods

Figure 7.4 Pictorial representation of a balanced diet.

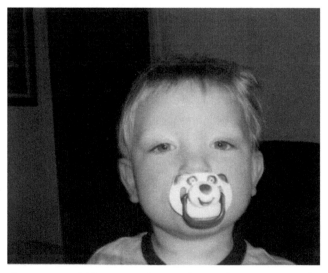

Figure 7.5 Child with comforter. The comforter must not be dipped in sugary foods.

This allergy may be revealed in the medical history, and should always be documented in the case record. Patients may also have intolerance to certain foods, leading to symptoms of arthritis, irritable bowel syndrome, headaches and hyperactivity. Such food intolerance may only be detected by an elimination process until symptoms no longer exist. The following are foods known to cause food intolerance: gluten, wheat, dairy produce and food colourings and flavourings.

The elderly

The energy requirements of individuals will vary according to their lifestyle and state of health. The housebound and frail elderly will be most at risk from malnutrition. From an oral perspective, as more elderly people retain their natural dentition, dietary advice is an important aspect in disease prevention. Economic problems, loneliness and lack of agility can all lead to the tendency to eat a diet high in refined carbohydrates, which is easy to prepare and chew. This, accompanied by hyposalivation, decreased oral clearance time, decreased manual dexterity for plaque removal and exposure of root surfaces, can lead to the development of primary carious lesions in the individual. This group is second only to children in caries incidence. This may also go undiagnosed due to lack of regular attendance at the dentist. Subsequent loss of teeth brings renewed problems, not only in inefficient mastication of food, but the teeth affected may support a denture, in which case both function and aesthetics may be compromised. These factors can lead to social isolation in the elderly, where eating is one of life's remaining pleasures!

Vegetarianism and veganism

This is the principle of restricting the diet, for health or humanitarian reasons, to foods of fruit or vegetable origin. Vegetarians exclude meat, fish and foods of animal origin. Veganism is a strict form of vegetarianism which excludes dairy produce, eggs and cheese.

Vegetarians must find alternative sources of protein such as soya and iron. B12 deficiency can also be a problem. Glossitis, aphthous ulceration and angular cheilitis can be signs of such deficiencies. Vegetarians may have objections to certain medications, derived from animal sources, such as bovine gelatine used in **Periochip**.

The effect of ethnicity and culture on nutrition

In a multicultural contemporary society, the health educator must have an understanding of the culture and religious practices which affect food choices. The selection and preparation of certain foods is an important aspect of religious beliefs, for example in Judaism, Christianity, Islam, Hinduism and Buddhism. These religions include days of fasting and feasting during which the religious laws must be followed. **Ethnicity** refers to culturally distinct groups, and it is different from race, which is genetically determined. Certain dietary preferences are associated with identified ethnic groups and the educator should be aware of the differences between their own culture and that of the client to whom dietary advice is being offered. Amongst the main Asian groups, for example, chapattis or rice are the staple cereal and ghee the main fat source. Certain meats, such as beef or pork, are prohibited and Muslims eat Halal meat only. Pulses are a major protein source and dairy products and vegetable curries are important. The reader is advised to refer to specific texts which cover dietary preferences and ethnicity in more detail (Kouba, 2005).

Dietary needs in specific states of disease

Diabetes mellitus

In both type 1 and type 2 diabetes the intake of dietary sugar has to be controlled. In type 1, it is important that carbohydrate intake is balanced with therapeutic insulin, otherwise the patient becomes hypoglycaemic. For this reason diabetic patients are advised to carry food and drink with them that can liberate glucose quickly when required. This should not be a problem in causing dental caries, because it is an occasional rather than a regular occurrence. Diabetics are encouraged to maintain a stable blood glucose level and monitor this for themselves.

The hospitalised and terminally ill

When individuals are unable to have their nutritional requirements fulfilled by a traditional diet, commercial supplements are available. These may be in liquid or powder form to prevent the consequences of malnutrition. These are known as essential multivitamin supplements and are used as sip feeds and as tube feeds. They supply all the macronutrients, energy, protein, fat, carbohydrates, vitamins and minerals and trace elements required.

Examples of patients who may need these supplements are cancer patients, who may be suffering from malabsorption due to radiotherapy or chemotherapy; patients with chronic neurological diseases, such as motor neurone disease; patients with chronic inflammatory bowel disorders; stroke patients; acquired immune deficiency syndrome patients; and the sick and elderly. The sip feeds, such as Fortisip (BNF, 2009), contain 300 kcal/200 ml, and the patients are encouraged to sip these throughout the day. The frequent exposure in the diet to the high sugar content of these drinks is a primary cause of dental caries in these individuals, who are least able to tolerate dental treatment.

The principles behind the dietary control of dental caries

The disease of dental caries has a multifactorial aetiology, requiring a dynamic interaction between the factors to result in the lesion of dental caries affecting the tooth surface. One of these factors is the substrate for the growth and metabolism by the bacteria. The substrate is referred to as **fermentable carbohydrates** because of the ability of cariogenic bacteria to metabolise them quickly, resulting in a rapid drop in plaque pH, with a potential to cause demineralisation of tooth enamel over time. Whilst in theory, removal of any of the aetiological factors will prevent dental caries, the control of the bacterial substrate is the most feasible and potentially manageable (Moynihan et al., 2003). These low molecular weight carbohydrates, the sugars (especially sucrose), are readily available in processed foods and as table sugars and are an integral part of Western diet. It is the role of the health educator to inform the public about potential harmful effects, and to motivate behavioural change based on scientific evidence. The evidence is produced as a result of studies with which the reader is advised to be familiar in order to substantiate the oral health messages.

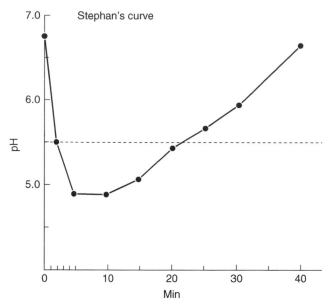

Figure 7.6 Stephan's curve. Rinsing with a 10% glucose solution produces a fall in pH which is plotted against time. The pH of 5.5 is known as the 'critical pH', below which the enamel has the potential to dissolve. (Reproduced with permission from Rugg-Gunn and Nunn (1999) *Nutrition, Diet and Oral Health*, Oxford University Press.)

The sugars diffuse readily into the plaque, causing a drop in pH within 2–5 minutes, which takes 30–60 minutes to be neutralised by the buffers in saliva. *Streptococcus mutans* strains are cariogenic because they synthesise extracellular polysaccharides from dietary sugars which add bulk and adherent properties to the plaque. This therefore increases the time component of the aetiological factors, in that, because the neutralisation effect of the saliva is prolonged, the potential for demineralisation by acids is increased. This forms the basis of the message that frequent consumption of sugar has the potential to cause dental caries. **Stephan** described this in 1944, in studies in which subjects rinsed with glucose and the pH was plotted against time (Figure 7.6).

In Stephan's studies different response rates were noted in subjects with sound occlusal surfaces, compared with those with inactive and active carious cavities. Lower pH values were recorded for longer in plaque within cavities, compared with plaque on inactive lesions or sound surfaces. Subjects with existing lesions therefore have the potential to develop additional lesions (Johansson and Birkhed, 1994).

Studies substantiating the role of sugars in dental caries

Various types of investigations have been undertaken to contribute to the evidence linking dietary sugars to dental caries. In summary, the following types are cited:

- **Clinical trials**: these are epidemiological studies in which the diets of groups of people are purposefully altered and the effect observed. These trials provide the most reliable source of evidence.
- **Observational studies**: these are epidemiological studies in which the relationship between the disease and the possible factors is observed. These are the second best source of evidence and often carried out because interventional studies are difficult to undertake due to the fact that they are ethically unacceptable and lengthy.
- **Animal studies**: rats, hamsters and monkeys have all been used to study the effect of sugar on the dentition but the difficulties lie in extrapolating the findings to humans because of plaque flora, saliva composition and the dry state in which the food is fed to the animals.
- **Laboratory experiments**: these use slabs of enamel from extracted teeth which are held in the mouth of human volunteers in a removable plate. The subjects may eat the diet in the usual way. The slabs are then analysed in the laboratory for the effect of the dietary components on the enamel. These studies are not as reliable as the previous types listed.

The Vipeholm study

The Vipeholm studies, reported by Gustafsson *et al.* in 1954, were human interventional studies carried out from 1945 to 1953 in Sweden. It was probably the biggest single study in the field of dental caries ever undertaken. It would not meet with ethical approval now because it was carried out in the Vipeholm Hospital on patients who had a mental deficiency. The purpose of the study was to investigate how dental caries activity was influenced. There was a control group and six main test groups to investigate ingestion of sugar either at meal times or between meals, in either a sticky or non-sticky form. All participants had the same basal carbohydrate intake, which was then supplemented by sugar in its various forms. Examinations to determine the decayed missing and filled teeth (DMFT) were conducted annually and the dental caries activity was the sum of all the new primary and secondary carious lesions and new filled surfaces. (For a detailed account of the study the reader is referred to Rugg-Gunn, 1993.)

The most marked rise in dental caries was seen in the 24-toffee group in which the toffees could be eaten throughout the day. The rise was 70% higher in females than males, with a DMFT of 14.1 at baseline, rising to 21 when the issue of toffee was stopped and replaced by fat (Figure 7.7). Consumption between meals was no longer allowed. This was accompanied by a dramatic fall in dental caries increment to near the level before the start of the study.

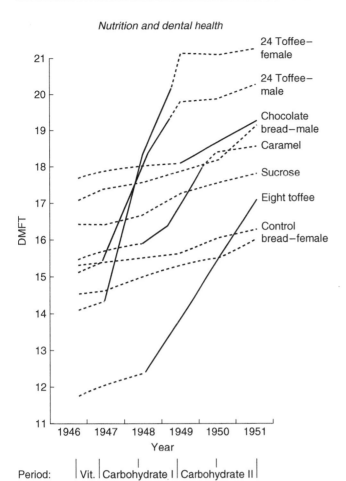

Nutrition and dental health

Period: | Vit. | Carbohydrate I | Carbohydrate II |

Figure 7.7 Vipeholm study results (Reproduced from The Vipeholm Dental Caries Study by Gustaffson *et al.* from *Odontologica Scandinavica*, www.tandf.no/actaodont, 1954, 11, 232–364 by permission of Taylor & Francis).

The conclusions of the Vipeholm study were as follows (Gustafsson *et al.*, 1954):

The risk of sugar increasing caries activity is greatest if the sugar is consumed between meals and is in a form in which the tendency to be retained on the surfaces of the teeth is pronounced with a transiently high concentration of sugar on these surfaces.

Human observational studies

Evidence can be taken from worldwide epidemiological studies. The dental caries experience of the population of the island of Tristan da Cunha is such an example. The island is 1500 miles west-south-west of Cape Town and the 200 inhabitants have only occasional contact with the outside world. Prior to 1940 the diet was low in sugar, but since 1940 sugar was available for sale on the island. The recording of the experience of dental caries in the islanders shows an increase from 1937 to 1966, rising faster in the children than the adults (Fisher,

1968). The increase in caries correlates with the increase in consumption of sugar and flour. Sugar consumption increased from 1.8 g/person/day in 1938 to 150 g/person/day in 1966. Sweets and chocolates increased from zero in 1938 to 50 g in 1966.

Hopewood House is a home in rural New South Wales Australia, in which about 80 children of low socio-economic background were brought up from birth to 12 years. They had a lactovegetarian diet, and sugar and flour products were virtually absent. The fluoride intake was low and oral hygiene measures absent. Up to the age of 12 years the presence of dental caries was low; 46% of 12-year-olds were caries-free compared to 1% in state schools. Once the period of close supervision ended the children developed the same caries rate as children in state schools. Harris (cited in Rugg-Gunn, 1993) concluded that the diet received up to 12 years did not protect the children from developing dental caries in subsequent years.

There are many studies of populations during and after World War II, which relate the lack of availability of sugar during wartime with the increased consumption post war. The dental caries rate in first permanent molars in 6–7-year-olds in Norway, Finland and Denmark, in relation to the sugar consumption in prewar, war and postwar periods was reported by Toverud in 1957.

Classification of sugars in relation to dental caries

The Committee on the Medical Aspects of Food Policy (COMA) is a committee in the Department of Health which has reported on dietary reference values for food energy and nutrition for the UK. In 1989 COMA produced a report on *Dietary Sugars and Human Diseases*. The sugars most responsible for dental caries were classified as **non-milk extrinsic sugars** (NMES) (Figure 7.8). This refers to sugar molecules outside the plant cell and includes sugars which are added to food and drinks during processing and preparation. It also includes sugars naturally present in fresh fruit juices, honey and syrups. Sugars inside the cell structure of the plant are intrinsic sugars and as such are not fully released into the mouth during eating, and are not considered to be cariogenic.

The committee proposed that the population's average intake of NMES should not exceed 60 g per day and 10% of total dietary energy intake. For children in the UK, NMES provide 17% of total dietary energy intake, much of which is hidden sugar (Figure 7.9). Fresh fruit juices and dried fruits should only constitute one of the recommended five daily portions of fruits. These foods have a high concentration of sugars and frequent consumption between meals could increase the risk of caries. Lactose (milk sugar) is virtually non-cariogenic.

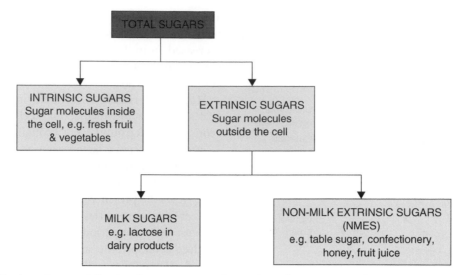

Figure 7.8 Classification of sugars following the COMA report (Reproduced from the *Scientific Basis of Oral Health Education*, 2004, p. 20, by Levine RS and Stillman Lowe CR, by permission of BDJ Books).

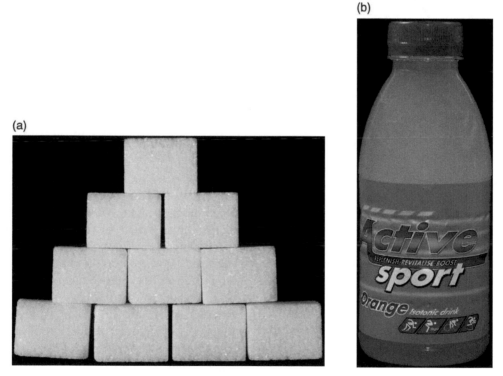

Figure 7.9 Sugar in fruit drink – the amount of sugar in a bottle of sports drink.

NMES with the potential to cause dental caries are:

- Sucrose.
- Glucose.
- Maltose.
- Fructose.

A safe level for sugar concentration in food and drink cannot be recommended because it is linked to the physical consistency of the sugar.

The role of starch

Starch is converted by salivary amylase to maltose and glucose.

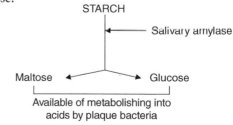

(a)

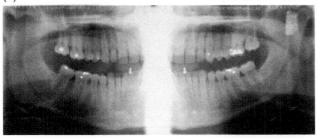

(b)

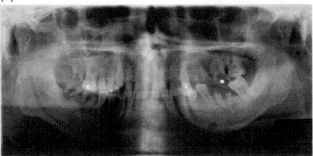

Figure 7.10 (a) Radiograph of healthy adult dentition. (b) The same dentition after a change to a diet of daily carbonated soft drinks.

This is a slow conversion and hence dietary starch alone is much less important than dietary sugars as a cause of dental caries.

Frequency

The frequency and timing of intake of sugary foods and drinks are important determining factors in caries levels (Figure 7.10). Such foods should be consumed with main meals because the oral clearance time is quicker and the salivary flow is increased. Salivary flow rate is reduced during sleep and therefore bedtime is the worst time to consume sugary products. A survey of 600 children who consumed both sugary drinks and a snack in the hour before bed found the children to have four times the number of decayed teeth compared to children who consumed neither (Levine, 2001).

Key points

- The frequency and amount of consumption of sugars in drinks and foods are the most important risk factors in dental caries.
- Sugar-sweetened snacks and foods should be avoided between meals and especially at bedtime.
- Sugar-free medicines should be presented for children whenever possible.

Alternative sweeteners

Non-nutritive sugar substitutes have been developed to restrict the consumption of sucrose both in manufactured foods and that used by the consumer. The COMA report on dietary sugars (1989) contains the recommendation that food manufacturers produce low-sugar and sugar-free alternatives to existing sugar-rich products, particularly those for children. Non-sugar sweeteners are beneficial in the control of dental caries and obesity.

Intense sweeteners

These artificial sweeteners are so called because they can be up to 3000 times sweeter than sucrose. The following are permitted for use by manufacturers of food in the UK:

- Saccharin.
- Acesulfame K.
- Aspartame.
- Thaumatin.

These substitutes do not contribute to the production of energy and most are excreted unchanged in the urine. They have been classified as 'safe for teeth'.

Bulk sweeteners

These are modified sugars or alcohol derivatives of sugars (polyols), for example:

- Sorbitol.
- Isomalt.
- Mannitol.
- Xylitol.
- Hydrogenated glucose syrups.

Sorbitol and mannitol are commercially used in chewing gum and sugar-free confectionery. They are only half as sweet as sucrose on a weight basis. The negative heat of dissolution gives a cooling taste. Large intakes of sorbitol can cause a laxative effect because it is only partially absorbed and there is osmotic transfer of water into the bowel. These bulk sweeteners do not require insulin for their metabolism and are therefore incorporated into foods for diabetics.

Sorbitol

At least 11 studies have been reported comparing the effect of sorbitol with the effect of sucrose on the development of dental caries in animals (cited in Rugg-Gunn, 1993). Some dental caries occurred when rats were super-infected with *Streptococcus mutans*, but little caries occurred when they were not super-infected with the organism. Rugg-Gunn (1993) states that dental caries would occur in individuals with very high *S. mutans* counts who consumed sorbitol to the exclusion of other dietary sugars.

Xylitol

Xylitol has sweetness approximately the same as sucrose. It produces less laxative effect than sorbitol or mannitol. It is found naturally in some fruits and vegetables and is extracted commercially from birch trees. It is more expensive than sucrose and sorbitol and is used in chewing gum, toothpaste and confectionery. Xylitol is non-cariogenic. The Turku Sugar Studies (cited in Rugg-Gunn, 1993) tested the development of caries over 2 years in adults by substitution of normal dietary sugars with xylitol. When precavitation lesions were included in the caries score, caries increment was zero in the xylitol group. Xylitol may be positively anticariogenic. Studies have been carried out in Finland using xylitol chewing gum to assess the reduction in *S. mutans* and hence the amount of plaque. The action of chewing gum will stimulate salivary flow and aid remineralisation. Isokangas *et al.* carried out a 3-year study published in 2000, in which mothers in Finland used the reduction of mutans colonisation as one method of targeting and reducing caries in their preschool children. Chewing xylitol products reduced *S. mutans* transmission from carer to child.

The relationship between diet and erosion

'Erosion is the physical result of a pathological, chronic localised loss of dental hard tissue that is chemically etched away from the tooth surface by acid and/or chelation without bacterial involvement' (ten Cate and Imfield, 1996). It is classified as a cause of tooth tissue loss and may present as a stand-alone condition, but is frequently seen in combination with other causes of tooth loss, such as abrasion and attrition. This arises because calcified tissue softened by acid is brushed away by the use of a toothbrush and abrasive paste, or worn away by mastication. Whilst tooth erosion was described in 1892 among Sicilian lemon pickers, there has been an increased prevalence in the last 10 years and there are several epidemiological studies to support this (for example Jarvinen *et al.*, 1992). In the 2003 children's Dental Health Survey, 53% of 5-year-old children had tooth surface loss on one or more primary incisors (National Statistics Online).

Causes of erosion

Erosion is a chronic disease caused by the repetitive contact of the tooth surface with the causative acids. These may arise from:

- Diet (extrinsic) (Table 7.7).
- Stomach (intrinsic).
- Environmental (extrinsic).

Table 7.7 Dietary source of acids that can lead to erosion.

Citrus fruits, fruit juices
Acid carbonated drinks
Acidic sports drinks
Wine
Cider
Vinegar and pickled produce
Acidic fruit
Flavoured sweets
Iron medicines
(Acidic mouthwashes)
Vitamin C

The type of acid varies. For example, phosphoric, citric and malic acids are found in fruit and fruit juices; ascorbic acid is added to sweets and sports drinks, and has been identified as a significant cause of erosion (Sorvari, 1989). In tooth tissue destruction from intrinsic causes the hydrochloric acid from the stomach causes the erosion. The lesions, at microscopic level, are similar to the pattern of mineral loss in the acid-etch restorative technique. The effect is due to the low pH of the acid and also its chelation effect which is the binding to calcium and removing it from the tooth surface. Whilst the pH of a drink is an indicator, a measure called the **total titratable activity**, which gives the capacity of a liquid to dissolve mineral, is a better guide. Enamel is gradually lost in layers and dentine is lost at a greater rate. The loss is irreversible, giving a characteristic appearance to the lesions. The remaining tissue is softened, and *in vitro* investigations suggest this is 1–5 µm for enamel and 1–2 µm for dentine, dependent upon the characteristics of erosion. Avoidance of tooth brushing after an 'acid attack' is based on preservation of this softened tooth tissue.

Clinical appearance

The clinical appearance of the lesions depends upon the source of the acid and the way the acid is moved around the mouth before swallowing. Drinking through a straw or sports drinks cup will result in loss of enamel from the palatal surface of the upper teeth. Consumption of citrus foods and wines, beers and ciders tends to affect the labial surfaces of the upper anterior teeth and the occlusal surfaces of molars.

The severity of the lesions will also be dependent upon the length and frequency of the acid being in contact with the teeth. A reduced salivary flow will result in a considerable reduction in the salivary buffering capacity and the maintenance of a lower pH for longer. The lesions should be observed after air drying as early lesions appear frosted. The tooth surfaces then become

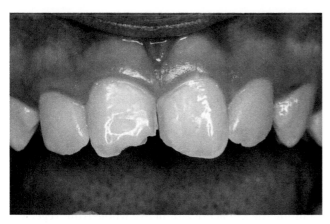

Figure 7.11 Acid erosion of anterior teeth.

smooth, shiny and rounded, and normal development lines in the enamel are lost. The surfaces become more concave and as dentine becomes lost there is often a 'halo' of enamel that remains as a rim around the eroded dentine. The incisal edges and cusps become thin and then translucent, and then the edges become worn away and chip easily (Figure 7.11). The teeth gradually darken as the enamel is lost and the yellowish dentine predominates. The incisal edges of eroded incisors may take on a greyish hue due to their translucency. Tooth surface loss in deciduous teeth results in cup-shaped defects on molars, and incisors are reduced in length. Loss in deciduous teeth can be more rapid due to thinner enamel.

Symptoms

Symptoms will vary according to the severity of the loss of tissue. Early loss of enamel may not give the patient any discomfort, but sensitivity to cold, hot and sweet fluids is a frequent complaint. In severe palatal erosion, the cusps of the teeth may be reduced to gingival margin level and the pulps may become non-vital.

Recording and monitoring of erosion

The most commonly used index for recording tooth wear is the tooth wear index of Smith and Knight, 1984 (Rugg-Gunn and Nunn, 1999). The problem with erosion monitoring is that subtle changes occur over time and would be difficult to record using this index, but it is useful as a baseline. Clinical photographs and study models cast from silicone impressions will aid in recording the baseline status and in patient evaluation.

Prevention

Prevention of erosion involves the following:

- Identify the aetiology.
- Educate the patient.
- Empower the patient to bring about lifestyle changes.

Whilst medical expertise will obviously be required in identifying cases of erosion caused by hiatus hernia, alcoholism and anorexic and bulimic states, the dental therapist has an important role in identifying dietary factors and advising changes in the consumption of erosive food and drinks. A dietary analysis sheet may be required to identify all the factors and personalise the advice.

Advice given to the patient would include:

- Inform the patient of the food and drinks in the diet that are likely to be erosive.
- Advise the patient to limit the intake of acid drinks to meal times and drink water or milk at other times.
- Discourage swishing and frequent sipping of acidic/fizzy drinks.
- Eating cheese and drinking milk will help to neutralise the acid.
- Avoid tooth brushing for an hour after eating erosive food and drink.
- Use fluoride toothpaste to strengthen the remaining enamel and the use of fluoride mouthwash may be appropriate.

The relationship of diet to periodontal diseases

The primary aetiological factor in gingivitis is the accumulation of microbial plaque over time. The published data on the effect of nutritional deficiencies on periodontal health indicate that deficiencies of vitamins A, B, D and E and also calcium are of no significance. The effect of deficiency of vitamin C, however, has been substantiated, beginning with the report by James Lind in 1747, following deaths of sailors from scurvy on voyage ships. In his experiment, the sailors with scurvy who were given two oranges and a lemon recovered. The vitamin C in the citrus fruit was essential to the prevention of disease. Vitamin C is essential for the maturation of collagen and acute deficiency results in oedema and haemorrhage of the periodontal ligament and tooth mobility, as the alveolar bone is also affected. Vitamin C is also required for wound healing.

The only other micronutrient reported to have any beneficial effect in the gingival tissues is folate. Both systemic and topical administration trials have been undertaken using folic acid mouth rinse. The mouth rinse produced a significant improvement in the gingival health of pregnant women in months 4–8 of pregnancy (Pack and Thompson, 1980). The principle behind the supplementation is possible 'end tissue deficiency' in the gingival tissues during pregnancy. Folic acid is required for DNA synthesis and tissues with the highest cell turnover (e.g. crevicular epithelium), may be affected by this deficiency.

The only macronutrient worthy of discussion in this section on nutrition and periodontal disease is carbohydrate. It is well documented that increasing the sucrose content of the diet will increase the bulk of supragingival plaque. This is due to the formation of extracellular polysaccharide by cariogenic bacteria. There is a strong positive correlation between the amount of supragingival plaque and the subsequent development of gingivitis. The bacteria dominating in supragingival plaque provide the nutrients and gaseous requirements for the colonisation of the subgingival environment by the anaerobic, Gram-negative organisms that initiate gingivitis.

Antioxidants and periodontal disease

During the inflammatory disease process polymorphonuclear leucocytes (PMNLS) produce reactive oxygen species (ROS or free radicals) via their respiratory burst. This is part of the normal host response system to infections but in periodontitis patients the process becomes dysregulated. Peripheral blood neutrophils from periodontitis patients have been shown to overproduce ROS in both unstimulated and stimulated states and this may give rise to oxidative damage to cells and vital molecules directly, as well as altering the expression levels of genes that control inflammation by cytokine production (for review see Chapple and Matthews, 2007). Various studies have been undertaken in recent years involving foods and micronutrients known to have antioxidant properties, to investigate their effect on the progression of periodontal tissue destruction. Antioxidant micronutrients appear important for limiting tissue damage caused by ROS and also in preventing oxidative stress and subsequent cytokine production by epithelial, as well as inflammatory immune cells.

A large scale epidemiological study investigated the relationship between serum levels of α-carotene, β-carotene, selenium, lutein, uric acid, β-cryptoxanthine, vitamins A, C, E, bilirubin and total antioxidant capacity (TAOC) in over 11 000 North American volunteers and found that vitamin C, bilirubin and TACO were significantly lower in periodontitis patients (Chapple et al., 2007). Other studies have demonstrated this is also the case for vitamin C (Amarasena et al., 2005; Amaliya et al., 2007) in European and Japanese populations.

In another human study the serum levels of arytenoids were investigated in a sample of men aged 60–70 years. The aim of the study was to correlate the level of antioxidants in those men with periodontitis. The levels of alpha and beta carotene were significantly lower in those with periodontitis (Linden et al., 2009).

Flavanoids are a group of naturally occurring phenolic compounds, many of which are plant pigments. Cocoa is an example of a flavanoid which was trialled in rats with a cocoa-enriched diet. The investigation was to study the effect on gingival oxidative stress; Tomofuji et al. (2009) concluded that such a diet could diminish oxidative stress which may suppress the progression of periodontitis.

Pomegranate juice has been trialled as a mouthwash in young adults and was found to increase the activity of an antioxidant enzyme (DiSilvestro et al., 2009). Coenzyme Q with vitamin E has also been proven to have a beneficial effect on the periodontal tissue for patients who took this substance for two months (Matthews et al., 2007).

Most recently, the first dietary intervention study to examine the impact of adjunctive whole fruit, vegetable and berry extracts, taken during periodontal therapy, reported significantly improved pocket depth reduction in supplemented groups than in a placebo group at 3-months. In this randomised double-blind trial, crevicular fluid volumes also reduced more significantly in the whole food supplement group relative to the placebo group 3-months post-treatment (Chapple et al., 2010).

Early data from rodent studies shows potential for omega-3 polyunsaturated fatty acids (PUFAs), derived from fish oils, in reducing bone loss and inflammation during experimental periodontitis (Kesavalu et al., 2006), but human studies are needed.

The effect of fibrous foods on gingival health

To date there is no evidence to support the hypothesis that the physical characteristics of the diet are related to the health of the periodontal tissues in man. Wilcox and Everett 1963 (cited in Rugg-Gunn, 1993) showed that the area of plaque, which accumulates along the gingival margins in humans, is not subjected to friction from food during mastication. Whilst chewing apples or carrots is more beneficial to the dentition than eating foods high in refined carbohydrates, there is no health gain in the prevention of gingivitis.

The relationship of the diet to conditions of the oral mucosa

The tongue, lips and oral mucosa may also show signs of nutritional deficiencies. They are relatively uncommon in the UK apart from aphthous ulceration or angular cheilitis (see Chapter 3, p. 55). Tables 7.5 and 7.6 give an overview of micronutrient deficiencies and the possible effects on the oral mucosa.

Oral cancer and nutrition

Alcohol is the most important dietary influence on the occurrence of oral cancer. There is reported to be a synergistic interaction between the consumption of alcohol and tobacco use – a relative risk of 15:6 compared with non-smokers and non-drinkers. Alcohol can facilitate the entry of tobacco carcinogens into cells and both factors have the potential to damage DNA. Unrepaired DNA damage can then be reproduced in subsequent generations of cells. A diet containing a daily intake of adequate fruit and vegetables has been associated with a 50% decreased risk of cancer of the mouth and pharynx. It has been estimated that almost 87% of the incidence of cancer of the mouth and pharynx can potentially be reduced by not smoking, reduced alcohol intake and increasing the consumption of vegetables and fruits (Rugg-Gunn and Nunn, 1999).

The role of the dental hygienist/therapist in dietary advice and counselling

Dental hygienists and therapists are educated to identify target groups and individuals who may benefit from preventive dietary advice and support. A method of classifying preventative intervention is to consider:

- **Primary prevention**: when there is no disease present and the advice is related to potential health issues, e.g. to mothers who care for young children.
- **Secondary prevention**: in dentistry this relates to the prevention of the development of existing disease by minimising its severity and reversing its progress (see also Chapter 11, p. 220). Secondary prevention requires behavioural change on the part of the recipient, and an understanding on the part of the adviser, of the complexity and diversity of the lifestyle which may influence motivation to change. Dietary messages must be based on sound clinical evidence and communicated effectively to the individual. This not only involves selective use of appropriate body and verbal language but personalisation of the advice. To bring about behavioural change, the recipient may need to change their opinions, perceptions and actions. An essential role of the dentist, hygienist and therapist is to recognise risk factors for disease and inform the patient or carer of the consequences. Failure to do this can be regarded as negligent in both an ethical and legal sense. How the individual responds will depend on many factors, some of which are outside the remit of the dental clinician.

What influences dietary habits?

Individuals do not eat and drink merely to satisfy nutritional requirements. Intake may vary according to mood or occasion and it is important to be mindful of cultural, religious, social and moral factors which influence choice (Table 7.8). Economic status also has

Table 7.8 Some of the circumstances that can affect dietary habits.

Cultural factors: ethnicity, religion, vegetarianism
Unemployment
Occupation (e.g. in food industry)
Working unsocial hours (e.g. shift work or long hours)
Excessive travelling to work or school
Unsatisfactory accommodation (e.g. bedsit, overcrowding)
Poor food storage facilities, no refrigerator
Poor cooking facilities (e.g. shared)
Inability to cook
Remoteness from shops (e.g. lack of transport, personal or public, reliance on mobile shops)
Poor choice and quality of foods in available shops
Poor choice or dependence on workplace or school for meals
Financial problems
Stress, e.g. divorce, illness
Lack of desire to cook/eat (e.g. elderly, single people)

From Rugg-Gunn and Nunn (1999) *Nutrition, Diet and Oral Health*. Reproduced with permission of Oxford University Press, Oxford.

an important influence on the buying and preparation of food. In the younger age groups in particular, peer pressure is a significant factor and may be a barrier to behavioural change.

Will the individual be receptive to advice?

This will vary accordingly to the personal circumstances of the individual and their particular frame of mind at the time the advice is given. The clinician must demonstrate sensitivity and empathy and be mindful that any suggestions to change will have an effect beyond the dental environment. The oral cavity may not be top priority! The advice will need to be frequently repeated, but not in a manner which can be interpreted as 'nagging'. Selecting the appropriate time during the appointment, and knowing when not to proffer advice, are both important skills of the counsellor. Advice is best given in 'small packages with perhaps one or two take-home messages'.

Broadly speaking, a person can only retain seven facts at any one time. If some of this information is given visually, as well as being given orally, the total retention increases. There must be a time for the individual to reflect and consider the advice before deciding whether or not to act upon it. Reinforcements on subsequent visits, followed by praise for modifications undertaken, will help to develop a rapport with the patient and lay the foundation for permanent behavioural change (see Chapter 6, p. 128).

Specific dietary advice for high-risk patients

Patients who have been identified as having a high caries experience or who have extensive dental erosion must be considered for detailed dietary advice. A method of personalising the advice is to ask the patient to complete a diet diary. An example of a dietary analysis record can be seen in Chapter 12, p. 251. This can be easily modified for use with adults. A suggested approach follows.

Appointment 1

After determining the medical, social and personal history and reviewing the clinical evidence, a dietary form is given to the patient. The reason for completion must be given, together with an explanation as to how to complete the form. The 3 consecutive day record is generally the accepted version in which the patient or carer enters everything eaten and drunk, including medicines, over the given period. One of the days must be a weekend day, to account for variation in dietary habits.

Appointment 2

The second appointment should ideally be a week later, and the patient is thanked for the efforts made in recording. It is important to remember that not all entries will have been made, whether through lapse of memory, insufficient time or avoidance of the whole truth! The clinician should go through the form with the patient highlighting omissions and seeking clarification. For caries analysis, the hidden sugar in drinks and cereals can easily be overlooked.

Appointment 3

Dietary analysis followed by feedback. The analysis is best done away from the patient to allow for full consideration of the dietary habits and the recommendations which will follow shortly afterwards. The analysis will:

- Separate the meals from the snacks.
- Identify foods which contain a significant amount of NMES.
- Identify the time of the last sugar snack in relation to bedtime.

The analysis will give an overview of the frequency of refined carbohydrate intake. If the analysis is for erosion, one should identify extrinsic acids and their frequency.

Feedback should be given in terms of general nutritional advice, as well as specific advice for prevention of oral diseases. An action plan will need to be drawn up in consultation with the patient to achieve 'realistic' goals. It is important that these are recorded for the patient to take home and refer to. The advice is as much about what can be eaten as what is to be restricted, therefore alternatives should be suggested, such as:

- Milk or water or sugar-free diluted squash.
- Cheese.
- Fresh fruit.
- Sandwiches containing cheese spread, salad or Marmite.

It is important to be aware of any sensitivities to specific foods, which if eaten or drunk could lead to a hypersensitivity reaction. Children in particular may have an acute allergic reaction to milk or nuts.

Recapitulation and reinforcement will be needed at subsequent appointments if behavioural change is to be achieved in the long term.

If the hygienist/therapist unveils dietary problems which are beyond their expertise, it is important to discuss this in the first instance with the prescribing dentist. The dentist may then need to liaise, with the patient's permission, via the patient's medical practitioner, with other health and social care professionals, such as a dietician, psychiatrist or social workers.

References

Amaliya, Timmerman, M.F., Abbas, F., Loos, B.G., *et al.* (2007) Java project on periodontal diseases: the relationship between vitamin C and the severity of periodontitis. *Journal of Clinical Periodontology*, **34**, 299–304.

Amarasena, N., Ogawa, H., Yoshihara, A., Hanada, N. and Miyazaki, H. (2005) Serum vitamin C-periodontal relationship in community-dwelling elderly Japanese. *Journal of Clinical Periodontology*, **32**, 93–97.

British National Formulary 58. (2009). p893. British Medical Association, Royal Pharmaceutical Society of Great Britain, London.

Chapple, I.L. and Matthews, J.B. (2007) The role of reactive oxygen and antioxidant species in periodontal tissue destruction. *Periodontology*, **43**, 160–232.

Chapple, I.L., Milward, M.R. and Diuetrich, T. (2007) The prevalence of inflammatory periodontitis is negatively associated with serum antioxidant concentrations. *Journal of Nutrition*, **137**, 657–664.

Chapple, I.L., Milward, M.R., Ling-Mountford, N., *et al.* (2010) Adjunctive effects of a dietary supplement comprising dried whole fruit, vegetables and berry juice concentrates on clinical outcomes of treatment of periodontitis. *Federation of American Societies for Experimental Biology Journal*, **24, 540.10.**

Committee on Medical Aspects of Food Policy (1989) *Dietary Sugars and Human Diseases*. HMSO, London, p. 41.

Department of Health (2009) *Delivering Better Oral Health. An evidence based toolkit for prevention*, 2nd edition. Department of Health, London, p11, p37–38.

DiSilvestro, R.A., DiSilvestro, D.A. and DiSilvestro, D.A. (2009) Pomegranate extract mouth rinsing effects on saliva measures relevant to gingivitis risk. *Phytotherapy Research* **23** (8), 1123–1127.

Fisher, J. (1968) A field study of dental caries, periodontal disease and enamel defects in Tristan da Cunha. *British Dental Journal*, **125**, 447–53.

Food Standards Agency www.food.gov.uk. Cited in Levine, R.S. and Stillman Lowe, C.R. (2004). *The Scientific Basis of Oral Health Education*. BDJ Books, London. p64. ISBN 0-904588-84X.

Gustafsson, B.E., Quensel, C.E., Lanke, L.S., *et al.* (1954). The Vipeholm Dental Caries Study. The effect of different levels of carbohydrate intake on caries activity in 436 individuals observed for five years. *Acta Odontologica Scandinavica*, **11**, 232–364.

Health Education Authority (1992) *Scientific Basis of Nutritional Education: a Synopsis of Dietary Values*. Health Education Authority, London.

Health Education Authority (1995). *Diet and Health in School Age Children*. Health Education Authority, London.

Isokangas, P., Söderking, E., Pienihäkkinen, K. and Alanen, P. (2000) Occurrence of dental decay in children after maternal consumption of xylotol chewing gum, a follow up from 0–5 years of age. *Journal of Dental Research*, **79**, 1885–1889.

Jarvinen, V., Rytomaa, I., Meurman, J.H., (1992) Location of dental erosion in a referred population. *Caries Research*, **26**, 391–396.

Johansson I. and Birkhed D. (1994) Diet and the caries process. In: *Textbook of Clinical Cariology*, Thylstrup A., and Fejerskovo, O. (eds). Munksgaard, Copenhagen.

Kesavalu, L., Vasudevan, B., Browning, E., *et al.* (2006) Omega-3 fatty acid effect on alveolar bone loss in rats. *Journal of Dental Research*, **85**, 648–652.

Kouba, J. (2005). Impact of environment, ethnicity and culture on nutrition and health. In *Nutrition and Oral Medicine*. Chapter 4. Touger-Decker, R., Sirosis, D. and Molbey, C. (eds). Humana Press Inc. Totowa NJ.

Levine, R.S. (2001) Caries experience and bedtime consumption of sugar sweetened foods and drinks – a survey of 600 children. *Community Dental Health*, **18**, 228–231.

Levine, R.S. and Stillman Lowe, C.R. (2004). *The Scientific Basis of Oral Health Education*. BDJ. Books London. Fig. 3.1 p 20.

Linden, G.J., McLean, K.H., Woodside, J.V., *et al.* (2009) Antioxidants and periodontitis in 60–70 year old men. *Journal of Clinical Periodontology*, **36** (10), 843–849.

Macpherson, G. (1995) *Blacks Medical Dictionary*, 38th edition. A&C Black, London.

Matthews-B.T., Kurhanstia, F.A., Wyganowska, S.M., *et al.* (2007) Healing of periodontal tissue assisted by Coenzyme Q/Sub10/with vitamin E. Clinical and laboratory evaluation. *Pharmacological Reports*, **59** Suppl 1, 257–260.

Moynihan, P., Lingström, P., Rugg-Gunn A.J. and Birkhed, D. (2003) The role of dietary control. In: *The Role of Dietary Control in Dental Caries. The disease and its clinical management*. Chapter 14. Ferjerskov, O. and Kidd, E. (eds) Blackwell Munskgaard, Oxford.

Naidoo, J. and Wills, J. (1998) *Health Promotion Foundations for Practice*, 5th edition. Baillière Tindall, London.

National Statistics Online – Children and Young People – Dental Health. [Online.] Available from www.ons.officefornationalstatistics.gov.uk/childdentalhealth.

Pack, A.R.C. and Thompson, M.E. (1980). Effects of topical and systemic folic acid supplementation on gingivitis and pregnancy. *Journal of Clinical Periodontology*, **7**, 402–414.

Rugg-Gunn, A.J. (1993) *Nutrition and Dental Health*. Oxford University Press, Oxford.

Rugg-Gunn, A.J. and Nunn, J.H. (1999) *Nutrition, Diet and Oral Health*. Oxford University Press, Oxford.

Scientific Basis of Nutrition. a Synopsis of Dietary Reference Values. (1996) 2nd Ed. p14–31. Health Education Authority, London.

Sorvari, R, (1989) Effects of various sports drink modifications on dental caries and erosion in rats with controlled eating and drinking pattern. *Proceedings of the Finnish Dental Society*, **85**, 13–20.

ten Cate, J.M. and Imfield, T. (1996) Etiology, mechanisms and implications of dental erosion. *European Journal of Oral Science*, **104**, 149–244.

The G I Guide (2005). The Sunday Times Publishing Group, London.

Tomofuji T., Ekuni D., Irie K., *et al.* (2009) Preventative effects of a cocoa-enriched diet on gingival oxidative stress in experimental periodontitis. *Journal of Periodontology*, **11**, 799–808.

Toverud, G. (1957) The influence of war and post war conditions on the teeth of Norwegian school children II and III. *Millbank Memorial Fund Quarterly*, **35**, 127–196, 373–459.

Further reading

Fejerskov, O. and Kidd, E. (2008) *Dental Caries. The Disease and its Clinical Management*. Blackwell Munksgaard, Oxford.

Touger-Decker, R., Sirois, D. and Mobley, C. (2004) *Nutrition and Oral Medicine*. Humana Press Inc., New Jersey.

8

Microbiology and infection prevention and control

Mary J. O'Donnell, Denise MacCarthy and David C. Coleman

Summary

This chapter covers:

- A requirement for a formal infection prevention and control policy
- An overview of potential transmissible pathogens of relevance to dentistry
- Practical guidance on the potential sources of infection in the dental environment and how to minimise cross-contamination and cross-infection risks
- Instrument decontamination, transportation and storage
- Effective waste management
- The dental chair unit as a vehicle for cross-contamination and cross-infection

Introduction

In the twenty-first century, should the prevention of transmission of infectious diseases be considered less important than dental treatment of patients? All dental healthcare professionals have a duty of care to their patients that includes the implementation of effective infection prevention and control (IPC) procedures designed to minimise the risk of transmission of pathogenic or potentially pathogenic microorganisms.

Dental healthcare personnel include all members of the dental team: dentists, dental hygienists, dental therapists, dental nurses, dental laboratory technicians (both working on-site in dental practices and hospitals and in commercial laboratories), students, contractors and other individuals not directly involved in patient care but potentially exposed to infectious agents

(e.g. administrative, clerical, housekeeping and especially maintenance personnel). The purpose of IPC in the dental clinic setting is to reduce cross-contamination and to minimise risks associated with the transmission of infectious or potentially infectious microorgansisms. Preventative practices are used to minimise exposure to reservoirs of pathogenic microorganisms and environmental microorganisms, many of the latter of which are potentially pathogenic or behave as opportunistic pathogens, and to body fluids, particularly percutaneous (penetrated through the skin) exposures to blood. Such practices include:

- Careful handling of sharp instruments and equipment.
- The use of rubber dams and high-volume suction.
- Correct hand hygiene techniques.
- Appropriate use of protective barriers (e.g. gloves, masks, protective eyewear, gowns and surface barriers).
- Effective decontamination of contaminated surfaces, instruments and equipment.

Requirement for a formal infection prevention and control policy

All dental practices should have an effective IPC programme that includes the development and implementation of policies, procedures and practices to prevent work-related injuries and illnesses among dental healthcare personnel and support staff, as well as healthcare-associated infections among patients (Kohn *et al.*, 2003). All dental team staff (including non-clinical staff) who may be subject to occupational exposure should receive regular and appropriate IPC training; they should be

---

Clinical Textbook of Dental Hygiene and Therapy, Second Edition. Edited by Suzanne L. Noble.
© 2012 John Wiley & Sons, Ltd. Published 2012 by John Wiley & Sons, Ltd.

aware of the associated infection risks with all aspects of patient care, the proper maintenance, cleaning and disinfection of dental equipment and instruments and waste segregation. The effectiveness of the IPC programme should be evaluated by audit on an ongoing basis and reviewed periodically to ensure that the practices are effective and efficient and that the policy is implemented. These policies require the commitment and accountability of all staff concerned.

Microorganisms

It is beyond the scope of this chapter to provide a comprehensive overview of microorganisms and microbiology. There are numerous excellent textbooks and more general microbiology books available and we wish to encourage the interested reader to familiarise themselves with the more general aspects of microorganisms (Murray *et al.*, 2009; Lamont, and Jenkinson, 2010). Microorganisms consist of bacteria (e.g. *Escherichia coli* and *Staphylococcus aureus*), fungi (e.g. *Candida albicans* and *Aspergillus fumigatus*), viruses (e.g. influenza virus and hepatitis B virus), protozoa, amoebae, mycoplasmas and rickettsiae. In relation to cross-infection in the dental clinic, the most significant microorganisms are bacteria, viruses and to a lesser extent fungi, the latter of which also include yeasts. Microorganisms are ubiquitous and occupy virtually every habitat, environment and niche in nature. Most of these organisms are totally harmless to humans and never cause us any problems. They are too busy just making a living (Figure 8.1).

Every individual comes into contact with numerous microorganisms every day, in the air, in water, in food and on both natural and artificial surfaces. Not surprisingly, a vast range of microorganisms is associated with the human body, the majority of which are usually harmless. In fact, many microorganisms that live on or in our bodies provide many beneficial effects and can be considered *friendly* microorganisms. These microorganisms are often referred to as **commensals** or the **normal microbial flora** and are present in enormous numbers on the skin, in the oral cavity and in the alimentary tract.

Microorganisms have always existed and evolved in close association with humans and we have developed complex and intricate specific (e.g. cell-mediated and humoral immunity) and non-specific (e.g. skin and epithelial barriers, and antimicrobial secretions such as saliva and tears) defence mechanisms to protect ourselves from becoming infected with microorganisms (Delves *et al.*, 2011). Even when our bodies do become infected with microorganisms, our immune defence systems usually quickly eradicate the invaders. A relatively small

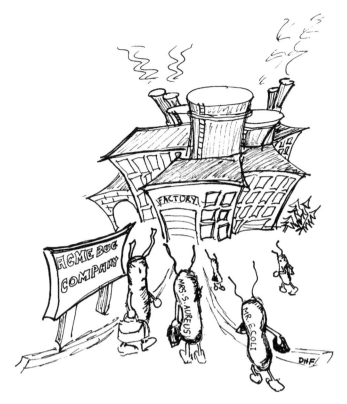

Figure 8.1 The majority of microorganisms present in nature never cause infection. They are usually too busy just making a living.

number of microorganisms have developed specific mechanisms to exploit weaknesses in host defences that enable them to establish infections and cause disease. These organisms are known as pathogenic microorganisms or **pathogens** because they may cause disease in healthy individuals once they have gained access to the body. Examples include influenza virus, which causes flu; the bacterium *Staph. aureus*, which can cause skin infections and abscesses; and various strains of the bacterial species *E. coli*, which can cause diarrhoea. Many pathogenic microorganisms have evolved mechanisms to avoid or evade host defence systems and many in addition produce **toxins** (e.g. cholera toxin produced by the bacterial species *Vibrio cholerae* and diphtheria toxin produced by the bacterial species *Corynebacterium diphtheriae*) that, for example, can cause local tissue damage and/or more widespread systemic effects.

Another group of microorganisms can only cause infection and disease following a local or general defect(s) in host defence mechanisms. These microorganisms are sometimes referred to as **opportunistic pathogens** and frequently are naturally occurring environmental microorganisms found in air, water, soil, vegetable matter and on food. The normal commensal flora can behave as opportunistic pathogens following impairment in host defence (e.g. oral thrush caused by the oral yeast *C. albicans* following antibiotic treatment).

Recent advances in medical science and patient treatment have dramatically improved the quality of life and lifespan of countless individuals. Thus in recent decades there has been a significant increase in the proportion of individuals with compromised or impaired host defences, including human immunodeficiency virus (**HIV**)-infected and acquired immune deficiency syndrome (**AIDS**) patients, cancer patients and organ transplant recipients. These individuals are more susceptible to infection than normal healthy people and frequently become infected with opportunistic pathogens. Furthermore, many microorganisms, including human-derived and environmental organisms, have adapted to colonise a wide variety of medical devices used in patient treatment (e.g. urinary catheters, indwelling venous lines, oral prostheses, dental chair unit waterlines) and may give rise to serious and even life-threatening infections.

Infection prevention and control is a rational process that is implemented in the healthcare environment to minimise infection risks to patients and staff. The process, which has many aspects, centres on management of all aspects of the dental clinic environment, managing and minimising cross-contamination risks and thus minimising the potential for cross-infection. It is important to emphasise that cross-infection risks cannot be totally eliminated as we live in a world teeming with microorganisms. However, effective IPC programmes will dramatically reduce opportunities for cross-infection, thus providing a safe environment for patients and dental team staff and works best when all the aspects are implemented appropriately and meticulously (Smith *et al.*, 2009).

Blood-borne viruses

The transmission of particular viral agents in blood and blood products has been identified as a serious and potentially fatal risk to healthcare workers, including dental healthcare professionals. These viruses include HIV, hepatitis B virus (HBV) and hepatitis C virus (HCV). Transmission of blood-borne viruses in the dental healthcare setting is relatively uncommon but does occur (Shah *et al.*, 2006; Redd *et al.*, 2007). Exposure to virus-infected blood can result in transmission from patient to dental healthcare staff, from dental healthcare staff to patient and from patient to patient. The potential for transmission is greatest from patient to dental staff. The risk of exposure to blood-borne viruses by dental healthcare staff depends on the prevalence of the viruses in the patient population and the nature and frequency of contact with blood and saliva through percutaneous or sharps injury (e.g. needlestick injury). The risk of infection following exposure to a blood-borne virus depends on the inoculum size (i.e. the number of infectious virus particles to which an individual is exposed), the route of transmission (e.g. percutaneous injury with a needle contaminated with blood) and the susceptibility of the exposed healthcare worker.

Hepatitis B virus

HBV is transmitted by percutaneous and sharps injury or mucosal exposure to blood, saliva or other body fluids of individuals with either acute or chronic HBV infection. Blood contains the highest proportion of infectious HBV particles and is the most significant body fluid responsible for transmission in the healthcare setting. Infectious HBV particles have been shown to survive in dried blood at ambient temperature on environmental surfaces for up to a week (Bond *et al.*, 1981). There is some evidence to suggest that some cases of HBV infection resulted from inoculation of HBV into cutaneous scratches, abrasions, other lesions, or on to mucosal surfaces. Fortunately, the incidence of occupational HBV infection among healthcare workers has decreased significantly over the last two decades because of vaccination and the implementation of effective IPC procedures. Safe and effective recombinant (i.e. genetically engineered) HBV subunit vaccines have been available for many years and all dental healthcare personnel should be vaccinated during training and before they are exposed to blood. These vaccines consist of viral protein purified from yeast cells and do not contain HBV particles.

Hepatitis C virus

HCV does not appear to be efficiently transmitted through occupational exposure to blood compared to HBV (Mitsui *et al.*, 1992; Puro *et al.*, 1995; Dement *et al.*, 2004). Nonetheless, cases of transmission of HCV infection to healthcare workers including dental staff following exposure to HCV-infected blood have been reported following needle-stick injury or blood splashes (Shah *et al.*, 2006). Currently there is no vaccine available for HCV.

Human immunodeficiency virus

In developed countries, the risk of HIV transmission in the dental clinical environment is very low. Prospective studies worldwide indicate that the average risk of HIV infection following a single percutaneous exposure to HIV-infected blood is 0.3%, and even lower following an exposure of mucous membranes in the mouth, nose or eye (Bell, 1997). Furthermore, the possibility of HIV transmission via saliva is remote (Navazesh *et al.*, 2010). Currently there is no vaccine available for HIV but effective antiviral treatment regimens are available to treat HIV infection (British HIV Association, 2008).

Transmissible spongiform encephalopathies

Transmissible spongiform encephalopathies (TSEs) are fatal degenerative brain diseases that occur in humans and several animal species (Goldfarb and Brown, 1995). They are caused by altered forms of naturally occurring **prion proteins** (PrP) that are normally present in human and animal brain tissue. In TSEs, these altered prion protein forms (PrPSc) accumulate in the brain and subsequently are responsible for the characteristic features of TSEs. These altered prion proteins are extremely resistant to inactivation by standard thermal, chemical, and other means used routinely for destroying microorganisms. The best-known human TSE is **Creutzfeldt–Jakob disease** (CJD). Person-to-person transmission of TSEs through direct contact does not occur. Iatrogenic (clinical treatment-associated) transmission via contaminated medical devices has been documented on rare occasions. In 1995 a new form of TSE was described in the United Kingdom called **variant CJD** (vCJD) (Hullard d'Aignaux *et al.*, 2001). A link has been established between vCJD and bovine spongiform encephalopathy (BSE) in cattle and vCJD appears to have arisen through the consumption of BSE-infected animal products. There have been several probable cases of vCJD derived from transfusion of whole blood (Llewelyn *et al.*, 2004) and blood products (Chohan *et al.*, 2010). In humans, prion proteins have been detected in tonsilar tissue, but the majority of oral tissues examined were negative, with the exception of the trigeminal ganglia (Head *et al.*, 2003). However, a recent study showed that following intestinal infection using a murine model with a prion agent related to vCJD, infectivity was widely disseminated in tissues of the murine oral cavity, including salivary glands, dental pulp and gingivae at a higher level than previously described, during the preclinical and clinical stages of the disease (Walker *et al.*, 2009; Walker, 2010). The study also provided evidence for the potential transmission of the disease from contaminated instruments by contact with the gingival margin.

No iatrogenic cases of CJD have been linked to dental procedures and there *currently* is no evidence of TSE infectivity, including vCJD, in dental tissues. Dental procedures can be considered low risk, assuming optimal standards of IPC and instrument decontamination are maintained (Walker, 2010). For patients who do not have a known or suspected TSE, Standard Precautions (see below) are sufficient for dental procedures. However, procedures that are likely to involve contact with neurovascular tissue should, if possible, be scheduled for the end of the treatment session, to allow time for appropriate cleaning and decontamination of instruments. Although there is no evidence of increased risk associated with performing dental procedures on known or suspected TSE patients, the following precautions are recommended:

- Single-use instruments should be used and destroyed following use by incineration.
- Dental handpieces should not be attached to dental chair unit (DCU) waterlines as there is a small possibility that potentially infected clinical material could be drawn into the water supply line due to antiretraction valve failure (see below). If irrigation is required, it should be provided using a disposable syringe.
- A portable suction unit, with disposable reservoir and suction tubes, should be used.
- Patients should rinse their mouth during and following dental treatment into a disposable bowl, rather than the DCU cuspidor.

For the interested reader, more comprehensive overviews on TSEs are provided elsewhere (Hullard d'Aignaux *et al.*, 2001; Taylor, 2004; Bennett *et al.*, 2007; Department of Health, 2007).

Immunisation

Immunisation or vaccination is an essential part of IPC programmes for dental healthcare workers, and a comprehensive immunisation policy should be implemented and monitored for all dental healthcare facilities. It is important to appreciate that vaccinations do not always result in immunity and that there are some diseases for which vaccination does not yet exist (e.g. HCV and HIV). For all dental healthcare personnel, the immunisation policy should incorporate current legislation and the guidelines and recommendations provided by national healthcare authorities. Immunisations should be carried out before the dental healthcare worker is placed at risk, preferably during training and prior to exposure to patient-derived clinical material (e.g. contaminated dental instruments). Immunisation should also be considered for non-clinical staff who, because of their duties, may be placed at risk of acquiring infections (e.g. maintenance, clerical, domestic and cleaning personnel). Routine childhood vaccinations include immunisation against poliomyelitis, tetanus, diphtheria, pertussis (whooping cough), measles, mumps and rubella. Vaccinations against meningococcal group C meningitis and septicaemia and *Haemophilus influenzae*

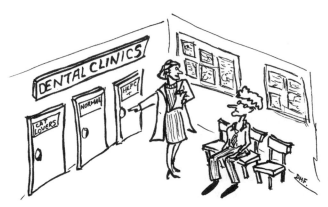

Figure 8.2 Standard Precautions should be applied to all patients regardless of their known or unknown infection status and medical history.

type B are also available. In addition to these vaccines, the dental healthcare worker should receive HBV vaccination and a follow-up blood test(s) to determine adequate serum antibody titre levels (consult your national guidelines with regard to recommended response levels). Annual immunisation should also be considered for influenza viruses, provided this is consistent with the indications of national regulatory authorities. The predominant influenza virus strain(s) circulating during any particular year is monitored by the **World Health Organization** (WHO) and they recommend the most appropriate vaccine for annual use (World Health Organization, 2010).

Standard precautions

In 1996, the USA Centers for Disease Control and Prevention (CDC) expanded the concept of Universal Precautions for IPC and changed the term to Standard Precautions. Standard Precautions integrate and expand the elements of Universal Precautions into a standard of care designed to protect healthcare personnel and patients from transmission of microorganisms from blood or any other body fluid, excretion or secretion. Standard Precautions apply to contact with all blood, body fluids, secretions and excretions (except sweat), regardless of whether they contain blood (Kohn *et al.*, 2003) (Figure 8.2).

They are also applied in relation to contact with non-intact skin (i.e. damaged or injured skin) and with mucous membranes. In addition to Standard Precautions, other measures may be necessary to prevent transmission of specific infectious diseases (e.g. tuberculosis, influenza and varicella (cause of chickenpox)) that are transmitted through airborne, droplet or contact (e.g. sneezing, coughing and contact with skin). In reality, patients who are acutely ill with these diseases rarely seek routine dental outpatient care. However, a general understanding of precautions for diseases transmitted by all routes is necessary as patients may not always be aware of their disease status (i.e. they may be asymptomatic) or they may deliberately conceal an existing condition from the healthcare worker. Necessary transmission-based precautions might include treating the patient in isolation, adequate room ventilation, respiratory protection (e.g. staff treating a patient with active tuberculosis should wear facemasks designed to exclude tuberculosis-causing bacteria), or indeed a postponement of non-emergency dental procedures.

A combination of Standard Precautions, personal protective clothing and equipment, surgery design and administrative controls is the best means to minimise occupational exposures. Written policies and procedures to facilitate prompt reporting, evaluation, counselling, treatment and medical follow-up of all occupational exposures should be available to all dental healthcare workers. These policies and procedures should be consistent with international and national guidelines and legislation, and local requirements and should address education and training, post-exposure management and exposure reporting. Dental training programmes based in dental schools and hospitals have the advantage of being able to coordinate with departments that provide personnel health services. However, the majority of dental practices are in settings that do not have direct access to comprehensive on-site health service programmes. In this regard, it would be prudent for the dental team leader(s) or practice manager(s) to ensure that appropriate IPC and referral arrangements are in place before any dental healthcare worker is placed at risk of exposure to infectious or potentially infectious microorganisms. The personal health of each member of the dental team is also important. Under certain circumstances, it may be necessary to exclude a member of the team from undertaking or assisting with invasive procedures (e.g. a dental team member colonised by methicillin-resistant *Staphylococcus aureus* (**MRSA**) should not be involved with invasive procedures (e.g. surgical procedures) until the MRSA has been eradicated). Exposure occurs most frequently during percutaneous and needlestick injuries. Other exposure methods are through contact with potentially infectious non-intact skin, other body fluids and mucous membranes.

Hand hygiene

Hand hygiene is one of the primary disease prevention procedures for all healthcare workers (Boyce and Pittet, 2002; Kampf *et al.*, 2009). It assists with reducing the numbers of resident microorganisms, predominantly bacteria, and also eliminates the majority of transient microorganisms that are acquired on a daily basis by handling and touching surfaces, instruments and equipment. Hand washing is a procedure where microorganisms and debris are removed with mechanical action and should be undertaken using a liquid soap preparation that conforms to hand washing efficacy standards and dermatological criteria. A liquid soap preparation containing an antimicrobial agent (e.g. **chlorhexidine**) is recommended for preoperative surgical procedures. Non-antiseptic soap bars or liquid soap should not be used in the dental clinic as these readily become contaminated with bacteria from skin and contaminated sinks and/or water and can therefore act as reservoirs and disseminators of infection (Hegde *et al.*, 2006; Rabier *et al.*, 2008). Liquid soap should be provided in disposable cartridges as refillable soap containers can become contaminated during the refilling process.

The duration of the hand-washing procedure depends on the procedure that is going to be performed: preoperative surgical hand scrub (2–6 minutes), social or antiseptic hand hygiene (15–30 seconds). A hand-washing technique that includes all surfaces of the hand should be used and these have been well described in the literature (World Health Organization, 2009).

Hands should be thoroughly dried after washing as wet surfaces encourage proliferation of bacteria and fungi. Good-quality disposable paper towels should be used for this purpose, as there is a significant risk of contamination when hands are dried using hand towels or roller towels. Poor-quality paper hand towels can cause abrasion or damage to the skin when used repeatedly. Hands should be dried using a patting rather than a rubbing action. Warm air dryers are not appropriate in the healthcare setting as the drying cycle time is often inadequate and they can be a source of cross-contamination (Boyce and Pittet, 2002).

There is considerable evidence in the literature that overall compliance with hand-washing procedures in healthcare settings is less than ideal (Kuzu *et al.*, 2005; Mathai *et al.*, 2010). There are many reasons for this, including lack of education, knowledge or motivation, perceived lack of need, lack of appropriate role models, general inconvenience, insufficient time between procedures or patients, inadequate or inaccessible wash basins and harsh hand-washing products that may cause contact dermatitis or eczema. There is also the potential for hands to become contaminated from microorganisms resident in hand-washing sinks (Coleman *et al.*, 2010). Therefore, dedicated sinks should be assigned and maintained for hand-washing procedures only, and should be regularly cleaned, disinfected and maintained. Furthermore, hands-free taps are also recommended.

In recent years, decontamination of hands by rubbing with alcohol-based solutions or gels has been advocated for use instead of hand washing when hands are visibly clean. Alcohol is more efficient and faster acting than antiseptic soaps and the use of alcohol-containing hand hygiene products helps to improve overall hand hygiene. Alcohols exhibit wide antimicrobial activity against bacteria (including mycobacteria), viruses and fungi, but poor activity against bacterial spores (World Health Organization, 2009). Alcohol alone has no residual effect and to counteract this, biocides such as chlorhexidine, triclosan or quaternary compounds have been added to some hand hygiene products, which increases the persistence of antimicrobial activity on the skin. Alcohol hand gels have many advantages:

* They have a wide antimicrobial spectrum.
* They act rapidly, they evaporate quickly.
* They spread easily on the skin.
* There is no need for a sink or drying facilities.
* They save time compared to conventional hand washing.

There is also evidence that healthcare workers are more likely to use them than to wash hands with soap and water. However, it is important to ensure there is adequate time to allow the hands to dry prior to putting on gloves. Use of towels or tissue to dry hands after application of alcohol hand gels may lead to recontamination. Alcohol hand gels may cause drying of the skin after repeated use and some products have added emollients to counteract this. Finally, a sticky residue may build up on the hands following several successive hand gel applications and some manufacturers recommend that hands should be washed periodically with soap and water to remove this.

Finger nails, hand and wrist jewellery

All wrist and hand jewellery should be removed prior to performing clinical procedures and before performing hand hygiene or donning gloves. Bacterial densities on hands are higher when rings are worn, particularly those containing stones or ridges. Wrist and hand jewellery interfere with thorough hand washing and make putting on gloves more difficult and increase the likelihood of gloves becoming damaged in the process and should not be worn. Nails, especially the underside, harbour the highest densities of microorganisms so they should be kept short, filed smoothly and free of varnish. Artificial nails (of any kind) increase microbial load and discourage vigorous hand washing and should not be allowed in a healthcare environment.

Aseptic techniques

Medical or clean asepsis is used in an effort to keep patients as free from exposure to microorganisms as possible. It is used to prevent contamination of wounds and other susceptible sites by microorganisms that could cause infection. Surgical or sterile asepsis includes procedures to eliminate microorganisms from an area. This is particularly applicable to theatre suites. Sterile equipment and fluids are used during invasive procedures. Medical or clean asepsis reduces the number of microorganisms present and prevents their spread. In the dental clinic, before patient treatments, it is important to check that instrument packs and kits are sterile and that packs are intact. Before setting up for a procedure in the dental clinic, work surfaces should be clean and dental staff should carry out hand hygiene and wear the appropriate protective clothing and equipment (see below). Staff should not lean or reach over the set-up area. Sterile packs should be opened only from the corners by peeling back and tipping the instruments gently on to the centre of the pre-prepared set-up area or sterile field. Air movement near the set-up should be minimised. Do not allow others to use your treatment area as a passageway.

In dentistry, it is necessary to recap local anaesthetic dental needles, as local anaesthetic may have to be readministered during the treatment session. This should be carried out using a single-handed bayonet or scoop technique (Figure 8.3). Alternatively, there are some commercially available devices that hold the needle cap firmly in position. The needle can then be recapped by inserting the needle into the prepositioned cap.

Protective clothing

Protecting dental healthcare personnel from potential exposure to microorganisms requires a combination of controls, one of which is the use of **personal protective equipment** (PPE) (Kohn *et al.*, 2003). The wearing of PPE helps to prevent contact with infectious microorganisms or body fluid by creating a barrier between the worker and the infectious material. National health and safety authorities require workers, including healthcare professionals, to wear PPE when there is a risk of exposure to potentially infectious diseases. PPE should *never* be worn outside the clinical environment.

Gloves

Gloves protect the dental healthcare worker's hands from exposure to microorganisms while performing dental procedures. However, they do not protect against percutaneous injuries. A variety of disposable gloves are available for this purpose, the majority of which are

(a)

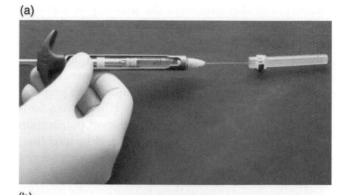

(b)

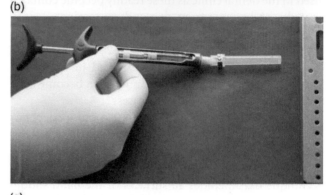

(c)

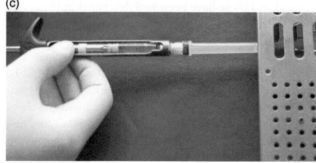

Figure 8.3 Recapping of local anaesthetic dental needles using a single-handed bayonet or scoop technique. (a) & (b) Place the needle cap on the work-top and 'fish' it up with the needle when you are ready to recap. Make sure you keep your free hand out of the way of the needle. (c) Push the recapped needle against a firm flat surface to secure the needle cap in position.

made of latex, vinyl or nitrile. Non-sterile, ambidextrous, disposable, latex examination gloves are the most frequently used type of glove in modern dental surgeries. The use of powdered gloves has been discontinued in many healthcare institutions to reduce exposure to latex powder that can cause allergy (Korniewicz *et al.*, 2005). If latex gloves are used, they should be powder-free and low protein gloves (Health and Safety Executive, 2008). Sterile surgical gloves are worn for surgical procedures. Auxiliary dental staff frequently wear disposable latex gloves when cleaning environmental surfaces in the dental clinic; however, they are not suitable or intended for this purpose. Reusable heavy-duty gloves made of latex

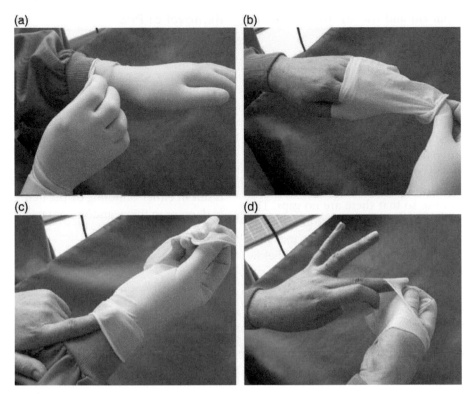

Figure 8.4 The correct way of removing contaminated disposable gloves used during dental procedures. (a) Remove gloves by grasping the outside edge of the glove closest to the wrist. (b) Peel the glove away from the hand and in so doing, the glove will be turned inside out. (c) & (d) Then slide an ungloved finger under the cuff of the remaining glove and peel off from inside.

or nitrile are more appropriate and individual pairs should be provided for each worker concerned and not used by many different individuals.

It is important to appreciate that gloves *only* protect you provided you do not touch environmental surfaces, face or hair with contaminated gloves. Care should be taken to ensure not to touch and thus cross-contaminate items such as pens, case notes, X-ray films, telephones, computers (screen, keyboard and mouse, etc.) with contaminated gloves. Gloves should be changed after each patient and should *never* be washed or reused. Gloves should also be changed if they become heavily soiled, even if being used during treatment of the same patient, or torn during use. Gloves should also be worn when handling or cleaning items or surfaces contaminated with body fluids (e.g. used clinical gowns and the DCU spittoon). Hand hygiene procedures should be undertaken before putting on and after removal of gloves. Care should be taken to limit self-contamination when removing gloves. Remove gloves by grasping the outside edge of the glove closest to the wrist; peel the glove away from the hand and in so doing, the glove will be turned inside out. Then slide an ungloved finger under the cuff of the remaining glove and peel it off from inside (Figure 8.4) (World Health Organization, 2009). Discard used gloves into a contaminated waste bin.

Gowns

Clean gowns should be worn to prevent cross-contamination of the clothes of dental healthcare staff during dental procedures. It is important to emphasise that uniforms (e.g. dental nurses' or dental hygienists' uniforms, etc.) are *not* protective clothing and protective gowns should be worn over uniforms during dental procedures. There are many different views regarding whether gowns should have long or short sleeves; however, long-sleeved gowns protect the forearms from contamination and are recommended. Gowns should protect the torso and be long enough to cover the knees of operators while in the seated position. Gowns should also be fluid resistant and, in the case of reusable gowns, be able to withstand high-temperature washing with a good-quality detergent. Gowns should be changed if they become visibly soiled. Gowns should be removed by loosening the ties or snap fasteners at the back of the gown, which should be uncontaminated, and then peeling the gown away from the neck and shoulders. During this process the contaminated outside part of the gown should be facing away from the wearer. The gown may then be rolled into a bundle and placed in a designated laundry bin in the case of reusable gowns, or a designated contaminated waste bin as appropriate. Gowns are the first item of PPE to be put on and the last to be removed before leaving the patient treatment area.

Facemasks

Standard facemasks are used to protect the mucous membranes of the mouth and nose from spray, splashes, spatter and aerosols. However, they only offer limited protection against respiratory pathogens like influenza virus. They are secured in place with either string ties at the back of the head and base of the neck or by adjustable elastic tapes. The mask should be adjusted to fit snugly against the face and nose so that there are no gaps. The mask should *not* be touched during procedures to prevent contamination from gloves. Face shields may also be worn and should protect the forehead, extend below the chin and also wrap around the sides of the face. Masks should be changed after each patient or if visibly soiled or wet. Facemasks should not be worn around the neck as a necklace as this serves no useful purpose. Masks should be removed by untying the strings from the bottom first and then the top and then discarding into a designated waste bin.

Protective glasses

Protective glasses or goggles should be worn during dental procedures by both dental healthcare workers and patients to prevent physical injury and transmission of microorganisms to the eyes. Eyes are particularly vulnerable to injury by high-velocity particles/debris generated during use of high-speed handpieces and scalers. Prescription glasses do not usually provide sufficient protection, so protective goggles or glasses should be able to fit snugly over the top of them. The goggles or glasses should be optically clear, be close fitting and have top and side shields to provide best possible eye protection. They should be washed with soap and water after each use. If glasses are disinfected, care should be exercised to ensure that they are thoroughly rinsed, as chemical residues may cause irritation to the skin and eyes of the wearer. Contact lenses do not protect the eyes and can increase the risk of exposure to microorganisms if contaminated fluids gain access beneath the lens. Protective glasses should not be pushed up on to the head as this may result in cross-contamination of the hair.

Shoes

The wearing of open-toed sandals and shoes made from fabric is to be discouraged in the dental clinical environment to minimise the potential for contamination or physical injury from dropped instruments, other items or chemicals falling on to the exposed foot.

Removal of PPE

1 Gloves.
2 Mask (or respirator), or a visor if worn and then mask.
3 Protective eyewear (goggles).
4 Followed by hand hygiene.

Topping up

Topping up boxes containing consumable items such as gloves or masks in the dental clinic should not occur. Many items are machine packed and topping up will result in either bundling of the items, possibly resulting in damage to them, and/or contamination of the storage boxes.

Processing and handling of dental instruments

The majority of instruments used in dentistry are double ended and can also be very sharp. For this reason they should be handled with appropriate care and attention. All instruments should be used only for the purposes for which they are intended.

Instrument decontamination

Several studies have identified significant deficiencies in the management of dental instrument decontamination and in the decontamination process (Scottish Executive Health Department, 2004; Letters *et al.*, 2005; Smith *et al.*, 2009). In 2009 the United Kingdom Department of Health published Health Technical Memorandum (HTM) 01-05, which provides detailed guidance on decontamination of instruments in primary care dentistry and was targeted at English and Welsh healthcare workers involved in instrument decontamination (Department of Health, 2009). This guidance supersedes all previous guidance on dental instrument decontamination in England and Wales. Scotland and the Republic of Ireland have also published detailed guidance on dental instrument decontamination (Health Protection Scotland, 2007; Department of Health and Children, 2007). It is beyond the scope of this chapter to provide an in-depth review of the guidance detailed in HTM 01-05 or in other guidance documents on dental instrument decontamination because of space constraints. To understand and effectively implement the dental instrument decontamination process, it is imperative that individuals engaged in this process receive adequate training and support. The principal features of current best practice for dental instrument decontamination are outlined below in the following paragraphs and sections.

All reusable medical devices, including dental instruments, must be decontaminated following each use. Dental surgeries should have dedicated space allocated for instrument decontamination and processing. The purpose of the designated area is to minimise opportunities for cross-infection of patients and clinical staff and cross-contamination of the working environment. The designated area should be made up of receiving, cleaning, decontamination, packing, sterilisation and storage areas. The area for processing of contaminated instruments should be segregated into contaminated and clean areas and contaminated instruments should be processed unidirectionally from the contaminated to the clean area to avoid recontamination of clean items. Enough space should be provided in the decontamination area to accommodate equipment, sinks and work benches.

It is vital that the *appropriate* method of decontamination is applied to all dental instruments and equipment. Generally, dental instruments and equipment may be divided into three risk categories: high, medium and low risk, according to the risk of infection associated with the subsequent use of each item of equipment. For **high-risk items** (e.g. instruments that become contaminated with blood), cleaning followed by heat sterilisation is the method of choice. For dental procedures it is best to use only instruments that will tolerate sterilisation by the moist heat method (i.e. autoclaving), as this is one of the safest and easiest to monitor and validate. **Medium-risk items** consist of instruments or equipment used in contact with mucous membranes in the oral cavity, such as light-curing units, that are not suitable for heat sterilisation and should be barrier protected prior to use. For reusable medium-risk items, the appropriate means of decontamination is cleaning followed by high-level disinfection or sterilisation. **Low-risk items** include instruments, equipment or other items/surfaces in the dental clinic that come into contact with a patient's healthy intact skin, and equipment that does not have close contact with the patient. For these items, cleaning is sufficient. However, disinfection may be necessary if there is a known infection risk. Examples of low-risk items include door handles and surfaces, including floors and walls.

Instrument collecting and transportation

After use in dental procedures, contaminated dental instruments have to be removed from the surgery and transported to the designated processing area for cleaning, decontamination and sterilisation. Steps in the collection and transportation process are outlined below:

- Instruments should be removed from the surgery or clinical environment using a defined procedure.

- To prevent injuries during transportation and during the decontamination process, instruments should be arranged in kits or cassettes for set procedures, e.g. examination kit, scaling kit, etc.
- Instruments should not be transported uncovered, as there is the likelihood of dropping the instruments en route or, indeed, colliding with patients or staff.
- Depending on how long the instruments are stored prior to cleaning, it may be necessary to store them in a disinfectant solution. Instrument manufacturer's instructions should be followed as some commercial disinfectant products recommended for this purpose cause corrosion if in contact with instruments for prolonged periods. Ideally, instruments should be cleaned and disinfected immediately or shortly after use. In the case of heavily contaminated instruments it is best to adopt a policy of removing as much of the contamination as possible prior to collection for transport to the decontamination area, e.g. instruments heavily contaminated with blood should be wiped in damp gauze using a single-handed technique.
- Remove all disposable items from the kit prior to dispatch, e.g. disposable needles, cartridges, polishing cups.

Hand washing of instruments

Cleaning should remove all visible blood, dirt, dust or other foreign materials from instruments following use. Hand washing of instruments should be avoided due to the high risk of percutaneous injury during cleaning and because hand washing of instruments cannot be validated. Unfortunately this hazardous approach is still widely used.

Ultrasonic cleaning

Ultrasonic cleaners can be used to decontaminate dental instruments and their use is far safer than hand washing instruments (Whitworth and Palmer, 2010). Contaminated instruments in an open basket or tray are immersed in an enzymatic solution designed to digest biological material. Ultrasonic waves are then passed through the solution resulting in the removal of contaminating material on the surface of instruments by a process called **cavitation**. Ultrasonic cleaning is suitable for stainless steel instruments but not suitable for plastic items. There are many different types of ultrasonic baths available ranging from the small bench-top variety to larger baths used more frequently in hospitals. Some important considerations concerning the use of ultrasonic baths are outlined below:

- The ultrasonic cleaning units or bath should be operated with a well-fitting lid to prevent release of aerosols.

- Fill the bath with the enzymatic detergent solution recommended by the manufacturer and drain and rinse twice daily or more often, as heavily contaminated cleaning solutions can transfer contaminants to later batches of instruments.
- The unit should be thermostatically controlled (43–45 °C: 3–4 minutes) to prevent coagulation of proteins on to instrument surfaces.
- Ensure that all items to be treated are fully immersed and hinged instruments should be opened.
- Baskets containing instruments must not be overloaded.

Washer disinfector

This is an automated machine that is specially designed to clean, decontaminate and thermally disinfect instruments and equipment. Washer disinfectors should conform to approved standards (e.g. International Standards Organization (ISO) 15883, parts 1 and 2; ISO, 2004a, b). The washer/disinfector runs a washing cycle, followed by a disinfection phase. Disinfection is performed by flushing with hot water of approximately 90 °C for 1–10 minutes. The machine renders equipment clean, disinfected, dry and safe for further handling. The machines are fast and are easy to operate. They usually have set, validated programmes for different types of loads and allow for minimum instrument handling. However, they are unsuitable for use with heat-sensitive items. Care should be taken not to over-fill the washer disinfector as this can cause some items to be shielded and result in them not being cleaned or disinfected properly.

Handpieces

After each patient use, any dental handpiece, ultrasonic scaler or air scaler that is connected to the DCU air/water system should be operated to discharge water and/or air for at least 30 seconds; care should be taken not to inhale the aerosol. This procedure is designed to dislodge any patient-derived material that may have been retracted into the air and/or waterlines due to failure of antiretraction valves. These valves are designed to prevent material or fluids from being retracted or siphoned back into air and/or waterlines. An Italian study of 54 DCUs, comprising 18 different models by six different DCU manufacturers reported an antiretraction device failure rate of 74% (40/54 DCUs tested) (Berlutti *et al.*, 2003).

Following air and waterline purging, handpieces and scalers should be detached, cleaned, decontaminated and sterilised according to the manufacturer's instructions and local policy. Scaler tips should be carefully detached, processed through a washer disinfector and

sterilised in a vacuum autoclave. Automated presterilisation cleaning is the preferred method of handpiece and scaler decontamination. However, where manual cleaning is used, clean the outside of the handpiece or scaler with detergent and warm water (follow the manufacturer's instructions with regard to type of detergent or other agent advised). If recommended by the manufacturer, lubricate the handpiece with pressurised oil until clean oil appears from the chuck (wear protective clothing including gloves, glasses and a facemask). Cover the working end of the handpiece with disposable paper towel to absorb the residual oil and clean away any excess oil. Following cleaning, sterilise handpieces and scalers in a vacuum autoclave.

X-ray

Intraoral films and digital imaging plates should always be barrier protected prior to insertion into the oral cavity. The barrier should be disposed of in contaminated waste after removal. Bite-blocks and film-holders should be autoclavable and a sterilised block and holder should be used for each patient. Similarly, used digital imaging plates should be decontaminated according to the manufacturer's instructions.

Single-use and single-patient-use items

If an item is marked *single-use*, it means that it must *only* be used on a single occasion and then it should be discarded into contaminated waste or a sharps box, as appropriate. Single-use item products should be labelled with the symbol ②. A single-use item or device *must not* be used on multiple occasions either on a single patient or on a different patient. Examples of single-use items include plastic syringes used for irrigation, suction tips, polishing cups and endodontic files. The use of *single-use* items is recommended where possible. Before using a prepacked sterile single-use item, check that the packaging is intact and the product is within its use-by date. Prior to use these devices must be stored in clean, designated areas where there is no risk of exposure to moisture or to aerosol and droplet contamination. It should be noted that only reusable medical devices should be reprocessed. Never reprocess medical devices designated for single-use only.

Packaging of instruments

After cleaning and decontamination, dental instruments have to be appropriately packaged prior to sterilisation. Instruments should be packed before sterilisation, because otherwise as soon as they are removed from the autoclave, they become recontaminated with dust and microorganisms from the environment.

Prior to packaging instruments should be dry and carefully examined for defects, the presence of residual contamination and/or corrosion. Packaging allows the instruments to be safely stored and transported within the clinical environment following sterilisation. The packaging material should be compatible with the sterilisation process (i.e. allow passage of air and steam) and should provide an effective barrier against recontamination by microorganisms (i.e. the packaging should be robust and permit handling and transportation while maintaining the sterility of the packaged instruments). Primary packaging consisting of sterilisation pouches or bags is generally sufficient for the dental clinic environment. Alternatively, instruments in kits or cassettes may be packaged as required. Packaging should also contain clearly visible chemical indicator strips that give a colour change when sterilising conditions have been achieved during autoclaving. Finally, packaging should be appropriately labelled so that the packaged instrument(s) is clearly identified.

Sterilisation of dental instruments

Sterilisation of instruments should be undertaken using a vacuum autoclave. Steam sterilisation is the recommended method of sterilisation for heat-tolerant dental instruments and should be undertaken using equipment that conforms to ISO 17665 (ISO, 2006). The manufacturer's instructions for correct use of equipment should always be followed and the equipment should be used by trained and competent personnel.

When loading the autoclave, instruments and other items to be sterilised should be arranged to permit free circulation of steam and care should be taken not to over-fill the autoclave chamber. This also facilitates proper drying during the drying phase of the cycle as wet packs are deemed unsterile. Autoclaves have to be monitored and validated to ensure they are working correctly and produce a sterile load (Harte and Miller, 2003). Professionals normally undertake validation and this service is usually provided by appropriately accredited commercial companies. Individual autoclave cycles (i.e. packaged instruments, laboratory glassware, etc.) are usually validated separately and autoclave validation should be undertaken at least once a year.

Sterilisation monitoring usually includes a combination of process controls, including mechanical, biological and chemical controls (Figure 8.5):

- Mechanical methods for monitoring sterilisation include assessing cycle time, temperature and pressure by observing parameter displays on the steriliser and recording these for each load. Many autoclaves are supplied with integral recording equipment that print

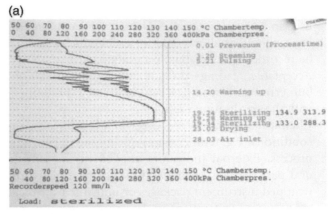

(a)

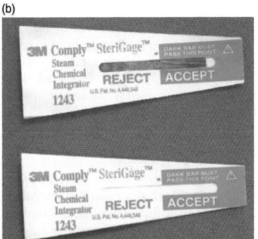

(b)

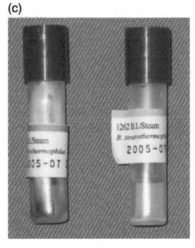

(c)

Figure 8.5 Examples of mechanical, chemical and biological controls for the sterilisation process. (a) A parameter printout from an autoclave following a sterilisation cycle. (b) Examples of chemical indicator strips used within instrument pouches to show that steam penetration has occurred; the upper strip has been exposed to steam within a pouch whereas the lower strip has not. (c) Examples of spore strip biological indicators. The indicator on the left has been subject to a sterilisation cycle and all of the spores have been killed (indicated by the blue colour). The indicator on the right has not been subject to a sterilisation cycle and the spores are viable (indicated by the yellow colour).

out this information. Larger autoclaves, such as those used in hospitals, may also have a remote data archiving facility that allows data for each autoclave run to be recorded in a database on a networked computer. Acceptable readings do not guarantee sterilisation, but erroneous readings can indicate a problem(s) with the sterilisation cycle.

- Chemical indicators are used to evaluate physical conditions (e.g. temperature) during the sterilisation process. External indicators applied to the outside of a package (e.g. chemical indicator tape placed on wrapped instrument packages or imprinted chemical markings on instrument packaging pouches) change colour rapidly when exposed to high temperature. Chemical indicator test results can be read by examining the autoclaved packages for the appropriate colour changes on indicator tape or imprint mark when the sterilisation cycle is completed. If chemical indicators or the autoclave parameter readout data indicate inadequate processing, the load should be reprocessed.
- Biological indicators (i.e. spore tests) can also be used for monitoring the sterilisation process. These usually consist of highly resistant bacterial spores (e.g. spores from *Geobacillus* or *Bacillus* species) that are only killed when adequate sterilisation conditions (i.e. time, temperature and steam pressure) are reached. If the high-density spore preparations found in biological indicators are killed following a sterilisation cycle, this indicates that other microorganisms present in the load have also been destroyed.
- Steam penetration tests such as the Bowie and Dick test are recommended as part of the validation process for steam sterilisers. Because dental instruments such as dental handpieces are lumened devices, an alternative steam penetration test such as the helix test may be appropriate. A more detailed overview of indicators and their use for monitoring the efficacy of sterilisation cycles is provided by Kohn *et al.*, 2003.

It is important that water supplied to autoclaves is of good quality to prevent the formation of residue on instruments during the sterilisation process. Residues can result from chemical compounds dissolved or suspended in the supply water or indeed from supply water heavily contaminated with microorganisms. Furthermore, water reservoirs within autoclaves should be drained and cleaned regularly. A variety of approaches for processing autoclave supply water is available, such as reverse osmosis and ion exchange. The autoclave manufacturer's instructions should be followed in relation to proper maintenance of the equipment, including the quality of the supply water.

Storage of sterilised items

Sterilised instruments, other items and disposable single-use items contained in wrapped packages or pouches should be stored in a dry enclosed area, preferably in closed cupboards, cabinets or drawers. They should not be stored under sinks or adjacent to taps or other locations where they may become damp or wet. All sterilised packages should contain the sterilisation date and, if there are multiple autoclaves in a particular facility, the autoclave used. The shelf life of sterilised packages is event related and can be influenced by the packaging materials, storage and handling conditions, the likelihood of product material deterioration and package design. In general, sterilised packages can be stored for up to 6 months. All sterilised packages should be examined prior to use to ensure they are dry and that the packaging is intact. If packaging is compromised, the instruments should be reprocessed.

Surgery design

Good dental surgery design is critical for effective IPC. Spending time at an early stage on developing an appropriate surgery design can help dramatically to improve the effectiveness of IPC programmes. A list of some of the essential features in a well-designed dental surgery is outlined below:

- Proper ventilation and temperature control in the dental clinic is important for the comfort of patients and dental healthcare staff. It also helps to minimise the environmental conditions that encourage growth of microorganisms. Minimise the entry of outside dust into the dental clinic; this is critical in reducing air-borne contaminants, particularly bacterial and fungal spores.
- Materials used in the construction of work surfaces should be able to withstand repeated disinfection. Surfaces should be smooth, without joins and be non-porous.
- There should be curved intersections between the vertical and horizontal components of the surgery furnishings to facilitate ease of cleaning and to prevent accumulation of debris in unsealed cracks and joins.
- A designated sink should be provided for hand washing only.
- All parts of the dental clinic and adjoining areas should be easily accessible for cleaning and disinfection.
- There should be clearly delineated clean and contaminated areas or zones. Zoning defines the areas that may become contaminated during patient treatment. Separate areas designated for instrument reprocessing should be divided into *contaminated* and *clean* areas.

- There should be a separate area for writing up patient charts or notes.
- Do not store unnecessary equipment (e.g. stock items, etc.) within the patient treatment environment to prevent contamination from spatter, droplets and aerosols.
- Disinfectant dispensers should dispense rather than spray disinfectant to minimise aerosol generation. Wash and dry the disinfectant dispenser bottles before replacing with fresh solutions of disinfectant.
- DCUs should have smooth, seam-free upholstery that is made of non-absorbent material.
- DCUs should have foot-operated controls that can be wiped clean on a daily basis.
- DCU manual controls must be able to withstand regular cleaning and disinfection without causing damage to the electrical components. Light handles, dental chair and instrument control buttons should be covered with impervious coverings and changed between patients. The instrument set-up area should be covered with plastic-backed paper. Care should be taken when removing these self-adhesive barriers to prevent contamination of the area that it is protecting.
- DCU operating light handles should be able to be easily removed for cleaning and autoclaving.
- DCUs should have a facility for waterline disinfection.
- Carpeting is only suitable for public areas of dental healthcare facilities and should be vacuumed regularly.
- Upholstered furniture in the public areas should be well maintained.
- If necessary, a pest-control strategy should be in place to deal with insects or vermin.

General surface cleaning and disinfection

Appropriate protective clothing should be worn prior to cleaning and disinfection of surfaces. Prior to cleaning, all instruments and other items should be removed. The surface should be physically wiped with a disposable paper towel saturated with detergent and allowed to dry. The paper towel should be discarded into a contaminated waste container. Following cleaning, the surface should be disinfected with a product with proven efficacy against viruses, bacteria and fungi. Care should be taken during disinfection of the DCU and surrounding areas to prevent recontamination. A strategy should be developed for cleaning that involves all aspects of the DCU and the surrounding areas. It is important to emphasise that there is no ideal disinfectant; the effectiveness of a particular product depends on the dilution factor, and the mode and speed of action in a particular environment. The interested reader should consult the CDC guidelines for IPC in dentistry for a more comprehensive overview on surface cleaning and disinfection (Kohn *et al.*, 2003).

Waste management

All dental hospitals and dental practices should have a formal clinical waste management policy that should be subject to periodic review (Kohn *et al.*, 2003). All dental healthcare personnel and support staff should be familiar with the policy and strictly adhere to it. Segregation of waste is always the responsibility of the waste producer and should take place as close as possible to where the waste is generated. Disposal of clinical waste from dental clinics must follow the guidelines and recommendations provided by the national registration authority, dental healthcare professional organisation and national healthcare authorities (e.g. Department of Health, 2006; Department of Health and Children, 2010). Clinical waste is defined as any human tissue, disposable items and materials that have been used on patients that may be contaminated with blood, saliva or body fluids (e.g. gauze, cotton wool rolls, wipes, gloves, gowns, facemasks, etc.). This waste may be potentially infectious to any person coming in contact with it and should be placed in appropriate bins or containers. Bags and containers for infectious waste should be marked with the international biohazard symbol. Within the European Union, clinical waste from healthcare institutions has to be disposed of by licensed waste management companies that have to comply with very strict regulations. The European Agreement concerning the International Carriage of Dangerous Goods by Road (ADR) (United Nations Economic Commission for Europe, 2010) governs transport of all hazardous waste, including clinical waste that may be contaminated by infectious agents. For this reason, clinical waste has to be streamed into UN-approved bags or containers that are clearly labeled with the appropriate UN waste category number. The ADR regulations are very detailed and contain specific requirements for packaging different kinds of clinical waste prior to transport. An in-depth overview of the aspects of ADR that relate to dental clinics is beyond the scope of this chapter because of space constraints. However, most clinical waste from dental clinics belongs to ADR Class 6.2 (infectious substances), subdivision I3-UN 3291 (clinical waste) and Category B. The specific requirements of packaging waste to be transported as Category B are detailed in ADR instruction P621 (for further details see Department of Health, 2006; Department of Health and Children, 2010; United Nations Economic Commission for Europe, 2010).

Key aspects of effective waste management

Key aspects of effective waste management in the dental clinic are outlined below:

- All waste should be segregated into clinical and non-clinical waste.
- Appropriate containers or waste-bag holders should be placed in all locations where clinical and non-clinical waste is generated.
- Instructions on waste segregation and identification should be posted at each waste collection point to remind staff of the procedures.
- UN-approved clinical waste bags should be closed with a cable tie or tape when they are two thirds full. Each bag of contaminated waste should have an individual tracing tag or label.
- Waste should not be allowed to accumulate at the point of generation.
- Waste should be collected daily (or as frequently as required) and transported to a designated secure central storage area.
- Waste bags or containers should be replaced immediately with new ones of the same type.
- Protective clothing should always be worn when handling waste, e.g. apron, overalls, gloves and safety shoes (if necessary).
- All staff that handle or transport waste should be vaccinated against HBV and tetanus.
- If general and hazardous wastes are accidentally mixed, the mixture should be treated as hazardous healthcare waste.
- Do not throw or drop clinical waste bags/containers.
- Re-bag split or leaking bags/containers into new bags/containers of the same type.
- Material spilled or leaked from clinical waste bags should be regarded as potentially hazardous. Spillages should be cleared according to local procedures.

Disposal of sharps

Sharps include syringes, needles, cartridges and small amounts of broken glass generated in dental clinics (Department of Health, 2006; Department of Health and Children, 2010). All of these items should be disposed of by placing in UN-approved yellow rigid, leak-proof and puncture-resistant sharps containers that should be available in the dental clinic. All dental healthcare personnel should take responsibility for their own sharps and dispose of them according to local policy (i.e. disposal by licensed waste management company). Non-clinical glassware or other uncontaminated used glassware should not be disposed of as healthcare risk waste sharps. Needles should never be bent or broken because this practice requires unnecessary manipulation of the needle and could result in percutaneous injury. Never fill a sharps box to more than three quarters of its capacity. Sharps boxes should be closed when not in use. Broken instruments should not be placed in sharps boxes. Separate arrangements should be made with your licensed waste management company to dispose of broken instruments. In some hospital trust areas in the United Kingdom, partially used local anaesthetic cartridges are regarded as hazardous waste and are subject to additional disposal controls. Refer to your local healthcare agency for guidelines in this regard.

The dental chair unit as a vehicle for cross-contamination and cross-infection

DCUs are complex medical devices designed to provide the equipment and services necessary for the provision of a wide variety of dental procedures. Because DCUs are used in the treatment of successive patients throughout the day, microbial contamination of specific component parts is an important potential source of cross-infection. Of particular concern are parts of DCUs that come into direct contact with the patient's oral cavity, including dental unit handpieces and suction hoses. Dental unit output water is also of concern as a source of potential cross-infection as it emanates directly from the DCU and enters the oral cavity of the patient during treatment (see below). There are a number of sources of microbial contamination of DCUs, including patient-derived, dental staff-derived and environmental sources. Because of the problem of microbial contamination of DCUs, a variety of standard procedures and guidelines have been proposed to minimise the potential for DCU-associated cross-infection. For example, sterile handpieces and suction tips are used for each patient.

Microbial contamination of dental unit waterlines

Dental unit waterlines (DUWLs) are an essential component of modern DCUs and supply water as a coolant and irrigant to ultrasonic scalers, turbine handpieces, three-way air/water syringes, as well as supplying water for the patient rinse cup filler and the cuspidor (also known as the spittoon). Water is required to cool and irrigate rotary handpieces, scalers and tooth surfaces, for oral rinsing and to flush the cuspidor bowl. Many studies have shown that output water from DUWLs is often contaminated with very high densities of bacteria. This is a universal problem and virtually all DUWLs in standard DCUs are likely to be contaminated (Coleman et al., 2009, 2010).

Bacterial contamination of DUWLs originates primarily in the water supplied to DCUs, which usually contains low numbers of microorganisms. The main reason for the extensive contamination observed in DUWLs is the complex design of the water delivery system from the water inlet junction within the dental chair to the point where water is delivered to the handpieces, three-way syringes and patient rinse cup fillers. This complex network of waterlines consists of several metres of plastic tubing with an internal diameter of a few millimetres in which water stagnates when the equipment is not being used. Microorganisms in water entering DUWLs, mainly aerobic heterotrophic Gram-negative environmental bacteria, and to a lesser extent protozoa, amoebae and fungi, attach themselves to the internal surfaces of the waterlines where they form microcolonies and eventually build up to form multispecies biofilm (Figures 8.6 and 8.7).

In nature, the majority of microorganisms persist attached to surfaces within a structured biofilm ecosystem and not as planktonic (free-living) organisms. Biofilms are mainly composed of bacterial exopolysaccharide, a slimy complex polysaccharide material produced by bacteria, which is highly hydrated and contains either single cells or microbial microcolonies interspersed heterogeneously with pores or channels. Biofilm forms because the water at the edges of the narrow-bore DUWL tubing flows more slowly than water at the centre of the tubing and therefore there is little or no disruption to the microorganisms present on the inside of the waterline. This allows the microorganisms to proliferate before eventually continuing on through the water supply as planktonic forms where they may be deposited at other sites within the tubing or are delivered directly in to the mouths of patients during dental procedures. Thus the biofilm provides a reservoir for ongoing contamination of dental unit output water. Furthermore, microorganisms and fragments of biofilm present in DUWL output water can be aerosolised by ultrasonic scalers and turbine handpieces, which can subsequently be inhaled by patients and dental healthcare staff.

Biofilms exhibit resistance to disinfectants due to failure to penetrate the polysaccharide matrix adequately. The presence of Gram-negative bacteria in waterline biofilm can also result in the presence of bacterial endotoxin in DUWL output water. Endotoxin consists of lipopolysaccharide (LPS) released from the cell walls of Gram-negative bacteria following cell death. Bacterial endotoxin levels >1000 units/ml may be present in DUWL output water. In comparison, the permissible levels of endotoxin permitted for sterile water for injection in the USA is 0.25 units/ml. Significant doses of endotoxin may cause adverse effects in susceptible individuals.

The presence of large numbers of microorganisms in dental unit water presents a risk of infection for dental

Figure 8.6 Confocal micrograph of a section of the inside of a dental chair unit waterline showing extensive biofilm (magnification ×60). Areas stained green are populated by living microorganisms, whereas areas stained red contain predominantly dead microorganisms. Good quality dental unit output water requires regular disinfection of waterlines with a disinfectant that efficiently removes biofilm.

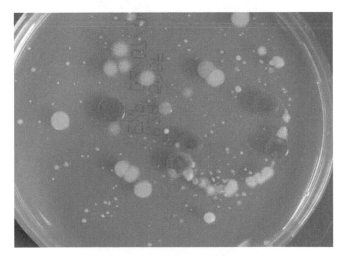

Figure 8.7 Colonies of bacteria from dental chair unit waterline output water following growth on R2A agar medium. The different size and colours of the colonies represent different bacterial species and reflect the multi-species population of microorganisms usually found in dental chair unit waterline biofilm.

patients and staff and is incompatible with good IPC practices. DUWL contamination is of particular concern in the treatment of medically compromised and immunocompromised individuals. Some of the bacteria found in dental unit water are known to cause disease in humans; of particular concern are *Pseudomonas*, *Legionella* and non-tuberculosis *Mycobacterium* species (Coleman *et al.*, 2009, 2010). Although only a few cases of disease transmission related to DUWLs and related biofilm have been documented in the literature, there is considerable potential for infection with bacterial pathogens such as *P. aeruginosa* and *Legionella pneumophila* as well as other organisms. *P. aeruginosa* is a well documented cause of opportunistic infection and is often responsible for cross-infection from contaminated medical devices. *Legionella* species (*L. pneumophila* and approximately 30 other species) are frequently found in water distribution systems in buildings and cause legionnaire's disease (pneumonia resulting from inhalation) and Pontiac fever (non-pneumonic legionellosis) in healthy individuals (Figure 8.8). Occupational exposure to aerosols of waterborne bacteria, generated by dental unit handpieces, can also lead to a higher prevalence of antibodies to *Legionella* in dental staff (Fotos *et al.*, 1985). Furthermore, a temporal association between occupational exposure to contaminated DUWL output water and development of asthma in a subgroup of dentists in whom asthma arose following the commencement of dental training has been reported (Pankhurst *et al.*, 2005). Approved codes of practice for the control

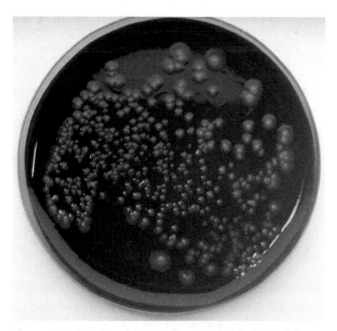

Figure 8.8 Colonies of *Legionella pneumophila* isolated from a hospital water supply grown on buffered charcoal yeast extract agar.

of *Legionella* bacteria in water systems are available (Health and Safety Commission, 2000; World Health Organization, 2007; Health Protection Surveillance Centre, 2009; BSI Publication 8580, BSI, 2010).

Atypical *Mycobacterium* species have also been recovered in large numbers in dental unit water and have potential for infection. *Burkholderia cepacia*, an organism frequently responsible for pulmonary disease in cystic fibrosis patients, and *Stenotrophomonas maltophilia*, a nosocomial (hospital-related) pathogen with significant virulence in debilitated patients, as well as other more harmless organisms, have also been isolated from dental unit water.

Currently there are no official standards or legislation that regulate the microbial quality of DUWL output water (Coleman *et al.*, 2007, 2009). In 1995, the American Dental Association (ADA) established a goal for the year 2000 of ≤200 colony forming units (cfu) per ml of aerobic heterotrophic bacteria for dental unit output water (Anon., 1995), but this has largely not been achieved in practice. The current potable water standard for aerobic heterotrophic bacteria in the European Union does not specify an upper limit, although water sold in bottles or containers should not exceed 100 cfu/ml (Anon., 1998). The CDC guidelines for infection control in dental health care settings recommend a maximum level of aerobic heterotrophic bacteria in DUWL output water of ≤500 cfu/ml (Kohn *et al.*, 2003). The current consensus from experts in the field of DUWL biofilm management is that the quality of DUWL output water should be maintained at ≤200 cfu/ml (Coleman and O'Donnell, 2007).

Disinfection of dental unit waterlines

The most efficient and effective means of maintaining good-quality DUWL output water is regular or residual disinfection of the waterlines with an approved disinfectant that removes biofilm, resulting in output water containing ≤200 cfu aerobic heterotrophic bacteria per ml (Coleman *et al.*, 2007, 2009). Biofilm regrowth can occur within a week following disinfection and so DUWLs should be disinfected at least once weekly with an appropriate disinfectant. For individual DCU models, the advice of the manufacturer should be sought in relation to the type of disinfectant that should be used for DUWL disinfection as well as the most appropriate disinfection protocol that should be used and the frequency of disinfection (Coleman *et al.*, 2007). Some DCU manufacturers have developed DCU models with integrated and semiautomated DUWL cleaning systems that facilitate the regular cleaning of DUWLs with effective disinfectants that eliminate biofilm (O'Donnell *et al.*, 2006, 2007). More recently, fully-automated biofilm management systems capable of consistently maintaining the quality of DUWL output water at better than potable quality simultaneously in large numbers of DCUs have been developed (O'Donnell *et al.*, 2009; Boyle *et al.*, 2010).

Water may be supplied to DUWLs from a number of sources. These include connections to the public water supply mains, water storage tanks and independent reservoirs within the DCU. Disinfectant can be introduced into DUWLs from independent reservoir bottles, or from disinfectant delivery devices connected to the DCU water supply inlet. In the case of DCUs connected to a public water mains supply, it is imperative that the connection is turned off prior to DUWL disinfection to prevent contamination of mains water with disinfectant. The water distribution systems in some DCU models are fitted with an air gap system that physically separates the water within the DUWLs from the supply water, thus preventing backflow of disinfectant or contaminated water into the supply water network. In the United Kingdom, the law requires that an air gap must be incorporated into the water supply to a dental surgery to prevent backflow into the mains supply (Department for Environment, Food and Rural Affairs, 2002). After disinfection, DUWLs should be thoroughly flushed with clean water before DCUs are used for patient treatments.

Microbial contamination of dental chair unit suction systems

The DCU suction system is another important potential source of cross-contamination and/or cross-infection. DCU suction systems are designed to remove blood, saliva and other debris generated during dental procedures from the oral cavity. Use of the suction system reduces the levels of aerosols, spray and spatter generated during dental procedures. It is important to emphasise that the use of ultrasonic scalers is the greatest source of aerosol contamination in the dental clinic. High-volume suction should always be employed when using an ultrasonic scaler as this has been shown to reduce aerosol formation by >90% (Harrel and Molinari, 2004).

In many modern DCUs the suction system consists of a vacuum source supplied to the body of the DCU to which two suction hoses are attached. The high-volume suction hose is used to remove debris and dental unit water and to reduce spray, spatter and aerosols, whereas the low-volume suction hose, or saliva ejector, is mainly used to remove excess fluids from the patient's mouth, especially if the operator is working unassisted. In a dental hospital or clinic equipped with many DCUs, a central vacuum plant provides the suction to the DCUs

through a network of pipework. The high- and low-volume suction hoses attached to each DCU are connected to a common suction pipe within the pedestal unit of each DCU through which waste fluids are passed to a central collection vessel. Each DCU is also equipped with an amalgam trap to remove pieces of dental amalgam, and a coarse filter to remove particulate matter. Both of these components are connected to the suction system pipe-work within each DCU.

By its very nature the DCU suction system, including suction hoses, becomes contaminated with microorganisms from the oral cavities of patients and from DUWLs. Furthermore, because the suction system hoses and pipework are frequently wet, they provide an environment conducive to the growth and proliferation of biofilm (O'Donnell *et al.*, 2005). For these reasons, DCU suction systems have to be disinfected regularly. Dentists or practice managers should consult with DCU manufacturers concerning the type of disinfectant recommended for particular DCU models. In general, DCU suction systems should be disinfected following each clinical session (usually following the morning and afternoon sessions) with the disinfectant(s) approved by the DCU manufacturer. One recent study described the presence of extensive bacterial biofilm throughout the suction systems of DCUs in a modern dental hospital equipped with one particular brand of DCU, despite twice-daily disinfection with the approved phenolic disinfectant (O'Donnell *et al.*, 2005). Similar findings were found in a range of other DCU models.

A small number of studies has demonstrated that microorganisms present in low-volume suction hoses can be retracted into a patient's mouth during use when a partial vacuum is created by a patient closing lips around the suction hose tip (Mann *et al.*, 1996; Barbeau *et al.*, 1998). This indicates that retraction of oral fluids and biofilm-derived microorganisms from contaminated suction hoses could potentially be an important source of cross-contamination and cross-infection. This potentially potent source of cross-infection in the dental clinic needs to be investigated further.

High- and low-volume suction hoses usually are equipped with special fittings or connectors into which sterile suction tips (high-volume) or single-patient-use saliva ejector tips (low-volume) are fitted before each patient treatment. These connectors may be equipped with intricate valve components to regulate suction strength and may also have metal or plastic adaptors to connect them to the suction hoses. Suction hose connectors frequently harbour resident biofilms that are shielded from disinfectant during routine suction system disinfection and these constitute another potential source of cross-infection and cross-contamination in the dental clinic environment (O'Donnell *et al.*, 2005; Coleman *et al.*, 2010).

Disinfection of dental chair unit suction systems

Disinfection of DCU suction hoses is usually undertaken by aspirating disinfectant solution through the suction hoses, a process that takes approximately 1–2 minutes. This is a relatively short contact time, particularly if biofilm is present in the suction hoses. All DCU suction systems operate in a similar manner to a domestic vacuum cleaner, in that material, including disinfectants, is sucked rapidly through the suction hoses to a central receptacle; it is very likely, therefore, that many DCU suction systems harbour bacterial biofilm due to inadequate disinfectant contact time. DCU manufacturers should be able to provide independent, published evidence that the disinfectant they recommend for particular DCU models is effective at controlling microbial contamination in DCU suction systems. This concerns the entire DCU suction system and not just the suction hoses, as dental team staff and maintenance personnel may be exposed to microorganisms in other suction system locations during routine maintenance and cleaning or while cleaning or changing filters and emptying amalgam traps. Finally, it is important that suction hose connectors are dismantled and cleaned and disinfected separately from the suction hoses as parts of these connectors can be shielded from disinfection if disinfection is attempted while they are attached to suction hoses (Coleman *et al.*, 2010).

Portable suction units

Many dental clinics use independent or portable units to provide suction during dental procedures. With these units, waste fluids and debris from the oral cavity are aspirated into a receptacle container that has to be emptied after use. These suction units are not recommended, as disposing of the waste contents can be hazardous and constitutes an additional source of potential cross-contamination. Theatre suction units are fitted with disposable suction tubing and waste materials are collected into a disposable bag that can be disposed of into contaminated waste after use.

The dental laboratory

Dental artifacts, including impressions and prostheses, come into direct contact with patient mucous membranes, saliva and possibly blood and should be decontaminated. Equally, any appliance or prosthesis delivered to a patient from the dental laboratory should be free of contamination. Impressions, prostheses or other dental appliances should be disinfected as soon as possible after removal from the patient's mouth and before drying of contaminating saliva and blood can occur. Particular materials or products may have different requirements in relation to disinfection time and compatibility with disinfectants and the manufacturer should be consulted as to what disinfectants and disinfection conditions are appropriate.

After removal from the oral cavity, impressions should be examined to ensure that they have captured the required information. Wearing appropriate protective clothing, the impression or artifact should be washed under running mains water using a designated sink, where possible. Care should be taken to avoid splashing. Washing with water from a tank-supplied water outlet should be avoided, as tank water is often heavily contaminated with microorganisms (especially bacteria and fungi) originating from tank sludge, sediment and/or biofilms (O'Donnell *et al.*, 2009; Coleman *et al.*, 2010). After rinsing, the impression or artifact is transferred to a denture dish or other suitable receptacle and transported to the disinfection area. Depending on the disinfection product used, it may be possible to immerse the impression or artifact completely in the disinfectant solution. Disinfectants must not be sprayed on to the surface of an impression or appliance as this diminishes the effectiveness of the disinfectant and can be harmful if the aerosol created is inhaled. Depending on the disinfectant product used, it may be necessary to remove the disinfectant from the impression or artifact by rinsing under running water, as leaving impressions and artifacts in disinfectant solutions for long periods of time may result in distortion. Contaminated dental impressions and prostheses should not be transported to the production laboratories as this could pose an infection risk.

In the laboratory, separate receiving and disinfecting areas should be designated to reduce contamination in the production area. Environmental surfaces should be barrier protected or cleaned and disinfected in the same manner as in the dental treatment area. Items that do not normally come in contact directly with patients, but which may get contaminated during use on a patient (e.g. articulator), should be cleaned and disinfected between patients according to the manufacturer's instructions. Dental prostheses and artifacts produced by the laboratory should be disinfected prior to dispatch to the dental clinic using disinfectants and conditions recommended by the manufacturers of the materials concerned. These items should be rinsed thoroughly under running cold mains water prior to insertion in the oral cavity. Laboratory waste may be regarded as general waste, as impressions and other artifacts received by the laboratory *should* have been disinfected prior to delivery. However, if this is not the case, dental laboratory waste should be treated as contaminated clinical waste and treated in the same manner as the waste generated in the dental treatment area. Personnel should dispose of sharp items (e.g. burs, disposable blades and orthodontic wires) in puncture-resistant containers in the same manner as the waste generated in the dental treatment area.

Diagnostic specimens

Specimens taken from patients in the dental clinic for diagnostic or investigational purposes may contain pathogenic microorganisms that could pose a risk of infection if not adequately packaged for posting to diagnostic laboratories. Within the European Union, the transport and packaging of diagnostic specimens should comply with the United Nations European Agreement ADR regulations (United Nations Economic Commission for Europe, 2010), as well as with local requirements. A summary of ADR packaging require-

ments (ADR Packaging Instruction P650) for diagnostic specimens (UN 3373) is outlined below:

- Packaging materials should be strong enough to withstand the impacts and loadings normally encountered during carriage and postage.
- The diagnostic specimen should be placed in a primary container that is leak-proof and watertight.
- The primary container should be wrapped in absorbent material capable of absorbing all liquid in case of breakage.
- The primary container should then be placed in a watertight, leak-proof rigid secondary container.
- Secondary containers should be secured in a durable outer shipping packaging with suitable cushioning material. The external surface of the outer packaging should be labeled with a square symbol positioned at 45 degrees containing the letters UN3373. The phrase 'BIOLOGICAL SUBSTANCE, CATEGORY B' should be located adjacent to the square symbol (Figure 8.9).
- Several secondary containers may be placed in one outer shipping package.

(a)

(b)

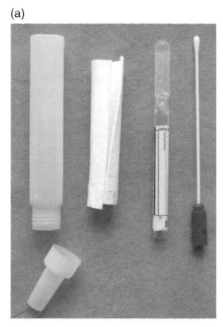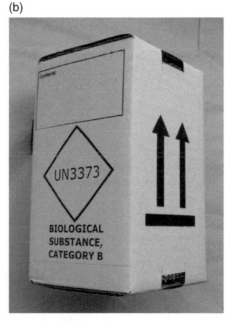

Figure 8.9 Examples of approved containers for packaging a diagnostic swab specimen for posting to a diagnostic laboratory. (a) On the right is a cotton wool swab stick typically used in dental practice. Immediately to the left of the swab is the primary container into which the swab stick is placed and secured by pushing the blue cap firmly so that the container is sealed. The primary container is then wrapped with the absorbent paper (shown to the left of the primary container) and the whole assembly placed in the secondary container shown to the left of the absorbent paper and the cap secured. (b) The secondary container is then placed in the outer packaging box shown. A box of this size can contain several secondary containers. The outer packaging box is clearly marked 'Biological Substance, Category B' beneath the UN3373 symbol. Within the European Union the transport and packaging of diagnostic specimens should comply with the United Nations European Agreement ADR regulations (United Nations Economic Commission for Europe, 2010), as well as with local requirements.

References

Anonymous (1995) ADA statement on dental unit waterlines. Adopted by the ADA Board of Trustees, December 13, 1995 and the ADA Council on Scientific Affairs, September 28, 1995. *Northwest Dentistry*, **75**(2), 25–26.

Anonymous (1998) Council Directive 98/83/EC of 3 November 1998 on the quality of water intended for human consumption. *Official Journal of the European Communities*, **L330**, 32–54.

Barbeau, J., Ten Bokum, L., Gauthier, C. and Prevost, A.P. (1998) Cross-contamination potential of saliva ejectors used in dentistry. *Journal of Hospital Infection*, **40**(4), 303–311.

Bell, D.M. (1997) Occupational risk of human immunodeficiency virus infection in healthcare workers: an overview. *American Journal of Medicine*, **102**(5B), 9–15.

Bennett, P., Grove, P., Perera, L. and McLean, I. (2007) Potential vCJD transmission risks via dentistry: an interim review. [Online]. Available from: http://www.dh.gov.uk/en/Publicationsandstatistics/Publications/PublicationsPolicyAndGuidance/DH_081170 (accessed 8th December 2010).

Berlutti, F., Testarelli, L., Vaia, F., Luca, M.D. and Dolci, G. (2003) Efficacy of anti-retraction devices in preventing bacterial contamination of dental unit water lines. *Journal of Dentistry*, **31**(2), 105–100.

Bond, W.W., Favero, M.S., Petersen, N.J., Gravelle, C.R., Ebert, J.W. and Maynard, J.E. (1981) Survival of hepatitis B virus after drying and storage for one week. *Lancet*, **1**(8219), 550–551.

Boyce, J.M. and Pittet, D.; Healthcare Infection Control Practices Advisory Committee; Society for Healthcare Epidemiology of America; Association for Professionals in Infection Control; Infectious Diseases Society of America; Hand Hygiene Task Force (2002) Guideline for hand hygiene in health-care settings: recommendations of the Healthcare Infection Control Practices Advisory Committee and the HICPAC/SHEA/APIC/IDSA Hand Hygiene Task Force. *Infection Control and Hospital Epidemiology*, **23**(12 Suppl), S3–40.

Boyle, M.A., O'Donnell, M.J., Russell, R.J. and Coleman, D.C. (2010) Lack of cytotoxicity by Trustwater Ecasol™ used to maintain good quality dental unit waterline output water in keratinocyte monolayer and reconstituted human oral epithelial tissue models. *Journal of Dentistry*, **38**(11), 930–940.

British HIV Association (2008) *Guidelines for the treatment of HIV-1-infected adults with antiretroviral therapy*. [Online]. Available from: http://www.bhiva.org/PublishedandApproved.aspx (accessed 8 December 2010).

British Standards Institution BS8580 (2010) *Water quality – Risk assessments for Legionella control – Code of practice*. BSI, London.

Chohan, G., Llewelyn, C., Mackenzie, J., Cousens, S., Kennedy, A., Will, R. and Hewitt, P. (2010) Variant Creutzfeldt–Jakob disease in a transfusion recipient: coincidence or cause? *Transfusion*, **50**(5), 1003–1006.

Coleman, D.C. and O'Donnell, M.J. (2007) Guest editorial. *Journal of Dentistry*, **35**(9), 699–700.

Coleman, D.C., O'Donnell, M.J., Shore, A.C., Swan, J. and Russell, R.J. (2007) The role of manufacturers in reducing biofilms in dental chair waterlines. *Journal of Dentistry*, **35**(9), 701–711.

Coleman, D.C., O'Donnell, M.J., Shore, A.C. and Russell, R.J. (2009) Biofilm problems in dental unit water systems and its practical control. *Journal of Applied Microbiology*, **106**(5), 1424–1437.

Coleman, D.C., O'Donnell, M.J., Boyle, M. and Russell, R.J. (2010) Microbial biofilm control within the dental clinic: reducing multiple risks. *Journal of Infection Prevention* **11**(6), 192–198.

Delves, P.J., Martin, S.J., Burton, D.R. and Roitt, I.M. (2011) *Roitt's Essential Immunology*, 12th edn. John Wiley & Sons, Ltd, Chichester.

Dement, J.M., Epling, C., Ostbye, T., Pompeii, L.A. and Hunt, D.L. (2004) Blood and body fluid exposure risks among health care workers: results from the Duke Health and Safety Surveillance System. *American Journal of Industrial Medicine*, **46**(6), 637–648.

Department for Environment, Food and Rural Affairs (2002) Environmental protection (UK), 2002. *Water Supply (Water Fittings) Regulations 199.9* [Online]. Available from: http://archive.defra.gov.uk/environment/quality/water/industry/wsregs99/index.htm (accessed 29 September 2011).

Department of Health (2006) Health Technical Memorandum 07-01: Safe management of healthcare waste. [Online.] Available from: http://www.dh.gov.uk/prod_consum_dh/groups/dh_digitalassets/documents/digitalasset/dh_073328.pdf (accessed 20 November 2010).

Department of Health (2007) *Potential vCJD transmission risks via dentistry: an interim review* [Online]. Available from: http://www.dh.gov.uk/en/Publicationsandstatistics/Publications/PublicationsPolicyAndGuidance/DH_081170 (accessed 29 September 2011).

Department of Health (2009) Health Technical Memorandum 01-05: Decontamination in primary care dental practices. [Online]. Available from: http://www.dh.gov.uk/en/Publicationsandstatistics/Publications/PublicationsPolicyAndGuidance/DH_109363 (accessed 10 December 2010).

Department of Health and Children (2007) Code of Practice for Decontamination of Reusable Invasive Medical Devices: Parts 5: Recommended Practices for Dental Services. (2007) [Online.] Available from: http://www.hse.ie/eng/services/Publications/services/Hospitals/Code_of_Practice_for_Decontamination_of_Reusable_Invasive_Medical_Devices_.html (accessed 14 December 2010).

Department of Health and Children (2010) Healthcare risk waste management: segregation packaging and storage guidelines for healthcare risk waste, 4th edition. DoH, London.

Fotos, P.G., Westfall, H.N., Snyder, I.S., Miller, R.W. and Mutchler, B.M. (1985) Prevalence of *Legionella*-specific IgG and IgM antibody in a dental clinic population. *Journal of Dental Research*, **64**(12), 1382–1385.

Goldfarb, L.G. and Brown, P. (1995) The transmissible spongiform encephalopathies. *Annual Review of Medicine*, **46**, 57–65.

Harrel, S.K. and Molinari, J. (2004) Aerosols and splatter in dentistry: a brief review of the literature and infection control implications. *Journal of the American Dental Association*, **135**(4), 429–437.

Harte, J.A. and Miller, C.H. (2003) Sterilization update. *Compendium of Continuing Education in Dentistry*, **25**(1 Suppl), 24–29.

Head, M.W., Ritchie, D., McLoughlin, V. and Ironside, J.W. (2003) Investigation of PrPres in dental tissues in variant CJD. *British Dental Journal*, **195**(6), 339–343.

Health Protection Scotland (HPS) (2007) [Online.] Available from: http://www.documents.hps.scot.nhs.uk/hai/decontamination/publications/ldu-001-02-v1-2.pdf (accessed 15 December 2010).

Health Protection Surveillance Centre (2009) *National guidelines for the control of legionellosis in Ireland*. [Online.] Available from: http://www.hpsc.ie/hpsc/A-Z/Respiratory/Legionellosis/Publications/File,3936,en.pdf/ (accessed 29 September 2011).

Health and Safety Commission (2000) *Legionnaires' Disease. The Control of Legionella Bacteria in Water Systems. Approved Code of Practice and Guidance*. Her Majesty's Stationery Office, Norwich.

Health and Safety Executive (2008) I work in a dental practice. [Online.] Available at: http://www.hse.gov.uk/skin/faq/dental.htm (accessed 29 September 2011).

Hegde, P.P., Andrade, A.T. and Bhat, K. (2006) Microbial contamination of 'in use' bar soap in dental clinics. *Indian Journal of Dental Research*, **17**(2), 70–73.

Hullard D'Aignaux, J.N., Cousens, S.N. and Smith, P.G. (2001) Predictability of the UK variant Creutzfeldt-Jakob disease epidemic. *Science*, **294**(5547), 1729–1731.

International Organization for Standardization. ISO 15883-1:2004 (2004a) *Washer-disinfectors – Part 1: General requirements, definitions and tests*. International Organization for Standardization, Geneva.

International Organization for Standardization. ISO 15883-2:2004 (2004b) *Washer-disinfectors – Part 2: Requirements and tests for washer disinfectors employing thermal disinfection for surgical instruments, anaesthetic equipment, bowls, dishes, utensils, glassware, etc*. International Organization for Standardization, Geneva.

International Organization for Standardization. ISO 17665-1:2006 (2006) *Sterilization of health care products – Moist heat – Part 1: Requirements for the development, validation and routine control of a sterilization process for medical devices*.

Kampf, G., Löffler, H. and Gastmeier, P. (2009) Hand hygiene for the prevention of nosocomial infections. *Deutsches Arzteblatt International*, 2009, **106**(40), 649–655.

Kohn, W.G, Collins, A.S., Cleveland, J.L., Harte, J.A., Eklund, K.J. and Malvitz, D.M.; Centers for Disease Control and Prevention (CDC) (2003) Guidelines for infection control in dental health-care settings – 2003. *Morbidity and Mortality Weekly Report. Recommendations and Reports*, **52**(RR-17), 1–61.

Korniewicz, D.M., Chookaew, N., Brown, J., Bookhamer, N., Mudd, K. and Bollinger, M.E. (2005) Impact of converting to powder-free gloves. Decreasing the symptoms of latex exposure in operating room personnel. *American Association of Occupational Health Nurses Journal*, **53**(3), 111–116.

Kuzu, N., Ozer, F., Aydemir, S., Yalcin, A.N. and Zencir, M. (2005) Compliance with hand hygiene and glove use in a university-affiliated hospital. *Infection Control and Hospital Epidemiology*, **26**(3), 312–315.

Lamont, R.J. and Jenkinson, H.F. (2010) *Oral Microbiology at a Glance*. John Wiley & Sons, Ltd, Chichester.

Letters, S., Smith, A. J., McHugh, S., Bagg, J. (2005) A study of visual and blood contamination on reprocessed endodontic files from general dental practice. *British Dental Journal*, **199**(8), 522–525.

Llewelyn, C.A., Hewitt, P.E., Knight, R.S., *et al.* (2004) Possible transmission of variant Creutzfeldt-Jakob disease by blood transfusion. *Lancet*, **363**(9407), 417–421.

Mann, G.L., Campbell, T.L. and Crawford, J.J. (1996) Backflow in low-volume suction lines: the impact of pressure changes. *Journal of the American Dental Association*, **127**(5), 611–615.

Mathai, E., Allegranzi, B., Seto, W.H., *et al.* (2010) Educating healthcare workers to optimal hand hygiene practices: addressing the need. *Infection*, **38**(5), 349–356.

Mitsui, T., Iwano, K., Masuko, K., *et al.* (1992) Hepatitis C virus infection in medical personnel after needlestick accident. *Hepatology*, **16**(5), 1109–1114.

Murray, P.R., Rosenthal, K.S. and Pfaller, M.A. (2009) *Medical Microbiology*, 6th edn. Elsevier-Mosby, Oxford.

Navazesh, M., Mulligan, R., Kono, N., *et al.* (2010) Oral and systemic health correlates of HIV-1 shedding in saliva. *Journal of Dental Research*, **89**(10), 1047–1049.

O'Donnell, M.J., Tuttlebee, C.M., Falkiner, F.R. and Coleman, D.C. (2005) Bacterial contamination of dental chair units in a modern dental hospital caused by leakage from suction system hoses containing extensive biofilm. *Journal of Hospital Infection*, **59**(4), 348–360.

O'Donnell, M.J., Shore, A.C. and Coleman, D.C. (2006) A novel automated waterline cleaning system that facilitates effective and consistent control of microbial biofilm contamination of dental chair unit waterlines: a one-year study. *Journal of Dentistry*, **34**(9), 648–661.

O'Donnell, M.J., Shore, A.C., Russell, R.J. and Coleman, D.C. (2007) Optimisation of the long-term efficacy of dental chair waterline disinfection by the identification and rectification of factors associated with waterline disinfection failure. *Journal of Dentistry*, **35**(5), 438–451.

O'Donnell, M.J., Boyle, M., Swan, J., Russell, R.J. and Coleman D.C. (2009) A centralised, automated dental hospital water quality and biofilm management system using neutral Ecasol maintains dental unit waterline output at better than potable quality: a 2-year longitudinal study. *Journal of Dentistry*, **37**(10), 748–762.

Pankhurst, C.L., Coulter, W., Philpott-Howard, J.N., Surman-Lee, S., Warburton, F. and Challacombe, S. (2005) Evaluation of the potential risk of occupational asthma in dentists exposed to contaminated dental unit waterlines. *Primary Dental Care*, **12**(2), 53–59.

Puro, V., Petrosillo, N. and Ippolito, G. (1995) Risk of hepatitis C seroconversion after occupational exposures in health care workers. Italian Study Group on Occupational Risk of HIV and Other Bloodborne Infections. *American Journal of Infection Control*, **23**(5), 273–277.

Rabier, V., Bataillon, S., Jolivet-Gougeon, A., Chapplain, J.M, Beuchée, A. and Bétrémieux, P. (2008) Hand washing soap as a source of neonatal *Serratia marcescens* outbreak. *Acta Paediatrica*, **97**(10), 1381–1385.

Redd, J.T., Baumbach, J., Kohn, W., Nianan, O., Khristova, M. and Williams, I. (2007) Patient-to-patient transmission of hepatitis B virus associated with oral surgery. *Journal of Infectious Diseases*, **195**(9), 1311–1314.

Scottish Executive Health Department (2004) NHS Scotland: Sterile Services Provision Review Group: survey of decontamination in general dental practice. [Online.] Available at: http://www.scotland.gov.uk/Publications/2004/11/20093/45220 (accessed 10 December 2010).

Shah, S.M., Merchant, A.T. and Dosman, J.A. (2006) Percutaneous injuries among dental professionals in Washington State. *BMC Public Health*, **6**, 269.

Smith, A., Creanor, S., Hurrell, D., Bagg, J. and McCowan, M. (2009) Management of infection control in dental practice. *Journal of Hospital Infection*, **71**(4), 353–358.

Taylor, D.M. (2004) Resistance of transmissible spongiform encephalopathy agents to decontamination. *Contributions to Microbiology*, **11**, 136–145.

United Nations Economic Commission for Europe (2010) *ADR applicable as from 1 January 2011*. United Nations, (ECE/TRANS/215, Vol. I and II). [Online.] Available from: http://www.unece.org/trans/danger/publi/adr/adr2011/11ContentsE.html (accessed 20 December 2010).

Walker, J.T. (2010) Decontamination in dentistry-the times they are a changing. *Journal of Infection Prevention*, **11**(6), 188–191.

Walker, J.T, Budge, C., Vassey, M., *et al.* (2009) vCJD and the cleanability of endodontic files: a case for single use. *ENDO, Endodontic Practice Today*, **3**(2), 115–120.

Whitworth, C. and Palmer, N. (2010) Decontamination in primary care dentistry. *Journal of Infection Prevention*, **11**(6), 200–204

World Health Organization (2007) *Legionella and the prevention of legionellosis*. [Online.] Geneva. Available from: http://www.who.int/water_sanitation_health/emerging/legionella.pdf (accessed 28 November 2010).

World Health Organization (2009) Guidelines on hand hygiene in health care. [Online.] Available from: http://whqlibdoc.who.int/publications/2009/9789241597906_eng.pdf (accessed 29 September 2011).

World Health Organization (2010) Recommended viruses for influenza vaccines for use in the 2010–2011 northern hemisphere influnza season. [Online.] Available from: http://www.who.int/influenza/vaccines/en/index.html (accessed 29 September 2011).

Further reading

British Dental Association (2009) Infection control in dentistry, Advice sheet A12. BDA, London.

Pankhurst, C.L. and Coulter, W.A. (2009) *Basic Guide to Infection Prevention and Control in Dentistry*. John Wiley & Sons, Ltd, Chichester.

9

Materials in restorative dentistry

Paul Franklin and Paul Brunton

Summary

This chapter covers:

- The properties, chemistry and clinical handling of materials for direct tooth restoration
  - Amalgam
  - Resin composite
  - Glass ionomer cements
  - Resin-modified glass ionomer cements
- Bonding to enamel and dentine
- Pulp protection regimes
- An overview of impression materials in common usage

Introduction

The purpose of this chapter is to consider the restorative materials available for the direct restoration of permanent and deciduous teeth. The chemistry and physical properties, as they relate to modern-day restorative practice, will be discussed, and the advantages, disadvantages, indications and contraindications of the materials will be outlined. To assist the reader further, hints and tips that relate to the successful use of these materials will be described.

Amalgam

Amalgam is one of the oldest direct restorative materials that are still in regular use. Relatively few changes have occurred in the recipe for amalgam since G.V. Black described a formulation that was durable and reliable, although the changes that have been made have significantly improved the physical properties of amalgam. For the most part of its historical use in dentistry, there have been few alternative direct placement materials, and even today amalgam is still considered by many to be the best available material to fill large cavities in load-bearing teeth.

An **amalgam** is a metal alloy containing mercury and one or more other metals. In the case of **dental amalgam**, the other metals are typically silver, tin and copper (Table 9.1). There may be traces of other metals included to modify the properties of the material, or aid in its manufacture.

The powdered alloy is mixed with liquid mercury, which readily reacts with the metals incorporated into the powder. Mercury is liquid at room temperature, and will give off a vapour which is potentially hazardous. To prevent inadvertent exposure it is usual for the powdered alloy and liquid mercury to be packaged in predetermined amounts in a sealed capsule (Figure 9.1). The powder and liquid are kept apart during storage by a thin membrane that is broken on activation. Alternatively, the powder and liquid could be stored in two hoppers in an **amalgamator**, which are then dispensed in a ratio and amount that are controllable by the operator. Amalgamators require the topping up of powder and mercury from time to time and this process increases the chance of mercury spillage. The mercury needs to be very pure and is usually triple distilled to eliminate impurities.

The final set material should contain 45–50% mercury; however, when there is less than 50% mercury in the amalgam mix it can prove too dry and difficult to work with. The more mercury in the mixed material, the softer the material is and the easier it is to pack and carve, but the set restoration will be weaker and more

Clinical Textbook of Dental Hygiene and Therapy, Second Edition. Edited by Suzanne L. Noble.
© 2012 John Wiley & Sons, Ltd. Published 2012 by John Wiley & Sons, Ltd.

prone to corrosion. To reduce the amount of mercury in the final restoration, the amalgam should be vigorously condensed, as this causes excess mercury to rise to the surface where it can be carved away and discarded in a safe manner. For this reason amalgam should always be placed to overfill a cavity.

Types of amalgam

Amalgam may be classified by the shape of the particles that make up the powder, or the constituent metals of the particles. The particles of alloy that make up the powder can either be **spherical** in shape or an irregular shape known as **lathe-cut** (Figure 9.2). The shape of the particles determines how the material handles. Spherical

Table 9.1 Typical composition of a modern amalgam powder.

Component	Percentage composition
Silver	60–70
Tin	27
Copper	13
Zinc	0–2

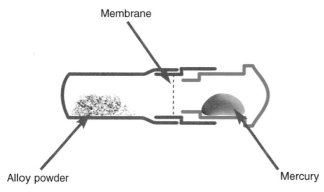

Membrane

Alloy powder

Mercury

Figure 9.1 Schematic diagram of an amalgam capsule. The capsule is activated by pressing in the plunger shown in green. This breaks the membrane, allowing alloy and mercury to be mixed together. The end of the capsule containing the powder is detachable, and can be used as a receptacle for the set material.

particles are formed by spraying molten alloy into an inert atmosphere. As it falls spheres form and solidify. The other method of creating the powder is to grind small particles from a solid block of alloy, hence the name lathe-cut. It gives more resistance when packing into cavities than spherical amalgam, but is not as prone to slump when building up a large restoration.

One of the most popular types of amalgam in current usage is dispersed phase or **admixed** amalgam, consisting of spherical silver/copper particles and lathe cut silver/tin particles. Combined together, they give good handling characteristics. With spherical amalgams being more easily condensed, less mercury is needed to wet the particles, which in turn leads to a final material with lower mercury content and better physical properties.

Setting reaction

The silver/tin phase, Ag_3Sn or γ phase, in the powdered alloy reacts with mercury when mixed. The mercury will dissolve the outer layer of particles, allowing the release of the metal ions within. Smaller particles will completely dissolve, but larger particles often keep their cores intact. The metal ions released join to form grains which grow until eventually the material becomes solid (Figure 9.3).

The set material contains unchanged particle cores consisting of the gamma (γ) phase, surrounded by a matrix of γ_1 and γ_2. The γ_2 phase is associated with increased corrosion, creep (plastic change over time) and lower strength. Modern amalgams have low γ_2 content due to the presence of higher amounts of copper. The copper acts to convert the γ_2 phase to γ_1 and the formation of a silver–copper alloy, Cu_6Sn_5, by the reaction:

$$Ag + Cu + \gamma_2 \rightarrow \gamma_1 + Cu_6Sn_5$$

The copper can either be mixed with the alloy powder, so that the particles contain silver, tin and copper, or silver–copper particles can be added to a traditional amalgam powder. For this reason modern amalgams are known as 'high copper' amalgams or 'non gamma-2'. On initial set, the material is quite weak and prone to fracture if

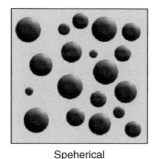
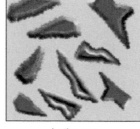
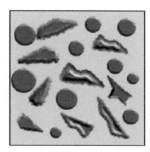

Speherical   Lathe-cut   Admixed

Figure 9.2 Types of particles available in common usage.

$$Ag_3Sn\ (\gamma) + Hg \longrightarrow Ag_3Sn\ (\gamma) + Ag_2Hg_3\ (\gamma_1) + Sn_7Hg\ (\gamma_2)$$

Figure 9.3 The setting reaction for traditional dental amalgam. There will be an amount of γ phase remaining in the final material, as not all of each particle is dissolved into the mercury. The γ_2 phase has adverse effects on the properties of the material.

heavy occlusal forces bear down on it, and it takes up to 24 hours for the material to reach its optimal strength.

Properties of amalgam

Good compressive strength gives amalgam the ability to withstand the forces of biting and chewing. It is hard wearing, yet kind to the tooth it is placed in and causes very little wear on the teeth opposed by it, due to low abrasivity (Jagger and Harrison, 1995).

Corrosion is reduced with the addition of copper but is still responsible for tarnishing giving a dull appearance and fatigue particularly at amalgam margins leading to marginal breakdown. Corrosion products however can be beneficial as they have been shown to seal the interface between the amalgam and the tooth reducing microleakage.

Clinical usage

Cavity preparation

Amalgam does not chemically bond to tooth surface but requires tooth preparation to create a shape of cavity that contains both retention and resistance forms to prevent dislodging of the restoration. This is carried out by creating undercuts, dovetails, pits and grooves in the dentine of the tooth. This inevitably requires more tooth tissue to be removed than is necessary to remove the caries alone and can lead to unnecessary destruction of precious tooth tissue. In addition to this, amalgam is weak in thin section, so cavities need to be created that are at least 1.5 mm deep and where the cavo–surface angle is never below 90°.

During the condensation stage of placing amalgam, the material is firmly pressed into all recesses of the cavity preparation. The act of vigorous condensation also brings any excess mercury in the material to the surface. As each successive increment is added the mercury can be encouraged to rise successively. The final increment should overfill the cavity and the now mercury rich top layer is removed during the carving process and discarded safely.

Carving should be carried out while the material is soft, using hand instruments to recreate the anatomical features of the tooth. It is important to remove any excess material overlying the enamel surrounding the margins of the cavity otherwise once set it will come under occlusal load and being in thin section will fracture and

leave a positive margin to the restoration ultimately acting as a plaque retention factor and area of stagnation. The amalgam–margin angle following carving should be no less than 70° to avoid thin sections as the material tapers out towards the edges of the cavity which could in time fracture off leaving a negative restoration margin with similar consequences.

Burnishing the material can improve the marginal adaptation and achieve a surface smooth enough without the need for polishing which is carried out less frequently than it was in the past. Detractors of polishing claim that shiny spots caused by heavy occlusal contacts are less easily recognised on a polished surface.

Amalgam bonding

The major drawbacks of amalgam are its very poor aesthetics and the fact that it does not bond to the tooth; hence its use does not encourage conservation of tooth tissue or prevent marginal microleakage. Recent developments in bonding techniques using materials that can both bond to the tooth and bond to the amalgam itself have reduced the need for dentine pins in larger cavities. There are several materials commercially available suitable for bonding amalgam. They contain chemically active resins such as 4-methacryloyloxyethyl trimellitate anhydride (4-META). The use of bonding systems, whilst potentially advantageous, adds a further step to the restoration process and the materials are highly technique sensitive. On top of this there is no clear evidence that bonding reduces the incidence of secondary caries or improves the longevity of the restoration. A simpler method of bonding amalgam using RMGIC is described later in this chapter.

Indications for amalgam restorations

Amalgam has a high compressive strength, but offers poor aesthetics and so is best suited to restorations of premolar and molar teeth, where heavy occlusal forces are experienced and where the cavities are not suitable for composite resins. Due to their durability, amalgam restorations are often used to rebuild badly broken down teeth prior to final restoration with crowning.

Recent changes in the National Health Service and pressure from patients to use alternative materials that are more aesthetic, or who have concerns about the mercury content of their restorations, may well see an end to the widespread use that amalgam has in today's dentistry.

Resin composite

Resin composites are a combination of a resin matrix, which is polymerisable, and an inorganic filler. Both components play a part in the final material's properties

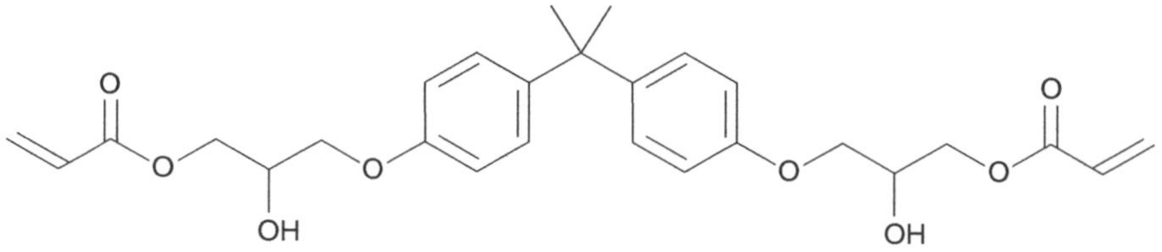

Figure 9.4 The formula for bisphenol A-diglycidylether methacrylate (Bis-GMA).

and both have been varied in their composition to attain desirable properties for differing situations. Composites are in fact a family of materials that can be utilised in many situations in dentistry where aesthetics, bonding ability and strength are the prime requirements.

Resin matrix

The setting reaction of a resin composite involves the polymerisation of the resin matrix. This is the process whereby small components, termed **monomers**, combine to form large-chain molecules. The longer the chain, the more viscous the material becomes until it reaches a solid state. The polymerisation process is often described as the **setting reaction** or **curing process**. The setting reaction is initiated by the production of **free radicals**, which are highly reactive charged substances within the material. These initiate the chain reaction of polymerisation. Free radicals can be created in one of two main ways with modern resin composites: by chemical reaction or by light.

Self-curing resin composites, sometimes known as chemically cured or autopolymerising resin composites, set without the need for a light. They are usually presented as two pastes both containing resin and filler. A tertiary aromatic amine has been added to the base material paste, and dibenzoyl peroxide is added to the other (the catalyst). When the amine and peroxide meet, the peroxide is cleaved to form two molecules each with a free radical.

For **light-curing materials**, there is a single paste containing resin, filler and camphorquinone. The camphorquinone has a breakable bond within it that is broken when exposed to light of about 470 nm. The result of this is the production of free radicals to initiate polymerisation.

Both methods of free radical production have their advantages and disadvantages. Light curing allows the operator to be in control of the working time. The greatest problem with light curing is that sufficient light of the correct wavelength needs to satisfactorily penetrate the material in order to get a high enough degree of polymerisation for the resin composite to have optimal properties. They also can become difficult to handle as they begin to polymerise under the glare of the dental light. In deep cavities and underneath crowns and veneers, chemically cured materials have the advantage in that they will optimally polymerise whatever the depth or availability of light. The largest disadvantage of chemical curing is that there is no control over working time and materials may set sooner than expected.

To try to overcome the problems with both types of curing, '**dual-cure**' materials were developed. These are partially set by light cure so that control of the working time is maintained but they will undergo a slower chemical cure to permit full curing of the whole restoration.

During polymerisation heat is produced and the resin shrinks as the monomer molecules join together. The shrinkage of pure acrylic resin alone can be up to 21%. This amount of shrinkage would have devastating consequences for a tooth, as it would lead to stresses within the enamel and dentine as both sides of a cavity were pulled together. If the bond to tooth tissue was not maintained there would be considerable marginal microleakage, leading to sensitivity and secondary caries. Shrinkage can be reduced by utilising higher molecular weight monomers. The predominant substance used as a monomer in dental resin composites is Bis-GMA (Figure 9.4). Bis-GMA produces a viscous, sticky resin; to help the material flow, smaller molecular weight monomers are added, such as TEGDMA (triethyleneglycol dimethacrylate). These are referred to as diluent monomers.

Larger methacrylate monomers, such as Bis-GMA, help reduce the shrinkage to a certain extent, but that alone does not reduce it sufficiently for the material to be clinically acceptable. It is the filler particles that reduce the overall amount of shrinkage to a degree that is acceptable, currently about 2%. In addition it is the amount and size of the filler particles that define the categorisation and intended applications for resin composites.

Filler particles

As a general rule, the more filler present, the stronger and harder wearing the resin composite will be, whilst also being less affected by shrinkage. Too much filler, on the other hand, may affect the optical properties and polishability of the material, also more filler makes the material less flowable.

(a)
(b)

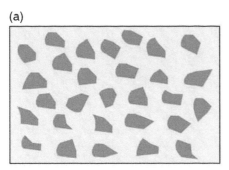
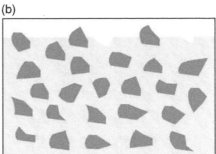

Figure 9.5 Macrofilled resin composite. (a) The gross structure shows the filler particles embedded within the resin matrix. (b) After wear has occurred, the surface of the material is rough, with particles protruding from the surface and small voids where some particles have been lost.

(a)
(b)

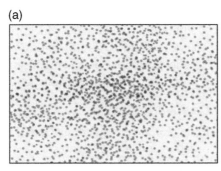
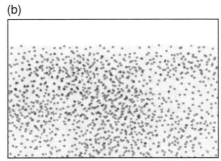

Figure 9.6 (a) A single-phase microfilled resin composite containing colloidal silica filler. (b) Following wear, the surface is still smooth and will not stain so readily as the macrofilled resin composite.

Early resin composites were filled with quartz particles of relatively large size. These are known as **macrofilled resin composites**. They are strong, but give poor long-term aesthetic results due to the size of the filler particles providing a surface that is not readily polished and which easily takes up staining (Figure 9.5). Filler particles in present use are composed of glasses often containing barium or strontium; these give the material radio-opacity, which helps in the detection of secondary caries.

Macrofilled resin composites have a high proportion of filler particles, about 86% loading by volume, which improves wear resistance and increases strength, although, due to the relatively poor aesthetic properties, they are really only suitable for posterior restorations. In order to produce a material that could be polished and retain better aesthetics, a later development was to introduce smaller particles composed of colloidal silica. These are known as **microfilled resin composites** (Figure 9.6).

During manufacture of microfilled resin composites, difficulty is encountered in obtaining a high enough filler content, to the effect that the resin is only about 50% loaded with filler. This low filler loading has an adverse impact upon the material's long-term strength and wear resistance. Lower percentages of filler also mean more polymerisation shrinkage with the problems which are associated with it. To try to overcome the problems with both macro- and microfilled resin composites, a hybrid of the two has been developed, containing both larger quartz particles and the smaller silica particles (Figure 9.7a).

Hybrid resin composites are in common usage as 'all purpose' materials, meaning they are suitable for both posterior and anterior teeth. The problem of having larger crystals that can protrude from the surface or be lost still remains, and has recently been addressed by nanotechnology, replacing the larger particles with clusters of nanoparticles (Figure 9.7b). These act together to give the material the strength of a hybrid, but, as wear occurs, they do not leave large voids, allowing the restoration surface to remain polished and stain free.

In all composite materials, to ensure that the resin and filler work together to strengthen the material and avoid loss of surface particles, the two components are joined together by a **silane coupling agent**.

Flowable resin composites

Flowable composites are a relatively recent addition to the composite family. They have a lower filler content of about 50–70% by volume and are thus less viscous and

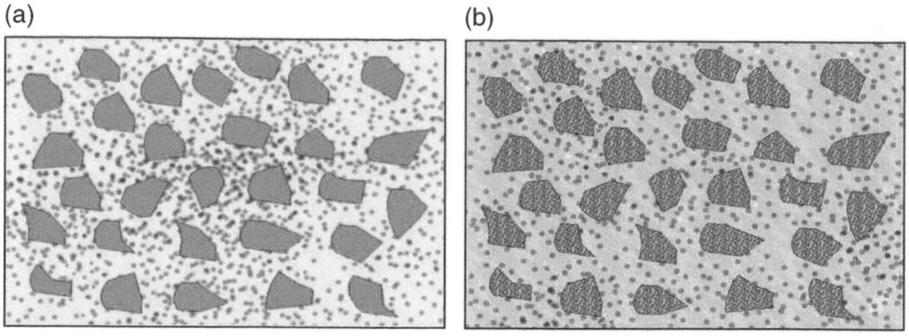

(a)   (b)

Figure 9.7 A hybrid resin composite containing both larger quartz particles and smaller colloidal silica particles (a) compared with the newly developed 'nano' composite (b) which, like the hybrid, has larger particles for improved strength and wear resistance; however, each large particle is a cluster of nano-particles that act together, but as the surface becomes worn will separate out individually, leaving a smooth, more stain-resistant surface.

are able to flow easily into cavities, though their wear resistance is low. The utilisation of monomers with elastic properties has led to the practice of using them to line cavities in posterior teeth prior to restoration with a more conventional composite. The inherent elasticity may to some degree absorb the stresses created during polymerisation shrinkage of the regular composite. Having a lower filler content means that polymerisation shrinkage will be increased. Efforts to reduce the stresses that this increased shrinkage would create upon the tooth include the addition of a modulator that controls polymerisation stress, allowing materials such as Dentsply's SDR™ to be able to be used as a bulk filler in larger restorations prior to veneering the occlusal surface with a more highly filled material.

Advantages of composite materials

Modern day resin composite restorative materials have considerable advantages for the practitioner and patient, which include the following:

- Used in conjunction with a dentine adhesive system, they can be placed with minimal or no tooth preparation. This is a distinct advantage over amalgam which requires a more destructive cavity design to gain retention and resistance form for the cavity. In this respect the utilisation of composite materials facilitates preservative preparation of teeth when a lesion requires operative management, and also non-destructive management of tooth wear.
- Light curing allows for command cure, which permits immediate finishing and polishing.
- The restoration, if placed correctly in suitably selected teeth, seals the tooth–restorative interface, reducing marginal leakage which can lead to staining, secondary caries and tooth sensitivity.
- It is possible to add material to cured increments, which allows for incremental build-up and further

additions at a later date, which means that practitioners can refinish, refurbish and/or repair restorations. Followed to its natural conclusion this will result in a more conservative, less destructive pattern of care.

Disadvantages

Resin composite materials suffer certain limitations, which include the following:

- Polymerisation shrinkage of typically 2–3% can disrupt the marginal adaptation of the material, fracture weakened cusps, notably in premolars, and produce postoperative sensitivity. This can be compensated for to a certain extent by correct placement procedures (see Chapter 13, p.286).
- Bonding to dentine can be problematical, especially at the margins of a preparation (for example, the floor of the box when the floor is below the cemento–enamel junction (CEJ) in proximal preparations).
- Water absorption with surface and marginal staining after some years of clinical service.
- Patient and operator sensitivity to the components of adhesive resins, in particular HEMA.
- Poor radiographic definition (unlike amalgam) making diagnostic interpretation more difficult.

Indications for resin composites

Current indications for resin composites include:

- Small, medium and large occlusal restorations in posterior teeth.
- Small, medium and large proximal restorations in premolar teeth and small to medium proximal preparations in permanent molar teeth. Where the proximal margins are below the CEJ, a bonded-base approach is indicated.
- Cervical lesions in all teeth.
- Incisal edge restorations.
- Fissure sealants and preventive resin restorations.

Contraindications

It is suggested that resin composite should not be used in the following situations:

- Large proximal preparations in permanent molar teeth in patients or areas where they would be subjected to high occlusal loads.
- Where it is not possible effectively to isolate the operative field (for example, distal preparations in third molars).
- Restoration of root caries lesions, which are better dealt with using glass ionomer cements.
- Where patients have a proven allergy to one or more of the numerous constituents of the resin-based restorative materials, including the adhesive systems.
- In deep interproximal boxes, because of the increased distance from the light source.

Hints and tips on the use of resin composites

Unlike amalgam, resin composites are technique sensitive. They are not tolerant of poor placement techniques, yet the results achieved are generally excellent in carefully selected cases. Success is more likely if attention is paid to the following:

- Resin composites should not be packed or condensed into cavities. They are not 'white' amalgam and should not be handled in the same way as amalgam. They should be adapted and contoured to the preparation. Packing of resin-based products has been shown to increase the formation of voids within the set material.
- In proximal preparations it is advantageous to build up the marginal ridge of the restoration in the first instance. Further build-up can be as for an occlusal preparation, which simplifies the process.
- Try not to connect two opposing walls when an increment is placed as it places the opposing walls under stress when the increment is cured. A clinical example of this is bulk curing of a large mesio-occlusal–distal resin composite placed in premolar teeth where cracks are often noted at the base of a cusp after curing. Oblique increments are recommended for this reason; they also facilitate easier contouring of the restoration (see Chapter 13, p.288).
- Transparent matrix bands offer no advantage over metal matrices. Apart from the difficulty of using them, they are so thick that they may lead to under-contouring of the contact area. Metal matrix bands, especially sectional metal matrices, have been shown to be equally effective for the placement of proximal resin composites, provided additional trans-tooth curing is done in the form of 20-second curing from either side of the embrasure after the band is removed. The use of metal bands allows for better contact formation and permits wooden wedges to be used. Sectional matrices are especially useful for forming contact points in proximal resin composite restorations.
- Use separate instruments for resin composite. Several manufacturers produce non-stick instruments especially for use with resin-based restorative materials. These should not be contaminated by using them with amalgam as this can lead to discoloration of the resin composite.
- The curing of resin composite is inhibited by oxygen, which is helpful on the one hand, in that each cured increment has uncured monomer on the surface to which additional increments can be added. On the other hand, this is undesirable for the final increment placed and for that reason it is preferable to overbuild the restoration slightly and cut it back during finishing and polishing. An alternative would be to contour the final increment anatomically and then apply an **air-block**, which excludes oxygen before curing. Petroleum jelly is effective in this situation.
- The use of a wedge is important when proximal preparations are restored. It creates a potential space for the interdental papillae and allows for tight contact point formation, especially when resin composite restorations are placed. Do not simultaneously wedge the tooth mesially and distally, as this will extrude the tooth by pressure on the periodontal ligament. This would result in the restoration being overcontoured when the occlusion is checked.

Glass ionomer cements

Conventional glass ionomer cements

Glass ionomer cements (GICs) were first introduced in the 1970s. In dentistry they have many applications including restorations, lining and bases, endodontics sealers and fissure sealants. Glass ionomers have two significant advantages: they adhere chemically to enamel and dentine and they release fluoride. They also adhere to base metals and so may be used as luting cements.

They do not have the compressive strength of amalgam, and do not have the flexural strength or aesthetics of resin composite, and so, as a primary restorative material, their use is limited to that of a temporary restoration material, or they can be used to restore class V and class III cavities, where aesthetics are not crucial. They are also widely used as a restorative material for primary (deciduous) teeth and in the **atraumatic restorative technique** (ART), as they do not require any cavity modification other than caries removal. There have been many modifications to the standard glass ionomer; however, at the heart of each type of glass ionomer is the same basic setting reaction.

Setting reaction

The essential constituents of glass ionomer cements are a polyalkenoic acid and an ion-leachable glass. The glass particles can vary in size, and the size can determine the properties of the material, and are therefore graded for the various applications for glass ionomers. The acids involved originate from the polyalkenoic family of acids, which includes, amongst others, polyacrylic acid, polyitaconic acid and polymaleic acid (Figure 9.8).

The glass particles commonly are a calcium-aluminosilicate glass and contain calcium or strontium and fluoride. Restorative glass ionomers tend to contain larger particles than luting cements or lining materials; the setting reaction is, however, essentially similar.

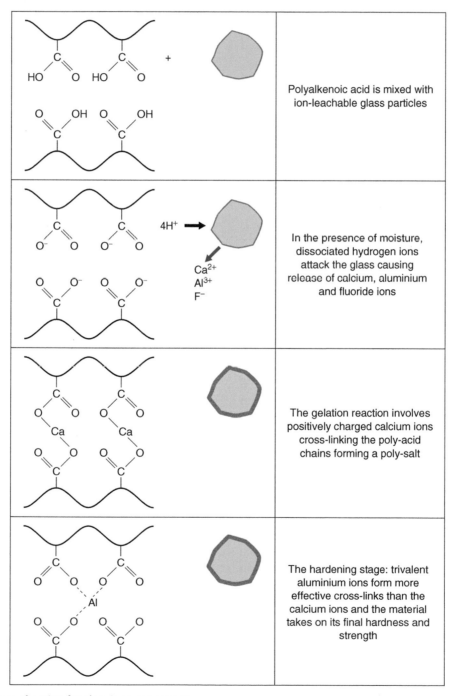

Figure 9.8 The stages of setting for glass ionomer cements.

The setting reaction undergoes three main stages: dissolution, gelation and hardening.

In the **dissolution stage**, the polyalkenoic acid, in the presence of moisture, releases protons which attack the surface of the glass, causing the release of fluoride, calcium and aluminium ions. The outer surface of the glass becomes gel-like as the lost ions are replaced by hydrogen from the carboxylate groups from the polyacid chains.

The **gelation reaction** occurs over a few minutes, where the freed divalent calcium ions form ionic bonds with the negatively charged carboxyl ions on the polyacid chains. They form cross-links if they connect to two adjacent chains or they may join two adjacent carboxyl groups on the same chain. During this stage, the material firms to the touch. Shaping of the restoration should be done quickly, as the material becomes friable as it hardens, making it very difficult to achieve a smooth shape.

The **hardening phase** may take several days to complete, and only then does the material reach its final strength. During this phase, trivalent aluminium ions form more effective cross-links between adjacent chains (Figure 9.9).

Other components of the glass ionomer cement include tartaric acid, pigments and radio-opacifiers. The tartaric acid, when used in the correct concentration, will cause the setting to be sharpened; that is, the material remains workable for a sufficient amount of time to be placed and shaped, and then hardening occurs more rapidly. The final set material is porous enough to allow the free movement of small molecules, such as hydroxyl and fluoride ions, in and out of the material.

Bonding to tooth substance

There are several theories on how glass ionomers bond to tooth substance. What is generally accepted is that the carboxyl groups bioreact with apatite in the tooth structure in a similar way to how they react with the glass particles: by causing dissociation of calcium and phosphate ions from the apatite and then the negatively charged carboxyl groups bonding with the charged surface of the enamel or dentine, so called '**ion exchange**'. In dentine, however, there is a much lower inorganic content, and adhesion is thought to be mainly due to the creation of hydrogen bonds with collagen within the dentine.

The bond strength to dentine is relatively weak and has been estimated to be about 5 MPa. The failure of the glass ionomer bond, however, tends to be cohesive (i.e. there is a failure within the glass ionomer itself). Thus if a restoration is lost, there is usually a thin layer of GIC left on the dentine, and the pulp–dentine complex will remain protected. The bond to dentine has been described as a dynamic bond, which breaks and reforms as the organic component of the dentine itself undergoes natural turnover. This is in contrast to that of resin-based adhesive materials that adhere to tooth via micromechanical interlocking, which is not able to adapt to natural collagen turnover within the dentine, and which tends to fail adhesively. The failure occurs between the resin and the dentine and therefore the pulp–dentine complex is not protected.

Handling

The original glass ionomers were presented as a glass powder and a viscous polyacid liquid. These were spatulated by hand to produce a smooth mix of material. More recently, polyacids have been added to the powder in crystalline form which, when mixed with water, become activated and the setting reaction occurs as outlined above. It is crucial that the powder:liquid ratio is correct for acceptable material properties and effective bonding to tooth tissue to take place. When dispensed by hand this ratio can be widely variable. To overcome this, it is more common for the materials to be pre-encapsulated in the correct proportions. The capsules are mixed at high speed in a regular amalgamator, and usually have nozzles through which the prepared material can be extruded directly into a cavity.

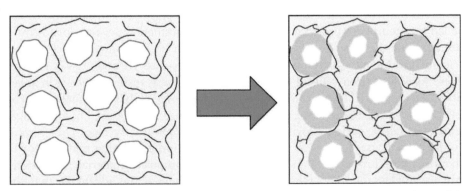

Figure 9.9 Glass ionomer materials before and after setting has occurred. In the set material, the outer layer of the glass has formed a gel, and calcium and aluminium released from the glass have cross-linked the poly-acid chains shown in red.

The prepared cavity should first be conditioned with a dentine conditioner, the most common one being 10% polyacrylic acid. The conditioner removes the **smear layer** and debris from the prepared cavity walls, allowing a clean surface to bond to, but leaves smear plugs intact so as to prevent contamination of the cleaned dentine surface with dentinal tubular fluid. The acids used for the bonding of resin composite should not be used for conditioning prior to glass ionomer placement, as the low molecular weight of these acids would demineralise the dentine, leaving less calcium available for the ion-exchange bonding mechanism. The polyacrylic acid conditioning agent should only be applied for a short time, about 10 seconds, and should be washed off thoroughly before drying without desiccating the dentine.

During the gelation phase and until hardening is complete, conventional glass ionomers are adversely affected by moisture contamination; it can cause the aluminium ions to be lost and so final hardening is adversely affected. During this phase the material is also more prone to dissolution. In the first few days following placement, a glass ionomer restoration should be protected with either a varnish, or alternatively coated with an unfilled resin material once initial shaping has been carried out. Final shaping should not be carried out at the time of placement.

Finishing should not take place until final hardening has occurred; to ensure this, finishing should be delayed for about a week after placement. Fine polishing of GICs is difficult to achieve and it is better to use a matrix to shape the restoration correctly at the time of placement, with the restoration taking on a smooth surface from the matrix.

Biocompatability

GICs are very biocompatible materials with little evidence of toxic or allergenic effects. Experimental evidence indicates that when placed directly on pulpal tissue following traumatic exposure of the pulp, the response is positive, including healing via dentine bridge formation. Some concerns over the possible toxic effects of aluminium have led to attempts to produce aluminium-free glass ionomers, but these have so far proved unsuccessful in terms of producing a material suitable for clinical use. There have also been reports of post-treatment sensitivity when using GIC luting cements for crowns on vital teeth; this is associated with the removal of smear plugs but is not usually experienced with resin-modified glass ionomer cement usage.

Fluoride ions can move freely throughout the set material, and thus freshly placed glass ionomers release large amounts of fluoride into the surrounding enamel and dentine, although this falls to a low level in a relatively short time. As fluoride ions from the environment can also enter the GIC, they act as fluoride reservoirs and can prolong the effects of fluoride therapy and tooth brushing by taking up some of the fluoride and releasing it over a period of time. Acidulated fluoride therapies, however, may cause degradation to the surface of GIC restorations. The fluoride released is believed to be cariostatic, though the evidence for any clinical benefit is poor; however, it has been shown that plaque bacteria and those bacteria associated with dental caries do not thrive on the surface of GICs.

Resin-modified glass ionomer cements (vitremers)

Resin-modified glass ionomer cements (RMGICs) have been developed to overcome some of the problems inherent within conventional GICS, these being the inability to control the working time, problems created by moisture contamination of freshly placed restorations and low flexural strength.

RMGICs have a similar acid–base setting reaction to conventional GICs but polymerisable groups are present on the polyacid chains as well as HEMA monomers that take part in the polymerisation reaction. These are activated in the presence of the same wavelength of light as resin composites. Once the polymerisation reaction has taken place, the material is protected from moisture contamination by the saliva, and so the final properties of the set material are more predictable and the special measures taken to protect GICs during the hardening phase can be safely omitted. The materials will set fully even in the absence of light curing due to chemical initiators of polymerisation being included.

Once the RMGIC material has been light cured it behaves much more like a composite in terms of it's capacity for ion exchange and bonding to the tooth surface, hence it is wise to leave it uncured for as long as possible, some authorities have suggested three minutes as being the optimal time to allow maturation of the GIC structure and ion exchange to take place.

The aesthetics are superior to conventional GICs and they can be recommended for use as aesthetic restorations for class III and class V restorations, but are not as effective as resin composite in areas of occlusal stress.

Reinforced GICs are usually presented in an encapsulated form that is mixed in an amalgam mixer and used in an applicator syringe. They have found a particular application as a lining material for both amalgam and resin composite materials; for resin composite placement there is the advantage that they have an elastic property that to some degree absorbs the stresses placed on the tooth during resin composite shrinkage.

HEMA has a tendency to absorb water and RMGICs should not be used as luting cements for brittle non-metallic crowns or for cementing posts into root canals, as the water absorption that takes place will cause the material to expand with the possible consequence of root or porcelain crown fracture.

RMGICs are typically available as a hand-mixed powder and liquid or pre-encapsulated for aesthetic restorations, and as powder–liquid or paste–paste systems for use as linings and luting cements.

Advantages

GICs have the following advantages:

- They develop self-adhesion to tooth tissue through bioreacting with the tooth surface. This process is enhanced if the tooth surface is conditioned and left moist but not wet prior to application of the material.
- The resin-based systems are command cured, although it is important to understand that the acid–base reaction for the traditional glass ionomer cement proportion of the material (about 80%) is really how the material cures and sets. This reaction is dependent on water absorption and takes several days for the process to be complete. More correctly, therefore, RMGICs are initially photostabilised rather than light cured.
- Fluoride release, although the clinical benefit of this has not been quantified.

Disadvantages

GICs have disadvantages linked to their inferior physical properties when compared with resin composites. These disadvantages include:

- Poor fracture strength and wear rates compared to composite or amalgam.
- Water absorption in RMGICs makes them unsuitable for use as luting cements for all ceramic restorations, as there is a net expansion of 4%, which places all ceramic restorations under undue stress.
- Poor strength in thin section can lead to marginal chipping of traditional GICs, particularly when they have been used to restore occlusal preparations.
- Traditional GICs tend to be more opaque and less aesthetic than RMGICs.
- Exogenous stain build-up is common with traditional GICs.

Indications for glass ionomer cements

GICs generally are indicated for use in the following circumstances:

- Liners and bases for direct and indirect restorations.
- RMGICs are indicated for bonded-base restorations and temporary restorations, especially between appointments in endodontic therapy.
- For rapid stabilisation of a dentition where there are multiple cavities in a patient with a high caries risk.
- Atraumatic restorative technique (ART).
- Cementation of cast indirect restorations.
- Traditional GICs are useful for the restoration of root caries in the elderly patient.

Contraindications for glass ionomer cements

GICs are not indicated in the following situations:

- Definitive restorations in the adult dentition, except for the treatment of root caries.
- Resin-modified glass ionomer luting cements are not suitable for luting of all ceramic restorations as they expand due to water absorption, the expansive force of which can result in fracture of the restoration. For the same reason they should not be used to lute posts in root canals as the expansion can cause root fracture.

Cermets

Cermets are traditional GICs in which metals, such as silver particles, have been incorporated into the glass powder, either sintered to the glass or simply added. The result is an unaesthetic, opaque grey material, and as such cermets are not suitable as an aesthetic restorative material. They have been advocated as a core build-up material for badly broken down teeth and as an alternative to amalgam for primary tooth restorations. They are not mechanically superior to conventional GICs, but have inherent radio-opacity which makes them suitable as a lining material and they may have improved abrasion resistance.

Compomers

Compomers, or polyacid–modified resin composites as they are otherwise known, are essentially resin composite materials that have an ion-leachable glass filler and monomers that will polymerise to create a matrix, on to which some acidic side chains are grafted. These will take part in an acid–base reaction as per GICs when moisture has been absorbed into a placed restoration, but this is not the initial setting reaction. They are used in a similar manner to resin composite, with the advantage of fluoride release. The amount of fluoride released, however, is less than for GICs. They have found particular popularity in the restoration of primary teeth, but have found little advantage over resin composite or glass ionomers in adult dentistry.

Compomers, like resin composites, require an adhesive agent to create a micromechanical bond to tooth structure as there is insufficient acid present for ion exchange with tooth surface to take place, nor is there enough acid or base for an acid–base setting reaction to cure the material and light is always needed.

Together the family of glass ionomers and resin composites form a continuum of materials. Figure 9.10 shows the essential differences between resin composites and GICs, and how RMGICs and compomers effectively blur the distinction between the two.

Advantages

Compomers and resin composites share the same advantages. Additional advantages include fluoride release and ease of handling. Manufacturers have suggested from time to time that these materials can be placed without the use of a dentine adhesive system, which is difficult to reconcile with the material's chemistry. It is recommended, therefore, that if a compomer is used, a dentine adhesive agent be used as well.

Disadvantages

These are similar to the disadvantages of resin composites.

Indications for compomers

There are no clear indications for the use of compomers. Indeed, it is difficult to identify an indication where the use of a compomer would confer an advantage over the use of a resin composite. Consequently, it has been argued that they are a redundant class of materials. The only situation where the use of a more hydrophilic resin system (i.e. a compomer) might be advantageous is in the restoration of non-carious and carious cervical lesions

where moisture control can be problematical. The hydrophilic nature does not mean that the material can tolerate excess moisture in the form of saliva and, as with all resin-bonded restorations, the use of a rubber dam during the placement of these materials is strongly recommended.

The modulus of elasticity of compomers is lower than resin composite and the material is less rigid as a consequence. This might confer some advantage in non-carious cervical lesions if tooth flexure is responsible for the lesion. The rigidity of particularly hybrid resin composite might explain the poor retention rates recorded for restorations of such materials. Further research is indicated to determine if compomer restorations have increased retention rates in this clinical situation.

Contraindications for use of compomers

These again are similar to those for resin composites.

Materials for the protection of fissures

Fissure sealants are materials that are used to protect vulnerable fissures in high caries risk patients. They are also used in preventive resin restorations when minimal tooth preparation of the fissure system is carried out to 'biopsy' early suspected caries.

The properties required of a fissure sealant are that it adheres to enamel, flows into fissures and is resistant to occlusal wear. The most common fissure sealants in use are lightly filled resin-based materials. They are presented in either a transparent or opaque white formulation. Each has their proponents; transparent sealants allow visual inspection of the underlying fissures but opaque sealants can be more easily detected and replaced if the seal to the tooth is defective.

Glass ionomers, compomers and flowable composites have also been produced for use as fissure sealants. Fissure sealants are only effective if they provide a complete seal of the fissure system. A partial break of the seal could lead to caries developing that is hidden from detection. Glass ionomer fissure sealants may have an advantage over resins in this respect as if they become debonded, they leave a protective layer on the enamel. However, their long-term success remains to be confirmed.

To ensure optimal adhesion to the tooth surface, the enamel should be cleaned thoroughly with pumice or an oil-free prophylaxis paste. Ideally they should be placed with the protection of a rubber dam.

Adhesion to tooth substance

Adhesive dentistry is revolutionising clinical practice. With the advent of adhesive procedures, practical dentistry is moving from a mechanistic domain to a more biological one. Improvements in adhesion are

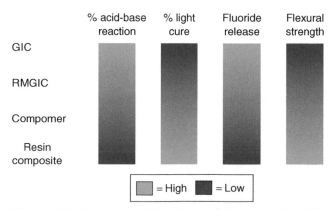

Figure 9.10 Some essential features of the composite–GIC continuum.

allowing preparations for direct placement restorations to be more conservative, reducing the need to modify preparations for retention or resistance or to increase the bulk needed for brittle materials. Adhesion means that dentine can be effectively sealed from the oral environment, reducing postoperative sensitivity and reducing the risk of secondary caries. Cast restorations require less tooth preparation, and aesthetics can be restored or improved with often very little destruction of healthy tooth tissue.

The hard tissues of the tooth that are potential adhesion sites (i.e. enamel and dentine), are very different materials (Table 9.2), and so the strategies for achieving successful adhesion to each need to be considered separately.

Bonding to enamel

Enamel is very highly mineralised. Unlike most other bodily tissues there is no turnover or repair mechanism for enamel; however, there is movement of mineral ions into and out of it, which plays an important role in both the progression of caries and also the remineralisation process that occurs when conditions are favourable. The mineral content is mainly hydroxyapatite crystals. These are packed together to form prisms that run outwards from the amelodentinal junction (ADJ) to the outer surface of the enamel (Figure 9.11). The prisms have an inner core and outer sheath.

Buonocore (1955) was the first to describe the effects of applying acid to the surface of enamel to create a surface on to which acrylic resins could be adhered. In the presence of 37% phosphoric acid, the prisms partially dissolve. Silverstone *et al.* (1975) described different patterns of etching, describing areas where the core was destroyed more than the sheath, areas where the sheath was most affected and areas where a mixture of both effects was seen. Figure 9.12 shows an electron micrograph of clean unetched enamel and an area from the same tooth which had been etched for 15 seconds with 37% phosphoric acid and thoroughly washed. What is evident is the increase in surface area. To the naked eye the etched enamel appears frosty when it is dried after thorough washing.

The etched surface is highly reactive, and any moisture present will quickly wet the surface particularly if blood or saliva are present. For this reason it is best to carry out the acid-etch technique with highly effective moisture control; this can best be achieved by use of a rubber dam. Bonding to enamel is described as micromechanical bonding rather than true adhesion, as the resin-based adhesive agents flow into the etched, porous surface and form a mechanical lock.

Adhesion to dentine

As has been shown in Table 9.2, dentine has a higher organic and water content than enamel. Dentine is also a living tissue that has fluid flow from the pulp via dentinal tubules to the surface.

Early attempts at gaining an adequate bond strength to dentine were flawed by using hydrophobic materials

Table 9.2 Comparison of the relative constituents of enamel and dentine expressed as a percentage of total weight.

Percentage content by weight	Enamel	Dentine
Inorganic	96	20
Organic	1	70
Water	3	10

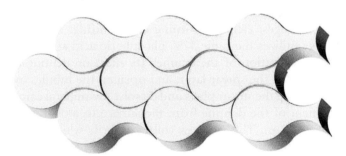

Figure 9.11 Enamel prisms. Each one is created by organisation of hydroxyapatite crystals.

(a)   (b)

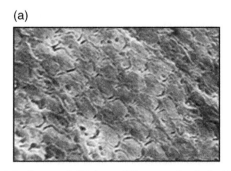 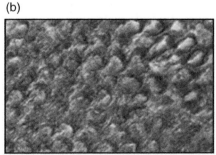

Figure 9.12 (a) Unetched enamel. (b) Area of the same tooth that had been etched for 15 seconds with 37% phosphoric acid.

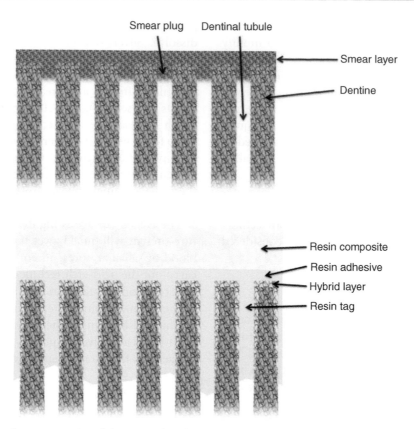

Figure 9.13 Diagrammatic representation of dentine surface following cavity preparation (top) and restoration placement (bottom).

and failing to remove the smear layer which then interfered with the bond.

Current techniques of adhesion to dentine involve three stages: etching, priming and bonding. The etch stage utilizes the same 37% phosphoric acid as is used for preparation of the enamel. Its effect on dentine is to remove the smear layer, and opening the tubules by removing the smear plugs and dissolve the mineral component of the dentine from the surface to a depthe of about 5 μm. This exposes collagen fibrils which stand proud of the surface with a spaghetti-like appearance. The etch must not be left in place for more than 15 seconds, and must be thoroughly washed off before gently drying. Over drying will cause the collagen fibrils to collapse flat to the surface, so a maximum of about 5 seconds drying is considered adequate.

The second stage of the adhesion process is **priming**. In this stage a bifunctional monomer such as HEMA dissolved in a solvent is applied to the surface. The solvent carried the HEMA in and around the collagen fibres as well as down into the exposed dentinal tubules. The HEMA has a hydrophilic terminal that interfaces intimately with the exposed dentine surface and a hydrophobic terminal that can be co-polymerised with resin restorative materials.

During the priming stage a small amount of moisture is desirable on the dentine surface to allow the primer to flow in and around the collagen fibrils. The primer will drive off the moisture before the hydrophobic bond is applied. If too wet, however, the primer will be ineffective and the subsequent bond weakened. Before application of the bond the surface should be gently air dried to encourage evaporation of the solvent. it is important that vigorous use of the 3-in-1 at this stage is avoided.

The third stage of the **adhesion** process is to apply a lightly filled resin adhesive to the primed dentine. This resin attaches to the hydrophobic terminal of the HEMA and upon light activated polymerization the resin adhesive interlocks around the collagen fibres forming what has been termed the 'hybrid layer' (Nakabayashi *et al.*, 1991). The process of bonding to dentine is summarised in Figure 9.13. The three stages of dentine bonding (etch – prime – bond) remain the gold standard in achieving high bond strength to dentine; however, in order to simplify the process for in surgery use, manufacturers have combined the steps into two- or even one-bottle systems. These are summarised in Table 9.3. With each modification of components into fewer steps, the bond strengths as measured in the laboratory decrease; however, there are fewer opportunities for mishandling

Table 9.3 Summary of recent trends in dentine adhesive components.

Number of components	Generation			
	4th	5th	6th	7th
1	Etch	Etch	Etch + Primer	Etch + Primer + Adhesive
2	Primer	Primer + Adhesive	Adhesive	
3	Adhesive			

of materials, and in the hands of the average practitioner the reliability increases.

Hints and tips for the successful use of dental adhesive systems

To maximise the results achieved with an adhesive system it is recommended that careful attention is paid to the following:

- Follow the manufacturer's directions for use.
- Use an adhesive system and resin composite from the same manufacturer, as the resin chemistry will be compatible.
- Do not over-etch dentine. Treatment times in excess of 15 seconds will result in post-operative hypersensitivity due to nanoleakage. Nanoleakage occurs when resin uptake is less than the depth of the etchant penetration, leaving a gap that allows fluid movement.
- Apply dental adhesive systems to proximal preparations before the matrix band is applied so that the cervical margin is adequately treated prior to the application of the first increment of resin composite.
- Whilst it is important to evaporate the solvent from the dentine adhesive agent, it is critical that this process is gradual. Aggressive use of a three-in-one syringe will thin the resin layer and result in poor film thickness, remembering that the resin's secondary function is to seal the dentine.
- When the restoration is finished, apply a further layer of adhesive resin to act as a surface treatment. Surface treatment resin penetrates surface cracks and strengthens the surface layer.

Pulp protection regimes

Bacterial contamination of dentinal tubules and subsequently the pulp is the principal cause of pulpal inflammation. The direct toxic effects on the pulp of restorative materials have been shown to be mild and transitory.

The pulp may have been inflamed prior to a restoration being placed but this inflammation will largely resolve following treatment (reversible pulpitis) provided further bacterial contamination is prevented. The pulp may also be damaged due to sudden and excessive rises in temperature generated during the restorative procedure, caused by inadequate water cooling of burs, use of worn burs and/or inadequately maintained handpieces and excessive dehydration of the pulp during operative procedures.

It has been demonstrated that thermal stimulation of dentine is not normally a problem clinically and that routine basing of preparations for amalgams, to prevent thermal stimulation, inherently weakens the restoration without benefit to the continuing vitality of the tooth. It is also accepted that dentine can be etched without deleterious pulpal effects and therefore routine lining of preparations for resin composites is now contraindicated.

All preparations should have some form of sealer applied and some preparations (usually deep) will require a liner and/or base. There is some merit in etching preparations prior to placing a sealer, liner or base, as etching will remove the smear layer, which is contaminated with bacteria. Removal of the smear layer in this way affords gross debridement of the preparation and will also improve the quality of the interface between the sealer/liner and the dentine substrate.

Sealers

A preparation sealer is a material that seals the dentinal tubules and provides a protective coating for freshly cut dentine. Examples of sealers include copal ether cavity varnish and dentine desensitisers.

Liners

Preparation liners also seal freshly cut dentine but have additional functions, such as adhesion to tooth structure, fluoride release and/or antibacterial action. Preparation liners are applied in thin section (<0.5 mm) and materials currently used include: RMGICs, dentine adhesive systems, flowable resin composites and hard-setting calcium hydroxide cements. It has been suggested that RMGICs have greater resistance to microleakage than dentine adhesive systems.

It has been recommended that the RMGIC liner should be applied to the preparation and not cured with the amalgam packed directly on to the liner. The rationale behind this approach is that the liner will chemically cure whilst developing adhesion both to the tooth and the amalgam restoration, further enhancing restoration retention. To date there is no evidence in the form of well-conducted clinical trials to demonstrate the benefit of lining amalgam preparations in this way.

If a dentine adhesive system is used it is recommended that a filled resin system (i.e. one that contains filler particles), should be used, as it is easier for the operator to ensure that all dentine is covered, sealed and lined with a somewhat thicker layer. The thickness of the layer is important in that it provides an elastic interface between the tooth and the restorative material, which allows for relief of stresses generated by curing contraction.

The direct application of dentine bonding agents and glass ionomer material to exposed pulp is contraindicated due to poor pulpal reparative responses and the possibility of sensitizing the patient to componenets in the materials such as HEMA. Hard-setting calcium hydroxide and mineral trioxide aggregate are both suitable materials for direct pulp exposure coverage; however, both have poor mechanical properties and will need protection prior to subsequent restoration placement.

Bases

Bases are dentine replacements, which reduce the bulk of directly placed restorative material, for example, amalgam. They are also used to block out preparation undercuts when indirect restorations are prescribed. Traditional and resin-modified GICs are examples of bases. Historically, zinc oxide eugenol and zinc phosphate have also been used as bases. It is difficult, however, to recommend their continued use given the superior properties of traditional and resin-modified GICs. The routine basing of restorations to prevent thermal shocking of the pulp through metallic restorations is contraindicated, as thermal stimulation of the pulp through metallic restorations has not been shown to be problematical. The use of RMGIC in an open sandwich type restoration where the principal restorative material is composite, but the cavity extends subgingivally interproximally have reasonable longevity with survival rates of up to 7 years reported (Andersson-Wenckert *et al.*, 2004).

Indications for sealers, liners and bases

Amalgam restorations

In the case of simple amalgam restorations two coats of a dentine desensitiser are recommended and sufficient to prevent microleakage and postoperative sensitivity. Current indications would seem to suggest that dentine desensitisers have largely replaced cavity varnish as a preparation sealer for amalgam restorations.

For deeper cavities where there is less than 2 mm of remaining dentine, a preparation liner should be placed in the deepest aspects of the preparation. It is usual to place a small increment of hard-setting calcium hydroxide cement in the deepest aspects (but only if a pulp exposure is evident or a micro-exposure suspected) and then place RMGIC over all remaining dentine. This is termed **direct pulp capping**. In very deep cavities in which the pulp is nearly exposed, hard-setting calcium hydroxide cement is applied to this area only and then a RMGIC liner is placed. This is termed **indirect pulp capping**.

Resin composite restorations

Dentine adhesive systems should be routinely used under all resin composite restorations. Dentine adhesive systems primarily retain the restoration but have another function, sealing the dentinal tubules, preventing postoperative sensitivity and bacterial contamination of the tubules. It is important that when dentine adhesive systems are applied, all dentine surfaces of the preparation are covered by a sufficient thickness of the agent. Multiple applications are often required, along with prudent use of the three-in-one syringe to evaporate the solvent and spread the film. This can be problematic if the three-in-one syringe is contaminated with water, which can be checked by blowing air from the three-in-one syringe into a tissue.

If pulpal exposure or near exposure is suspected then hard-setting calcium hydroxide cement should be used as described above as a direct or indirect pulp capping agent. It is important to minimise the extent and thickness of the hard-setting calcium hydroxide cement, as extensive application of the material will limit the area of dentine available for bonding, also sixth generation bonding systems should not be applied directly to calcium hydroxide as the acidic primers in the bonding system will dissolve it. It should first be protected by a layer of RMGIC.

Temporary dressing materials

The use of temporary dressings is often a necessity. Circumstances such as allowing a period of time for healing to occur, in between visits when treatment on a tooth cannot be completed at one visit and emergency restorations often require a tooth to be temporised. Classically, simple cements have been used for this purpose such as zinc oxide eugenol, zinc polycarboxylate and zinc phosphate. Whilst these materials are simple and quick to use they exhibit poor resistance to wear, occlusal loads and are quite soluble.

It has always been held that eugenol-containing restorative materials are contraindicated as temporary restorations for resin-bonded indirect restorations. This is because the eugenol is absorbed into the resin composite restorative material or retained in the dentinal tubules, resulting in plasticising of the monomer, and subsequent softening and discoloration of the resin composite restoration and/or luting cement. The issue of residual eugenol in dentinal tubules has recently been investigated and it has been shown that the routine use of an etchant on dentine will remove residual eugenol from the dentinal tubules.

The advent of glass ionomer materials has provided us with a material that can offer the simplicity of the cements with a durable and bonded restoration. New developments using intensely coloured glass ionomer materials has also lead to improved ability to remove the material from a cavity without undue removal of adjacent tooth tissue.

Impression materials

The ideal properties of a material to create an impression of the teeth would include; flowable before set and able to pick up the finest detail of each tooth. It should be have a sufficient working time for it to be correctly seated, be pleasant tasting, easy to use and hydrophilic. Once set, the material must be able to be withdrawn from undercut areas without distortion or tearing, and be dimensionally stable. It must have no adverse effect on the plaster or stone subsequently used for the creation of models. When taking impressions of edentulous areas the need for elasticity may not be so great and the viscosity of the material may have an effect on the compression of the soft tissues being recorded. Impression materials may therefore be grouped into elastic and non-elastic types.

Elastomers

These are indicated when accuracy is paramount, such as for crown and bridge work and implants.

Silicone impression materials are subdivided into **condensation-** and **addition-cured silicones**. Condensation-cured silicones, for example Xantopren and Optosil, are relatively cheap compared with other elastomers, but they are prone to some shrinkage and should be cast immediately. Addition-cured silicones are therefore to be preferred.

Addition-cured silicone impression materials, for example Aquasil, President and Dimension, are very stable, which means that impressions can be sent through the post or stored prior to casting. A perforated tray is advisable as the adhesives supplied are not very effective. Up to five viscosities are manufactured, allowing a range of impression techniques. The more viscous that material the higher it's dimensional stability but poorer the ability to record surface detail. Lighter-bodied materials have the opposite properties. For this reason silicones are often used in a combination of viscosities within the same impression, with heavy bodied materials filling the impression tray and lighter bodied materials forming a thin layer over the surface of the teeth.

It should be noted that powdered latex gloves (now rarely used) can retard setting of putty materials.

Polysulphide impression materials, for example Permalastic, are messy to handle, but are useful when a long working time is required. They should be used with a special tray and, although stable, should be cast within 24 hours due to their inherent inaccuracy. They are not consequently recommended.

Polyether impression materials, for example Impregum, are popular impression materials because they use a single mix and a stock tray and can be mixed mechanically. The set material is stiff and removal can therefore be stressful in cases with deep undercuts or advanced periodontitis. The material absorbs water and therefore impressions should not be stored with alginate impressions. These impression materials are routinely used for implant cases and crown and bridge work, especially when there are multiple preparations.

Hydrocolloids

Reversible hydrocolloid impression materials are accurate, but liable to tear. To use these materials requires the purchase of a special water bath and are difficult to disinfect. Consequently these materials are not widely used today in the UK.

Alginate is an **irreversible hydrocolloid** impression material. Its setting reaction is a double decomposition reaction between sodium alginate and calcium sulphate. It is very popular because it is cheap and can be used with a stock tray. However, it is not sufficiently accurate for crown and bridge work.

After an alginate impression has been taken, the material is highly prone to moisture loss or gain from its environment. Water is lost if left uncovered by a process known as **syneresis**. The impression will rapidly shrink and change shape rendering it useless. Likewise if an alginate impression is stored in water it will swell by a process called **imbibition** and again distort. The recommended method of handling an impression is to disinfect immediately and then wrapped in a damp gauze or tissue and placed in a sealed plastic bag.

Impression compound

This is available in either sheet form for recording preliminary impressions, or in stick form for modifying trays. The sheet material is softened in warm water (55–60 °C) and used in a stock tray to record the edentulous ridges.

The viscosity of compound results in a well extended impression, which frequently lacks detail.

Zinc oxide pastes

These are a mixture of zinc oxide and eugenol. Typically they are dispensed in a ratio of 1:1 and mixed to give an even colour. They are used for recording edentulous ridges in a special tray or in the patient's existing dentures, but cannot be used where there are undercuts because of the material's rigidity. Setting time is decreased by warmth and humidity.

Key points

- Amalgam, though still a suitable material for withstanding heavy occlusal forces, is declining in popularity as resin composite materials are developing.
- Adhesive techniques minimize the unnecessary removal of tooth substance for retention purposes.
- Moisture control is critical with adhesive techniques.
- For successful adhesion, the manufacturers instructions should be carefully followed.
- Flowable and nano-filled resin composites have increased the range of uses for composite materials.
- Glass ionomer materials form a chemical bond to dentine and are largely seen as dentine replacements, and as restorative materials where the load is low and moisture control difficult to achieve (for example root caries).
- Glass ionomers make excellent temporary restorations.
- The main factor when protecting the pulp is the exclusion of bacteria.
- Silicone materials are the most accurate and dimensionally stable, they are also the most expensive.

- Alginate is accurate enough for most applications, but must be carefully stored before pouring the model.

References

Andersson-Wenckert, I.E., van Dijken, J.W. and Kieri, C. (2004) Durability of extensive class II open-sandwich restorations with a resin-modified glass ionomer cement after 6 years. *American Journal of Dentistry*, **17**, 43–50.

Buonocore, M.G. (1955) A simple method of increasing the adhesion of acrylic filling materials to enamel surfaces. *Journal of Dental Research*, **34**, 849–853.

Jagger, D.C. and Harrison, A. (1995) An in vitro investigation into the wear effects of selected restorative materials on dentine. *Journal of Oral Rehabilitation*, **22**, 349–354.

Nakabayashi, N., Nakamura, M. and Yasuda, N. (1991) Hybrid layer as a dentin-bonding mechanism. *Journal of Esthetic Dentistry*, **3**, 133–138.

Silverstone, L.M., Saxton, C.A., Dogon, I.L. and Fejerskov, O. (1975) Variation in the pattern of acid etching of human dental enamel examined by scanning electron microscopy. *Caries Research*, **9**, 373–387.

Further reading

Anusavice, K.J. (2003) *Phillip's Science of Dental Materials*. W.B. Saunders, London.

Brunton, P.A. (2002) *Decision-making in Operative Dentistry* (Quintessentials: Operative Dentistry). Quintessence Publishing, New Malden.

Hilton, T.J. (1996) Cavity sealers, liners, and bases: current philosophies and indications for use. *Operative Dentistry*, **21**, 134–146.

Kugal, G. (2000) The science of bonding: from first to sixth generation. *Journal of the American Dental Association*, **131**, 20–25.

Van Noort, R. (2002) *An Introduction to Dental Materials*. Mosby, St. Louis.

10

Pharmacology and pain control

Margaret Kellett

Summary

This chapter covers:

- Prescribing regulations, access and use of the BNF
- The dental application and use of antibiotics
- Management of patients at risk of infective endocarditis
- Use of anticoagulants, adrenocorticosteroids, cardiovascular drugs, psychotherapeutic agents
- The relevance of other drugs that may affect oral health and dental treatment
- Drugs, techniques and complications of local anaesthesia

Introduction

In the practice of clinical dentistry, it is essential for all of the dental team to understand the role of patient medication and how existing medication may complicate delivery of dental care, may predispose the patient to oral diseases and how drugs may be applied in dental care to both control infection and manage pain.

Every patient's medical history must be checked on every occasion they attend the dental surgery.

Where there is any doubt about the risks associated with medical status or pharmacotherapy interactions do seek guidance from a supervising dentist or the patient's medical practitioner.

The dental team have a duty to support patients in preventing oral disease through active involvement in smoking cessation activity.

As clinical guidance changes it is important to constantly update our knowledge. The National Institute for Clinical Health and Excellence has made significant change to guidance on risk of infective endocarditis.

Prescribing regulations and the use of the BNF

The **British National Formulary** (BNF) details all medicines that are prescribed in the UK, with special reference to their indications, cautions, contraindications, side effects, dosage and relative cost. Compiled with the advice of clinical experts, the BNF provides authoritative and practical information on the selection and clinical use of medicines for use in the NHS. Updated every 6 months, published in both paper-based and web versions (http://www.bnf.org/bnf/), it reflects current best practice, in addition to legal and professional guidelines in relation to the use of medicines.

Regulation of prescribing

The **Medicines Act 1968** was introduced by the Department of Health and Social Security after a review of legislation prompted by the incidence of severe birth defects that were caused by the drug thalidomide. The Act consolidated previous legislation regarding medicines and introduced a number of new provisions for the control of prescribing of medicines. The legislation established three categories of drugs depending upon the danger which they posed and the associated risk of drug abuse. The categories are:

- **Prescription only medicines**, which may be sold or supplied to the public only through the provision of a prescription signed by an approved practitioner. Approved practitioners include doctors and dentists.

Clinical Textbook of Dental Hygiene and Therapy, Second Edition. Edited by Suzanne L. Noble.
© 2012 John Wiley & Sons, Ltd. Published 2012 by John Wiley & Sons, Ltd.

With the exception of controlled drug preparations below certain strength (defined in schedule 5 of the Misuse of Drugs Regulations 2001); all controlled drugs are prescription only medicines.

- **Pharmacy medicines** are those which, subject to certain exceptions, may be sold or supplied only from registered premises by, or under the supervision of, a pharmacist.
- **General sales list medicines** may be sold or supplied direct to the public in an unopened manufacturer's pack from a lockable premises. No controlled drugs are on general sales list.

Current regulation limits the prescribing of medication to doctors, dentists, pharmacists and some nurses. Dental hygienists and dental therapists may, if appropriately trained, dispense medication (most frequently local anaesthetic agents) to patients under the direction of prescribing dental practitioners. The requirement for an individual written prescription for administration of local anesthesia has been simplified by legislation (Statutory Instrument 2000a, www.hmso.gov.uk/acts.htm) permitting Patient Group Directives. In effect this allows specific drugs to be delivered by a defined group of healthcare professionals with the approval of a registered prescriber.

Many patients attending for dental care are taking prescription medication, and the dental hygienist and dental therapist therefore require a knowledge and understanding of such medication and the potential complications which this may cause, either as part of the delivery of dental care or in relation to the patient's susceptibility to oral disease.

Accessing and using the British National Formulary

The BNF is jointly published by the British Medical Association and the Royal Pharmaceutical Society. The Dental Advisory Group produces advice on drugs in relation to oral and dental conditions. In addition to twice yearly updated printed versions the BNF can be accessed on line at www.BNF.org. The main text contains classified notes on clinical conditions, drugs and preparations. These are divided into 15 chapters, each of which is related to a particular system of the body or aspect of medical care. Each chapter is then divided into sections which begin with *appropriate notes for prescribers*. These notes are intended to provide healthcare professionals with information to permit selection of suitable treatment. Further information on drug therapy relating to dental treatment can be obtained in the UK by contacting **UK Medicines Information** (telephone numbers can be found on the UKMi website http://www.ukmi.nhs.uk/).

Guidance on dental and oral conditions is identified by means of a relevant heading (e.g. Dental and Orofacial Pain) in the appropriate sections of the BNF. The notes are followed by details of relevant drugs and preparation. Preparations which can be prescribed by dental surgeons using NHS form FP10D (GP14 in Scotland, WP10D in Wales) are identified within the BNF by means of a note headed Dental Prescribing on the NHS.

The section *Guidance on Prescribing* includes information on prescription writing, controlled drugs and dependence, prescribing for children and the elderly. Advice is given on the reporting of adverse reactions. The BNF also includes advice on medical emergencies and other medical problems in dental practice, together with a review of the oral side effects of drugs.

Medicines should be prescribed only when clinically necessary and, in all cases, the benefit of administering medication should be considered in relation to the risk involved. In particular, patients should be advised of the potential side effects and complications of prescribed medication. Difficulties in compliance with drug treatment occur regardless of age. Factors contributing to poor compliance with prescribed medicines include:

- Prescriptions not collected or dispensed.
- Purpose of medication not clearly explained.
- Perceived lack of efficacy by the patient.
- Real or perceived side effects.
- Instructions for administration not clear.
- Complicated regimen.
- Unattractive formulation, e.g. unpleasant taste.

Emergency Treatment of Poisoning provides information on the management of acute poisoning when first seen in the home.

Appendices and Indexes include information on interactions, liver disease, renal impairment, pregnancy and breast feeding, and cautionary and advisory labels for dispensing medicines. The Dental Practitioners' List and the Nurse Prescribers' List are to be found in this section. The indices contain the manufacturers and the main index.

Prescribing by dental surgeons

Until new prescribing arrangements are introduced for NHS prescriptions, dental surgeons should use form FP10D to prescribe only those items listed in the Dental Practitioners' Formulary. The Act and Regulations do not set any limitations upon the number and variety of substances which the dental surgeon may administer within the dental surgery or may order by private prescription. Provided the relevant legal requirements are observed, the dental surgeon may use or order whatever is required to manage the clinical situation. Dentists are not required to communicate with the patient's doctor when prescribing for dental care; however, in any situation where a complex medical condition or therapy may lead to patient risk, then it is essential to do so.

When prescribing the following principles should be applied:

- Never prescribe a drug unless there is good clinical indication.
- Make prescriptions clear.
- Use approved drug names not brand names.
- Always make the source of the prescription clear.
- Always record the prescription details in the clinical notes.
- Avoid prescribing during pregnancy whenever possible.
- Avoid abbreviations; give the name of the drug in full.

The use of antibiotics and antimicrobials in dentistry

Microbial resistance to antimicrobial drugs is increasing and constitutes a major health problem contributing to deaths from hospital-acquired septicaemia. The indiscriminate prescribing of antimicrobials is considered to be a significant contributory factor in drug resistance. Antimicrobial drugs selectively kill sensitive microorganisms, resulting in the emergence of larger numbers of resistant microorganisms. These drug-resistant forms of bacteria can pass on genetic information, thus conferring acquired drug resistance to other commensal organisms and, in addition, to pathogenic species. The three main mechanisms of antibiotic resistance are reduced bacterial permeability, enzymatic alteration of antibiotics and altered target site.

Antibiotics are an important group of drugs in dental therapy. The decision to prescribe an antibiotic should be based upon a thorough history, physical examination, laboratory data and a diagnosis. It is important to record all information, including prescribed drugs, in the patient's clinical notes.

There are three main indications for the use of antimicrobial drugs in dental treatment:

- If there is a severe or potentially life-threatening infection which will not resolve without the use of antibiotics.
- If an antimicrobial can act as an adjunct to other mechanical therapy in controlling acute or chronic infection.
- When a patient is immunocompromised or is at risk because of a systemic condition, e.g. poorly controlled diabetes or previous use of bisphosphonates.

Potential problems arising from antibiotic use

In addition to the risk of resistant bacteria forms developing, the overgrowth of other organisms (e.g. oral *Candida albicans*), may be problematic.

Allergic drug reactions are common and range from simple itching and rashes to severe life-threatening conditions, such as **anaphylaxis**.

Drug interactions with serious consequences can occur with the use of antimicrobial drugs. It is important to check the BNF before prescribing antimicrobials if the patient is taking other medication (e.g. antimicrobials and oral contraceptives).

Antimicrobial drugs may fail to control infection if:

- The incorrect drug is selected (e.g. microorganisms are not susceptible to the chosen drug).
- An incorrect dose and/or duration of drug is prescribed.
- The patient does not comply with the prescription.
- The antibiotic is taken simultaneously with an interfering drug, e.g. an antacid with tetracycline.
- Drainage is inadequate or necrotic tissue has not been removed.
- Infection is with resistant species of bacteria, or there is emergence of resistant species of bacteria.
- The antibiotic fails to reach the infected site.
- There is a poor host response, such as malabsorption, as a result of systemic disease.
- A foreign body, e.g. an implant, is the focus of infection.

Dental use of antimicrobial drugs

Minor surgical care

Antimicrobials are sometimes prescribed for healthy patients when they are scheduled for minor oral or periodontal surgery. There is no evidence to support the routine use of antimicrobials in this way. Postoperative complications following minor oral and periodontal surgery are rarely serious and are readily managed should they arise. There is no evidence to suggest that antimicrobials can improve the outcome of regenerative periodontal surgery.

Although some authors do advocate routine antimicrobial therapy following removal of third molar teeth (to reduce the risk of dry socket, localised infective osteitis), such prescribing practice confers no advantage and current guidelines suggest prophylactic antimicrobials are not usually required. Following simple extraction in the permanent dentition, dry socket (alveolitis) occurs in only 3–4% of cases. Given the low risk:benefit ratio for use of antibiotic prophylaxis, current guidelines do not support the use of antimicrobial prophylaxis to avoid dry socket except in the case of a clear history of previous repeated dry socket following tooth extraction.

Management of infection

Dental infections which may require the use of antibiotics include:

- Pericoronitis.
- Acute dentoalveolar infection.
- Lateral periodontal abscess.
- Acute ulcerative gingivitis.

The principles that govern management of infection argue that it is not essential to prescribe an antimicrobial routinely for dental infection. The initial assessment of an infection is important; this permits the clinician to assess the patient for signs of spreading uncontrolled infection and consider the need for prescription of antibiotics and/or hospital referral. The features which indicate uncontrolled infection are:

- Grossly elevated temperature, lethargy, tachycardia (indications of septicaemia).
- Spreading cellulitis.
- Swelling involving the floor of mouth which may compromise the airway.
- Difficulty in swallowing.
- Dehydration.
- Failure to respond to treatment.

The treatment process in the management of dental infection should be:

- Identify the cause of infection.
- Define the extent of the spread of infection.
- Record the temperature (normal 36.5 °C).
- Establish drainage and where possible eliminate the cause of infection.
- Consider taking microbiological samples to determine the antibiotic sensitivity of infecting organisms.
- Ensure the patient drinks plenty of fluid to remain hydrated.
- In the event that it is not possible to obtain drainage and the patient's condition is worsening, seek specialist advice.

When antibiotics are considered as an adjunct to the management of dental infection, it is important to review the patient 2–3 days after prescribing to ensure resolution has occurred.

Amoxicillin, 250 mg three times per day, for up to 5 days, is the drug of first choice. Alternatives are amoxicillin, 3 g as two doses 8 hours apart, or **phenoxymethylpenicillin**, 500 mg four times per day for up to 5 days. **Metronidazole**, 200 mg three times a day for up to a maximum of 3 days, is an alternative drug, indicated in particular for anaerobic infections. **Erythromycin**, 250 mg four times a day for a maximum of 5 days, or 0.5–1 g every 12 hours, is a further alternative.

Antimicrobials in periodontal therapy

Systemic administration

Given that gingivitis and periodontitis are for the most part plaque-induced diseases, rarely associated with systemic disorders, it is not surprising that a great deal of research has been undertaken to assess the role of systemic antimicrobials in the management of periodontal diseases.

The use of a systemic drug has not been shown to give any long-term benefits in the management of chronic periodontitis. Chronic periodontitis is characterised by poor oral hygiene and a complex, Gram-negative anaerobic microflora. Microorganisms, often commensal in the mouth, elicit local opportunistic infection in an otherwise healthy patient. The variation in site and rate of progression of disease may be explained by the virulence of the microorganisms, the toxicity of their metabolic by-products and, in addition, the considerable individual host variation in defensive reaction.

Systemic antimicrobials should be reserved for that small proportion of patients who have aggressive forms of periodontitis. This is characterised by low plaque and calculus levels in conjunction with either local or generalised rapid and extensive loss of connective tissue attachment and a failure to respond to conventional non-surgical therapy. The microbial flora in this type of periodontitis is considered to be more aggressive and has a high proportion of periodontal pathogenic species. The use of systemic adjunctive antimicrobial therapy as part of an intense non-surgical programme of care can be beneficial.

Tetracycline is considered a useful drug since not only is it antibacterial but, in addition, it reduces host-mediated bystander damage and enhances tissue healing. Alternatives include a combination of metronidazole with amoxicillin. The use of low-dose long-term tetracycline has been advocated for patients with aggressive periodontitis but there are concerns regarding the risk of the emergence of bacterial drug resistance within the oral flora. The recognised periodontal pathogens are present not only in deep pockets but also in the saliva, on the tongue, palate and other non-pocket sites. These bacterial reservoirs can reinfect treated pockets, hence the indication for a systemic antimicrobial drug to eliminate the whole oral environment of periodontal pathogens.

Topical administration

It is recognised that local pocket response may vary in chronic periodontitis, dependent upon factors including pocket depth, root morphology, furcation involvement and operator skill. A range of topical antimicrobial agents has been developed for specific use in the management of local pockets which have failed to respond to root surface debridement.

Local antimicrobial delivery systems should only be considered as an adjunctive treatment, not an alternative to instrumentation. Thorough debridement should precede any consideration of local therapy. It is important to follow instructions in the product literature carefully at all times.

Topical antibiotics agents lack substantivity as they are washed out of the pocket by the flow of crevicular fluid and so repeated application may be required. An alternative to topical antibiotics is the use of biodegradable gelatin shields containing chlorhexidine which maintain antibacterial levels of the active agent for 10 days.

Current guidance on prophylaxis against infective endocarditis

Antimicrobial prophylaxis is the prevention of infection by the administration of antimicrobial agents. In principle, the administration of antimicrobial drugs should reduce morbidity and mortality. The issue is by no means clear in relation to the indications for and efficacy of the prophylactic use of antibiotics in dentistry. The incidence of infective endocarditis was and remained low despite the widespread use of antibiotic prophylaxis until recent times. It has been estimated that more people have been subject to damage as a result of adverse effects from the use of prophylactic antibiotics than have been prevented from developing infective endocarditis.

Historically in order to deliver a protective effect, prophylactic antibiotics were administered pre-operatively and time allowed for drug concentration in tissues to reach a therapeutic level prior to invasive dental treatment. Antibiotic prophylaxis was in the past routinely provided for patients deemed to be at risk of infective endocarditis.

Predisposing medical conditions and infective endocarditis

Infective endocarditis is a condition resulting from inflammation of the endocardium. The heart valves are especially at risk of damage. The infection is generally caused by bacteria (streptococci, *Staphylococcus aureus* and enterococci) but on occasion viral and fungal organisms can be associated with infective endocarditis. A rare condition with an annual incidence of 10 cases in a normal population of 100 000 infective endocarditis is, however, a serious life-threatening condition with a significant (20%) risk of mortality and morbidity.

Patients at risk of infective endocarditis include some, but not all, patients with a history of rheumatic fever who as a consequence may go on to develop heart valve damage. A cardiology assessment is required to confirm whether or not valve damage is present.

In the past, immunocompromised, renal dialysis and transplant patients were recommended to have prophylaxis. The Working Party of the **British Society for Antimicrobial Chemotherapy** (BSAC) advise that immunosuppressed patients (including transplant patients) and those with indwelling intraperitoneal catheters do not require antibiotic prophylaxis for dental treatment. Similarly the Working Party advised that patients with a prosthetic joint implant (including total hip replacement) do not require antibiotic prophylaxis for invasive dental procedures. Joint infections have rarely been shown to follow dental procedures and are even more rarely caused by oral streptococci. It is considered that it is unacceptable to expose patients to the adverse effects of antibiotics when there is no evidence that such prophylaxis is of any benefit. The advice is that patients who develop any infection require prompt treatment with antibiotics to which the infecting organism is sensitive.

Principles of treatment planning related to risk of infective endocarditis

Clinicians are expected to be familiar with and follow current clinical guidelines in relation to prophylaxis against endocarditis. It is vital to keep updated throughout your career as guidance may change.

National Institute for Health and Clinical Excellence (NICE) clinical guideline 64 'Prophylaxis against infective endocarditis' provides a framework for decision making. Healthcare professionals are however required to use the guidance in conjunction with clinical judgment when deciding on the care of individual patients. The recommendations made by the guideline are based upon a review of current evidence and literature. The removal of recommendation to provide antibiotic prophylaxis for patients who are known to be at risk of infective endocarditis recognizes that the incidence of infective endocarditis is not reduced by large-scale use of antibiotics and the antibiotics themselves are thought to cause more risk of harm to patients in terms of allergic reaction. Antibiotic prophylaxis does not completely eliminate bacteraemia following dental procedures although it has been shown to reduce the frequency of detecting bacteraemia after dental treatment. Patients at risk of infective endocarditis are best served by the introduction of preventive strategies to maintain oral health. These include oral hygiene instruction, dietary advice, fissure sealing and fluoride supplements. Patients benefit from regular assessment and reinforcement of oral health education.

Clinical Guideline recommendations

The 2008 NICE guidance recommends that healthcare professionals should continue to consider people with some cardiac conditions as being at risk of developing infective endocarditis. These include:

- Acquired valvular heart disease with stenosis or regurgitation.
- Valve replacement.
- Structural congenital heart disease, including surgically corrected or palliated structural conditions, but excluding isolated atrial septal defect, fully repaired ventricular septal defect or fully repaired patent ductus arteriosus and closure devices that are judged to be endothelialised.
- Previous infective endocarditis.
- Hypertrophic cardiomyopathy.

There will be many patients who have prior to 2008 been advised to routinely have antibiotic prophylaxis before dental treatment. It is important to communicate with this group and indeed all patients at risk of endocarditis in a clear and consistent manner. A strong emphasis on the need for prevention of dental diseases is vital.

Information provided to patients should include:

- The benefits and risks of antibiotic prophylaxis including an explanation of why antibiotic prophylaxis is no longer routinely recommended.
- The importance of prevention in avoiding dental and oral diseases.
- The symptoms that may indicate infective endocarditis and instruction as to how and when to seek expert advice.
- The inherent risks of undergoing invasive procedures, including non-medical procedures such as body piercing or tattooing.

It is important, that to reduce the risk of endocarditis developing, any episode of infection in a person at risk of developing infective endocarditis is investigated and treated promptly. Some invasive procedures involving the gastrointestinal and genitourinary tract where there is already suspected infection will still require antibiotic prophylaxis. In these cases drug selection requires an antibiotic which is effective against organisms known to cause infective endocarditis. It is best practice to ensure patients are examined, advised of the importance of oral health and rendered dentally fit prior to surgery for total hip replacement, commencing renal dialysis, organ transplant, endocardial surgery, chemotherapy and radiotherapy to the head and neck.

Chlorhexidine mouthwash

Chlorhexidine is an effective antibacterial mouthwash; however, when used as an oral rinse it does not significantly reduce the level of bacteraemia following invasive dental treatment. Therefore chlorhexidine mouthwash should not be offered as a form of prophylaxis against infective endocarditis.

The selection and administration of antibiotic prophylaxis

Should a medical practitioner make specific instruction that as an exception antibiotic prophylaxis for infective endocarditis be administered then specific principles must be followed. Before administering antibiotic prophylaxis, it is important to check that the patient has no history of allergy to the selected drug and that the same drug or other antibiotics have not been recently prescribed. The selected (**bactericidal**) antibiotic should be taken in the presence of a dentist, dental nurse, dental hygienist or therapist to ensure compliance.

Examples of suitable drug selection for invasive dental procedures in patients who have not received more than a single dose of penicillin in the previous month, is **oral amoxicillin**, 3 g 1 hour before the procedure. Patients who are either allergic to penicillin or who have received more than a single dose of a penicillin in the previous month should be prescribed **oral clindamycin**, 600 mg 1 hour before treatment.

For multistage procedures, a maximum of two single doses of penicillin may be given in a month; alternative drugs should be used for further treatment and the penicillin should not be used again for 3–4 months. If clindamycin is used, periodontal or other multistage procedures should not be repeated at intervals of less than 2 weeks.

The use of analgesics in dentistry

Analgesic use in dentistry includes the use of both oral and local agents. While the dental hygienist and therapist may not prescribe oral agents, they will frequently be required to treat patients who are using these drugs and should note this when recording medical histories and be aware of any potential effects of these drugs in relation to dental local analgesia and treatment. Prescribers should advise patients if treatment is likely to affect their ability to drive motor vehicles or manage machinery. This is especially important in relation to oral analgesics, which may also have a sedative effect. Patients should be warned that these effects are increased by alcohol.

Oral analgesics should be used judiciously as part of dental therapy. Analgesics offer only temporary relief from dental pain. A full investigation and diagnosis of the cause of pain should be undertaken. Dental pain of inflammatory origin will not be managed by oral analgesics alone. Pulpitis, apical infection, dry socket or pericoronitis are usually best managed by treating the local infection through drainage, endodontic treatment and other local measures. Where a patient has a raised temperature then paracetamol or ibuprofen are the analgesics of choice due to their antipyretic action.

Pain and discomfort associated with acute conditions of the oral mucosa (e.g. acute herpetic gingivostomatitis, erythema multiforme) may be managed using benzocaine mouthwash or spray. **Non-steroidal anti-inflammatory drugs** (NSAIDs) are frequently prescribed by medical practitioners and, in addition, millions of aspirin, paracetamol and ibuprofen tablets are purchased over the counter for self-medication of headaches, dental pain, musculoskeletal disorders, etc. This group of drugs has to varying degrees analgesic, antipyretic and, at higher doses, anti-inflammatory actions. NSAIDs are not effective against severe visceral type pain, such as renal colic.

Both therapeutic and toxic effects are related to the ability of this group of drugs to inhibit prostaglandin synthesis. The most common toxic effects are:

- Reduced prostaglandin production in the gastric mucosa results in damage which can cause not only dyspepsia, nausea and gastritis, but, more seriously, gastrointestinal bleeding and perforation.
- **Prostaglandins** PDE_2 and PGI_2 are powerful vasodilators synthesised in the renal medulla and glomeruli, respectively. The prostaglandins control renal blood flow and excretion of salt and water. Inhibition of renal prostaglandin synthesis may result in sodium retention, reduced renal blood flow and renal failure. In addition, NSAIDs may cause interstitial nephritis and hyperkalaemia (an increase in blood potassium level). Prolonged analgesic abuse over a period of years is associated with papillary necrosis and chronic renal failure.
- Allergies, skin rashes and bronchospasm occur especially in asthmatic patients.
- **Aspirin** has an important antiplatelet activity which, while beneficial in ischaemic heart disease and of value in prevention of strokes, poses risk of abnormal haemorrhage after minor dental surgery or simple extraction.

Aspirin (acetylsalicylic acid) is the longest-standing NSAID and is an effective analgesic with duration of action of about 4 hours. Aspirin is the drug of choice for mild or moderate pain. The drug is frequently associated with adverse effects, including bronchospasm, gastrointestinal irritation, gastrointestinal bleeding and tinnitus. Care should be taken when prescribing **aspirin** to patients with asthma, uncontrolled hypertension, and history of peptic ulceration or anticoagulants.

Aspirin is contraindicated in

- Children and adolescents under 16 years of age (Reye's syndrome).
- Active peptic ulceration.
- Haemophilia and other bleeding disorders.
- Warfarinised patients.
- Known hypersensitivity to other NSAIDs.

Ibuprofen, **fenbufen** and **naproxen** are propionic acid derivatives of aspirin and are associated with fewer serious adverse effects. **Indomethazone** is one of the indoleacetic acids. It is an effective agent frequently associated with adverse effects including ulceration, gastric bleeding, headaches and dizziness. It may also cause blood dyscrasias. **Piroxicam** has a long half-life and requires only a single daily dose but in the elderly often causes gastrointestinal bleeding. **Phenylbutazone** is an extremely potent anti-inflammatory agent but has serious toxicity, being associated with the risk of aplastic anaemia. **Paracetamol** has no significant anti-inflammatory component. It is well absorbed and does not cause gastric irritation. It has the disadvantage of inducing hepatoxicity in overdosage. The effect of paracetamol is limited to analgesia with some affects against pyrexia; it has no significant anti-inflammatory property.

Opioid analgesics act centrally to modify pain perception; they interact with multiple opiate receptors and mimic endogenous opioid type peptides, endorphins, enkephalins and dynorphins. This class of drugs produces sedation and euphoria which assist with anaesthetic properties in pain management. Oral opioids used for acute dental pain include: codeine, hydrocodone, oxycodone, and dihydrocodeine. Synthetic opioids such as tramadol, propoxyphene and meperidine are also effective in management of acute dental pain. Common adverse effects include nausea, dizziness and drowsiness. Use should be short term to avoid the risk of tolerance and addiction.

The relevance of other drugs that may affect oral health and dental treatment

Anticoagulants

Warfarin is an oral anticoagulant, which is frequently prescribed to reduce blood clotting following venous thrombosis and pulmonary embolism and for patients with prosthetic heart valves. Anticoagulants are one of the classes of medicines most frequently identified as causing preventable harm and resulting in hospital admission. Oral anticoagulants act by interfering with the activation of clotting factors. It takes several days before clotting factors already present are degraded and the full effects of doses are seen. The drug action may be enhanced by a wide range of drugs including NSAIDs, antibacterials, antidepressants, antidiabetogenics, antifungals, antivirals and corticosteroids.

Patients who are anticoagulated require frequent measurement of the level of anticoagulation in effect. These patients carry a record card showing haematology results for measurement of the International Normalised Ratio (INR). The normal therapeutic range for INR is 2.5 to 3.5. It is safe to provide dental treatment for patients provided the INR is less than 4. Should the INR exceed 4 dental treatment should be delayed and the patient's haematology clinic or medical practice should be contacted to ensure the INR is below 4 for the next scheduled appointment.

Adrenocorticosteroids

The adrenocorticosteroids are natural proteins produced in the adrenal cortex. There are two categories the glucocorticosteroid that affect intermediate carbohydrate metabolism and mineralocorticosteroids which affect the water and electrolyte composition of the body. The major steroid in the body is cortisol. Normal adult secretion of cortisol is 20 mg per 24 hours. Stress induces a tenfold increase in cortisol production.

Steroid medication is used because of an anti-inflammatory and anti-allergenic response. They are used for a wide range of medical conditions including asthma, ulcerative colitis, rheumatoid arthritis and autoimmune diseases. Dental use of steroids includes: aphthous ulceration, mucocutaneous conditions, temporomandibular joint (TMJ) arthritis and pulpal dressings.

Drugs designed for inhalation, topical application and oral preparations are all easily absorbed and hence cause systemic effects.

There are a wide range of complications arising from use of systemic steroids. These include gastrointestinal effects, hypertension, glaucoma, behavioural changes, osteoporosis, infection and delayed wound healing.

The major dental implication arises as a result of adrenal suppression and risk of adrenal crisis. When subject to stress the body produces adrenocorticotrophic hormone (ACTH) in the hypothalamus, which causes the adrenal cortex to produce cortisol. Where steroids have been supplied in drug form they inhibit the production of ACTH and cortisol in response to stress. Suppression of the hypothalamic–pituitary–adrenal axis is dependent upon the potency of the drug, dose and the duration of administration. Even after drug therapy is stopped it can take months for the adrenal gland to recover normal function.

Lack of cortisol may induce adrenal crisis which is exacerbated by dehydration, infection, abrupt cessation of medication, surgery and trauma. Adrenal crisis is a serious medical event which presents with features including low blood pressure, rapid heart beat, confusion, loss of consciousness, seizure, sweating and vomiting. Adrenal crisis can result in fatal circulatory collapse. Rapid hydrocortisone 100 mg IV is required to stabilise the patient.

Patients attending for treatment with a dental surgeon or dental therapist are not considered to be at risk of adrenal crisis. To reduce risk the dental team must always check the medical history carefully and ensure the patient takes routine drugs on the day of treatment, ensure a good standard of anaesthesia is obtained and check the blood pressure before treatment, commences.

Patients on high doses of prednisolone (>7.5 mg prednisolone per day) who are scheduled for minor surgical treatment under local anaesthesia should double the normal oral dose of prednisolone on the day of surgery. When steroid cover is advised by the medical practitioner 100 mg prednisolone IV should be given before surgery.

Cardiovascular drugs

Cardiovascular drugs have proven effective in extending the life span of a large proportion of the population. An up to date medical history is essential, where there is any doubt the patients medical practitioner should be contacted for guidance. The pulse and blood pressure should be checked for patients with a history of cardiovascular disease before each treatment commences.

Stable and managed cardiovascular disease is not a contraindication to delivery of dental therapy care. Epinephrine (adrenaline) vasoconstrictor should be limited to 0.04 mg in cardiac patients. Care must be taken to inject local anaesthetic slowly and use aspiration to prevent intravascular injection of the agent.

Common cardiovascular drugs include digitalis glycosides, angiotensin-converting enzyme inhibitors, angiotensin receptor blockers, β-adrenergic blockers, antiarrhythmics. Always ensure GTN tablets or oral spray are brought to appointments and easily accessed during the appointment.

In some circumstances dental treatment should be delayed until medical approval to proceed has been obtained:

- Acute or recent myocardial infarction.
- Unstable or recent onset of angina pectoris.
- Uncontrolled congestive cardiac failure.
- Uncontrolled arrhythmias.
- Significant uncontrolled hypertension.

Psychotherapeutic agents

Psychotherapeutic agents may be used to treat major psychiatric disorders (e.g. schizophrenia, bipolar and unipolar affective disorders, neurosis or minor conditions such as neurosis such as anxiety). **Antipsychotic drugs** used to manage major psychiatric disorders have side effects including

- Sedation.
- Extrapyramidal effects, acute dystonia, parkinsonism, akathisia, dyskinesia.
- Orthostatic hypotension.
- Cardiovascular effects, e.g. tachycardia.
- Seizures.
- Anticholinergic effects, blurred vision, xerostomia, constipation.
- Agranulocytosis is a risk with clozapine.

There are two classes of antipsychotic drugs, conventional (e.g. chlorpromazine, chlorprothixene, haloperidol) and atypical drugs such as aripiprazole and risperidone, which have fewer side effects.

When managing a patient known to be prescribed antipsychotic drugs the dental therapist should be aware to:

- Always check for xerostomia and instigate management to prevent increased oral and dental disease.
- Take care to use caution in all patient interactions as psychotic patients may misinterpret verbal and non-verbal communication.
- Understand that extrapyramidal side effects may limit jaw opening.
- Note that sedation may be increased by multiple drug therapy.
- Note that epinephrine (adrenaline) is safe to use in dental local anaesthetic.
- Bring patients slowly to the upright position after treatment to avoid hypotension.
- Remember that patient cooperation may be limited by extrapyramidal dyskinesis.

Antidepressant drugs are widely used to manage neurosis including depression and in some cases are also prescribed for chronic TMJ dysfunction. Current types of antidepressant drugs include tricyclic antidepressants (TCA), selective serotonin reuptake inhibitors (SSRI) and monoamine oxidase inhibitors (MAOI). Adverse reactions are similar to those reported for antipsychotic drugs.

The most serious effect of TCAs is cardiac toxicity resulting in congestive cardiac failure, arrhythmias and myocardial infarction. Xerostomia is a frequent finding. TCAs interact with other drugs including amphetamines and other central nervous system stimulants.

The dental therapist should always check for a full list of current medication as TCAs are often used in combination with other antipsychotic drugs. Remember TCAs are not always prescribed for depression. Take care to ensure any xerostomia is recorded and an effective preventive programme of dental care is established. Epinephrine (adrenaline) may cause an increased vasopressor response and so use of local anaesthesia should be adjusted to deliver a maximum of 0.04 mg if raised blood pressure is a concern.

SSRIs (e.g. Prozac) are a group of antidepressants often selected as they have fewer side effects than TCA drugs. Oral effects in addition to xerostomia include taste changes, aphthous ulceration, glossitis and occasionally increased salivation.

MAOIs have many adverse effects and toxicity can lead to severe toxic reaction. MAOIs react adversely with drugs such as amphetamines and food (e.g. cheese, wine, and fish) resulting in a hypertensive crisis. These are infrequently prescribed.

Oral side effects of drugs

Patients using prescribed medication may present with oral features and side effects. These may be due to local action on the mouth or to a systemic effect manifested by oral changes. Medications which are left in contact with the oral mucosa can cause inflammation or ulceration. **Aspirin** tablets, if allowed to dissolve in the buccal sulcus for treatment of toothache, can cause ulceration. There is a particular risk of oral ulceration in patients prescribed **cytotoxic drugs** (e.g. methotrexate). **Erythema multiforme**, a severe form of ulceration, may follow from the use of a wide range of medication including anticonvulsants, antibacterials and sulphonamide derivatives. White patches typical of lichenoid eruption are found in association with NSAIDs, methyldopa, chloroquine, oral antidiabetogenics, thiazide diuretics and gold.

Tooth staining may be intrinsic (e.g. tetracycline induced or **fluorosis**), or extrinsic, as associated with chlorhexidine mouthrinse.

Immunosuppressant drugs are used to prevent organ transplant rejection. These will reduce resistance to normal commensal organisms in the mouth, resulting in viral, fungal and bacterial infection.

Drug-induced **gingival hyperplasia** is a complication of calcium channel blockers (e.g. **Epanutin, nifedipine** and **ciclosporin**).

A wide range of drugs (e.g. antispasmodics and tricyclic antidepressants) may cause **xerostomia**, which subsequently predisposes to plaque retention and increased levels of dental caries and periodontal disease.

Candidiasis can be a complication of use of antibiotics, immunosuppressants and inhaled corticosteroids.

Non-prescription drugs and habits can have an adverse effect on the oral tissues. Perioral ulceration is associated with solvent abuse; Oral carcinoma risk is increased by smoking and alcohol consumption. Cannabis use is associated with gingival ulceration and periodontitis. Tobacco smoking produces oral features of fungal infection, smoker's palate, oral pigmented patches, leukoplakia, erythroplakia, periodontitis and necrotising ulcerative gingivitis.

Sugar-free medication in prescribing practice

Oral liquid medications that do not contain fructose, glucose or sucrose are described as 'sugar-free'. Preparations containing hydrogenated glucose syrup, mannitol, maltitol, sorbitol or xylitol are considered 'sugar-free' since there is evidence that they do not cause dental caries. When medication containing cariogenic sugars is prescribed it is important to advise the patient of appropriate dental hygiene measures. Sugar-free preparations should be used whenever possible, particularly in children if long-term medication is being prescribed.

Local analgesic agents

The two classes of local analgesic agents are **esters** and **amides**. These differ in their mechanism of metabolism. Esters are rapidly metabolised in plasma by **pseudocholinesterases**. The breakdown of amides is more complex and hence slower. Amides in general need to be transported to the liver for breakdown. Some metabolism of prilocaine occurs in the lungs. Articaine is the exception as it undergoes initial degradation in plasma by esterases.

The ester local analgesic agents are prone to induce allergy and are not generally used for dental injection, although some have use as topical agents. In general the amide agents have superior analgesic properties for application by infiltration.

Local analgesic agents are often used with a vasoconstrictor, which will:

- Reduce haemorrhage.
- Extend the duration of pulpal analgesia.
- Produce a more effective, deeper level of analgesia
- Reduce systemic toxicity

The vasoconstrictors used in dental analgesic solutions are **epinephrine** (**adrenaline**), a naturally occurring hormone, and **felypressin**, a synthetic octapeptide which resembles the pituitary hormone vasopressin. Use of epinephrine should be restricted in patients with cardiac problems, such as unstable angina or severe dysrhythmia. Epinephrine has superior vasoconstrictor

properties to felypressin. The agents present in a typical dental analgesic cartridge are summarised in Table 10.1.

Amide local analgesics

The amide local analgesic agents approved for used in dentistry are:

- Lidocaine.
- Prilocaine.
- Mepivacaine.
- Articaine.
- Bupivacaine and levobupivacaine.
- Ropivacaine.

Only lidocaine, prilocaine, mepivacaine and articaine are available in specific dental analgesic cartridges. The other drugs are required to be drawn up from standard vials and are not in general use.

Lidocaine (20 mg/ml) is the most frequently used local analgesic agent. First introduced in 1949, this amide derivative of xylidine has now replaced procaine. Procaine is now seldom used (despite being as potent as lidocaine); it has a much shorter duration of effect and considerably less ability to spread through the tissues. Lidocaine has a rapid onset of analgesia and spreads widely through the tissues. These features render the technique less sensitive to operator skill in depositing the drug into a localised target area. Lidocaine delivers profound analgesia of relatively long duration. In 2% solution with 1:80 000 epinephrine (adrenaline) vasoconstrictor, pulpal analgesia of up to 1–1½ hours and soft tissue analgesia of 3–4 hours are possible. Intraligamentary application will give approximately 15 minutes pulpal analgesia. Lidocaine is also an excellent topical anaesthetic agent.

Prilocaine is available in two forms: a 3% (30 mg/ml) solution with the vasoconstrictor felypressin (octapressin), and also as a plain 4% (40 mg/ml) solution. Prilocaine with felypressin has a similar activity to

Table 10.1 Contents of an analgesic cartridge.

Constituent	Example
Local anaesthetic	Prilocaine, mepivacaine (carbocaine), lidocaine
Vasoconstrictor	1:80 000 epinephrine (adrenaline), 1:2 000 000 felypressin
Vehicle	Isotonic Ringer's solution
Fungicide	Thymol
Preservative	Caprylhydrocuprienotoxin, methylparaben
Reducing agent	A reducing agent which prevents oxidisation of the vasoconstrictor

lidocaine with epinephrine (adrenaline) when used for infiltration and inferior dental block analgesia. When used during intraligamentary injection, the preparation is less efficient than lidocaine and is less effective in controlling haemorrhage. Prilocaine produces less vasodilatation than lidocaine and in plain presentation is a useful agent when a vasoconstrictor-free drug is required, for example when providing dental analgesia for patients who have had radiotherapy to the head and neck.

Prilocaine also has a potent topical anaesthetic effect and is presented in combination with lidocaine, both at a concentration of 2.5%, in **EMLA** (eutectic mixture of lidocaine and prilocaine). The formulation produces effective analgesia of skin and is of use prior to venous cannulation. EMLA is not licensed for intraoral application.

Mepivacaine is available in two formulations: a 2% (20 mg/ml) solution with 1:100 000 epinephrine (adrenaline) and a 3% (30 mg/ml) plain solution. The combination of mepivacaine with vasoconstrictor has a similar effect to lidocaine with vasoconstrictor. Mepivacaine produces less vasodilatation than lidocaine. A plain solution is of use in applications where it is essential to conserve a good blood supply to the operative site, for example in patients who have had radiotherapy to the head and neck and require tooth extraction.

Articaine is available as a 4% (40 mg/ml) solution, combined with 1:100 000 or, alternatively, 1:200 000 epinephrine (adrenaline). When used with a vasoconstrictor, the efficacy is similar to that of lidocaine with epinephrine (adrenaline). The metabolism of this drug commences in plasma, and as a result it has a much shorter duration of action, with a half-life of 20 minutes compared to 90 minutes for lidocaine. The risk of toxicity is therefore reduced using articaine.

Ester local analgesics

Benzocaine is an excellent topical agent, applied in a 20% gel. Since the drug is insoluble in water it cannot be injected. **Tetracaine** is toxic and cannot be injected; however, in 4% topical form it can be used to anaesthetise the skin prior to venepuncture for intravenous sedation or general analgesia. **Cocaine** was at one time used in dentistry but is now avoided due to its potential for misuse. Cocaine is a drug of addiction which causes central nervous stimulation. It may occasionally be used in topical form.

Techniques for local analgesia

Registered dental hygienists and dental therapists may deliver local analgesia by topical application and infiltration techniques, including inferior dental nerve block and intrapapillary injection. In accordance with General Dental Council (GDC) regulations they should treat patients following a treatment plan obtained from a registered dental surgeon who has examined the patient. The use of intraligamentary and intraosseous techniques is not currently within the remit of the dental hygienist and dental therapist.

The relevant anatomy and nerve supply of the oral region

In order to anaesthetise the teeth and oral mucosa for delivery of dental care the dental hygienist or therapist needs to be able to select and anaesthetise the sensory nerve supply. This is limited to two branches of the trigeminal nerve – i.e. the maxillary and mandibular divisions of the fifth cranial nerve. The anatomy and distribution of these nerves are described in detail in Chapter 1(p. 18–19), but a brief summary of the branches and the structures supplied relevant to local analgesia of the maxillary and mandibular teeth is given in Tables 10.2 and 10.3.

Table 10.2 The nerve supply of the maxillary teeth and supporting tissues.

Structures	Nerve supply
Second and third molars and adjacent buccal supporting tissues	Posterior superior alveolar nerve
First molar and adjacent buccal supporting tissues	Mesiobuccal pulp from the middle superior alveolar nerve, distobuccal and palatal pulp from the posterior superior alveolar nerve
Premolars and adjacent buccal supporting tissues	Middle superior alveolar nerve
Canines and adjacent supporting buccal tissues	Anterior superior alveolar nerve
Incisors and adjacent buccal supporting tissues	Anterior superior alveolar nerve
Palatal supporting tissue molar and premolar area	Greater palatine nerve
Palatal supporting tissue canine area	Greater palatine and nasopalatine nerves
Palatal supporting tissue incisor area	Nasopalatine nerve
Soft palate and uvula	Lesser palatine nerve
Skin and mucosa of the upper lip	Infraorbital nerve

Table 10.3 Nerve supply to the mandibular teeth and surrounding structures.

Structure	Nerve supply
Teeth and alveolus	Inferior alveolar nerve
Buccal gingival and mucosa opposite molars	Long buccal nerve
Buccal gingival and mucosa opposite premolars	Long buccal and mental nerve
Buccal gingiva and mucosa opposite canines and incisors	Mental nerve
Anterior two thirds of the tongue	Lingual nerve
Lingual gingiva, mucosa and floor of mouth	Lingual nerve
Skin and mucosa of the lower lip and chin	Mental nerve

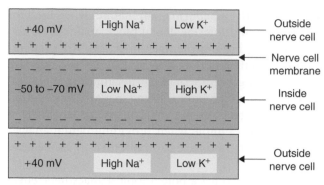

Figure 10.1 Nerve resting potential.

The pharmacology of local analgesia and its mode of action

In order to understand the mode of action of a local anaesthetic it is first necessary to understand the mechanism of normal peripheral nerve conduction.

How do nerves work?

The nerve cell or **neuron** consists of a cell body with a nucleus and projections from the cell body called **dendrites** which pick up messages or stimuli. An extension of the cell, the nerve fibre or **axon**, connects one cell to the dendrites of the next (separated by small gaps or **synapses**) and carries impulses away from the cell body. The conduction of stimulus along a nerve fibre is dependent upon changes in the electrophysiological status of the nerve membrane. When a nerve is unstimulated there is a negative 'resting' potential of −50 to −70 mV within the cell, compared with the exterior cell membrane surface (Figure 10.1). When stimulation occurs, a measurable transmembrane action potential occurs.

After stimulation the following sequence of events occurs. A relatively slow phase of depolarisation occurs during which the electrical potential within the nerve cell becomes progressively less negative. Eventually the potential difference between the interior and the exterior surface of the cell membrane reaches a critical level (threshold potential) when **depolarisation** reverses the potential so that the inner aspect of the nerve is positively charged in comparison to the exterior of the cell membrane (Figure 10.2). At the peak of the action, the intracellular positive potential reaches about 40 mV. Once the peak intracellular positive potential is reached, a process of **repolarisation** begins. The repolarisation overshoots the resting potential to about −90 mV. This

is called **hyperpolarisation** and restricts the nerve from receiving another stimulus during this period of time. After hyperpolarisation, during the so-called **refractory period**, the resting intracellular potential of −50 to −70 mV is gradually restored. The potential change is then propagated along the whole length of the nerve fibre (Figure 10.3). The nerve cell membrane becomes progressively easier to stimulate during the refractory period as the intracellular resting potential is restored; so it will take a slightly above threshold stimulus to cause an action potential near the end of the relative refractory period.

The interior peripheral nerve cell cytoplasm has a high concentration of potassium ions and a low concentration of sodium ions (Figure 10.1). This is the opposite of the extracellular fluids. At rest the inside/outside potassium ratio (K_j/K_o) is approximately 30; it is this gradient which produces a negative intracellular resting potential. While the resting nerve is resistant to ion passage, upon stimulation the cell membrane permeability increases and there is an initial influx of sodium ions into the cell (the **sodium channel**). This accounts for the depolarisation phase of the action potential. Once the cell reaches maximum depolarisation, the passage of sodium ions is arrested and potassium ions pass out of the cell; as a result the repolarisation of the cell membrane takes place.

While the movement of sodium and potassium during nerve stimulation is passive, the repolarisation events are active. Sodium is extruded by the sodium pump using energy derived from oxidative metabolism of **adenosine triphosphate**. A metabolic pump may also effect the restoration of the resting intracellular potassium ion concentration, since the necessary movement is also against the concentration gradient. Alternative potassium ion transport may be effected along the electrostatic gradient between the resting cell and its extracellular fluid. This does not require the expenditure of energy.

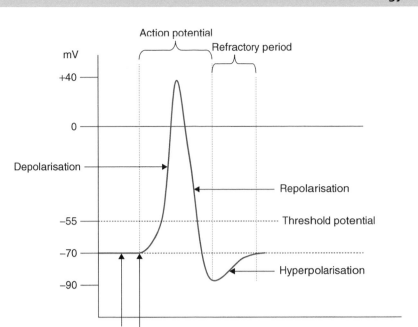

Figure 10.2 A nerve action potential.

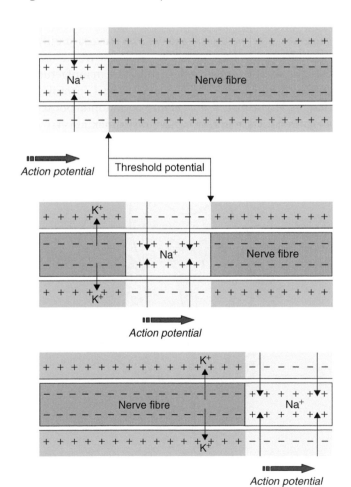

Figure 10.3 Diagram showing normal nerve transmission is the result of differential sodium ion concentration across the nerve membrane.

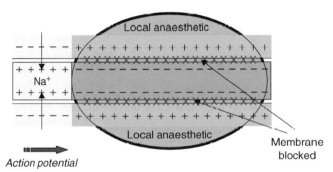

Figure 10.4 Diagram illustrating the action of local anaesthetic agents preventing sodium entering the cell, thus blocking nerve stimulation.

The mechanism of action of local analgesic agents

Nerve trauma, such as occurs to the inferior dental nerve sometimes during third molar removal or when alcohol injections are used to control intractable trigeminal neuralgia, may produce permanent local analgesia. In dental use it is desirable to obtain reversible local analgesia.

Reversible local analgesic agents work by inhibiting the passage of sodium ions into the nerve cell. As a result, the potential changes which allow the wave of depolarisation to travel along the nerve fibres are arrested. The mechanism is, in part, due to a non-specific expansion of the nerve cell membrane, which results in a physical barrier to sodium ion movement into the nerve cell (Figure 10.4). In addition, local analgesic agents bind in a reversible manner to specific receptors in the sodium channel. During the refractory period of the firing cycle of nerve impulse transmission, the binding site for local analgesic solution is exposed due to a change in conformation. During this period further stimulation of the nerve does not produce depolarisation. When the local analgesic binds to its receptor, the sodium channel remains in the refractory conformation.

Access to the local analgesic binding site is within the nerve cell. Local analgesic agents need to be soluble in fat to enter the cell, since the cell membrane is lipid rich. Lipid-soluble molecules are non-charged and hence local analgesics must be present in a non-charged state in the tissues. However, molecules that can then bind to the local analgesic receptor site need to be charged. In summary an active local anaesthetic must be uncharged to enter the cell and charged to bind to the receptors. Local analgesic agents have the desired property since they are weak bases. In solution there is an equilibrium in which a proportion of molecules are charged and others uncharged. These uncharged molecules traverse the cell membrane and immediately re-equilibrate to produce a mixture of charged and non-charged molecules. Agents that have a naturally higher proportion of uncharged molecules present when in tissue fluids pass through the nerve cell more rapidly and are more effective local analgesic agents. The pH of the tissue affects the proportion of non-charged molecules; this is lower at higher pH, such as occurs in tissues which are inflamed.

The other factor that determines efficacy of individual local analgesic agents is their effect on blood vessels. Those with a more effective vasoconstrictor property are retained at higher concentration for a longer period of time in the tissues; hence they provide better depth and duration of analgesia. The addition of a vasoconstrictor such as epinephrine (adrenaline) reduces local blood flow, slows down the rate of absorption of the local analgesic and thus prolongs the duration of analgesia. In dental formulations up to 1 in 80 000 epinephrine (adrenaline) (12.5 µg/ml) is used in local analgesic solutions.

Lidocaine 2% with 1 in 80 000 epinephrine (adrenaline) is a safe and effective formulation that has been used for routine dentistry for many years. In patients with severe hypertension or unstable cardiac rhythm the use of adrenaline in local analgesic solution is hazardous. In such patients it is usual to use prilocaine with or without felypressin (a vasoconstrictor related to octapressin). Both mepivacaine and articaine are available with and without adrenaline in their formulation.

Methods of application of local analgesic agents in dentistry

The methods currently available for delivering local dental analgesics are shown in Figure 10.5, and these include:

- Topical.
- Jet.
- Infiltration.
- Regional block.
- Intraosseous.
- Intraligamentary.

The dental hygienist and dental therapist are trained to use topical, infiltration and inferior dental block techniques. The dental surgeon need not be present. The dental hygienist and therapist may give local analgesic only to facilitate the delivery of their own care to the patient. They should not give local analgesic for the sole purpose of allowing another person (e.g. a dentist), to deliver treatment.

The ester type agents are used in topical preparations; these are in general more likely to produce allergy reaction than amide agents. Both lidocaine and benzocaine are effective topical agents. The mucosa should be dried and topical agents left in contact with the tissues for a period of time as indicated by the manufacturer's instructions (Figure 10.6). A new topical formulation designed to be placed as a gel into periodontal pockets is suggested for use in root surface instrumentation.

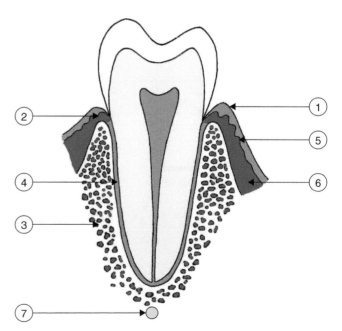

Figure 10.5 Diagram to show the various methods of application of dental analgesic. 1 topical; 2 intrapapillary; 3 intraosseous; 4 intraligamentary; 5 subepithelial; 6 infiltration; 7 nerve block.

Infiltration analgesia

Using modern local analgesic preparations, infiltration is a simple technique. The agent is deposited beneath the epithelium but above the periosteum within the mucosa. The analgesic is deposited around the terminal nerve endings and is therefore effective in a given site regardless of the source of the innervation.

In the maxilla, the cortical bone is thinner than in the mandible, and simple buccal infiltration can deliver pulpal analgesia. The ideal application is for a local site which is free from infection. Infection may be spread by injecting into the site and reduces the efficacy of analgesia. In the mandible, with the exception of the incisor teeth, the thick cortical layer of bone present precludes the use of an infiltration technique for molar analgesia in the adult dentition (however, see Chapter 12 and 14 for the child patient).

The needle should be introduced in the buccal fold within the reflected mucosa. By stretching the tissues, smooth penetration of the needle with minimal discomfort is assured. Injection into the epithelium produces blistering and pain, so the needle should be advanced into the mucosa before injection commences. Injection beneath the periosteum is painful and produces postanalgesic discomfort. Aspiration should be performed before injecting. A slow injection rate of 1 ml over 30 seconds is ideal. The technique takes approximately 2 minutes before analgesia is achieved. Pulpal analgesia lasts for 45 minutes (2% lidocaine with 1:80 000 epinephrine (adrenaline)), soft tissue analgesia lasts for a longer duration; approximately 1–2 ml of solution should be injected.

Occasionally there is an additional nerve supply in the maxilla to pulpal tissue from the greater palatine and nasopalatine nerves. In this case an additional palatal infiltration is required. The upper first molar has a nerve supply from both the posterior and middle superior alveolar nerves and, given that buccal access may be reduced due to the zygomatic buttress, a block of these nerves may be required as infiltration will be ineffective.

Palatal infiltration (Figure 10.7) can be used to anaesthetise palatal soft tissue for upper teeth distal to the canine. The injection should be placed just distal to the selected tooth, 10–15 mm from the gingival margin. Only a few drops of solution are required.

Regional block analgesia

The delivery of regional block analgesia in the maxilla is not permitted by the dental hygienist or dental therapist. Given the success of infiltration techniques, the dental hygienist or therapist will rarely have difficulty in delivering painless dental care using infiltration methods alone in the maxilla.

In the mandible, the choice of technique for analgesia delivery is dependent upon the age of the patient and the location of the tooth to be anaesthetised. Infiltration is successful in obtaining analgesia for mandibular primary teeth (see Chapter 14). In adults infiltration is preferable to regional block for pulpal analgesia of the mandibular incisor teeth due to its efficacy and as a result of supply from the contralateral inferior dental nerve to central incisor teeth.

Regional block methods in the mandible will produce a widespread area of analgesia from a single injection and have the advantage that the delivery of analgesic is at sites discrete from local areas of infection.

Regional block analgesia has the following disadvantages:

- The technique is more difficult than infiltration.
- Midline crossover of nerve supply is not managed.
- Patients dislike the excessively wide distribution of soft tissue analgesia.
- Deep tissue haemorrhage can cause infection and trismus.
- Although rare, direct nerve injury may occur.

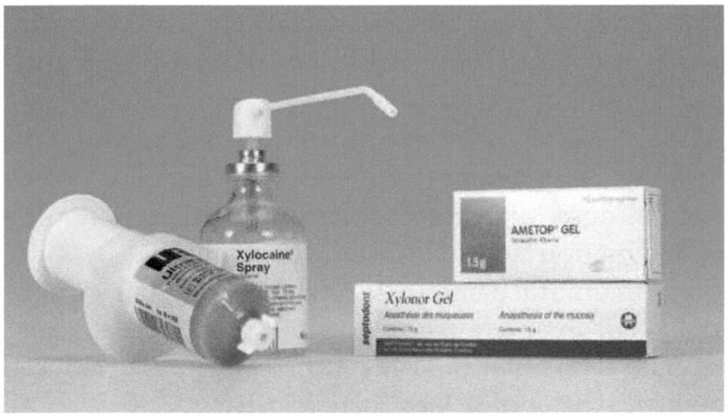

Figure 10.6 The range of topical analgesia preparations available for use in dental practice.

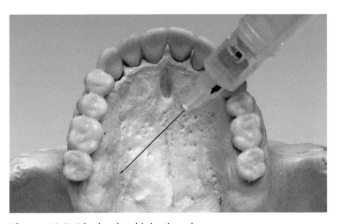

Figure 10.7 Ideal palatal injection sites.

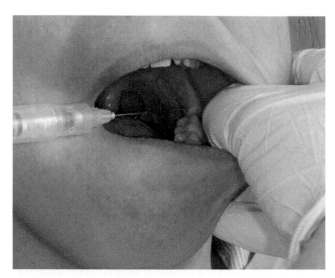

Figure 10.8 Direct method of inferior alveolar dental nerve block.

The dental hygienist and dental therapist are trained to deliver the inferior alveolar nerve block as a means of securing pulpal analgesia in adult mandibular canines, premolar and molar teeth. The technique aims to deposit local analgesic solution in close proximity to the mandibular foramen on the medial aspect of the mandibular ramus. The analgesic solution thus blocks nerve conduction where the nerve is accessible before it enters the inferior alveolar canal.

The direct technique uses simple anatomical landmarks to assist the operator in locating the mandibular foramen. The patient's mouth is opened wide and the ramus is held with the thumb on the retromolar area in the coronoid notch of the ascending ramus. The thumb palpates the internal oblique ridge of the mandible and stretches the overlying mucosa thus facilitating easy needle penetration (Figure 10.8). The index finger is placed exteriorly on the posterior aspect of the ramus at the same height as the thumb. In the adult the mandibular foramen is halfway between the operator's thumb and index finger. The syringe is placed across the premolars of the opposite side of the mouth and directed between the external oblique ridge and the pterygomandibular raphe. The technique is not always successful. Failure may be due to faulty technique, anatomical variation in the location of the mandibular foramen, bending of the needle or accessory nerve supplies.

Difficulties, complications and emergencies that can be associated with local analgesia

Despite the recognition that local analgesia has a safe record in dental applications, it is important to be familiar with potential complications. At greatest risk of complication from use of local analgesia are children,

the elderly and the medically compromised. It is vital to obtain a careful medical history including analgesic history before delivering local analgesic, since allergy, toxicity and drug interactions account for the most serious complications.

Adverse effects of local analgesics include:

- Trauma.
- Failure to achieve analgesia.
- Toxicity.
- Fainting.
- Hypersensitivity.
- Drug interactions.
- Facial nerve paralysis.

Trauma

The delivery of rapid injection or poor technique can result in direct nerve damage or haematoma formation. These can lead to pain and patient anxiety. Pain at the time of injection can be avoided by careful technique, including the use of a slow injection of isotonic solution. After-pain results from direct tissue trauma resulting in haematoma, infection or trismus.

Failure to achieve analgesia

Patient anxiety may lead not only to fainting but also to a reduced analgesic efficacy. In such cases it may be necessary to consider the use of conscious sedation to reduce anxiety. Provided they have had appropriate training, a dental hygienist or therapist may treat patients who are sedated in this way but only if a dental surgeon is present in the surgery. Inflammation in the site of injection will prevent adequate analgesia. In such circumstances, use of a regional block may be more successful. Anatomical variation in relation to bone architecture and nerve supply also accounts for failure to achieve analgesia.

Toxicity

The toxic effects associated with local analgesic drugs usually result from excessively high plasma concentrations; in normal use a single application of local analgesic does not generally result in systemic side effects. *As a general rule a volume of one tenth of a cartridge per kilogram body weight is the maximum safe dose.* When normal doses are exceeded there is a risk of sensation of inebriation and light-headedness followed by sedation, circumoral paraesthesia and twitching; convulsions can occur in severe reactions. Care should be taken, as patients with renal and hepatic disease will have reduced ability to metabolise local analgesic drugs.

It is best practice to use no more than one and a half cartridges to achieve infiltration analgesia in a quadrant,

Table 10.4 Maximum safe dose of local anaesthetics.

Concentration	Adrenaline	Maximum (mg) cartridges	*Octapressin
Lidocaine 2%	1:80 000	200	5
Prilocaine 4%	1:200 000	400	5.5
Mepivocaine 2%	1:20 000*	300	11
Articaine 4%	1:100 000	500	7

or one cartridge for a single nerve block application in the mandible. No more than two cartridges should be used in a fit healthy adult per dental visit. Table 10.4 shows the maximum safe dose of local anesthetic agents. Cartridges vary from 2.2 to 1.8 ml depending upon the standard or self aspirating formats and it is important to check the drug content, vasoconstrictor and dose along with the expiry date before using any local anaesthetic.

Should toxicity be caused by local analgesic agents, the patient should be laid flat and oxygen should be administered; intravenous fluids and anticonvulsants may be required along with basic life support. Epinephrine (adrenaline) toxicity associated with intravascular injection of the drug causes increased cerebral blood pressure and the patient is best placed in an erect rather than fully supine position. Oxygen should only be given if the patient is not hyperventilating. Recovery is rapid and the patient should be reassured.

To avoid a toxic reaction it is advisable to:

- Aspirate before injecting analgesic.
- Calculate the safe dosage considering the patient's age, renal and hepatic function and current drug therapy. Young children should be weighed to ensure correct maximum dose is not exceeded.
- Deliver the injection slowly.

Methaemoglobinaemia is a toxic effect most frequently associated with the use of prilocaine. **Methaemoglobin** is formed from haemoglobin when iron in ferric rather than ferrous form is present. The irreversible binding of haemoglobin causes cyanosis and responds to intravenous injection of methylene blue.

Intravascular injection, should it occur during dental injection, can result in convulsions and cardiovascular collapse. To avoid such complications aspiration syringes and a slow injection technique, with the patient in a supine position, are essential. Local analgesics should not be injected into inflamed or infected tissue, as not only is there a risk of spreading infection but rapid absorption into the blood may increase the possibility of systemic side effects.

Fainting

Fainting may occur before, during or after the administration of local analgesic. Typically the patient will become pale, sweaty and complain of nausea. Some patients describe a tingling sensation in the hands and feet prior to loss of consciousness; the pulse is first rapid then becomes slow and weak. Fainting is due to a reduction in cranial blood supply subsequent to a slowing of the heartbeat due to intense vagal stimulation. Fainting can be avoided by dealing with the patient in a calm, reassuring and confident manner. The delivery of local analgesia should always take place with the patient in a supine position. In the event of a faint, lay the dental chair flat to ensure a supply of blood to the brain. The patient should recover spontaneously and treatment can then continue (see Chapter 16).

Hypersensitivity

Hypersensitivity reactions occur mainly with the ester-type local analgesic agents, such as benzocaine, cocaine, procaine and tetracaine. Sensitivity reactions are less frequent with amide-type drugs, such as lidocaine, bupivacaine, prilocaine and ropivacaine. If a patient gives a history of allergic reaction to local analgesia it is essential this be investigated. Referral for specific testing to identify safe local analgesic agents for a patient with possible allergy is usually through the dermatology specialist service.

There is also the potential for allergic response in sensitised patients to **latex**, which is present in the plungers of some local analgesic cartridges. Life-threatening anaphylactic reaction may be induced. Confirmation of the material in specific cartridges should be made with the manufacturer.

Citanest 3% with octapressin (prilocaine hydrochloride and octapressin corresponding to felypressin) dental injection standard and self-aspirating in 1.8 ml cartridges has components that are latex-free. However, the manufacturers have warned that the product may come into contact with latex containing materials during the production process. The components of Oraqix 25/25 per g periodontal gel (lidocaine, prilocaine) are latex free and do not come into contact with latex during the manufacturing process.

Drug interactions

Drug reaction can be related to either the analgesic agent or the vasoconstrictor. Potential reactions can occur with a wide range of drugs, including:

- Anticonvulsants.
- Antimicrobials.

- Benzodiazepines.
- β-adrenergic blockers.
- Calcium channel blockers.
- Diuretics.
- Antidepressants.
- Social/drugs of abuse.

The interaction with anticonvulsants is unlikely to be more than a theoretical risk in normal dental practice. The other drugs listed are not considered a contraindication to the safe use of local analgesia which should, however, be used with caution. In the event of any concerns it is wise to seek advice from the patient's medical practitioner.

Facial nerve paralysis

If during inferior alveolar nerve block the analgesic solution is inadvertently deposited within the parotid gland then the facial nerve may be affected, resulting in hemifacial paralysis. The condition is alarming for patients but is reversible. In the event that the eyelid is paralysed the eye requires protection for the period of paralysis.

Equipment used in dental local analgesia

Syringes, along with attached needles and analgesic cartridges, are required for conventional delivery of local analgesic with simple hand pressure. Computerised delivery systems have a pump to control the pressure and hence the rate of injection. Current safe policy for the use of used needles precludes re-sheathing. Modern disposable syringe and needle combinations avoid the need to dismantle or re-sheath used needles, thereby reducing the risk of sharps injuries.

Needles for use with dental syringes have a stainless steel silicon tip with a bevelled edge and a plastic hub. Specialist dental needles (Figure 10.9) have a portion

adjacent to the butt, which protrudes. Standard Luer type needles are used in some systems. Luer type needles are supplied in sterile blister packs, whereas dental needles are supplied with individual sterile sheaths with seals indicating the needle size and date up to which the contents are sterile. If the seal is damaged the needle should be discarded.

Primarily, needles are supplied in varying lengths and two gauges. The gauge measures the external diameter of the needle. The 30 gauge needle is 0.3 mm and the 27 gauge is 0.4 mm diameter. The length of needles ranges

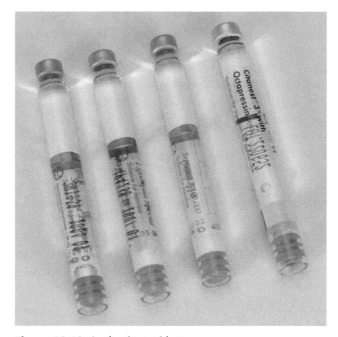

Figure 10.10 Analgesic cartridges.

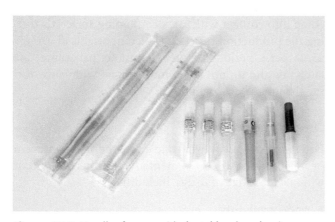

Figure 10.9 Needles for use with dental local analgesics.

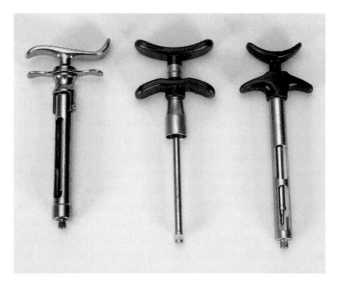

Figure 10.11 Dental syringe systems.

from 25 mm (short) to 35 mm (long). All dental needles are disposable single use; they should never be bent to improve access as this poses the risk of needle fracture.

Dental analgesic cartridges have three components:

- Cylinder.
- Plunger.
- Cap.

The cylinder (Figure 10.10) has information stamped on it indicating the contents, concentrations and expiry date, along with the manufacturer's name and batch number. Glass cylinders can be used for all dental applications. Plastic cylinders are produced but are not suitable for use in intraligamentary equipment. Before using a local analgesic cartridge the operator must confirm the drug and concentration present and check that the expiry date has not passed. The contents should be checked, to ensure there is no clouding of contents, large air bubbles, cracks or disturbance of the plunger.

The plunger is composed of rubber, although constituents do vary and some products contain latex. Both solid and hollow plungers are used in dental cartridges.

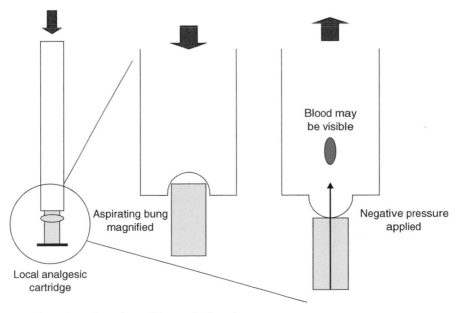

Figure 10.12 Safe dental syringe systems.

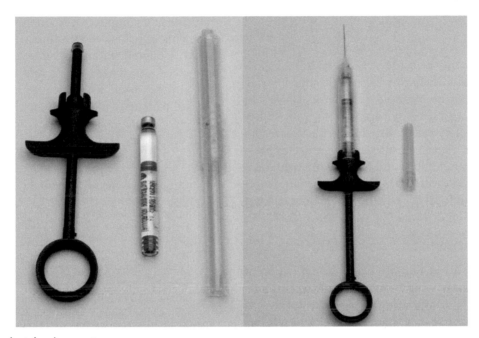

Figure 10.13 Diagram to show the action of a positive aspiration plunger.

Hollow plungers are designed to work with self-aspirating syringe systems.

Conventional syringes (Figure 10.11) for dental analgesia are made of metal or alternatively from disposable plastic. Reusable metal components should withstand sterilisation without sustaining damage. Although individual manufacturers' products do vary, the general design is composed of:

- A barrel.
- A viewing point.
- A threaded needle-mounting hub.
- A plunger rod.
- A handle or thumb ring or rest.
- Finger grips.

Products are now available which are fully disposable and designed to help prevent needle stick injuries. Figure 10.12 shows an example of a sterile, single use, disposable, self aspirating syringe system with a pre-mounted needle. The system provides both passive and active aspiration. The integral needle guard effectively prevents needle-stick injury and has a permanent locking position for safe disposal. There is no need to re-sheath this type of local anaesthetic system and hence it conforms to GDC guidance.

Aspiration

In order to avoid accidental intravascular deposition of analgesic solution, it is necessary to routinely aspirate before injecting. Non-aspirating syringes are not recommended for dental use as it is not possible to determine if the tip of the needle is in a vein. If an artery has been entered then simply removing the pressure will allow some blood to flow into the cartridge. However, this is a rare event and the risk is greater of accidental intravenous penetration.

Positive aspiration systems require the operator actively to apply negative pressure. A plunger hook or barbed plunger tip allows the plunger rod tip to engage the plunger rod. Pulling back the rod withdraws the plunger, thereby reducing the pressure in the cartridge. The technique is prone to error. In applying negative pressure the tip of the needle tends to move such that the site of aspiration may not correspond to the site of injection.

Passive aspiration is a superior system as it requires only minimal movement of the operator's thumb. An aspirating nipple is designed within the plunger (Figure 10.13) such that, provided pressure is simply released, a negative pressure is produced within the cartridge; if the needle tip is within a blood vessel this will be evident because of the presence of blood visible within the cartridge.

Conclusions

- The dental hygienist and dental therapist should always carefully check the medical history of patients for whom they provide dental care.
- The patient's medication may be of relevance to dental disease and complicate provision of dental treatment.
- Patients at risk of endocarditis will need a good preventive dental treatment plan to reduce the risk.
- Dental local analgesia is a safe technique but care should be taken when treating medically compromised patients, children and the elderly.

Further reading

British National Formulary, http://www.bnf.org/bnf/

Faculty of General Dental Practitioners (UK) (2000) *Adult Antimicrobial Prescribing in Primary Dental Care for General Dental Practitioners.* Royal College of Surgeons of England, London.

Haveles, E.B. (2007) *Applied Pharmacology for the Dental Hygienist.* Mosby Elsevier, St Louis.

Herrera, D., Alonso, B., Leon, R., Roldan, S. and Sanz, M. (2008) Antimicrobial therapy in periodontitis: the use of systemic antimicrobials against the subgingival biofilm. *Journal of Clinical Periodontology,* **35**(suppl. 8), 45–66.

Howe, G.L. and Whitehead, F.I. (1990) *Local Anaesthesia in Dentistry* (Dental Practitioner Handbook), 3rd edn. Wright Publishing Company, New York.

Meechan, J.G. (2002) *Practical Dental Local Analgesia.* QuintEssentials of Dental Practice 6. Oral Surgery & Oral Medicine 1. Quintessence Publishing, New Malden.

National Institute for Clinical Excellence (March 2008) NICE clinical guideline 64 *Prophylaxis against infective endocarditis.* www.nice.org.uk/CG064Neal, M.J. (1997) *Medical Pharmacology at a Glance,* 3rd edn. Blackwell Science Ltd, Oxford.

Newman, M. and Korman, K. (1990) *Antibiotic/Antimicrobial Use in Dental Practice.* Quintessence Publishing, New Malden.

Robinson, P.D., Pitt Ford, T.R. and McDonald, F. (2000) *Local Anaesthesia in Dentistry,* 7th edn. Wright Publishing Company.

Standing Medical Advisory Committee (SMAC) Department of Health (1998) *The Path of Least Resistance.* Department of Health, London.

11

Preventive dentistry

Sarah Murray and Baldeesh Chana

Summary

This chapter covers:

- Prevention
- Fluoride
- Life-long prevention
- Prevention for people with special needs
- Prevention and implantology
- Oral cancer, alcohol abuse, illegal drug abuse
- Smoking cessation
- The primary healthcare team

Introduction

Prevention of disease must be the foundation of all healthcare provision. To avoid invasive treatment, whether it is cardiac surgery or the provision of dental restorations, must be the goal of all healthcare practitioners. Oral health is essential to overall health and well-being and profoundly influences the quality of life, including speaking, eating, and self esteem and has the possibility to disrupt our ability to learn and work.

Oral diseases, particularly dental caries and periodontal disease, are common in the United Kingdom, affecting both children and adults. Most oral health problems are preventable. Oral health is not solely dependent on individual behaviours. Much can be done to reduce oral diseases by using a variety of approaches that include community-based initiatives, self-care, and professional care. There is also much that governments and other authorities can do to ensure that oral health continues to improve. Findings from the Adult Dental Health Survey (2011) show that edentulousness has decreased significantly over the past 30 years and the role of different members of the dental team in the prevention of oral diseases has no doubt played a huge part in the improvements to the health of the population. Surveys such as this one, undertaken every 10 years, are important as this enables the government to develop policies to provide targets and strategies for the promotion of oral health. The Department of Health produced *Delivering Better Oral Health: An evidence-based toolkit for prevention* in 2009 and this document was developed by a number of well-known experts who have provided contemporary evidence-based oral health prevention and promotion guidelines. The document identifies key areas and comments on how the main problem areas could be addressed by providing clear and simple messages for setting targets for improving the oral health of the individual.

Definitions of prevention

Prevention can be defined as preventing either the onset or the progress of a disease or to restore function lost due to disease. Prevention can be divided up according to the stages of disease prevention, and can be categorised into primary, secondary and tertiary prevention (Table 11.1). However, not all disease prevention strategies fall into a single category of primary, secondary or tertiary prevention; e.g. dietary advice could fall into either primary prevention to prevent dental caries from occurring in the first place, or secondary prevention to prevent dental caries that has already occurred in one or more teeth from progressing further.

Clinical Textbook of Dental Hygiene and Therapy, Second Edition. Edited by Suzanne L. Noble.
© 2012 John Wiley & Sons, Ltd. Published 2012 by John Wiley & Sons, Ltd.

Table 11.1 Primary, secondary and tertiary prevention applied to oral and general health interventions.

	Primary prevention	Secondary prevention	Tertiary prevention
Dental team interventions			
Individual Approach	Dietary advice Plaque control advice Advice on risks of smoking Alcohol cessation advice Dental examinations Screening for oral cancer Diagnostic radiography Fissure sealants Topical fluoride self medication & home care Periodontal probing Removal of local secondary factors, e.g. restoration overhangs Prophylaxis	Investigations, e.g. pulp testing, vitality testing Sealant restorations Minimal restorations Diagnostic radiographs to monitor disease progression Pulp capping Pocket chart probing Sub and supragingival scaling Smoking cessation advice	Complex dental restorations Removable and fixed prostheses Dental extractions Primary tooth pulpotomies Periodontal surgery Administration of antimicrobial agents
Community based approach	Water fluoridation Smoking cessation programmes School dental health screening Fissure sealant programmes Prevention of oral-facial injuries by mouth guard usage 'Brushing for Life' programmes	Smoking cessation – advice, e.g. T.V and radio Bottle-to-cup programmes	
General health interventions			
Individual Approach	Immunisation Dietary education	Screening for cancer	Providing continuing care and support for terminal illness
Community based approach	Immunisation programmes Campaigns for prevention of accidents 5-a-day healthy eating programmes	Alcoholics Anonymous Weight loss support programmes	

Primary prevention

Primary prevention protects individuals against disease, such as immunisation, and prevention of the initiation of the disease, as in dietary advice and plaque control within dentistry. Primary prevention is aimed at keeping an individual and a population healthy and to minimise the risk of disease or injury.

It is this stage that seeks to implement programmes, procedures, or measures to prevent a disease, before it actually occurs. Programmes designed to prevent people from starting to use tobacco (primary prevention) or to help them quit if they have already started (secondary prevention) can help prevent oral cancer and periodontal diseases, and also be an effective general health promotion strategy. Additionally, plaque control and diet are effective primary prevention methods for both the prevention of dental caries and periodontal disease. Other primary prevention methods include the provision of fissure sealants, water fluoridation and routine dental examinations and diagnostic radiographs.

Secondary prevention

Secondary prevention aims to limit the progression and effect of a disease at the earliest possible opportunity after onset. It refers to the cessation of the disease process and preventing its progressive activity to more advanced stages, as well as preventing the recurrence of the disease, with further primary prevention interventions and advice. Therefore, to stop disease progression and recurrence, once a condition has been recognised, actions are needed to control and eliminate the further spread of that condition.

Removing carious tooth tissue and restoring structure and function at an early stage of the caries process can prevent tooth loss or the need for more extensive treatment. This intervention may be in the form of preventive resin restorations or the placement of more extensive restorations. Secondary prevention measures to diagnose and treat periodontal diseases include periodontal probing and diagnostic radiographs, professional removal of hard and soft deposits, and the local application of antimicrobial agents. Oral examinations of the soft tissues, in addition to obtaining a comprehensive social history to assess past and present tobacco and alcohol use, are also effective measures for detecting oral cancer at its early, most treatable stages.

Tertiary prevention

Tertiary prevention is concerned with limiting the extent of disability once a disease has caused some functional limitation. At this stage, the disease process will have extended to the point where the patient's health status has changed and will not return to the prediseased state. Tertiary disease prevention refers to the rehabilitation of an individual, and with respect to oral disease, the re-establishment and maintenance of the integrity of the oral cavity.

In the dental caries process, tertiary prevention is aimed not only at restoring carious teeth but also must include further primary and secondary prevention in order to prevent further carious attack. This means that in addition to the placement of a restoration, the causes of caries must also be addressed as part of a clinically effective caries management programme. When considering periodontal disease, periodontitis can be treated by a variety of interventions, surgical procedures or by administering antimicrobial agents either locally or systemically but again the aetiology must be identified.

Prevention of periodontal disease

Mechanical plaque control

Effective plaque control is necessary to maintain oral health, as dental plaque is the main aetiological factor in both periodontal disease and dental caries. There are so many oral care products available on the market, that it is easy for consumers to feel overwhelmed by the choice on offer and not select the most appropriate product for their own needs. It is important for dental professionals to consider the manual dexterity, motivation and financial abilities of the individual, and to also consider the available research supporting an evidence base prior to recommending any dental product.

Regular toothbrushing with fluoride toothpaste is arguably the most widely employed method of home dental care. However, in the multicultural society in which we live, not all people use a toothbrush and toothpaste and caution should be exercised as some people may use more natural products such as a 'chewstick' or Miswak (tree twigs from the *Salvadora persica* plant). These products may be effective, although the evidence base is limited, but do not offer the additional benefit of the application of topical fluoride to the tooth surface so may be less effective at preventing caries.

Toothbrushing

The first mass-produced toothbrush was made by William Addis in England in around 1780. The toothbrush as we know it today was not invented until 1938; before then toothbrushes were made with bamboo handles and boar bristles. Nylon bristles made from nylon yarn were first introduced in 1938.

The aims of toothbrushing are to obtain a high standard of oral hygiene by the mechanical removal of plaque from accessible sites and to allow the application of fluoride and other agents to the tooth surface. The western diet, being relatively soft, does little to stimulate the maintenance of healthy keratinised gingivae. The frictional effect of toothbrushing on the attached gingivae, when managed correctly, provides an effective substitute for a more fibrous diet. In periodontal disease, removal of plaque assists in the reduction of the inflammatory process of the periodontal tissues. Twice daily brushing, particularly last thing at night when saliva is decreasing, therefore reducing the washing and buffer effect, is recommended as it plays a key role in the prevention and control of dental caries, periodontal disease and dental erosion.

Over the years, dental professionals have seen many designs of toothbrush on the market. Variations in design include the length, shape, diameter and angulation of the filaments, and heads that contain tongue brushing adjuncts. Oral care companies continue to produce innovative designs in an effort to increase sales and try and achieve the most effective toothbrush both for both plaque control and periodontal health. In reviewing these requirements, the following aspects should be considered:

The 'ideal' toothbrush should have

- A head size that is small enough to meet the needs of the individual for whom it is recommended; a toothbrush that is too large to be manoeuvred around the mouth may cause gagging and will not remove plaque more effectively; similarly, a toothbrush that has too small a head will also be ineffective as the individual may tire of brushing because of the excessive time requirement. It is the responsibility of the dental professional to recommend the brush to best fit the needs of the individual taking into account the mouth size, ability to gain access, muscular configuration, and dexterity.
- Toothbrush bristles should be soft or medium in texture and have round ended filaments with a compact arrangement of filaments as this causes less damage to the gingival tissues and reduces toothbrush abrasion at the cervical margins of the teeth. Bristles should also be of nylon texture and made from synthetic rather than natural materials, as natural bristles may be porous and therefore more likely to harbour bacteria and their texture is less predictable.

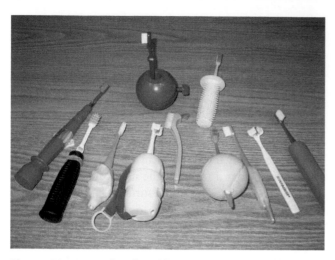

Figure 11.1 Examples of modified toothbrushes.

- The handle should have the correct length and thickness appropriate to the age and dexterity of the individual. It must be easy to use and provide for a firm and comfortable grip. Toothbrush handles can easily be modified if difficulty is experienced with a regular brush handle (Figure 11.1).

It is important to modify the patient's existing toothbrushing technique and encourage a systematic approach, so that all surfaces are cleaned; ensuring that the gingival margin area is cleaned by using the modified bass or mini scrubb technique is recommended if the existing technique is inadequate. Parents should be encouraged and shown how to brush children's erupting teeth, as the occlusal surfaces of erupting first and second molars are below the level of the arch during eruption and are prone to dental caries.

Patients need to be reminded to change their toothbrushes regularly at approximately 3 month intervals or when the bristles have become 'splayed' as the toothbrush will then cease to be effective in the removal of plaque.

An adjunct to toothbrushing is interdental cleaning as these are areas that are most covered with dental plaque, as regular toothbrushing appears to be less successful at removing plaque from these sites. There is a body of evidence to suggest that interdental brushes are more effective at plaque removal than dental floss, but the choice of interdental aid should be based on the size of the interdental space and the ability, motivation and compliance of the individual.

Powered toothbrushes

There are a variety of powered toothbrushes available on the market, with these being battery operated or electric rechargeable. They often have a small round head and the head movement is usually oscillating, rotating or counter-rotational. There have been a number of recent studies on the benefits of powered toothbrushes over manual ones and the evidence is equivocal but it has been found that generally manual toothbrushes are as good as electric toothbrushes, if used correctly. However, a systematic review by the Cochrane Collaboration concluded that powered toothbrushes with a rotation oscillation action reduce plaque and gingivitis more effectively than manual toothbrushing (Robinson *et al.*, 2005).

Instances where powered toothbrushes may be more appropriate than manual brushes include children who struggle to brush their teeth, either because of lack of dexterity or lack of motivation, which may be improved particularly if the brush has a timer. Other people who may benefit from powered brushes are the elderly and people with arthritis or other disabilities, who may find it difficult to manage effectively with a manual toothbrush. Additionally, people who have become institutionalised may rely on carers to brush their teeth and the carers may find a powered brush easier to manipulate. However, it must be noted that some powered brushes may be heavy for individuals to use, particularly for those people with hand related problems. Of course brushing of the teeth and supporting structures will only be really effective where the patient is well motivated and has received professional instruction on the appropriate use of the brush, whether manual or powered.

Dentifrices

The functions of a dentifrice are to:

- Assist in removing plaque and stain and polishing the teeth.
- Prevent and reduce dental caries by applying topical fluoride to teeth.
- Prevent gingivitis by the inclusion of antimicrobials.
- Achieve other effects such as desensitisation and whitening.
- Give the patient a feeling of well-being with a pleasant tasting mouth and fresh breath.

The principal constituents of toothpastes are outlined in Table 11.2.

Sodium monofluorophosphate and sodium fluoride are probably the most common fluoride formulations used by toothpaste manufacturers in concentrations from 525–1450 ppm F. Toothpastes containing fluoride were introduced during the 1970s, and the addition of fluoride to toothpaste has contributed greatly to the reduction in caries in UK with reductions of 20–40% over a 2–3 year period of use (Fejerskov and Kidd, 2003). Fluoride toothpastes currently represent more than 90% of the sales of toothpaste products in

Table 11.2 The constituents of toothpaste.

Agent	Examples	%	Effect
	Constituents of toothpaste		
Polishing/abrasive	Sodium bicarbonate Calcium carbonate Calcium sulphate Sodium chloride Silica particles Diatomaceous earth Dicalcium phosphate	30–40%	Clean and polish the tooth surface without damaging enamel, keeps pellicle thin, prevents accumulation of stain
Humectant	Glycerine Sorbitol Water	10–30%	Prevents evaporation of water keeping toothpaste moist
Binding agent	Carboxymethyl cellulose Hydroxyethyl cellulose Carrageenan Cellulose gum	1–5%	Holds all the ingredients together and assists in creating the texture of the toothpaste
Detergent/foaming	Sodium lauryl sulphate Sodium N-lauryl sarcosinate	1–2%	Lowers the surface tension & loosens debris which assists removal with a toothbrush
Preservative	Formalin Alcohols Sodium benzoate	≥ 1%	Prevent contamination by bacteria & to maintain purity of the product
Colour/flavouring	Peppermint/spearmint Menthol Eucalyptus Aniseed Saccharin	1–5%	Mask flavour of other ingredients, especially SLS, and promotes user compliance
Water			Solvent for some ingredients & provides consistency
	Therapeutic agents		
Fluoride	Sodium Monoflurophosphate, Sodium fluoride		Anticaries, remineralisation of early carious lesions
Desensitising agents	Strontium chloride Strontium acetate Potassium nitrate Potassium citrate		Reduce or eradicate dentine sensitivity by having a direct desensitising effect on the pulp nerve fibres.
Antiplaque agents Anticalculus	Triclosan Pyrophosphates Ureates Zinc citrate		Antibacterial reducing plaque formation Inhibits plaque mineralisation, Alteration of pH to reduce calculus formation
Bicarbonates			Suggested to reduce acidity of dental plaque

many EU Member States, such as Germany, France, Italy, Denmark and the UK.

When recommending fluoride toothpaste, dental professionals should consider an individual's caries risk; this should take into account previous caries experience, dietary habits, socio-economic status and whether fluoride is in the local water supply. Spitting out excess toothpaste, rather than rinsing immediately after brushing, will enable individuals to get an elevated effect of fluoride intra-orally and the full benefits of both the topical and systemic application.

- A family fluoride toothpaste (1350–1500 ppm fluoride) is indicated for maximum caries control for all members of the family over the age of 3, except for those children who cannot be prevented from eating toothpaste.
- Children under the age of 3 should use a toothpaste containing no less than 1000 ppm fluoride using a smear of toothpaste on their toothbrush.
- Parental involvement and supervision is needed to ensure that a small amount of toothpaste is used for children up to the age of 7 years and that the child spits out excess toothpaste.

- Toothpaste containing 2800 ppm or 5000 ppm fluoride is appropriate for adults who have a high risk of dental caries, especially the elderly who are more prone to root caries, those with xerostomia or patients undergoing head and neck radiation therapy.

Prevention of caries

Dental caries is an oral disease often found in young children due to the vulnerability of the tooth surface to acid attack by refined carbohydrates. It has been discussed already (Chapter 4, p. 72) that four factors are necessary for dental caries to occur: these are bacteria, a substrate, time and a tooth. Saliva also plays a role, as teeth are continually bathed in saliva and a reduction in this causes an increase in food retention and a decrease in buffer capacity; this has the potential to cause rapid carious attack.

Prevention of dental caries is by effective toothbrushing, reduction in refined carbohydrates through a healthy diet, use of fluoride and fissure sealants. These aspects are discussed in more detail in Chapters 4 and 7 and the section on Fluoride.

Identifying the 'at-risk' individual

Assessing caries risk is important for all patients and the process has to be repeated at regular intervals throughout life to be most effective, as an individual's circumstances and personal habits can change. People can move from a low-risk to a high-risk group; diet, medication, and radiotherapy can play a part. Assessing risk is important to dental clinicians as this will assist them in determining whether intervention is appropriate and what the recall periods for re-assessment should be for each individual.

Assessing the recall interval

The frequency of review for both the maintenance of oral health and the prevention of disease is currently a contentious issue since there is little scientific evidence on which to base a judgement. Some authorities argue that recall intervals should be relatively short to support a preventive approach to disease management whilst others argue that longer time intervals reduce costs with minimal impact on oral health (Pitts and Pendlebury, 2001). *The Scientific Basis of Oral Health Education* (Levine and Stillman Lowe, 2004) states that the period between oral examinations must be flexible and based on a professional assessment of the risk from oral disease.

The **National Institute for Health and Clinical Excellence** (NICE, 2004) recommends that the shortest interval between oral health reviews for all patients should be 3 months. The longest interval between oral health reviews for patients younger than 18 years should be 12 months and the longest interval for patients aged 18 years and older should be 24 months. The recall interval should be reviewed again at the next oral health review, to learn from the patient's responses to the oral care provided and the health outcomes achieved.

In children, the assessment of those individuals who are considered 'high risk' to dental caries ensures that fissure sealants are placed in those who would benefit most from them.

When assessing caries risk a number of factors need to be considered; risk factors will increase our patients' susceptibility to dental caries and by identifying these allows us to educate our patients on the best ways to manage them.

Aspects that need to be considered include:

- Medical history: cardiovascular disease; bleeding disorders; immunosupression; diabetes; cariogenic medication,
- Social history: socioeconomic status; high caries rate in parents and siblings; motivation towards dental treatment; attendance patterns.
- Dietary assessment: frequent intakes of fermentable carbohydrates.
- Fluoride use: use of fluoride toothpaste; exposure to fluoridated water.
- Dental caries status: presence of new lesions; past caries experience; exposure of root surfaces.
- Plaque control: poor oral hygiene; evidence of plaque retentive factors; presence of high levels of lactobacilli and *Streptococcus mutans.*
- Saliva flow: xerostomia.

Figure 11.2 indicates the caries imbalance; the balance between disease indicators, risk factors and protective factors determines whether dental caries progresses, halts or reverses.

Primary prevention of dental caries in high-risk children

The **Scottish Intercollegiate Guidelines Network** (SIGN, 2000) and the **National Guideline Clearinghouse** (NGC, 2009) have published evidence-based recommendations. Children identified as being at high caries risk should:

- Have individual oral health education at the chairside as this intervention has been shown to be beneficial.
- Have emphasised the need to restrict sugary food and drink to mealtimes only.
- Be encouraged to use non-sugar sweeteners, e.g. xylitol in food and drink.

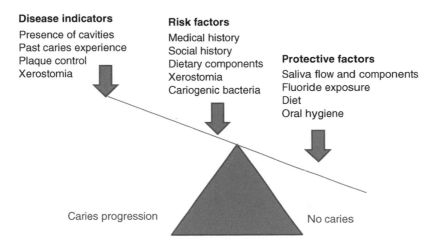

Disease indicators
Presence of cavities
Past caries experience
Plaque control
Xerostomia

Risk factors
Medical history
Social history
Dietary components
Xerostomia
Cariogenic bacteria

Protective factors
Saliva flow and components
Fluoride exposure
Diet
Oral hygiene

Caries progression

No caries

Figure 11.2 The caries imbalance (Adapted from Featherstone J.D.B (2004) The Continuum of Dental Caries-Evidence for a Dynamic Disease Process. J Dent Res 83 (Spec Iss C):C39–C42, 2004.)

- Be encouraged to use sugar-free chewing gum when this is acceptable.
- Have dietary analysis regularly reviewed and as previously described; fissure sealing should be considered.
- Be considered for a fluoride varnish, e.g. Duraphat applied professionally every 4 to 6 months.

Fluoride

History of fluoride in caries prevention

The first record of fluoride use dates back to the 1870s when **potassium fluoride** was advocated for use by pregnant women and children by Erharde who believed fluoride could play a part in the prevention of dental caries in a similar way to iron supplements for blood. At the time there was no scientific basis for this advice; it was only an opinion which appeared in a German publication for 'rational physicians'.

Sir James Crichton, who addressed the British Dental Association in 1892, emphasised the link between fluoride and dental caries. His address consisted of an inspired guess regarding the importance of fluoride in the diet. He claimed that the improved diet of white bread and food made from fine flour was to blame for the decrease in fluoride content that had previously been present in the population's diet.

However, it was only through Dr Frederick McKay's extensive research over 30 years in the early part of the last century that any evidence was produced to support these claims. As a recently qualified dental graduate in 1901, Dr McKay took up a position in Colorado Springs, USA. He soon noticed that many of the residents had a distinctive stain on their teeth, which was known to local residents as '**Colorado stain**'. McKay noticed that only the residents who had lived all their lives in Colorado

were affected by the stain. Even those inhabitants who had moved into the area when very young (2 or 3 years old) seemed to escape the minute white, yellow and brown flecks that gave their teeth a mottled appearance. On further investigation over a period of years, McKay established that occurrence of mottling was localised over a definite geographical area and was not influenced by home or environmental factors but all the areas affected all received their water supply from one source. In 1931 McKay, in collaboration with the US Public Health Service, and a chemist called Churchill, published his findings showing an increased level of fluoride in the water supply. However, Churchill emphasised the fact that no precise correlation between fluoride content and mottled enamel had been established, only that an unsuspected quantity of fluoride had been found in the endemic areas.

Chemistry of fluoride action on tooth enamel

Natural fluoride exists in two forms, inorganic and organic but it is only the inorganic form that yields the fluoride ion. Inorganic fluoride can be either ionic or non-ionic and it is only the former that is relevant to dentistry and measured in parts per million.

The mineral of tooth tissues exists as a carbonated apatite, which contains calcium, phosphate and hydroxyl ions in the form of hydroxyapatite $[Ca_{10}(PO_4)_6(OH)_2]$. Carbonated portions weaken the structure and render the tissue susceptible to attack. Food remnants and debris mix with saliva and adhere to tooth surfaces as dental plaque. Bacteria present in the oral cavity, particularly those considered cariogenic such as *Streptococcus mutans* and *Lactobacillus* species, metabolise dental plaque and produce acid that lowers the pH of the mouth. When the pH is below the critical level of 5.5 for hydroxyapatite, demineralisation occurs with an outward flow of calcium and phosphorus ions from the enamel surface into plaque and saliva. When the pH returns to 7.0, remineralisation occurs with an inward flow of ions into the enamel surface. If ionic fluoride is present during remineralisation it is incorporated in the enamel to form **calcium fluorapatite** $[Ca_{10}(PO_4)_6(F)_2]$ according to the following equation:

$$Ca_{10}(PO_4)_6(OH)_2 + 2F^- \rightarrow Ca_{10}(PO_4)_6(F)_2 + 2OH$$

Calcium fluorapatite is more stable and resistant to further attacks than calcium hydroxyapatite.

Fluoride toxicity

Excessive ingestion of fluoride can result in **fluorosis** (mottling), which presents as opaque or white areas, lines or flecks in the enamel surface and can be cosmetically disfiguring when they occur on anterior teeth. Fluorosis can occur at different times and varies in severity. Figure 11.3 shows very mild dental fluorosis (graded TF1) and Figure 11.4 shows more severe fluorosis (graded TF3) classified by the York review as being 'of aesthetic concern'. The most important time is when ingestion of excessive fluoride occurs during enamel formation of the aesthetically important permanent upper anterior teeth at between 15–30 months of age, although this period can be extended from birth to 6 years. More severe and cosmetically unacceptable cases of fluorosis are uncommon in the UK but these can result from the use of fluoride supplements in areas where the water is artificially fluoridated or where fluoride occurs naturally at the optimum level of 1 ppm. It has been estimated that about 20% of all enamel defects in the UK are attributable to fluorosis but mainly of the mildest form (TF1). Most of the staining in mottled enamel is confined to the outer 50–100 μm so if treatment is considered necessary this is usually by composite restorations or in severe cases (Figure 11.5) by crowning or veneers. More severe toxicity can result in systemic disease such as osteoporosis and skeletal deformity (Table 11.3).

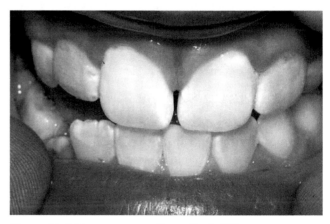

Figure 11.5 Very severe mottling – Grade TF4.

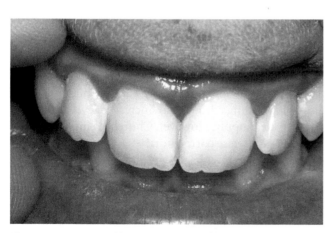

Figure 11.3 Very mild enamel mottling (fluorosis) – grade TF1.

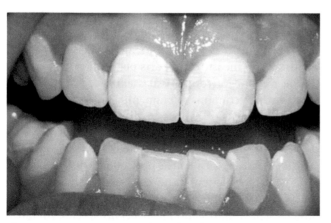

Figure 11.4 More severe mottling 'of aesthetic concern' – grade TF3.

Table 11.3 Potential toxicity of fluoride.

Exposure to fluoride (mg/1 drinking water)	Age	Effect
>2	Child	Dental fluorosis
>8	All ages	Skeletal fluorosis
>50 (12 hours)	All ages	Gastroenteritis
Pathological doses for exposures other than drinking water	Age	Effect
5–20 mg/m³ air (occupational)	Adults	Crippling fluorosis
2500–10000 mg oral	Adults	Lethal dose
>16 mg/kg oral body weight	Child	Lethal dose

Adapted from NHMRC, 1991.

The most extreme outcome of fluoride toxicity is death. The lethal dose is approximately 15 mg/kg body weight, although as little as 5 mg/kg may kill some children. The exact method that fluoride produces a toxic effect is not known. Symptoms of sublethal poisoning are salivation, nausea, and vomiting. A lethal dose of fluoride will result in death from cardiac or respiratory failure within 24 hours of the overdose. If the overdose is a result of ingestion, symptoms usually appear within 1 hour and therefore if this follows topical application, symptoms may not be seen until after the patient has left the surgery. However, to put this risk into perspective, a 5-year old child weighing 20 kg would need to ingest 0.9 ml (1/5 teaspoon) of sodium fluoride varnish (2.26% F) to have the effects of a sublethal acute poisoning dose, and 4 ml (4/5 teaspoon) for a potentially lethal dose (Kidd, 2005).

Drinking a large volume of milk will neutralise a small dose of fluoride but if the dose exceeds 5 mg/kg ingested or is unknown, medical attention must be sought immediately because of the rapid absorption of fluoride by the body.

It is suggested by some that the impurities in the water fluoridation process can lead to toxicity. Some of the possible impurities include heavy metals such as lead, aluminium and iron. However, the Water Fluoridation Act 1985 gives maximum limits for impurities. Despite this, toxicity from aluminium appears to pose the greatest of concerns to a significant proportion of the population. Aluminium and fluoride are mutually antagonistic in competing for absorption in the gut, therefore the more fluoride in the diet, the less aluminium is absorbed. Aluminium has been implicated as having an aetiological role in Alzheimer's disease. It follows that if absorption of aluminium is reduced by ingestion of fluoride, this condition may be less common in communities with fluoridated water (Foster, 1993).

Methods of delivery of fluoride

The water supply

Fluoride can occur naturally in the water supply, for example, the water supply of Hartlepool has a natural fluoride content of 1.2 ppm. All water contains fluoride at some concentration because of the natural minerals present (e.g. fluorspar – calcium fluoride – CaF_2). When this dissolves in water it releases fluoride ions:

$$CaF_2 = Ca^{2+} + 2F^-$$

Throughout the 1930s researchers discovered that people living in areas where drinking water contained naturally high levels of fluoride suffered less dental caries than in other areas. More extensive research demonstrated that, in a temperate climate, a water fluoride level of 1 part per million (1 ppm) was optimal for a significant reduction in dental caries. This led researchers to believe that the benefits of this naturally occurring fluoride could be replicated in areas where the level of natural fluoride was low, by artificially increasing the level to 1 ppm (Lennon, 2004). The concentration of fluoride in water is measured by a **fluoride ion specific electrode**, which measures free fluoride ions not fluoride bound to metals such as calcium, magnesium, etc.

In 1944, Dr **Trendley Dean** and his colleagues carried out a trial to test this hypothesis in a community in **Grand Rapids**, USA, followed by a number of other studies. Dean published his results in 1942 and established that mottling of the teeth was extremely rare at fluoride levels of 1 ppm or below, while the greater part of the caries preventive effect was to be seen at 1 ppm. These results were mirrored at about the same time by a number of other studies in Canada, East Germany, the Netherlands, New Zealand and the UK.

In 1953 the UK Medical Research Council recommended that the Government should send an expert committee to visit the North American trial sites used by Dr Trendley Dean and his colleagues. As a result of the committee's report, in the mid-1950s the Government established fluoridation schemes in Anglesey, Watford, Kilmarnock and Andover, with detailed reports being published after 5 and 11 years. These reports confirmed the findings of the earlier studies and shortly after their publication the local authorities in Birmingham and Solihull started schemes in 1964 followed by Newcastle a few years later. By the early 1980s approximately 10% of the UK's population were benefiting from water fluoridation; currently approximately 6 million people in the UK and around 400 million worldwide receive water with the fluoride level adjusted to the optimum level.

In the UK the fluoride compound most commonly added to the water supply is liquid hexafluorosilicic acid (H_2SiF_6). When this is added to water it releases fluoride ions according to the formula:

$$H_2SiF_6 + 4H_2O \Leftrightarrow 6F^- + Si(OH)_4 + 6H^-$$

Despite the success of fluoridation in the early implementation sites of Birmingham and Newcastle, further efforts to expand water fluoridation to other areas in the UK have been impaired by legislation and a small but vocal antifluoridation movement. The result is that dental caries remains an intransigent public health problem in socially deprived, non-fluoridated areas across the UK. It is estimated that by extending water fluoridation from the current 10% to 25–30% of the UK's population, targeted at communities with high levels of disease, there would be a substantial reduction in dental caries experience and a reduction in the large inequalities that exists in dental health.

In 1994 a World Health Organization (WHO, 1994) Expert Committee drew the following conclusions regarding water fluoridation:

- Community water fluoridation is safe and cost-effective and should be introduced and maintained wherever socially acceptable and feasible.
- The optimum fluoride concentration will normally be within the range 0.5–1.0 mg/l.
- The technical operation of water-fluoridation systems should be monitored and recorded regularly.
- Surveys of dental caries and dental fluorosis should be conducted periodically.

A systematic review was commissioned by the Chief Medical Officer of the Department of Health to 'carry out an up to date expert scientific review of fluoride and health' in 2000, known as the **York Review**. This was the largest assessment of evidence on the positive and negative effects of population wide drinking water fluoridation strategies. After reviewing 214 separate studies the review found no conclusive negative effects on health from water fluoridation.

In 2004 the British Dental Association collaborated with a number of other organisations including the **British Fluoridation Society** to produce a definitive document on water fluoridation called 'One in a Million, The facts about water fluoridation' (Lennon, 2004). This document aims to inform Strategic Health Authorities and Primary Care Trusts as they consider whether or not to take fluoridation forward in their localities as a result of new legislation (The **Water Industry Act**) in 2003.

Toothpaste

Fluoride toothpaste has been in general use since the early 1970s and is recognised as being the single most important development in the reduction of dental caries in the last 30 years.

A review of clinical trials going back more than 50 years firmly establishes that, in children, brushing with toothpaste containing fluoride results in 24% less cavity formation than does brushing with non-fluoridated toothpaste (Marinho *et al.*, 2003). High fluoride concentration toothpastes containing 2880 ppm or 5000 ppm fluoride are available on prescription for high caries risk patients (Table 11.4).

The formulations of toothpaste are described earlier in this chapter.

Acidulated phosphate fluoride gel (APF)

This may be used on high caries-risk patients, including patients undergoing orthodontic therapy. APF comes in the form of a gel that can be applied to the dentition

Table 11.4 Recommended level of fluoride in toothpastes.

Age	Fluoride Amount
Up to 3 years	1000 ppm – smear
3–6 years	1350–1500 ppm – pea size
7+ years	1350–1500 ppm
10+ years	1350–1500 ppm
	2800 ppm – prescription – high risk
16+ years	1350–1500 ppm
	5000 ppm – prescription – high risk

Table 11.5 Different types of fluoride varnishes.

Types of varnish	Concentration ppm	Manufacturer
Bifluorid	56 3000 ppm 5.6 % F	Voco Gmbh
Duraphat	22 600 ppm 2.2 %F	Colgate
Fluor Protector	8000 ppm 0.8 %F	Ivoclar Vivadent
Laweflour	22 600 ppm 2.2 %F	LAW

as a high-strength gel (1.23% = 12 300 ppm) by a dentist, dental therapist or hygienist; it is applied in trays for 4 minutes every 6 months. Gels may be flavoured to make them more palatable, although this form of fluoride application is not commonly used. Application is required with caution as the risk of toxicity is high.

Fluoride varnishes

Varnishes contain a high concentration of fluoride, they adhere to the tooth surface (Table 11.5).

There is a risk of toxicity, as with any high-concentration formula, and the varnish should be applied sparingly with a cotton bud. A small pea-size amount is usually sufficient for a full mouth application. The Cochrane Collaboration (Marinho *et al.*, 2003) and *Delivering Better Oral Health – an evidence-based toolkit* (DoH, 2009) both suggest a substantial caries-inhibiting effect of fluoride varnish in both the permanent and primary dentitions. It is therefore recommended for all children three years and above and all adults where applications may be repeated at either 3- or 6-month intervals depending on the risk status. Varnishes should not be applied where there is a possibility of contact with bleeding tissues because of the risk of contact allergy.

Fluoride mouth rinses

Daily and weekly mouth rinses are available, containing 0.05% fluoride (225 ppm) or 0.2% (900 ppm) respectively of sodium fluoride. It is advisable for patients to use a mouth

Table 11.6 Advised prescribing regime for fluoride tablets.

Age of child	Water content level		
	≤0.3 ppm	0.3–0.7 ppm	≥0.7 ppm
6m – 3 years	250 µg daily	Not advised	
3–6 years	500 µg daily	250 µg daily	Not advised
6 years and over	1 mg daily	500 µg daily	

From *Delivering Better Oral Health* (DoH, 2009).

rinse on a separate occasion to their usual toothbrushing regime to increase the number of fluoride exposures. All orthodontic patients should be advised to use a fluoride rinse to minimise the risk of demineralisation and white spot lesions at appliance margins. Mouth rinses are widely considered a safe method of fluoride application however caution should be taken with young children under the age of 6 where there is an increased risk of ingestion.

Fluoride drops and tablets

These have been reported to reduce caries from between 20 to 80%. However, the success of supplements depends largely on the compliance of the patient and this is usually poor in the high-risk groups who would benefit most. Supplementing the diet of children with fluoride is no longer considered to be an effective public health measure for this reason except in cases where the consequence of caries would pose a hazard to general health or where treatment would be difficult.

The doses of supplements vary throughout the world and are increasingly being held responsible for a rise in fluorosis. The dose is dependent on the age of the patient and level of fluoride in the local drinking water. Supplements should not be prescribed if the drinking water level is greater than 0.7 ppm (Table 11.6).

Alternative methods of fluoride intake

Fluoridated salt

The main advantages of salt as a vehicle for fluoride are that it does not require a community water supply and it permits individuals to accept or reject it. So far five countries have used salt as a vehicle for fluoride, including Switzerland who introduced it in 1955 and where it now constitutes 78% of sales. Non-fluoridated salt, like non-iodised salt, can be made available to the population.

The disadvantages of using salt as a vehicle are:

- Salt consumption is lowest when fluorides are most needed, i.e. in early years.
- There are large individual variations in salt intake.

- It could lead to excessive intake in water fluoridated areas.
- Its use in processed food products needs to be controlled.
- Advertising the preventive benefits of it may encourage high salt consumption resulting in associated systemic problems.

Fluoridated milk

It has been introduced widely in Russia and Chile and a number of studies with encouraging results have been undertaken in the UK (e.g. Scotland and Knowsley) where it has been introduced in schools. It has the advantage that it can make fluoride available in areas of social deprivation but when delivered to children it requires parental consent. The World Health Organization's Oral Health Unit is currently coordinating a 'demonstration programme' for fluoridated milk, which is being provided to 35 000 children attending nursery and primary schools in Bulgaria, Russia and the UK.

Fluoridated sugar

Although this would appear to be desirable in view of the relationship between sugar and caries, currently no studies have been published exploring this possibility. As a means of providing a regular daily supplement, sugar would not be ideal, as the daily consumption varies considerably and a high intake of sugar would be detrimental to general health.

Fluoridated chewing-gum

This is available in some countries. It may be recommended to patients at high caries risk particularly those with low saliva production because it tends to stimulate saliva secretion.

Tooth picks and floss containing fluoride

This is available in some countries. It may be recommended to patients at high caries risk, particularly those with low saliva production because it tends to stimulate saliva secretion.

General guidelines on the use of fluoride supplements based on the Department of Health (2009) *Delivering Better Oral Health – an evidence-based toolkit for prevention*, are included in Table 11.7.

Fissure sealants

The use of resin pit and fissure sealants is known to be an effective method of preventing caries in pits and fissures. Sealants protect the occlusal surfaces of molar

Table 11.7 General guidelines on the use of fluoride supplements.

Children aged up to 3 years	Smear 1000 ppm fluoride toothpaste
All children aged 3–6 years	Pea sized 1350–1500 ppm fluoride toothpaste
	Fluoride varnish every 6 months (2.2% F)
Children giving concern – those likely to develop caries, those with special needs	Pea sized 1350–1500 ppm fluoride toothpaste
	Fluoride varnish 3–4 times a year (2.2% F)
	Fluoride tablets/drops
All children aged from 7 years and young adults	Fluoride toothpaste 1350–1500 ppm
	Fluoride varnish every 6 months (2.2% F)
Those giving concern – those likely to develop caries, those with special needs	Fluoride toothpaste 1350–1500 ppm
	Fluoride varnish 3–4 times a year (2.2% F)
	8+ years with active caries – Daily fluoride mouthrinse – 0.05% – different time to brushing
	10+ years with active caries – 2800 ppm toothpaste
	10+ years with active caries – 5000 ppm toothpaste
Adults	Fluoride toothpaste 1350–1500 ppm
Those giving concern – those likely to develop caries, those with special needs	Fluoride toothpaste 1350–1500 ppm
	Daily fluoride mouthrinse – 0.05%
	Fluoride varnish every 6 months (2.2% F)
	Active caries – 2800 ppm fluoride toothpaste
	Active caries – 5000 ppm fluoride toothpaste

teeth, providing a smooth surface as the morphology of this surface makes it more susceptible to dental caries, favouring plaque stagnation and maturation.

The guidelines regarding the use of fissure sealants are described in Chapter 12, p. 252.

It has generally been considered that pit and fissure surfaces of molar teeth usually become carious within 3 years of eruption or not at all, unless the caries susceptibility of the individual changes. Fluoride has however influenced this judgement by effectively delaying the onset of early caries. Teeth that have shallow pits or fissures on the permanent molars or premolars, and individuals who have few risk factors for dental caries, would generally not benefit from sealants. Fissure sealants would also be contraindicated for teeth that have obvious caries on either the occlusal or interproximal surfaces which can be diagnosed clinically or by radiographs. Additionally, delaying the placement of sealants on partially erupted teeth may be recommended, due to poor access, poor moisture control and the close proximity to the gingival tissues.

Types of materials

The ideal sealant material should have good retention properties, low solubility within the mouth and be biocompatible with the oral tissues, and be easy to apply.

Resin composite: The longevity of resin based materials is based on the need for a tight seal between the tooth and the material, preventing leakage of nutrients to the microflora within the fissure. Acid-etch resin composite

sealants can be classified into two basic types, according to the method of polymerisation.

Self-cured resins: Self-cured materials are supplied in two parts, a catalyst and base, that are mixed together to chemically activate the polymerisation process. The working time is variable depending on the temperature of the environment and the proportions of the mix and can vary between 60–90 seconds.

Light cured resins polymerise when the initiator (camphorquinone) in the resin is activated by a light source that has a wavelength within the range of 400 to 500 nm. The working time is therefore under the control of the operator i.e. it is said to be **command set**.

Both types of resins may be either filled or unfilled and their resin chemistry is described in Chapter 9, p. 184; Resins can also be clear or opaque. Opaque resins are easier to identify if subsequent debonding has occurred. Filler particles, usually consisting of quartz or silica, are added to the resin to increase the resistance to abrasion and wear. Fluoride releasing resins have been developed to increase caries resistance and to remineralise early enamel lesions but their effectiveness requires further research.

Over the past few years, glass ionomer cements started to become more popular as a material for fissure sealing, particularly when it was difficult to achieve adequate moisture control, as this material is less sensitive to the presence of moisture. This material is easy to use on children, bonds well to enamel and releases fluoride providing a potentially cariostatic effect; however, currently their failure rate is higher than resin composites and more research is required to evaluate the long-term success of this material (Kuhnisch *et al.* 2011).

Failure of sealants

There are a number of reasons why fissure sealants may fail:

- Air bubbles may be present within the sealant, which may weaken the material. The sealant should be polished to expose the air bubble, and the bubble should then be filled or repaired with the same sealant material. If this is delayed, caries may develop.
- Porosities may develop in the sealant; this may happen if water contaminates the tooth during sealant placement.
- The sealant may debond. The sealant needs to be reapplied ensuring that the correct technique is followed to ensure longevity. Even if sealants debond, they may still provide some tooth protection, as some material may remain in the microporosities created in the tooth surface by etching. Sealants are commonly lost from lingual and buccal pits of mandibular molars; this may be due to the difficulty in achieving adequate etching and moisture control during placement.
- Caries left under the sealant. Sealants should not be placed if obvious caries is present; a more appropriate strategy would be a preventive resin or more extensive type of restoration (see Chapter 13).

Fissure sealants are an effective preventive measure but should be used in conjunction with other preventive regimes e.g. a low cariogenic diet and fluoride therapy.

Life-long prevention

Babies

Babies' mouths are sterile at birth (**gnotobiotic**) and bacteria are transferred to their mouths by contact from external sources such as kissing and finger poking. Dental caries can begin to develop as soon as the primary teeth erupt. Babies should not go to bed with a bottle, particularly if it contains juice or milk. Salivary flow diminishes at night and the saliva buffering capacity will be insufficient to counteract the effect of sugared liquids. Routine night time use of a bottle containing either of these can be habit forming and lead to early caries often called **nursing bottle caries** (see Chapter 12, p. 249).

Parents should start toothbrushing once the primary teeth have started to erupt. This may be with gauze with a spot of children's toothpaste and then later introducing a small-headed toothbrush, which is appropriate for the child's age. It is important to try and make toothbrushing a regular and fun activity, so that it becomes part of the baby's daily routine.

Parents should be encouraged to have infants drink from a cup as they approach their first birthday; weaning from the bottle should occur at about 12 to 14 months of age. Consumption of juice from a bottle should be avoided particularly at night when there is reduced salivary flow; a cup should be used when juice is offered.

It should be remembered that routines established during childhood form the basis of behaviours throughout life.

Toddlers

Children should be encouraged to start brushing their teeth with parental supervision from 2–3 years, using a toothbrush with an appropriately sized head. Due to the unintentional swallowing of fluoride toothpaste by children, which could cause fluoride mottling during tooth formation or toxicity, it should be recommended that a small amount of toothpaste is used and a smear of toothpaste across the length of the brush head is recommended. Children must be discouraged from licking or eating toothpaste from the tube and therefore must be supervised.

Schoolchildren

As children develop, toothbrush heads should become progressively larger and consideration should be made as to whether powered toothbrushes with a timer would provide increased motivation. As previously described, children should brush their teeth twice a day using toothpaste containing at least 1350–1500 ppm fluoride and spit away excess toothpaste. Children should be encouraged to attend their dental appointments with their toothbrush and toothpaste, as this will enable them to demonstrate their technique allowing for modifications to take place, but also to check the appropriateness of fluoride in their toothpaste and how much is used when placed on the brush.

Contact sports: The use of **mouth guards** to prevent orofacial injuries should be recommended if the individual plays contact sports. Mouth guards should be custom made to produce an accurate fit. Proprietary mouth guards, although cheaper, provide inadequate protection and because of their poor fit are infrequently worn.

Teenagers

Teenagers should be encouraged to use interdental aids to establish an effective plaque removal programme for life. They should be encouraged to modify their existing toothbrushing technique if it is assessed as being ineffective.

Orthodontic therapy: Many teenagers undertake orthodontic treatment and therefore require additional preventive advice. This includes:

- Appliances (both fixed and removable) tend to cause food and plaque stagnation therefore care must be given to brushing, flossing and using interdental or single tufted brushes effectively around brackets, wires and bands without causing damage.
- Removable appliances should be cleaned outside the mouth and over a basin half full of water to prevent damage if dropped.
- A removable appliance should not be worn when playing contact sports.
- If there is a risk from caries (although this is a contraindication to orthodontic therapy) then there may be benefit from daily or weekly fluoride mouthwashes and the application of fluoride varnish to early enamel lesions.
- A damaged or broken appliance should be reported to the orthodontist as soon as possible.

Habits such as smoking and binge drinking amongst teenagers may have been established and a strong preventive message emphasising the potential long-term general and oral health damage is advisable and should be reinforced throughout life.

Adults

Adults should continue with good plaque control that has been developed in their teenage years and any adverse changes in caries experience or periodontal health carefully monitored. Techniques may need to be adapted as gingival tissues recede and root caries and tooth loss become more prevalent. The size of interdental brushes may need to be reviewed to ensure they are at their most effective since teeth may drift and result in increased interdental spaces (see Chapter 5, p. 115). Single tufted brushes may be appropriate where interdental surfaces have become exposed due to tooth loss. Times of high stress such as bereavement or looking after an elderly relative can result in a detrimental change in oral hygiene habits or diet; medication resulting in xerostomia can quickly affect the oral cavity. Even if this is only temporary it can have long-term oral health implications.

Older adults

As more and more people live longer and retain most or all of their teeth throughout life, the role of prevention needs to be continued and adapted accordingly. The maintenance of good oral hygiene can be difficult with issues such as impaired manual dexterity, physical issues and mental health problems, and changes in eating habits to 'grazing' can mean an increase in the frequency of sugar intake. Older people can be challenging to motivate to change habits developed over a lifetime. It is important to emphasise the immediate outcomes (e.g. benefits) that can be expected if effective oral hygiene and dietary management is undertaken regularly. Because many older adults focus on immediate benefits as a source of motivation, it is important that the advice given is tied to specific and reasonable goals and personalizing any messages given.

Prevention for persons with special needs

For some individuals, preventive advice may need to be adjusted to suit individual special needs. These people may have a disability such as a learning difficulty or a physical impairment, which could significantly affect the delivery of oral care and the ability to undertake self maintenance. For people with disabilities, oral health problems have the potential to be greater than for the general population and this may further jeopardize the patient's general health. Conversely, people who have poor general health may have reduced resistance to oral infections.

In early years young children may not be referred to a dental practitioner until an oral health problem produces symptoms of pain or affects their overall general health. As these children have a number of other needs, which may be physical, developmental or emotional, understandably oral health may not be regarded as a high priority.

Over the past 50 years there have been numerous changes in our society with respect to the management and treatment of people with disabilities, in particular a trend towards acceptance of these individuals within our communities, with many of these individuals living at home rather than in long-term residential care. Therefore many depend on primary dental services for the provision of oral health care, rather than treatment within a hospital or institutional environment, and dental hygienists and dental therapists should be competent in providing effective and appropriate management.

These individuals present challenges to dental care professionals who may feel their training and lack of experience has not provided them with the necessary skills and knowledge to undertake appropriate oral health care. In addition, the treatment of patients with special needs frequently requires an increased time commitment which can generate conflicts in a busy practice environment. Behavioural aspects of patients may include limited understanding, uncontrolled movements, lack of dexterity, limited mouth opening, poor posture, limited mobility or poor treatment tolerance. These behaviours can interfere with the provision of effective prevention and oral care. It is therefore paramount to promote primary prevention to reduce invasive dental treatment, particularly if the individual is unable to communicate their problems. A team approach is invariably desirable and depending on the needs of the individual, involving carers and other health care professionals will be beneficial.

It is beyond the scope of this chapter to review individual preventive care regimes for the large number of medical conditions encountered in routine clinical practice and the reader is referred to a more comprehensive text (Nunn, 2004); however, the following are some important preventive care guidelines:

- Where there is loss of dexterity, toothbrushes can be adapted to the needs of the individual by enlarging the handles, providing additional grips or straps which will prevent the brush from being dropped (Figure 11.1). Extending the length of the toothbrush handle may assist those individuals who have reduced movements in their arms. Powered toothbrushes, which are not too heavy to hold, can often provide a more effective substitute.
- Many conditions result in xerostomia, e.g. Sjögren's syndrome, radiation therapy etc. increase the caries risk. Artificial saliva substitutes, e.g. Glandosane, Saliveze or salivary stimulants (**sialogogues**) can be useful.
- Adopting a team approach is often beneficial e.g. liaising with occupational therapists who could advise on specific aids and how they can be adapted.
- Where no self-maintenance is possible and the patient is dependent on carers, foam sponges can be useful to maintain the soft tissues and for the removal of dried mucous or crust from the palate, tongue or teeth. However, these should not be considered as effective for cleaning teeth so should be used as an adjunct to using a regular or soft-textured small-headed toothbrush.
- A low-foaming toothpaste may be advised if the individual is unable to tolerate the foaming action or unable to spit out; additionally dipping the toothbrush into a fluoride mouthwash, and then brushing the teeth in the usual way, will ensure that the teeth will benefit from the caries preventive effects of fluoride.

The maintenance of oral health has specific benefits for those individuals with special needs as it may provide a better quality of life, the ability to eat meals and maintain weight, and generate a feeling of well being without oral pain or discomfort.

Prevention and implantology

To a patient who has received dental implants it is important that regular monitoring, advice and maintenance is provided by the dental team. Whilst dental hygienists and therapists will not be responsible for the treatment planning or placement of implants, patients considering such a treatment option may wish to discuss potential problems of success and after care prior to surgery. It is therefore important that both dental hygienists and therapists have a comprehensive knowledge of implant dentistry to allow them to offer advice and guidance throughout the various stages of treatment, and maintain implants appropriately throughout the patient's life.

Implants are used to replace one or more missing teeth. There are basically two different types of implant:

Endosteal (in the bone): This is the most commonly used type of implant. The various types include screws, cylinders or blades surgically placed into the mandible or maxilla. Each implant supports one or more crowns. This type of implant is generally used as an alternative to the construction of bridges or removable dentures.

- **Subperiosteal** (below the periosteum, on the bone): These are placed on top of the jaw with the metal framework's posts protruding through the mucosa to hold the artificial teeth. These types of implants are used for patients who are usually edentulous and have insufficient bone available to support endosteal implants.

The success rate of implants has increased dramatically over the last 20 years such that in spite of their relatively high cost, they are now considered to be a very effective alternative to bridges or dentures. The success is, however, dependent on the skills of the operator, case selection, patient maintenance and professional care and monitoring. Implants in the mandible tend to be more successful than in the maxilla. Age should not be considered to be a contraindication unless the patient lacks the ability to provide good maintenance.

The contraindications to the placement of implants are:

- Patients showing evidence of poor plaque control: a high level should be achieved prior to embarking on the placement of implants particularly as patients are likely to have lost teeth due to periodontal disease in the past.
- Smokers: smokers are considered to be more than twice as likely to have an implant fail than a non-smoker (Bain and Moy, 1993).
- Patients with a history of periodontitis: the long-term success rates tend to be reduced.
- Lack of suitable supporting bone: although this can be improved by bone grafting or augmentation.

- Heavy alcohol consumption, which can increase the number of problems associated with initial healing and thereafter may negatively influence the long term health of the surrounding tissues.

Implants are normally made of titanium and when this is placed in direct contact with living bone tissue, the two literally grow together to form a permanent biological adhesion known as **osseointegration**. The implant is rigid within the bone so that, unlike natural teeth which have a periodontal membrane, there is no functional mobility.

The role of the dental hygienist and therapist

Prior to any consideration of dental implants, the dental hygienist or therapist may identify potential patients who have a high standard of oral health and should be free from any systemic illnesses or other factors that may delay healing. There must be adequate bone in which to place the implant. Additionally, the patient must understand the time, financial implications and long-term home care requirements of receiving dental implants.

Before implant placement

- Any active disease (periodontal disease and caries) needs to be treated and controlled.
- Chairside oral hygiene instruction should be given.
- The patient should be made aware of their essential contribution to the maintenance of a high level of oral hygiene.
- Any smoking or heavy drinking habits should be addressed.

Transitional treatment phase

Implants are usually surgically inserted and then temporarily covered with a provisional appliance for between 6 weeks and 6 months (although one stage techniques can also be undertaken) to allow osseointegration to take place. During this phase, the hygienist and therapist should monitor the oral health under any temporary appliance and provide appropriate advice to minimise post-operative inflammation and prevent secondary infection.

Completion of treatment

After placement, the patient should attend for regular maintenance and monitoring. When the patient attends the dental hygienist or therapist for review, the following features should be checked:

- **Mobility of the implant**: there should be no loose screws or detectable movement of the intrabony components. Percussion should give a characteristic hard

'ring'. If a dull noise is heard, this may suggest that the implant is not integrated with the bone and the patient should be referred back to the implantologist.

- **Signs of mucosal inflammation and peri-implantitis**. Assessment of tissue health can allow for early intervention in the disease process. Peri-implant connective tissue surrounding the implant is more vulnerable to infection due to lack of decreased vascularity and lack of true connective tissue attachment. Peri-implantitis affects the entire circumference of the implant creating bone loss and inflammatory tissue extending to the bone surface. Any periodontitis associated with natural teeth may have a detrimental effect on implants. It is possible that bacteria associated with periodontitis, e.g. *Porphyromonas gingivalis*, are also important pathogens in destructive inflammatory lesions around implants. Clinical assessment includes determining the presence or absence of bacterial plaque, bleeding on probing and exudate. There is limited evidence on whether probing should be carried out routinely around implants, or whether this should be undertaken when pathology is present such as bleeding and exudate. There is also limited evidence whether probing should be undertaken with metal or plastic probes, and further research is required in this area. However, probes should not be used to establish probing depths, as this would damage the delicate long junctional epithelial attachment of the mucosa surrounding the implant.

- **Treatment at maintenance appointments** should include removal of plaque and calculus deposits, using implant-safe instruments. If a patient is performing effective home care, supragingival and subgingival calculus should be light or non-existent. Plastic, gold or Teflon-coated scaling instruments are specifically available for implant management. An ultrasonic tip may be used only with a plastic covering that prevents gouging and disturbance of the titanium surface. It is important to avoid too much pressure when scaling implants, as calculus deposits are not as tenacious as calculus on natural teeth. Scaling needs to be gentle, using short working strokes, as the junctional epithelium and the peri-implant gingival tissues are fragile; the periodontal fibres are not multidirectional, as with natural teeth, but run in one direction only.

- Non-abrasive polishing pastes should be used for polishing, and polishing kits are specifically manufactured for implants. To avoid implant structures being damaged, it is advisable to polish the implant first with a new polishing brush or cup, as this would not have any contaminating residue from previous treatments, and to use an implant polishing paste. The prophylaxis can be completed with more traditional abrasive paste in the remaining areas of the mouth.

Although peri-implantitis is uncommon, treatment is difficult because of the bone destruction and a preventive approach must be adopted. Effective plaque control is essential and the following points should be noted:

- Toothbrushes with round ended nylon bristles or electric toothbrushes are recommended. When recommending interdental brushes, the wire should be plastic coated so that the wire does not damage the metal implant and scratch the surface of the titanium.
- Flossing is advised when cleaning around the implant superstructure and superfloss would be appropriate for this. Floss or superfloss should be inserted at the buccal surface and threaded around the lingual aspect, so that it completely surrounds the abutment; the floss can then be moved gently backwards and forwards to clean the surface effectively.
- Single tufted brushes can also be considered as they can access smaller spaces and bristles can be cut according to needs, to allow for a smaller tuft.

Oral cancer screening

Whilst there is no evidence that recalling patients specifically to screen (checking for disease when there are no symptoms) for oral cancer reduces the mortality, the dental hygienist and dental therapist are in a unique position to screen for early signs of oral malignant change during routine review or treatment visits for all patients. The clinical presentation of oral carcinoma is fully described in Chapter 3.

The risk factors associated with this disease are:

- Oral cancer most often occurs in those who use tobacco in any form.
- Alcohol use combined with smoking greatly increases risk.
- Prolonged exposure to the sun increases the risk of lip cancer.
- Age: oral cancer is more likely to occur after the age of 40.
- Exposure to human papillomavirus.

However, it should be noted that more than 25% of oral cancers occur in people who do not smoke and have no other known risk factors. Studies have also suggested that a diet high in fruits and vegetables may prevent the development of potentially cancerous lesions, and should be encouraged as they will also provide general holistic benefits.

The dental hygienist and dental therapist should undertake a systematic examination commencing with an extraoral examination checking for lymphadenopathy in the neck region. Intraorally, the clinician needs to check all the soft tissues including the tonsillar region for any possible signs of tissue change, such as red or white patches. It is also important to palpate the floor of the mouth with one finger placed under the tongue with the other hand placed under the chin to provide some resistance. The most common sites of occurrence are the lateral border of the tongue, floor of mouth and the retromolar region. These areas should be examined routinely by asking the patient to extend the tongue, then grasping the tip of the tongue by using a piece of dry gauze and gently pulling the tongue first to the one side and then the other and then raising the tongue to view both the sides of the tongue and the floor of the mouth.

A diagnostic kit (Orascreen) is available as an adjunct to physical examination which contains a dye (**toluidine blue**) designed to stain premalignant tissue and aid its identification (Figure 11.6). It is not intended to be used

(a)

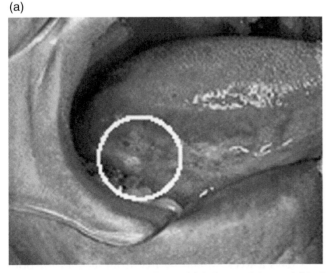

(b)

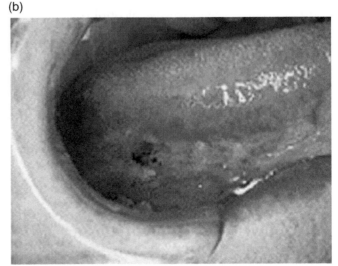

Figure 11.6 A premalignant lesion (a) before staining and (b) after staining with toluidine blue.

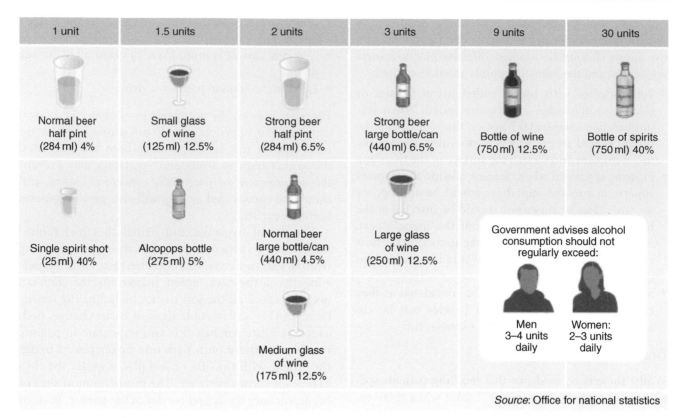

Figure 11.7 Units of alcohol. (*Source*: Office for National Statistics licensed under the Open Government Licence v.1.0.)

for screening in the general population but as an adjunct to clinical examination in patients at high risk.

Alcohol abuse

Alcohol abuse is one of the major avoidable health hazards Alcohol is associated with various forms of cancer including those involving the pharynx, larynx and oral cavity; when excessive alcohol consumption is combined with smoking the risk of oral cancer is significantly increased. The consumption of alcohol is on the increase especially in young adults. A high alcohol intake on a single occasion, as in the case of binge spirit drinking, leads to acetaldehyde accumulation in the oral mucosa which promotes the formation of carcinogenic, highly reactive, free radicals. Acetaldehyde seems to be a carcinogenic factor (Petti and Scully, 2005).

'Alcohol' in any social context relates to ethanol (C_2H_2OH). The percentage of ethanol by volume varies in different alcoholic drinks and the dental hygienists and dental therapists should be aware of this when advising patients. A unit of alcohol is 10 ml (1 cl) by volume, or 8 g by weight of pure alcohol. One alcohol unit is roughly equivalent to one measure of spirits, one 250 ml glass of wine or half a pint of ordinary strength beer. Units of alcohol is calculated more accurately by the percentage alcohol by volume (% abv) of any drink equals the number of units in one litre of that drink; for example

- Wine at 12% abv has 12 units in one litre.
- Strong beer at 6% abv has six units in one litre.

This calculation makes it easier for individuals to calculate their consumption and monitor their own health behaviour. It is an offence to drive with more than 80 mg of alcohol in 100 ml of blood, or 35 µg of alcohol in 100 ml of breath. As everyone metabolises alcohol at different rates, it is difficult to say how many units or drinks this represents (Figure 11.7). The national guidelines are to 'drink alcohol in moderation, if at all'. The recommended limits of drinking alcohol are:

- Up to14 units of alcohol a week for a woman, with a recommendation of no more than 2–3 units a day as women have lower level rates of metabolising alcohol then men.
- Up to 21 units of alcohol a week for a man, with a recommendation of no more than 3–4 units a day.
- 2 days a week should be free from alcohol for both women and men.

Someone who is described as alcoholic is said to be consuming alcohol to such a degree as to cause a deterioration in social behaviour or physical illness and the development of dependence from which withdrawal is difficult or causes adverse effects.

Treatment

Treatment is by brief interventions (e.g. advice on the risk of dependence), specialized treatment programmes (e.g. in residential settings) or psychosocial treatments (e.g. Alcoholics Anonymous).

Prevention

Dental hygienists and dental therapists can play a useful part in prevention by:

- Including questions regarding alcohol consumption during a social history; advice and support regarding appropriate referral can then be given, especially if the social history also reveals the patient smokes.
- Undertaking a thorough examination of the soft tissues at every opportunity, particularly in individuals who are considered high risk, and referring any suspicious lesions promptly.
- Highlighting the risks of heavy alcohol consumption particularly in younger patients.
- Encouraging pregnant mothers to decline from alcohol consumption during pregnancy as it has a detrimental effect on foetal development.
- Being prudent in the recommendation of mouthwashes which contain alcohol particularly among children and high-risk subjects, although there is limited evidence that mouthwashes containing alcohol have an increased effect regarding oral cancer.

Smoking cessation

Smoking is one of the greatest public health challenges the world faces. Every year 4.9 million deaths are caused by tobacco (WHO, 2002). In 2009, an estimated 81 400 deaths and 462 900 hospital admissions of those aged 35 and over in England, were attributed to smoking (NHS Information Centre, 2010). Smoking-related costs to the NHS were in the region of £5.5 billion (Allender *et al.*, 2009).

The clear link between oral diseases and tobacco use is alarming, with significant effects including oral cancer, premalignancy (e.g. leukoplakia, increased severity and extent of periodontal disease) and poor wound healing (Allard *et al.*, 1999). Smokeless tobacco use (e.g. chewing tobacco, paan, khat, zarda – similar to snuff) is also associated with a range of oral pathologies (Cogliano *et al.*, 2004). It has been estimated that between 63 000

and 190 000 smokers would stop smoking each year if all dental clinicians routinely offered smoking cessation advice (Levine and Stillman-Lowe, 2004).

At an individual level, dental professionals, unlike most other primary care workers, are in the unique position of seeing healthy patients on a regular basis when they are not preoccupied with other health concerns and motivation to stop smoking is likely to be higher. This provides the opportunity to frequently discuss attitudes and habits of smokers and those who use tobacco derivatives. At a professional level, dental associations have a role to play by lobbying the government to implement changes nationally. The 2011 Department of Health's white paper '**Healthy Lives. Healthy People**' advocates that all health professionals should identify smokers and provide brief smoking cessation advice, and refer patients to local NHS stop smoking services. This guidance has been specifically targeted at dental teams in two documents helping to change the face of modern dentistry; *Modernising NHS Dentistry* (DoH, 2000), and NHS Dentistry: Options for Change (DoH, 2002).

Smoking habits

In 2009, 21% of UK adults reported smoking (General Lifestyle Survey (GLS), 2011). There is an abundance of evidence to suggest that there are large socioeconomic differences in smoking and tobacco use habits in the UK. Between 1973 and 1994 the prevalence of smoking among adults with a higher socioeconomic status has halved, whereas the habits of people in the lower socio economic groups showed little change. Between 1998 and 2009, prevalence decreased by approximately a quarter among non-manual workers and a fifth among manual workers. In 2009, 26% of manual workers in England were cigarette smokers, compared with 16% of non-manual workers (GLS, 2011).

Reasons for starting to smoke

Starting smoking can be due to one or more of the reasons listed in Table 11.8.

Reasons for continuing to smoke

External influences can hinder an individual's motivation and commitment to smoking cessation (Table 11.9).

Smoking is associated with emotional dependence. The subconscious desire to smoke is often a way to deal with specific circumstances, for example smoking can provide an individual with breaks from boredom, it can provide 'thinking' time in stressful situations throughout the day or can even be used as a substitute for snacking. For confirmed smokers the action of smoking is often

Table 11.8 Reasons for starting smoking.

Environmental	Parents who smoke (children are twice as likely to start) Siblings and friends who smoke Media promotions targeted at young people Lower socio-economic class
Behavioural	Low academic ability and performance (linked to truancy and early drop out) Associated with other problem behaviours/addictions (e.g. alcohol and other drug misuse)
Personal	Low self worth and esteem Poor knowledge of the adverse effects Mental health problems (anxiety and depression)

Table 11.9 Reasons for continuing to smoke.

Family circumstances	Living with a smoker is likely to result in a relapse
Socioeconomic class	Stresses of living in poverty is likely to influence motivation and level of dependence
Psychological	Depressive illnesses are associated with low rates of cessation
Pharmacological	Daily dependence and how soon cigarettes are consumed after waking

an unconscious habit that they barely remember from one cigarette to the next. It is important to acknowledge the unique love/hate relationship that many smokers develop with their habit. Smokers often express a desire to stop despite never having made an attempt to do so. Cigarettes hold the unparalleled position of being used to stimulate and calm users, which adds to the strong psychological dependency that many people have. This strong psychological dependency is matched by the physical addiction that cigarettes foster. The receptors in the brain that register when an individual has smoked remain sedated by regular doses of nicotine. If nicotine falls below the individual's addiction threshold the receptors become stimulated and the individual will feel a craving. Once they have responded to the craving and the nicotine level rises, the receptors are sedated again and the cycle continues. One of the reasons that cigarettes are so addictive is the instant relief they provide for cravings. It takes approximately 7 seconds from the first inhalation of smoke for the nicotine to register with the brain receptors. This instant relief forms a powerful subconscious link between smoking and a feeling of well being.

All smokers are different and their motivation for stopping is equally unique. However, research has shown a considerable proportion of smokers successfully stop when given support to do so. Much of this success depends on recognising when an individual is ready to stop. It is important for members of the dental team to assess their patient's readiness to quit, and to realise many patients make several attempts before succeeding (see Chapter 6, p. 129). Whether or not a smoker is successful in their attempt to stop depends on the balance between motivation and dependence. In a clinical setting it's important for the clinician to spend time with the patient to assess both these characteristics.

The impact of smoking

Most smokers start during their adolescence. In England in 2009, 29% of 11–15-year-olds had tried smoking, and 6% were regular smokers (The NHS Information Centre, 2010).

Some two thirds of smokers want to stop, yet only about 40% attempt to do so each year. Just 3–5% of unaided quit attempts are likely to last a year or more (Hughes *et al.*, 2004), compared with approximately 15% of those made with NHS Stop Smoking Services (Ferguson *et al.*, 2005).

- It is estimated that the life span of a smoker if shortened by approximately 5 minutes for each cigarette they smoke. Smokers dying of related illnesses will have reduced their life span by 10–15 years on average (Royal College of Physicians Tobacco Advisory Group, 2000). The health risks of smoking are considerable and the following are important:
- Evidence has shown that there are at least 50 different diseases associated with smoking of which the most important oral diseases are carcinoma and periodontal disease.
- Healing among smokers is slower and less successful than non-smokers due to the effect that tobacco has on the vascular system causing peripheral vasoconstriction within the oral cavity.
- Smoking has an adverse effect on the healing process of extraction wounds (Meechan *et al.*, 1998).
- Often the poor aesthetic appearance caused by extrinsic staining of the teeth as a result of smoking is a strong motivating factor to giving up. Tobacco can cause yellow and brown darkening of the teeth through the penetration of tobacco into tooth enamel, restorations and dentures.
- Halitosis can be caused by smoking or chewing tobacco and as with staining can be reversed. The social impacts of these conditions can result in severe loss of confidence and a wish not to interact with others.

- Former smokers and those who have previously used tobacco in other forms report an improved sense of smell and taste. Reduced sense of smell and taste are among the first of the adverse health effects to be reversed once the habit has ceased.

Smoking cessation advice

The Cochrane Review on brief advice from health professionals and more intensive behavioural support have been shown to increase a smoker's chance of quitting (Fiore et al., 2000) There is strong evidence that smoking cessation advice by health care professionals in the clinical setting is effective (Gorin and Heck, 2003).

Telephone helplines reach a more representative sample of smokers in various states of readiness to quit than will attend a dental practice, and will therefore provide a service for a population not reached by clinics (Table 11.10).

The Department of Health's white paper 'Smoking Kills' (1998) outlined the **Stop smoking cessation service** (formerly the smoking cessation service) established in 1999 that is now available across the NHS in England. This service provides expert advice and support to smokers and professionals, who can refer patients directly. Smokers accessing this service have a fourfold greater chance of stopping relative to unassisted quitting, yet such support is used in approximately only 2% of all quit attempts. All members of the dental team should encourage smokers to stop and promote the use of this service. The document 'Smokefree and smiling: helping dental patients to quit tobacco' guidance document (DoH, 2007) is available to primary care dental teams on smoking cessation.

The Three As model

The three As model (Figure 11.8) of smoking cessation support is suitable for use within the dental surgery or clinic and can be easily incorporated into daily clinical practice. It's an easy method of identifying smokers who want to stop and how best to help them. The three As model has been modified over recent years with more emphasis now placed on brief advice.

Ask

It is important to establish patients smoking status on a regular basis as part of their medical history. Answers should be recorded in the patients' clinical notes. This will help to assess a smokers' motivation and where to place them in the behaviour change cycle (see Chapter 6, p. 128). The questions which should be asked are:

- Do you want to stop smoking?

Table 11.10 Telephone helplines and websites.

Country	Phone number	Website
England	0800 022 4332	www.smokefree.nhs.uk
Wales	0800 085 2219	www.stopsmokingwales.com
Scotland	0800 848 8484	www.canstopsmoking.com
Northern Ireland	0800 858 8585	

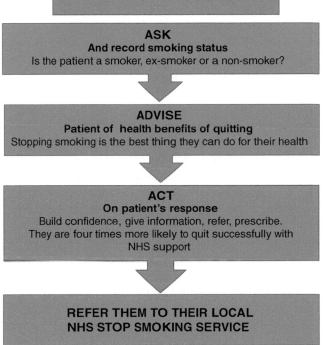

Figure 11.8 The Three As approach to smoking cessation.

- Are you interested in making a serious attempt to stop in the near future?
- Are you interested in receiving help with your quit attempt?
- How many cigarettes do you usually smoke per day?
- How soon after you wake up do you smoke your first cigarette?

Smokers who smoke within 30 minutes of waking or who smoke more than 15–20 cigarettes a day are displaying high levels of nicotine dependence.

Advise

Everyone who uses tobacco in any form should be advised of the health and social benefits of stopping and the increased risks of continuing with their habit.

It is important that advice is personalised to individual patients. Blanket advice will have little effect. All too often smokers are given advice that is little more than a list of health risks and this does little to motivate an individual. Everyone will respond to different motivating factors (e.g. stained teeth, halitosis or changes to the soft tissue, etc.). For example, young people are more likely to respond favourably to the immediate social benefits of lack of staining and halitosis than the long-term benefits of a reduced likelihood of carcinoma of the lungs. In the advice given it is important to explain the effect that tobacco use has on the oral cavity. Most people are aware through health promotion campaigns that smoking or tobacco use is harmful to general health and can cause lung cancer and heart conditions, etc. This is an area where the common risk factor approach can be used to integrate the risks to oral health with the risks to general health.

Act

Many patients will have considered giving up smoking or tobacco use but do not know how to seek help. They may have made one or more attempts to stop in the past but relapsed especially if they were trying to stop by themselves. The NHS Stop Smoking Service (see above) has a range of services available from one to one counselling to group sessions, in addition to effective pharmacotherapy (see below). Patients can also self-refer to the service for support. Details of local Stop Smoking Services can be found by contacting the local Primary Care Trust or Health Promotion Department or by accessing the web. By referring the patient to their local NHS Stop Smoking Service, they are four times more likely to quit successfully.

Nicotine replacement therapy (NRT)

NRT works by reducing craving and withdrawal symptoms. It delivers a lower dose of nicotine, and more slowly, relative to cigarettes, and without all the tar, chemicals and other harmful elements of tobacco smoke. NTR is available in the following forms; patches, gum, nasal spray, lozenges, inhalers, sublingual tablets, mouth spray, bupropion (Zyban – a prescription antidepressant) and varenicline (Champix).

Only in a small percentage of smokers with specific medical conditions is NRT contra-indicated; even smokers who are pregnant can use NRT. NRT will considerably increase the chances of cessation but motivation and willpower is still required and smokers will still need support with withdrawal symptoms although these will be reduced. Some smokers express concern that they may become addicted to NRT, although this is rare (approximately 5% of users, depending on product type). Smokers should be encouraged to continue using NRT at the recommended dose and frequency for 8–12 weeks. Combining two NRT products (typically patch and one other) is more efficacious than using only one form of NRT.

Zyban, and Champix are an alternative to NRT and do not contain nicotine. Both are available only on prescription. Zyban is thought to interrupt the areas of the brain that are associated with addiction and the pleasurable effects of nicotine. Champix is a partial agonist which both stimulates and inhibits the nicotine receptors in the brain, Similar to NRT, both Zyban and Champix help to relieve cravings and withdrawal symptoms. It is important to note that both these medications should be taken for approximately 7–14 days before stopping smoking. Bupropion is prescribed for a total of 9 weeks, and Champix for 12 weeks. The evidence suggests the different medications are of equivalent efficacy when combined with expert advice. Zyban and Champix should not be offered to young people under the age of 18, pregnant and or breast feeding women and people who have unstable cardiovascular disorders.

Illegal drug abuse

A history of substance abuse or drug dependency may be revealed when taking a routine medical history. Unfortunately this is not always the case since such patients are frequently very secretive about such habits for obvious reasons. Because of the risk of dental complications, where suspicion is aroused, every effort should be made to establish a history of drug abuse whilst at the same time respecting the patient's right to confidentiality. If this is revealed during a social history, the clinician needs to develop an honest rapport while not being judgmental, so that the patient is being treated in a supportive, clinical environment, and appropriate referral can be considered.

Drugs of abuse can be categorised into narcotics (e.g. cocaine and opium), antidepressants (e.g. benzodiazepine), stimulants (e.g. methamphetamine), hallucinogens (e.g. LSD and mescaline) or cannabis (e.g. marijuana).

Patients who are intravenous drug users have an increased likelihood of having hepatitis B, C or D or HIV infection. Even if drug abuse is suspected but not confirmed, all patients should be treated as if they are infective.

In order to institute effective prevention, the aetiology should be established and therefore the following are important oral or dental considerations:

- Cocaine can have a potentially lethal effect when combined with local anaesthetics containing epinephrine significantly increasing the likelihood of hypertension or a heart attack.
- Patients taking heroin crave sugars so consideration needs to be given to fluoride supplements to control and manage the dental effects.
- Patients can present with rampant caries directly as a result of taking the drugs, e.g. methamphetamine (or 'crystal meth'), which is acidic, or because of the associated xerostomia.
- Patients taking ecstasy may have severe erosion due to the drug induced dehydration and the consumption of compensatory carbonated drinks.
- Oral hygiene and general health may be neglected resulting in an increased likelihood of periodontal disease
- Many patients exhibit tooth grinding or clenching with associated attrition.

If illegal drug abuse is suspected but not elicited as part of the medical history, the referring dentist should be informed.

The primary health care team

It has been said that 'The mouth is the window of the body'. Oral health is intimately linked with general health and therefore not only does the dental hygienist and therapist have a role to play in the promotion of general health as described previously in this chapter, but also the converse is true. There are a large number of important members of the primary health care professions who have an important complementary role to play in preventing oral disease. They and the areas where their activity can overlap are listed in Table 11.11.

There are many opportunities for inter-referral and collaboration between these health care workers and dental care professionals. In addition there are another group of health professionals associated with complementary medicine (e.g. chiropractors and acupuncturists), who may make an important contribution to health promotion and disease prevention. Their potential contribution is described in Chapter 20.

Liaising with these professionals is not only important in highlighting the importance of preventing oral disease in the context of general health but also to make sure that preventive messages given by all

Table 11.11 Primary care providers.

Health care provider	Area of activity overlap
General medical practitioner	Drug interactions
	Medical history
	Sugar free prescriptions
	Oral diagnosis
	Alcohol and smoking cessation
Nurse practitioner	Diet advice
	Healthy options
	Sugar free prescriptions
Community midwives	Oral health education
	Dietary advice
Community psychiatric nurse	Anxiety and stress counselling
Dietician	Diet and general/oral health
Physiotherapist	TMJ pain
	Back pain and occupational problems
Practice nurses	Hypertension
	Smoking cessation
	Diet and oral health education
District nurses	Home visits
	Prevention of illness
	Health promotion
	Elderly care
Health visitors	Elderly health screening and advice, Home visits
	Family nutrition and child health
	Parenting advice
Midwives	Mother and baby feeding advice
Speech therapist	Speech and communication problems
Occupational therapist	Modified oral hygiene aids
	Improving dexterity

professionals are consistent and not contradictory – crisps might be recommended as an alternative to sweets to reduce the likelihood of caries but their high fat content may have adverse affects on the heart and vascular system.

When looking at the broader sphere of health in the community there are many professionals and organisations whose primary activity is not healthcare but who have a significant contribution to make e.g. teachers, education authorities etc. (see Chapter 6) Dental care professionals should appreciate that they have, and should take, advantage of opportunities to liaise with this larger sector of the community in raising public awareness of the importance of oral health and prevention. They can also provide a valuable contribution in informing opinion in the context of health structures and legislative changes.

References

Allard, R., Johnson, N., Sardella, A. *et al.* (1999) Tobacco and oral diseases: Report of EU Working Group. *Journal of Irish Dental Association* **46**, 12–23.

Allender, S., Balakrishnan, R., Scarborough, P., Webster, P. & Rayner, M. (2009). The burden of smoking-related ill health in the UK. *Tobacco Control*, **18**, 262–267.

Bain, C., and Moy, P.K. (1993) The association between implant failures and cigarette smoking. *International Journal of Oral and Maxillofacial Implants* **8**, 609–615.

Cogliano, V., Straif, K., Baan, R., Grosse, Y., Secretan, B. and Ghissassi, F. (2004) Smokeless tobacco and tobacco related nitrosamines. *Lancet Oncology*, **5**, 708.

Department of Health (2000) *Saving Lives: Our Healthier Nation.* [Online] Available from http://www.york.ac.uk/inst/crd/fluores.htm

Department of Health (1998) Smoking kills: a White Paper on Tobacco. [Online.] Available from http://www.archive.official-documents.co.uk/document/cm41/4177/4177.htm (accessed 17 October 2011).

Department of Health (2000) Modernising NHS Dentistry – Implementing the NHS Plan. [Online.] Available from www.doh.gov.uk/dental/strategy (accessed 17 October 2011).

Department of Health (2002) NHS Dentritry: options for change. [Online.] Available from http://www.dh.gov.uk/en/PublicationsandstatisticsPublications/PublicationsPolicyAndGuidance/DH_4008017 (accessed 17 October 2011).

Department of Health (2007) Smokefree and smiling: helping dental patients to quit tobacco
Available from: http://www.dh.gov.uk/en/Publicationsandstatistics/Publications/PublicationsPolicyAndGuidance/DH_074970 (accessed 28 September 2011).

Department of Health (2011) *Healthy Lives, Healthy People: A Tobacco Control Plan for England.* [Online.] Available from: http://www.dh.gov.uk/en/Publicationsandstatistics/Publications/PublicationsPolicyAndGuidance/DH_124917 (accessed 28 September 2011).

Department of Health and the British Association for the Study of Community Dentistry (2009) *Delivering Better Oral Health: An evidence-based toolkit for prevention*, 2nd edition. [Online.] Available from: http://www.dh.gov.uk/en/Publicationsandstatistics/Publications/PublicationsPolicyAndGuidance/DH_102331 (accessed 28 September 2011).

Featherstone J.D.B (2004) The Continuum of Dental Caries-Evidence for a Dynamic Disease Process. J Dent Res 83 (Spec Iss C):C39–C42, 2004.

Fejerskov, O. and Kidd, E. (2003) *Dental Caries: The Disease & its Clinical Management.* Blackwell Munksgaard, Oxford.

Ferguson, J., Bauld, L., Chesterman, J. *et al.* (2005) English smoking treatment services: long term outcomes. *Addiction*, **100**(Suppl 2), 59–69.

Fiore, M.C., Bailey, W.C., Cohen, S.J. *et al.* (2000) Treating tobacco use and dependence. Clinical Practice Guidelines. US Department of Health and Human Services, Rockville, MD.

Foster, H.D. (1993) Fluoride and its antagonists: Implications for human health. *Journal of Orthomolecular Medicine*, **8**,149–153.

General Lifestyle Survey (2011) Smoking and Drinking Report 2009. [Online.] Available from: http://www.ons.gov.uk/ons/rel/ghs/general-lifestyle-survey/2009-report/smoking-and-drinking-among-adults-2009.pdf (accessed 12 October 2011).

Gorin, S.S. and Heck, J.E. (2004) Meta-analysis of the efficacy of tobacco counseling by health care providers. *Cancer Epidemioliogy and Biomarkers Prevevention*, **13**(12), 2012–2022.

Hughes, J.R., Keeley, J. and Naud, S. (2004) Shape of the relapse curve and long-term abstinence among untreated smokers. *Addiction*, **99**, 29–38.

Kidd, E. (2005) *Essentials of Dental Caries.* Oxford University Press, Oxford.

Kuhnisch, J. *et al.* (2011) Longevity of materials for pit and fissure sealing-results from a meta-analysis. *Dent Mater* doi 10: 10.1016/j.dental.2011.11.002.

Lennon, M. (2004) One in a Million: The facts about water fluoridation. The British Fluoridation Society, London.

Levine, R.S. and Stillman-Lowe, C. (2004) *The Scientific Basis of Oral Health Education.* British Dental Journal Books, London.

Marinho, V.C.C., Higgins, J.P.T., Logan, S. and Sheiham, A. (2003) Fluoride toothpastes for preventing dental caries in children and adolescents. *The Cochrane Database of Systematic Reviews*, Issue 1. Art. No.: CD002278. DOI: 10.1002/14651858.CD002278.

Meechan, J., MacGregor, G.M., Rogers, S.M. *et al.* (1998) The effects of smoking on immediate post–extraction socket filling with blood and on the incidence of painful sockets. *British Journal of Oral Maxillofacial Surgery*, **26**, 402–409.

National Health and Medical Research Council (1991) *A Systematic Review of the Efficacy and Safety of Fluoridation.* NHMRC, Canberra.

National Guideline Clearinghouse (2009) Strategies to prevent dental caries in children and adolescents: evidence-based guidance on identifying high caries risk children and developing preventive strategies for high caries risk children in Ireland. [Online.] Available from: www.guideline.gov (accessed 29 September 2011).

NHS Information Centre (2010) *Statistics on Smoking in England.* [Online.] Available from: http://www.ic.nhs.uk/pubs/smoking10 (accessed 29 September 2011).

NHS Information Centre for Health & Social Care (2009) Adult Dental Health Survey. [Online.] Available from http://www.ic.nhs.uk/webfiles/publications/007_Primary_Care/Dentistry/dentalsurvey09/AdultDentalHealthSurvey_2009_ExecutiveSummary.pdf (accessed 11 October 2011).

National Institute for Clinical Excellence (2004) Dental recall: Recall interval between routine dental examinations. NICE Clinical Guideline No.19. London: National Institute for Clinical Excellence. [Online.] Available from http://guidance.nice.org.uk/CG19 (accessed 29 September 2011).

Nunn, J. (2004) Oral health education. In: *Special Care Dentistry: advanced dental nursing* (ed. Ireland, R.) Blackwell Munksgaard, Oxford, pp. 27–78.

Petti, S. and Scully, C. (2005) The role of the dental team in preventing and diagnosing cancer: 5 Alcohol and the role of the dentist in alcohol cessation. *Dental Update*, **32**, 454–460.

Pitts, N.B. and Pendlebury, M.E. (eds) (2001) *Clinical Examination and Record Keeping: Good Practice Guidelines.* Faculty of General Dental Practitioners, London.

Public Health Service (2000) AHRQ publication no. 00-0032. [Online.] Available from: http://www.surgeongeneral.gov/tobacco/ (accessed 29 September 2011).

Robinson, P.G., Deacon, S.A., Deery, C. *et al.* (2005) *The Cochrane Database of Systematic Reviews* Issue 2.

Royal College of Physicians Tobacco Advisory Group (2000) *Nicotine addiction in Britain.* Royal College of Physicians, London.

Scottish Intercollegiate Guidelines Network (2000) Preventing dental caries in children at high caries risk: targeted prevention of dental caries in the permanent teeth of 6–16 year olds presenting for dental care. A National Clinical Guideline No. 47. Scottish Intercollegiate Guidelines Network, Edinburgh.

World Health Organization (1994) Fluorides and oral health. WHO Expert Committee on Oral Health Status and Fluoride Use, WHO Technical Report Series, 846, Geneva.

World Health Organization (2002) *The Tobacco Atlas*. WHO, Geneva.

York Review, A Systematic Review Of Water Fluoridation. NHS Centre For Reviewing And Dissemination, Report 18.

Further reading

Boyle, S. and Griffiths, J. (2005) Holistic oral care-a guide for health professionals. Stephen Hancocks Ltd, London.

Callum, C. (1998) The UK Smoking epidemic: deaths in 1995. Health Education Authority, London.

Miribid, S.M. and Ahing, S. (2000) Tobacco-associated lesions of the oral cavity: malignant lesions. *Journal of the Canadian Dental Association*, **66**, 308 311.

12

Paediatric dentistry

Sharon M.G. Lee and George T.R. Lee

Summary

This chapter covers:

- Dental development and dental anomalies
- Dental caries – pathogenesis and prevention
- Tooth wear
- Treatment of caries in the primary dentition
- Soft tissue problems in children
- Anxiety and pain control
- Trauma in children

Introduction

Paediatric dentistry involves the oral and dental care of children from birth onwards and is concerned with all aspects of oral and dental development and problems that may arise. This chapter includes some of the important features and considerations that are presented to the clinician together with treatment modalities. It is, in effect, a multidisciplinary subject with the common theme being the care of children. Therefore it is not surprising that many aspects which are applicable to paediatric dentistry also appear elsewhere in this textbook (e.g. preventive dentistry, tooth notation, materials, etc.).

Dental development

The earliest evidence of dental development in the fetus occurs as early as 7 weeks *in utero* when there is a proliferation of the oral epithelium to form the **dental lamina**, which then goes on to form the **enamel organs**. The latter are ten discrete cellular condensations in the lower jaw and ten in the upper jaw and these are the beginnings of the **tooth germs**, which are destined to become the primary (deciduous, baby) teeth. At a much later stage there is an outbudding from each primary tooth germ and these form the tooth germs of the permanent teeth which will replace the primary predecessors. At the distal part of each, the dental lamina continues to grow backward and produces tooth germs for the permanent first, second, and third molar teeth.

Tooth notation

Tooth notation systems have been developed in order to provide a quick, accurate and standardised way of referring to particular teeth. Of over 32 different systems that exist, the two most commonly used in the UK are described below.

The Zsigmondy–Palmer system

This system, sometimes called the Palmer system, was first developed by Zsigmondy, an Austrian dentist, as early as 1861. The mouth is divided into four quadrants and each primary tooth is assigned a letter of the alphabet from A to E, starting at the midline with the central incisors (the permanent teeth are assigned the numbers 1 to 8). The letters are placed inside an L-shaped symbol used to identify the quadrant. Because of the problems of recording this information electronically and in printed text, a modification of this notation can be used which replaces the L quadrant indicator with the letters UL, UR, LR and LL, e.g. URE for upper right second primary molar, LLA lower left central incisor, etc.

The FDI notation

This was adopted by the Federation Dentaire Internationale (FDI) in 1971 and is used more internationally than the Zsigmondy–Palmer system. It is a two-digit code and again the mouth is divided into quadrants. The first of the two digits indicates the quadrant and the second the tooth position. The quadrants are numbered 1 to 4 in the permanent dentition and 5 to 8 in the primary dentition, such that the upper right quadrant is 1 or 5, upper left is 2 or 6, lower left is 3 or 7 and lower right is 4 or 8, depending on the dentition. For example, the lower left primary first molar is 74; however, it is not spoken as 'seventy-four', but rather 'seven four'. All the primary teeth in the mouth would therefore be:

55 54 53 52 51 61 62 63 64 65
85 84 83 82 81 71 72 73 74 75

Tooth eruption

The first tooth to erupt is the primary mandibular central incisor at 6 months of age (Table 12.1). This is soon followed by the maxillary central incisors and then all the lateral incisors. Thus all the incisors have erupted by about 9 months of age. There is then a quiescent period of 3–5 months until the next eruption phase when the primary first molars emerge at about 12–14 months of age. The second quiescent period of 3–5 months occurs after which is seen the eruption of the primary canines at 16–18 months. The third and longer rest period of 5–10 months then follows after which the last teeth, the second molars, complete the primary dentition at 24–30 months of age. There is then a long interval of about 4 years before the permanent molars start to appear at 6–8 years of age when the first permanent molars erupt together with the incisors. The next quiescent period of 2–3 years precedes the next phase of eruption of the premolars, second molars and canines at 10–13 years. The last teeth to erupt, if present, are the third molar or 'wisdom' teeth and this occurs at any time from about 18 years onwards.

The timing of eruption will vary greatly and it may not be unusual for teeth to erupt soon after birth or as late as 12 months and still be considered within the limits of normality. The important feature is the sequence of eruption of teeth. For instance, the normal eruption sequence of the maxillary permanent anterior teeth is central incisors first followed by the laterals. If, however, the lateral incisor appears before the central, then almost certainly it is an untoward situation and may indicate some pathology, such as a supernumerary tooth, retained primary tooth, damaged permanent central incisor, trauma, etc.

Morphological differences between primary and permanent teeth

There are numerous differences between the primary and permanent dentition, many of which give rise to considerations in relation to operative treatment, as discussed later in this chapter. Essentially, primary teeth have:

- A shorter crown.
- A lighter colour.
- Narrower occlusal surfaces.
- Broader and flatter interproximal contact areas.
- Thinner enamel and dentine.
- Longer pulp horns, particularly the mesial buccal.
- Relatively larger pulps.
- Enamel prisms which run slightly occlusally at the cervical margin.
- Curved roots (to accommodate the developing permanent successor).
- Roots which have open apices.
- More tortuous and irregular pulp canals.
- An abundance of accessory pulp canals at the furcation areas.

Disruption in the number of teeth

Hypodontia

If there is a failure of the dental lamina to form tooth germs, then the number of teeth that develop will be affected. A reduction in the number of teeth is known as hypodontia. In extreme cases, where no tooth germs at all develop, there will be a complete absence of primary and secondary teeth, a condition known as total hypodontia or **anodontia**. In these rare cases it is invariably an inherited disorder and is always associated with

Table 12.1 Approximate eruption dates.

Teeth	Approximate eruption date
A|A / A|A	6 months
B|B / B|B	7–9 months
EDC|CDE / EDC|CDE	12–24 months
6 21|12 6 / 6 21|12 6	6–8 years
7 543|345 7 / 7 543|345 7	10–13 years
8 | 8 / 8 | 8	18+ years

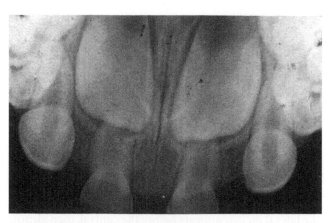

Figure 12.1 Occlusal radiograph of a three year old child showing bilateral congenital absence of the primary and permanent lateral incisors.

other problems which fall under the generic name of **ectodermal dysplasia**. Patients so affected, as well as having no or at least substantially fewer teeth than normal, may have a decrease in sweat glands and hair follicles, defects in finger nails, etc. Absence of a smaller number of teeth is relatively common and in the permanent dentition the third molar teeth are commonly absent. Less frequent is the congenital absence of maxillary lateral incisors (Figure 12.1) and second premolars.

The presence of teeth affords proper development and growth of the mandible and maxilla and, therefore, in cases of total hypodontia or anodontia, management is difficult owing to smaller jaws and a lack of alveolar bone growth, making the provision of dentures and subsequent use of intraosseous implants problematical. The management of one or two congenitally absent teeth is usually much easier. Often a primary tooth that has no permanent successor will remain in place as a functional tooth for many decades. Where the primary tooth with no permanent successor is lost then the resultant space may close either naturally with the adjacent teeth moving into the space or with orthodontic appliance therapy. Should this not be the case and the space needs to be managed, then a partial denture, bridge or, subsequently, an intraosseous implant will be required.

Hyperdontia

Should extra tooth germs of either the primary or secondary dentition occur, then extra teeth will appear, a condition known as hyperdontia. This may have arisen as a result of extra proliferations of the dental lamina or one of the normal tooth germs, at an early stage, actually splitting to form two tooth germs. These extra teeth are also called **supernumerary teeth** and can occur in any part of the mouth and may be related to a particular tooth group. Hence they can be incisoform, caniniform and molariform. However, they tend to be rare in the primary dentition but common in the permanent dentition. They are ten times more frequent in the maxilla than in the mandible and tend to be in the anterior region. Their form can vary from a normal-looking tooth to conical or tuberculated shaped teeth. The former is often the result of a permanent tooth germ splitting at an early stage and causing two identical teeth to form. Where the extra tooth is identical to the tooth of the normal series, then it is termed a **supplemental tooth**.

Occasionally an extra tooth causes no problems and is accommodated into the dental arch without disruption to the occlusion. More often than not it leads to localised crowding and this is remedied by the extraction of the tooth that is in the least favourable position.

Supernumerary teeth may cause no problems and may erupt in ectopic sites such as the palate and may be simply extracted. At other times supernumerary teeth may impede the eruption of permanent teeth or cause them to be deflected from their normal path of eruption. If this occurs, then a surgical extraction of the supernumerary tooth is required. Once a clear path of eruption has been established, the unerupted permanent tooth is likely to erupt uneventfully. Where it may be deemed that this tooth has impaired eruptive potential, then often the unerupted tooth is surgically uncovered and an orthodontic bracket and gold chain is attached. The tooth is recovered and the mucosa is sutured back in place. Subsequent gentle pressure via an orthodontic appliance will pull the errant tooth into a normal position. Occasionally, supernumerary teeth that have not led to problems may be left in order to avoid a surgical extraction. Where this occurs, as with any unerupted tooth left *in situ*, it will need to be monitored by having a radiograph taken at least every 2 years to ensure no pathological changes have occurred, such as resorption of adjacent teeth or cyst formation of the dental follicle.

Disruption of tooth form

The shape and size of a tooth are usually under genetic control and development of elements within the enamel organ is responsible for the resultant tooth form. In the enamel organ there are two layers of cells. The first layer is the **ameloblast layer** and this induces the second layer of cells, the **odontoblasts**, to form. The former cells are responsible for the formation of enamel whilst the odontoblasts lay down dentine. As these hard tissues form, the two layers of cells recede as the enamel and dentine layers become thicker. It is a continuous process and it has been shown that enamel is deposited at the rate of $4\,\mu m$ per day. It therefore can be considered

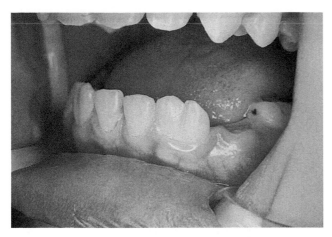

Figure 12.2 Geminated mandibular permanent left lateral incisors.

that the original position of the layer of ameloblasts and odontoblasts maps out what is the future junction between the enamel and dentine and once hard tissue is deposited this then establishes the future shape of the tooth. Therefore, it follows that if there is some sort of disturbance in this layer of cells prior to enamel and dentine formation, then the tooth form will change. Conversely, once the hard tissue is formed then the tooth form is 'fixed' and no changes can occur.

Double teeth

These can occur in both the primary and secondary dentitions and usually affect the anterior teeth. It may have arisen by two adjacent tooth germs that are in close proximity coalescing and forming a single but expanded tooth and this is termed **fusion**. When this occurs, since there are two tooth germs involved, there is one large tooth in place of two teeth, unless fusion has taken place between a tooth of the normal series and a supernumerary tooth. The other way in which double teeth arise is where there has been an expansion of a normal tooth germ before enamel and dentine has been formed. Presumably, if this was allowed to continue, the end result would be the formation of two tooth germs and subsequently two teeth as described above. However, before separation takes place, hard tissue is laid down and the resultant tooth, when it erupts, is very much wider than normal. This process is called **gemination** (Figure 12.2) and unlike fusion, the number of teeth present is normal.

Double teeth of either variety are generally characterised by a vertical labial groove which often becomes carious, and hence fissure sealing at an early stage would be beneficial. Where these teeth have separate roots and a substantial crown, the tooth can be split and allowed to continue as separate teeth. However, more often than

not, there is a single but somewhat expanded root, which makes separation impossible and, in view of the aesthetic and local crowding implications of having a much wider tooth in the dental arch, an extraction and management of the resultant space would be the usual treatment.

Dens in dente (dens invaginatus)

This literally means a 'tooth within a tooth' and is commonly seen in permanent maxillary lateral incisors. It arises due to prolific growth of the layers of ameloblasts and odontoblasts which are mapping out the palatal surface of the tooth. In order to accommodate the exuberant growth, there is a fold in the sheet of cells which causes an inward (towards the pulp) growth. Enamel and dentine are deposited in this new shape and essentially form a blind channel with an opening on the cingulum pit. Clinically this may be recognised as a deep pit or fissure in this area of the tooth. As with pits and fissures elsewhere in the mouth, this area is susceptible to caries. On other occasions, where the enamel and dentine in the depth of the channel have failed to form properly, the pit provides a direct opening into the pulp. When this happens and no preventive or remedial action has been taken, the patient will have problems owing to direct infection of the pulpal tissues from the oral cavity. It would therefore be important that this is diagnosed at an early stage, preferably as soon as the tooth erupts, and that the cingulum pit or fissure is fissure sealed. If there are signs of early caries then this must be treated accordingly.

Dilaceration

A dilacerated tooth is one in which the crown is bent at an angle to the roots. It occurs most commonly in the upper central incisors as a result of trauma from primary incisors.

Enamel pearls

These are small nodules of enamel which form typically on the buccal root surface.

Abnormalities of tooth structure

Enamel and dentine, as previously mentioned, are formed by ameloblasts and odontoblasts respectively. Although this is a continuous process, there are two distinct stages. The first is the formation of an organic matrix which acts like a framework for the second stage; the second stage is the mineralisation phase, whereby the hydroxyapatite crystals are deposited to form the hard tissue. Disturbance of matrix formation will lead to deficiencies in the enamel bulk and may result in **hypoplastic pits** or thin enamel (Figure 12.3).

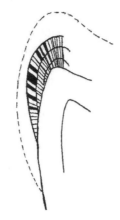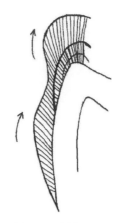

Normal enamel
development with enamel
prisms radiating from the
enamel-dentine junction

Shaded areas represent
loss or damage to the
ameloblast cells

Remaining ameloblasts continue
to form enamel prisms but their
change in orientation results in
a pit or groove formation
on the enamel surface

Figure 12.3 Development of hypoplastic pits in enamel.

Problems with mineralisation will affect the amount of enamel deposited in the matrix and, therefore, although there may be normal enamel thickness, there will be discoloured areas of **hypomineralisation**. These disturbances may be localised and affect only one or two teeth, or they may be generalised and affect most if not all the teeth. Inherited or acquired disturbances of tooth structure including **amelogenesis imperfecta** and **dentinogenesis imperfecta** are fully described in Chapter 3, p. 68–69.

Where a child suffers from an inherited condition, such as amelogenesis imperfecta, considerable restorative treatment is required to maintain function and appearance. In the young child interim measures, such as simple restorations, stainless steel crowns or composite veneers, may be required; these may progress to full-coverage crowns and porcelain veneers later.

Dental caries

Dental caries, despite being the commonest disease in humans, is a complex multifactorial phenomenon with three main factors which contribute to its pathogenesis (see Chapter 4).

Dental plaque is essentially a mucopolysaccharide film with elements derived from the saliva and micro-organisms which reside in the oral cavity. The plaque microflora, despite being derived from the oral flora, is a selection of different bacteria in type and quantity. Dental plaque contains bacteria that are acid producing, with *Streptoccocus mutans* being the most important member in terms of caries production. Lactobacilli are also implicated in the process and rapidly increase in number as the carious process becomes established.

Diet is the single most important factor in the whole process as a substrate is produced from fermentable carbohydrates. Diet is particularly significant in children since they have more taste buds than adults (the average adult has <10 000), and frequently demonstrate a particular craving for sweet things, although this diminishes with adolescence. Sugars such as sucrose are readily implicated, but other products such as starch can be broken down by plaque bacteria to form sugars, which in turn produce various acids, the chief one of which is lactic acid. The acids so produced dissolve the hydroxyapatite crystals that form the enamel structure. All fermentable carbohydrates can be converted to acids in plaque, but sugars such as sucrose are rapidly changed, whereas starch products involve an additional step in the conversion and therefore take longer.

Host factors play an important part in caries initiation and prevention as they alter the resistance of the individual to caries attack. The quality of enamel, dentine and cementum may differ from person to person which results in differing caries susceptibilities. The quality and flow of saliva are extremely important. Saliva contains biochemical complexes, which help to buffer plaque acids, thus reducing or eliminating demineralisation of the enamel. Saliva may also be rich in calcium and phosphate ions which help to remineralise areas almost immediately and therefore reverse the caries process. Also a good flow of saliva aids the removal of not only substrates from the mouth, but also any plaque acid that has been formed.

The interplay of these three factors leads to either demineralisation or remineralisation. Any fermentable carbohydrate challenge in the form of a snack, sucrose

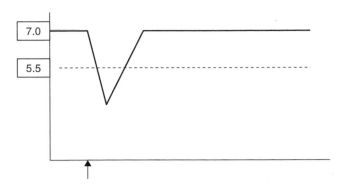

Figure 12.4 Stephan curve showing fall in plaque pH from a resting state of 7.0 to below the critical level of 5.5 (indicated by dotted line) following a single intake of fermentable carbohydrate as indicated by the arrow. The portion below the dotted line represents the amount of demineralisation that occurs.

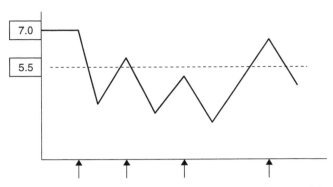

Figure 12.5 Stephan curve after multiple fermentable carbohydrate intakes. It can be seen that the plaque pH stays below the critical level of 5.5 for a long period and this amount of demineralisation is not reversible.

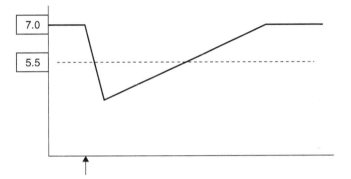

Figure 12.6 Stephan curve showing fall in plaque pH from a single fermentable carbohydrate but where it is retained in the mouth for a longer period than normal. The slower elimination of plaque acid leads to an increase in demineralisation.

drink, etc. will lead to plaque acid production, resulting in demineralisation initially at microscopic level. The calcium and phosphate ions that are released are held in the plaque and saliva and, should the acid environment in the plaque disappear within a short space of time, then the calcium and phosphate ions reform the crystalline structure of the enamel. Thus this system of damage and repair or, more strictly, demineralisation and mineralisation normally maintains a balance. Where the balance is disturbed with more demineralisation than remineralisation, then the resultant destruction produces the typical carious lesion and cavitation. The **Stephan curve** (Figure 12.4) illustrates the increase in plaque acidity (or fall in pH) following a single fermentable carbohydrate intake. After its consumption, there is an elimination of the acid and a return to normal plaque pH at which time any destruction of the microscopic enamel structure is repaired. If, however, fermentable carbohydrate intake is frequent throughout the day, then the acidic or low pH of the plaque is maintained for longer periods with considerable demineralisation occurring and this amount of destruction cannot be remineralised as before (Figure 12.5).

It should also be remembered that remineralisation and repair will only take place when the plaque pH rises to above 5.5 and the longer the period of acidic conditions, the more likelihood of caries developing. Where foods have a particular adherence, for instance sticky toffee, etc., or where there is a poor salivary flow as a result of medication (e.g. antihistamines) or treatment (radiotherapy), or a reduced salivary flow (during sleep), a single fermentable carbohydrate intake can tip the balance towards demineralisation (Figure 12.6).

Where the process is rapid it is often referred to as 'rampant caries'. This condition usually occurs in very young children where the sugar intake is both high and frequent. The causative agent is often fruit juices or similar containing sucrose, given in a feeding bottle. The drink is given over long periods on demand and often the child falls asleep with the feeding bottle in his/her mouth. Thus the upper anterior teeth are constantly bathed in the sucrose condition and, with the child falling asleep, there is even less opportunity for elimination of the drink or the plaque acid from the mouth. Because this usually occurs in very young children who are still using a feeding bottle, the condition has also been referred to as '**nursing caries**' (Figure 12.7).

Prevention of dental caries

Prevention is important for all patients, but there are certain factors which render individuals, especially children, very much more at risk, and it is perhaps prudent to target these individuals or groups. These may be general or local factors. General factors include:

- Low socioeconomic groups.
- Medically and physically compromised patients.
- Special needs children.

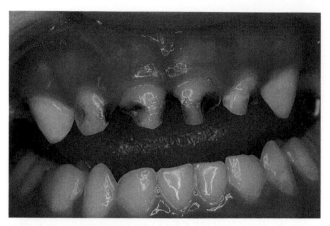

Figure 12.7 'Nursing caries' affecting maxillary upper primary teeth.

Local factors include:

- Existing caries experience.
- Excessive periods of sugar intake per day.
- Poor oral hygiene.
- Conditions where there is a poor salivary flow.
- Orthodontic appliance therapy.

Diet modification

By far the most important factor in caries initiation and propagation is the effect of diet, as described above. It is therefore not surprising that dietary analysis and modification form the mainstay of any caries preventative programme. Parents often fail to recognise the relationship of their child's diet and their caries experience and frequently dispute the fermentable carbohydrate intake. This may be because they assume that it is the consumption of sweets which is entirely responsible and are unaware that other foods, including snacks such as crisps, etc., are also implicated. In addition, most processed foods contain **hidden sugars**. The term 'hidden' is somewhat unfair in that the food manufacturers will argue that the amount of sugar is listed on the labelling. However, usually these are foods which parents do not readily consider as causing tooth decay. Another reason why parents underestimate the dietary effect relates to the importance of frequency of consumption rather than the total consumed. Thus a quantity of sweets consumed over a short period is less detrimental than a smaller amount spread over a longer time.

In order to be able to provide advice regarding the diet it is necessary to examine what is being consumed. This is achieved by the completion of a diet diary which records all food, drinks and snacks consumed over usually a period of 3 days. One of the days should be a weekend day as the eating pattern may be different

from a weekday or a school day. It is essential that the diet diary is filled in at the time that the food or drink is consumed. To complete the diary retrospectively at the end of the day or at the end of the 3-day period is likely to lead to omissions of between-meal snacks and drinks which may have become a subconscious routine but, of course, are very important in the analysis. Figure 12.8 illustrates an example of a diet diary.

There are many ways in which a dietary diary may be analysed. The simplest is to identify to the parent and child the good and bad aspects of the record, pointing out the decay-producing foodstuffs and the frequency. A more effective way is a more detailed analysis which differentiates mealtime and between-meal snacking, using a scoring system for acid attacks on the teeth as follows:

	Score
Main meal	2
Main meal + brushing	1
Between meal snacks	
Food or drink consumed within a 5-minute period (e.g. biscuits, sweets, fruit cordial, etc.)	1
Food consumed over longer than a 5-minute period	2

Table 12.2 illustrates the analysis of a typical caries-prone child for a single day using the above scoring system. It can be seen that there have been 12 acid attack episodes, which can realistically be reduced to the recommended maximum of five. This is a very simple way of analysing the data which produces targets which are easily understood and can be achieved. It is important that the whole process is conducted in an informative way and that neither the parent nor child are made to feel intimidated.

Fluorides

The use of topical and systemic fluoride is fully described in Chapter 11, p. 225–229.

Fissure sealants

Fissure sealing became popular from the early 1970s and the technique was made viable by the introduction of the acid-etch technique, which enabled materials, such as dental resins, to be attached to the enamel surface without the need for mechanical preparation of the tooth. The principle of fissure sealing is based on the concept that the occlusal fissure pattern of, particularly, first permanent molar teeth and, to a lesser extent, the premolars and second molars is very susceptible to becoming carious. Indeed, epidemiological studies have demonstrated the high caries prevalence of these clinical

DETAILS OF FOOD INTAKE

PATIENT'S NAME: ....
(please print)

Far more is known about dental decay today than was known a few years ago and we now understand how it can be controlled better. One of the most important factors that affects the dental decay rate is the diet. Therefore we would like an accurate and complete dietary history of your child's eating habits.

INSTRUCTIONS

1. A complete record of everything eaten or drunk for three consecutive days (which should include one weekend day) for three days.

2. Record every type of food consumed, solid or liquid, at mealtimes, between meals, while watching television, etc. Record also sweets and chocolates.

3. For each meal list the food preparation (fried, boiled, etc.) and amount (1 tsp, or 1 tbl, 1 cup, number of pieces).

4. Record the amount of sugar or sugar products and cream or milk added to cereal, beverages, or other foods.

5. Record foods in the order in which they are eaten.

6. Particular information on snacks is most important. Do not leave out the smallest detail.

Thank you

DAY 1

DATE.................... DAY..............................

TIME	FOOD	QUANTITY	PREPARED

DAY 2

DATE.................... DAY..............................

TIME	FOOD	QUANTITY	PREPARED

DAY 3

DATE.................... DAY..............................

TIME	FOOD	QUANTITY	PREPARED

Figure 12.8 Typical diet diary.

Table 12.2 Acid exposures of teeth.

	From diet diary	Recommended
Breakfast	1	1
Between meals	2	0
Lunch	2	2
Between meals	3	0
Dinner	2	2
Bedtime snacks	2	0
TOTAL	**12**	**5**

sites. By taking a sound tooth and covering the fissure system with a resin, this very vulnerable area of the tooth remains protected as it becomes much easier to keep plaque-free than before. Although fissure sealing has been regularly used for over 35 years, the idea of protecting a sound tooth is not new. Almost 50 years before the first fissure sealant had been developed, an American, Thadeus Hyatt, advocated a technique which he called **prophylactic odontotomy**. This essentially involved taking a sound tooth and preparing shallow occlusal cavities, predominantly in enamel, which eliminated the fissure system. The tooth was then filled with amalgam. Whilst prophylactic odontotomy had is proponents, it was not an idea that received much support, and in some ways it was rather illogical to place an amalgam filling in a tooth to prevent caries which, if it had occurred, would need an amalgam filling.

Not all children will develop fissure caries and therefore it would not be cost effective to carry out the procedure on all paediatric patients. The British Society of Paediatric Dentistry (2000) published guidelines regarding the use of fissure sealants. These are summarised below.

Patient selection indications include:

- Children with impairments, especially where the condition gives rise to problems as a result of developing dental disease or in providing treatment.
- Children who have caries experience, as judged by the existence of two or more cavities in the primary dentition. Susceptible sites on the permanent teeth should be sealed.

Tooth selection indications include:

- Deep fissures.
- Where caries exists in one or more of the permanent teeth. The other susceptible sites on the remaining permanent teeth should be sealed.
- A stained fissure that is not deemed to be carious by clinical and radiographic examination.

Modern fissure sealants may be Bis-GMA resins similar to composite resins, or they may be glass ionomer or a mixture of glass ionomer and composite resin. All these materials utilise the acid-etch technique, which creates microscopic pores in the enamel surface and into which the resin flows and provides the micromechanical retention that holds the sealant in place. The added benefit of sealants containing glass ionomer is that there is some fluoride in this material which in turn can cause further protection to the dental tissues. The long-term success for glass ionomers used as fissure sealants is, however, questionable.

The technique of fissure sealant application is fully described in Chapter 11, p. 230–231.

Regular review of the fissure sealant is important to ensure that:

- It remains intact. Where it is lost it will need to be replaced and where there is partial loss then it will need to be replenished.
- Caries has not been inadvertently sealed under the fissure sealant as demonstrated by colour changes observed through clear fissure sealants or by the use of bitewing radiographs.

Plaque control

Whilst diet modification remains the most important aspect in caries prevention, it has to be remembered that it is the microbiological activity in plaque that results in the conversion of sugars to acids. Therefore any removal of plaque will not only maintain good gingival health, but also have an effect in reducing caries. An example of the latter is the decalcification that occurs around orthodontic brackets when plaque removal has not been as thorough as it should have been.

Tooth brushing remains the main method of plaque control in children and, with the use of toothpaste as previously described, provides a very convenient vehicle for fluoride. However, it requires both a reasonable degree of manual dexterity and also motivation, two factors that young children below the age of 6 years probably do not possess. It is therefore important that parents carry out this routine for their children and, in so doing, not only effect efficient plaque removal but also instil the habit of good oral health for the future. Older children may have developed the skills but perhaps the motivation may be lacking and parental supervision is advisable.

Monitoring of the efficacy of tooth brushing is aided by the use of plaque-disclosing tablets or solutions which essentially are harmless vegetable dyes. Plaque will be stained usually red and give a clear indication to the child and parent of areas in which more concentration is required. The use of plaque indices as a method of quantifying the amount of plaque on the teeth can be quite helpful. The score is usually given as a percentage and whilst it lacks scientific validation, it nevertheless provides a target for the child and parents by which future improvement in tooth brushing may be measured. Other methods of plaque removal such as the use of floss are inadvisable in a young child, as injudicious use can lead to gingival damage.

Tooth wear in children

Gradual loss of the tooth surface has, in the past, been associated with an ageing process and therefore was considered to be related to advancing years. However, in recent years, this has become a recognised problem in children and was first included in the Children's Dental Health in the United Kingdom Survey in 1993 and was monitored again more recently in the 2003 survey.

There are three mechanisms that produce tooth wear:

- **Attrition**: wear due to tooth-to-tooth contact.
- **Erosion**: tooth loss due to chemical (usually acid) attack and not mediated through bacterial activity.
- **Abrasion**: tooth wear due to contact with a foreign body, e.g. toothbrush, etc.

There is no doubt the process of tooth wear is often the combination of two or all three factors and those that are more likely to occur in children are erosion and attrition. Acids in the mouth cause the surface of the tooth to be weakened which allows tooth-to-tooth contact during mastication to effect greater loss of the tooth surface than would otherwise be the case if erosion or attrition were occurring alone.

The source of the acid may be intrinsic, arising from gastric acid escaping from the stomach into the oesophagus and then into the mouth. This may be a result of a weakened or defective sphincter between the stomach and oesophagus leading to **gastro-oesophageal reflux disease** (GORD) with usually accompanying indigestion, heartburn and epigastric pain as well as dental erosion. Recurrent vomiting also has similar effects and this may be associated with irritable bowel syndrome or travel sickness, or it may be self-induced as occurs in the eating disorders of **anorexia** and **bulimia nervosa**. Extrinsic acids arise from dietary sources and whilst carbonated drinks and fruit juices are readily identified as being the cause, it should also be remembered that foods such as pickled vegetables, brown sauce and tomato ketchup do have erosive potential.

This erosion can affect any surface which comes into contact with the acid but it is more likely to occur on the occlusal and palatal surfaces of the maxillary teeth and to a lesser extent of the mandibular teeth. Figure 12.9

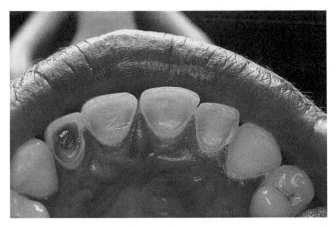

Figure 12.9 Severe surface tooth loss of the palatal aspects of the permanent maxillary incisors.

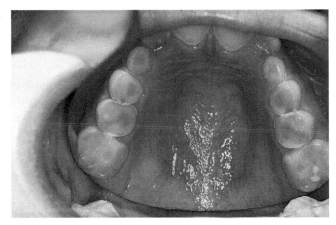

Figure 12.10 Erosion of occlusal and palatal surfaces of maxillary posterior teeth as a result of gastro-oesophageal reflux disease.

shows severe tooth surface loss as a result of excessive intake of carbonated drinks. The considerable erosion that has taken place is well demonstrated by the raised appearance of the amalgam restoration on the palatal surface of the maxillary right lateral incisor. The amalgam at the time of placement was flush with the enamel surface but now the latter is well below the original level. Figure 12.10 shows erosion as a result of gastro-oesophageal reflux disease.

It is important that the condition is recognised at an early stage when the aetiological factors may be identified. Where it is dietary in origin, diet analysis and counselling will prevent further deterioration in the condition. Patients with gastro-oesophageal reflux disease or eating disorders should be referred initially to their medical practitioner. Where the amount of tooth loss has been mild and in the absence of tooth sensitivity, the condition may be left and the situation monitored at regular intervals to ensure that the wear has stopped.

Where there has been a greater degree of surface loss, then restorative treatment by way of composite coatings, veneers or crowns may be required.

Treatment of dental caries in the primary dentition

The primary dentition should be restored because this will avoid:

- Pain in the future.
- Pulpal infections and sequelae.
- Extractions.
- A general anaesthetic for the extractions.

It will also maintain:

- An intact arch.
- Space in the arch for the permanent successor.
- Mastication.
- Speech.
- Aesthetics.

Whilst it would seem sensible from the above list to preserve the primary dentition until natural exfoliation occurs, there are some circumstances where primary teeth should not be restored. The contraindications to restoration are:

- The tooth or teeth are beyond conservation, for example where caries has extended into the root area.
- Extremely unco-operative behaviour.
- Multiple grossly carious teeth.
- Imminent exfoliation.
- There is danger from likely infection (e.g. immuno-compromised children).
- There is acute infection with facial swelling and/or pyrexia.
- There is poor parental motivation.

Restorative materials for children

Amalgam

Amalgam has been the most popular restorative material for posterior teeth for many years for adults and children. It is a hard-wearing material which is both economical and easy to use, but there is no adhesion to dental tissues and its retention relies on having cavities that have some degree of undercut. Furthermore, there have been concerns in recent years regarding the safety of the material, as mercury is one of the main constituents and in a number of countries its use in primary teeth has been limited (e.g. in Sweden, but for environmental reasons). Nevertheless amalgam still remains a durable and widely used material in children (British Society of Paediatric Dentistry, 2001).

Resin composite

This is a material that is likely to be the future replacement for amalgam as a posterior restorative material. Also because it is tooth coloured, it is the material of choice for anterior restorations. It has reasonable wear resistance and, when used with the acid-etch technique, has adhesive properties which obviate the need for mechanical retentive means as described for amalgam restorations. The earlier composite materials were a two-paste system of a base and catalyst, but nearly all modern versions are polymerised by use of a curing light giving the advantage that the setting of the material is under the control of the operator. The main disadvantage of composite resin is that it is technique sensitive and any contamination, such as by moisture, will prevent adequate adhesion. Also there is considerable polymerisation shrinkage on curing and therefore a large cavity needs to be filled and cured in a number of small increments.

Glass ionomer

Glass ionomer is a restorative material which comes in two main forms. As a cement it consists of a base and an acidic water soluble powder. The resultant combination is set by a chemical reaction to form a material that is susceptible to wear and fracture. It does have the benefit of adhesive properties and contains fluoride, thus providing some cariostatic effect on surrounding dental tissues. More recently introduced are the resin-modified glass ionomers which, as the name suggests, have a resin incorporated; this provides greater fracture and wear resistance as well as the ability to be polymerised by a curing light (see Chapter 9).

Cavity preparation in primary teeth

The modification that is required for cavity preparation in primary teeth as compared with the permanent counterparts is based on the differing tooth morphology. Primary teeth are small and hence the overall dimensions of cavities must be reduced accordingly. Furthermore, pulp horns tend to be more pronounced in primary teeth, thus creating an additional hazard.

The prevalence of pit and fissure caries in primary teeth is far less than the permanent counterparts because the fissures are shallower and less plaque retentive. Where it does occur, the class I cavity design reflects the difference in tooth size and depth compared with a permanent tooth.

After the administration of a local anaesthetic, gaining access to the carious lesion is by use of a medium rose-head high-speed or slow-speed bur to a depth of about 1.5 mm (i.e. just into dentine). Lateral movement of the bur at this depth removes caries at the enamel–dentine junction and any residual caries may be removed using a medium excavator, taking care where the cavity base is close to the pulp. Unsupported enamel must be removed and the cavosurface angle should be approximately 90°. If amalgam is the restorative material then it is essential for the cavity to be undercut in order to provide mechanical retention. It is no longer necessary to extend the cavity throughout the whole of the fissure system, provided it is caries-free, and therefore the occlusal extent of the cavity is determined mainly to ensure that adequate access is achieved for caries removal. A lining is necessary for deeper parts of the cavity but none is required where the cavity base is a minimal depth (i.e. just into dentine). Class V cavities for cervical buccal or lingual caries are approached in a similar way to a class I cavity.

The largest type of carious cavities in primary teeth are proximal lesions in molar teeth and their treatment involves the placement of a class II restoration (for definition see Chapter 13). Access to the carious lesion is via the marginal ridge if intact (Figure 12.11a). The proximal box should be extended towards the cervical margin, not only to remove the carious enamel and dentine, but also to take this part of the cavity below the contact area. Buccal and lingual margins should also be placed in relatively self-cleansing areas if possible and converge to the occlusal surface (Figure 12.11b). There should be a 90° cavosurface angle. The axial wall should be parallel with the outer contour of the tooth and should have a depth of approximately 1 mm. The width of the isthmus for an amalgam restoration should be approximately one half to one third of the intercuspal width and should reach a depth of 1.5–2 mm; the occlusal lock should only be sufficient to provide adequate resistance form. Overextension into the whole of the fissure system would invariably weaken the remaining crown (Figure 12.11c). As with a permanent tooth, the pulpoaxial junction should be bevelled in order to avoid stress build-up in the amalgam which could result in fracture of the restoration (Figure 12.11d). A lining prior to placement of the restoration in deep cavities is desirable to provide protection for the open dentinal tubules and also to act as a thermal barrier to prevent conducted temperature changes resulting in sensitivity or pulpal damage. Calcium hydroxide is a particularly good material for lining deep cavities that are close to pulpal exposure.

Preformed crowns

Where there has been more extensive loss of tooth tissue, an intracoronal restoration, such as an amalgam or composite resin filling, would not be strong enough; full coronal coverage provided by a metal preformed crown would be more appropriate. These are usually made from stainless steel, although other metals such as nickel–chromium have been used in the past.

Metal preformed crowns are indicated where the tooth has:

- Extensive caries with loss of two or more cusps.
- Weakened internal structure following pulp treatment.
- Cuspal fracture as a result of indirect trauma (sudden closure of the mandibular teeth against the maxillary teeth).
- Excessive tooth wear, e.g. due to bruxism or erosion.
- Defective enamel, e.g. enamel hypoplasia or amelogenesis imperfecta.

In addition, a preformed crown may be used to construct a space maintainer to prevent adjacent teeth moving into the area of a missing tooth.

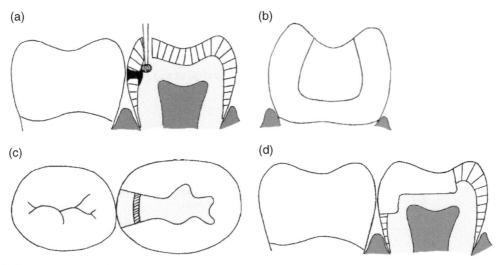

(a)　(b)　(c)　(d)

Figure 12.11 Clinical stages in class II cavity preparation in primary teeth.

Metal crowns are prefabricated for each primary molar tooth. Thus they may be maxillary or mandibular, first or second molar tooth, and either left or right. For each of these eight teeth there are usually six different sizes to cater for the variation in mesiodistal diameters of most teeth encountered.

After the administration of a local anaesthetic, the primary molar crown is reduced on all aspects in order to provide sufficient space to accommodate the stainless steel crown. This is usually achieved in a systematic way with the occlusal surface first being reduced by 1.5 mm (Figure 12.12a). It is important that an even layer is removed as the preparation should reflect the original contour of the tooth. Simply flattening the occlusal surface usually involves the removal of the cuspal areas with very little, if any, tooth tissue removed from the fissure areas. Such a preparation would lead to a crown that would be too high and severely interfere with the occlusion. The proximal surfaces are reduced next using a high-speed tapering fissure bur to create a sloping preparation approximately 15° to the long axis of the tooth (Figure 12.12b). The finish at the gingival margin is a shoulderless preparation and it is important that a shoulder is not inadvertently created. Should this occur then it will prevent the stainless steel crown from seating properly in the cervical region. Care should also be exercised to avoid damaging the adjacent tooth (**iatrogenic damage**). The reduction of the lingual and buccal surfaces is the same as for the proximal surfaces, again taking care not to inadvertently create a shoulder at any part around the cervical margin of the tooth. The last part of the procedure is to eliminate any sharp angles to ensure a smooth rounded preparation (Figure 12.12c).

A crown is now selected and, as mentioned previously, there will be six different sizes for any particular tooth. A crown is chosen to provide the best fit, particularly at the cervical margin. A crown which is too small will not seat into position whilst an oversized crown will give rise to overhanging margins, resulting in plaque retention and ultimately poor gingival health. An ideal crown should be a reasonably tight fit as it is pushed into place

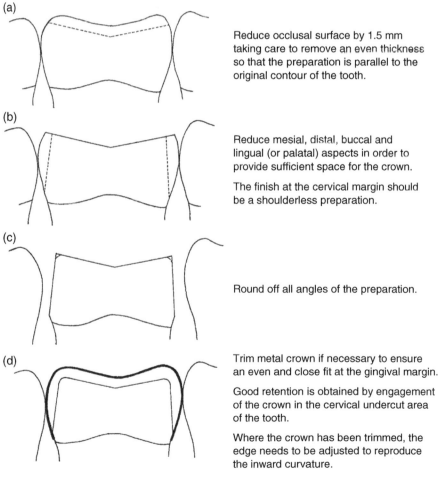

(a) Reduce occlusal surface by 1.5 mm taking care to remove an even thickness so that the preparation is parallel to the original contour of the tooth.

(b) Reduce mesial, distal, buccal and lingual (or palatal) aspects in order to provide sufficient space for the crown.

The finish at the cervical margin should be a shoulderless preparation.

(c) Round off all angles of the preparation.

(d) Trim metal crown if necessary to ensure an even and close fit at the gingival margin.

Good retention is obtained by engagement of the crown in the cervical undercut area of the tooth.

Where the crown has been trimmed, the edge needs to be adjusted to reproduce the inward curvature.

Figure 12.12 Clinical stages of preparation of primary molar tooth for a preformed crown.

to engage the undercut just beyond the shoulderless preparation (Figure 12.12d).

It can now be appreciated why a shoulder anywhere would be detrimental, as the edge of the preformed crown would merely sit on the shoulder and no amount of reasonable force would move the crown into the cervical area. Most crowns will seldom be the correct height and invariably, without adjustment, would stand above the occlusal level. Crowns can be trimmed around the cervical margins with a pair of Beebe scissors or shears until the crown seats at the correct occlusal height. Any sharp edges need to be reduced and polished using a green stone and rubber wheel in a slow handpiece. Once a preformed crown has been trimmed in this way, the margins no longer curve inwards and, to restore this contour, the crown needs to be crimped using a pair of orthodontic pliers (e.g. Adams pliers). This involves gripping the edge of the crown and bending the margin inwards and working along the whole perimeter. Having carried out this procedure, the stainless steel crown will have a minimal overhang at the gingival margin. Having first protected any deep areas with calcium hydroxide, the crown can then be cemented with an appropriate luting cement, taking care to remove any excess material which might otherwise cause gingival irritation and plaque stagnation. The occlusion should be checked again when the crown is seated to confirm that there is no premature contact.

Hall technique for preformed crowns

More recently the Hall technique has been introduced for the management of carious primary molar teeth. It is a simplified method of applying preformed crowns with no local analgesia, caries removal, nor tooth preparation. This procedure is a departure from the concept that caries removal is essential and very much depends on completely sealing the carious lesion leading to an arrest of the process or, at the very least, slowing of its progress. No preparation of the tooth invariably results in an oversized preformed crown being used and therefore occlusal interference after application is very common. Fortunately, children adapt very quickly to such occlusal problems and very few complain of persistent symptoms. Where there is lack of interproximal spacing it is often difficult to apply the preformed crown at that visit and therefore it would be necessary to use separators for a week in order to create the slight space that is required for adequate placement. The advantage of the Hall technique is that it can be used to treat multicarious dentitions where perhaps previously extractions may have been considered. Furthermore, the need for local analgesia and tooth preparation is obviated, and therefore this technique may be more acceptable to young and/or dentally anxious children.

The Hall technique is an established procedure and randomised control clinical trials have shown a high degree of acceptability by patients and greater favourable outcomes in terms of pulpal health and restoration longevity compared with conventional restorations.

Strip crowns for anterior primary teeth

The upper anterior primary teeth are particularly vulnerable to 'nursing' caries, where not only are the interproximal surfaces affected, but also the labial. As these teeth are relatively small, the incisal edge becomes quickly involved and results in an extensive carious lesion. Despite the advent of adhesive materials, such a cavity would be difficult to restore and therefore a strip crown may provide the solution.

Strip crowns are cellulose acetate crown formers, which are designed for primary central or lateral incisors, and for left and right teeth. For each particular tooth there is a number of sizes and the one that matches the contralateral tooth is usually the one that provides the best fit, i.e. if an upper left central incisor is being restored, the best size of crown will be the size that matches the upper right central incisor.

Following the administration of a local anaesthetic and, preferably, the application of dental dam, the tooth is reduced in a similar way to the preparation for a preformed crown on a posterior primary tooth. Caries is removed and any deep parts should be lined with calcium hydroxide.

The incisal edge is reduced by 2 mm using a fine high-speed tapering diamond bur and then the proximal surfaces are reduced in order to produce a 15° taper with a shoulderless finish at the gingival margin (Figure 12.13a and b). The labial and palatal surfaces are prepared in the same way and the whole preparation is rounded to avoid any sharp angles (Figure 12.13c). The strip crown is usually too long and needs to be trimmed at the cervical margin with a sharp pair of fine curved scissors. Application of the strip crown to the preparation should result in the cervical part of the crown being trimmed to the gingival margin whilst at the same time the incisal edge should be level with the contralateral tooth. Using a straight probe, the strip crown is pierced at the mesial and distal incisal angles. This will form a vent in order to assist air and excess composite material to escape, thus preventing air pockets developing in the material. The tooth is etched, irrigated and dried followed by the application of a bonding agent. The strip crown is filled with composite and is pushed firmly over the preparation. Excess material is expressed through the incisal vents and also at the cervical margin. The latter may be removed prior to curing using a probe or Wards wax carver (Figure 12.13d). After polymerisation the

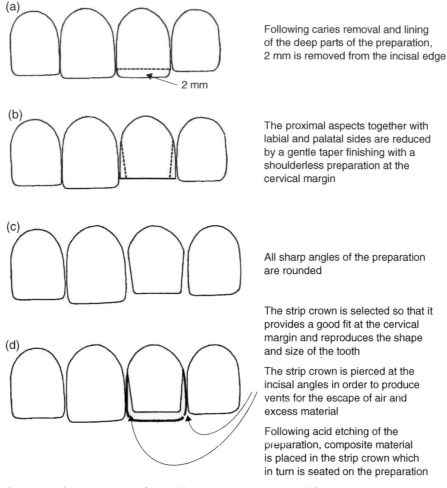

(a) Following caries removal and lining of the deep parts of the preparation, 2 mm is removed from the incisal edge

2 mm

(b) The proximal aspects together with labial and palatal sides are reduced by a gentle taper finishing with a shoulderless preparation at the cervical margin

(c) All sharp angles of the preparation are rounded

(d) The strip crown is selected so that it provides a good fit at the cervical margin and reproduces the shape and size of the tooth

The strip crown is pierced at the incisal angles in order to produce vents for the escape of air and excess material

Following acid etching of the preparation, composite material is placed in the strip crown which in turn is seated on the preparation

Figure 12.13 Clinical stages in the preparation of a maxillary anterior primary tooth for a strip crown.

strip crown can easily be removed by inserting a probe or excavator between the crown and composite material which enables it to peel away from the composite, leaving a very smooth composite surface. The hardened excess composite at the cervical margin and at the incisal angles can be smoothed using rotary finishing and polishing instruments. Finally the occlusion should be checked for premature occlusal contacts. The end result is a restoration which not only restores function and eliminates caries, but also restores aesthetics.

Pulp treatment in primary molar teeth

Pulpal exposures due to caries are much more likely in primary teeth than permanent teeth because the thickness of dentine is relatively less and hence the carious process can traverse this tissue much more rapidly. In addition, primary molar teeth have a much larger contact area and interproximal caries is much more difficult to detect clinically unless it has reached a fairly advanced stage. Once overt clinical changes can be observed, such as the breakdown of the mesial or distal marginal ridge, the caries process will probably have reached the pulp and pulp treatment may be the only alternative to an extraction. There are different types of procedures that can be carried out, depending on the extent of the changes within the pulp (Ranly and Garcia-Godoy, 2000).

Indirect pulp cap

Indirect pulp capping is appropriate where a tooth has been asymptomatic and caries removal has revealed a deep cavity, at the base of which is a thin layer of dentine covering pulpal tissue. This layer of dentine may be reasonably hard but not entirely caries free, but it is preferable to leave this intact rather than create an exposure. The indirect pulp cap using **calcium hydroxide** has two benefits: firstly the material induces secondary dentine to form on the pulpal aspect, thus providing a natural barrier to the caries process; and secondly the high alkalinity of the calcium hydroxide has a bactericidal effect on the microorganisms on the affected dentine. The success rate of indirect pulp capping is high if used under the correct circumstances and can obviate the need for more complex treatment.

Direct pulp cap

Where a carious exposure has occurred, any attempt at just applying a pulp cap using calcium hydroxide will invariably result in failure. Primary teeth have a lesser ability to resist the spread of pulpal infection compared with permanent teeth, and the child will return after a few weeks with symptoms of pulpal necrosis. Perhaps the only circumstance where a direct pulp cap may be justified is when pulp exposure has occurred as a result of a traumatic exposure during cavity preparation. There will have been less opportunity for bacterial contamination in this instance.

Pulpotomy

This procedure is indicated where there is a pulpal exposure but the tooth is asymptomatic or exhibits signs of reversible pulpitis. The latter is characterised by pain of short duration or where the tooth is sensitive to temperature changes. Thus a cold drink may elicit some discomfort which disappears quickly. This indicates that the pulp has undergone inflammatory changes but this is probably confined to the coronal part only and the radicular pulp tissue is likely to remain unaffected. The vital pulpotomy therefore involves the elimination of the coronal pulp, which allows the remainder of the pulp to be retained.

In addition to the general indications and contraindications for restoring primary teeth mentioned earlier, more specific considerations in respect of pulp treatment of primary molar teeth are listed below:

Indications

- Extensive caries with loss of one third or more of the marginal ridge.
- At least two thirds of the root remaining.
- Absence of abscess or sinus.
- No radicular bone loss.
- No evidence of internal resorption.

Contraindications

- Bi- or trifurcation involvement.
- Less than two thirds of root remaining.

The tooth (Figure 12.14a) is anaesthetised and with isolation under a dental dam, all remaining caries is removed together with the roof of the pulp chamber. This exposes the coronal pulpal contents, which then may be removed by a slowly rotating rosehead bur leaving the floor of the pulp chamber bereft of all pulp tissue except for the apertures of the root canals (Figure 12.14b). Care

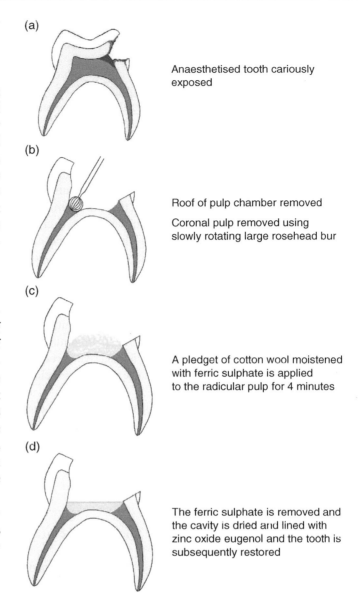

(a) Anaesthetised tooth cariously exposed

(b) Roof of pulp chamber removed

Coronal pulp removed using slowly rotating large rosehead bur

(c) A pledget of cotton wool moistened with ferric sulphate is applied to the radicular pulp for 4 minutes

(d) The ferric sulphate is removed and the cavity is dried and lined with zinc oxide eugenol and the tooth is subsequently restored

Figure 12.14 Pulpotomy clinical stages.

is required to avoid inadvertent perforation of the floor of the pulp chamber with the rosehead bur. The vacant pulp chamber is irrigated with water using the triple syringe and dried with a cotton pledget. The bleeding from the radicular pulp should have stopped so as to leave a clear, dry pulp chamber floor.

Ferric sulphate (15.5% concentration) is now applied to treat the remaining pulp; this is applied for 30 seconds with a lightly moistened cotton pledget (Figure 12.14c). The ferric sulphate is an astringent and therefore reduces any bleeding that might occasionally occur from the radicular pulp. The pledget is removed and the floor of pulp chamber and the radicular pulp are covered with a lining of zinc oxide eugenol (Figure 12.14d) and the tooth is restored in the appropriate way. Should a composite resin be the restorative material then an additional lining, such as zinc phosphate, is required to prevent the adverse effect of the zinc oxide eugenol on the setting of the composite resin.

An alternative to ferric sulphate as a pulpotomy medicament is mineral trioxide aggregate (MTA). This material is relatively new but clinical trials have indicated that its success rate as assessed by clinical and radiographic criteria is at least comparable to ferric sulphate.

In cases where there is evidence of irreversible pulpitis, characterised by constant pain exacerbated by thermal changes, the assumption is that inflammatory changes extend throughout the pulpal tissue, including the radicular pulp. Application of ferric sulphate as before would be unsuccessful as this would be placed on inflamed tissue. Where there is an irreversible pulpitis, the coronal pulp is removed under local anaesthesia as described above, and **Ledermix** is placed over the radicular pulp. This is a proprietary paste which contains a corticosteroid (1% triamcinolone) and an antibiotic (3% chlortetracycline). The former is effective in reducing the inflammation whilst the latter has bactericidal properties.

The success of a pulpotomy procedure is indicated clinically by:

- The absence of pain and swelling.
- No tenderness to percussion.
- No pathological mobility.

It is indicated radiographically by:

- The absence of pathological radiolucency at the furcation area of the root.
- Normal root resorption as part of the exfoliation process.

Should failure occur as demonstrated by these signs and symptoms, then an extraction is usually indicated.

Soft tissue problems in children

Teething

Discomfort and associated problems occurring at the time of the emergence of teeth in the mouth are experienced more in the primary dentition than in the permanent dentition. The pathogenesis is the same for both dentitions, but where it occurs in younger children with the eruption of the primary dentition, the level of tolerance of the symptoms is far less than with adults due to their immaturity; young children are likely to seek a greater degree of attention from their parents.

The changes that occur during tooth movement into the oral cavity can cause the surrounding gingival tissues to be inflamed. This leads to some soreness, which in turn provides difficulty in keeping the area clean, which can further exacerbate the inflammation. Fortunately, this is only a transient problem and will resolve spontaneously when eruption of the tooth is further advanced. In young children, this problem is described as 'teething'. Very often the local problems are associated with systemic involvement, such as accompanying diarrhoea, raised temperature and sleepless nights. It is difficult to explain how local problems of teething can cause systemic problems as described. One explanation is that they are not linked and they are purely coincidental – i.e. there is an association but not a cause and effect. Teething is almost a continuous process from the age of 6 months to 2½ years, and any of the systemic problems that occur during this period may be conveniently attributed to 'teething' in the absence of any other obvious cause. Another explanation is that eruption of teeth causes local soreness as previously explained and there is a tendency for the child to place his or her fingers in the mouth. As young children go through a phase of crawling as their main mode of getting around prior to learning to walk, it would not be unreasonable to assume that infections may be picked up this way and transferred to the gastrointestinal tract which might explain the symptoms experienced.

Usually a mild **analgesic** for the discomfort and an **antipyretic** for the raised temperature may be given. Paediatric paracetamol suspension (e.g. Cupal, Panadol, Calpol) has both these qualities and is usually the drug of choice. There are various proprietary teething gels (Dentinox) which can provide analgesic and anti-inflammatory properties to the local area.

Chronic gingivitis

Most chronic gingivitis in children is plaque induced and therefore poor or inadequate oral hygiene is the most common aetiological factor. There may be predisposing factors which make plaque removal more difficult (e.g. lack of manual dexterity in tooth brushing, irregular teeth, overhanging margins of restorations, presence of orthodontic appliances, etc.) or increased sensitivity of the gingival tissues to plaque toxins (e.g. hormonal changes during puberty).

The main line of treatment is to improve oral hygiene and plaque control, concentrating on any areas frequently missed, for instance the lingual aspect of the lower incisors or around orthodontic brackets. Any overhanging margins of restorations should be corrected. The use of a plaque index accompanied by regular toothbrush instruction is extremely useful as an aid to achieving acceptable levels of plaque control.

Acute herpetic gingivostomatitis

This is a relatively common infection affecting usually preschool children but it can occur in older children and adults. It is a viral infection which is passed usually by direct contact, and the usual scenario is that the young child has come into contact with an adult who has active **herpes labialis** or 'cold sores'. After a short incubation period the child becomes unwell with a high temperature. Shortly afterwards the mouth becomes sore and small vesicles appear on the tongue, gingivae and hard palate. These vesicles burst to leave ulcers which are very painful. Despite these acute symptoms, the infection is self-limiting and within 2 days the ulcers start to heal and the whole episode subsides in about a week or 10 days.

Usually no treatment is required apart from reassurance to the parents and a high fluid intake. Analgesics and antipyretics in the form of paracetamol suspension may be given for the discomfort and the high temperature. Where the painful ulcers are causing prolonged problems, a topical application of 1% **chlorhexidine gluconate** (Corsodyl Gel) or 0.15% **benzydamine hydrochloride** (Difflam Spray) to the ulcers may be required to make them more comfortable. On occasions a systemic antiviral drug such as **aciclovir** (Zovirax) is used, but by the time the child presents in the dental surgery, the vesicles on the oral mucosa have normally progressed to ulcer formation, which is the start of the healing process and therefore the drug would have only a very limited effect. However, it may be advocated in babies who may have a habit of putting their fingers in their mouths and immediately rubbing their eyes. As the vesicles break down to form ulcers, the virus is released into the saliva and this infected material may be transferred to the eyes, resulting in an ocular infection and the use of aciclovir may prevent this spread of infection. Also children who are immunocompromised are at great risk of developing very serious complications from the acute herpetic gingivostomatitis and therefore the administration of aciclovir at an early stage is important.

Herpes labialis

Once the primary herpetic infection has subsided, the virus is not eliminated from the body but lies dormant in the tissues. At times when the body resistance is lowered (e.g. having a cold, etc.), then the virus reactivates. These secondary lesions appear on and around the lips initially as vesicles but they coalesce to form larger lesions. These, like the primary infection, are self-limiting and disappear within about 10 days. Topical aciclovir may be used at the early stages to prevent or limit this local infection. As mentioned before it is the virus in these secondary lesions in the adult which may be passed to a young child, which in turn gives rise to the primary herpetic gingivostomatitis.

Traumatic ulcers

These are quite common in children and arise as a result of trauma to the mucosa. An accident such as a fall or inadvertent lip or cheek biting are the usual causes. Children who have had a local anaesthetic may be susceptible to lip biting whilst the numbness is wearing off and therefore it is always advisable to warn the child and parents to take particular care during this recovery period.

The surface of the mucosa is damaged and after a day or so the surface layer breaks down to form a typical ulcer. The size and shape are governed by the area traumatised and, logically, the larger the ulcer, the longer it will take to heal. The base of the ulcer has nerve endings which make the area particularly painful to touch or to hot or spicy foods. The ulcers heal within a week or 10 days without any treatment, although if they are particularly uncomfortable topical use of benzydamine hydrochloride (Difflam) or chlorhexidine (Corsodyl) may be considered.

Recurrent aphthous ulcers

These are ulcers that, as the name suggests, occur on a regular basis. They are more likely to occur in older children and young adults and the aetiology is unknown, although it has been reported that predisposing factors may be stress or deficiencies in the blood such as folate, serum iron or vitamin B12. There can be a familial history (see Chapter 3, p. 55). The presentation of these ulcers can be varied but usually they fall into one of three groups (Field et al., 1992):

- **Major aphthous ulceration**: large ulcers usually greater than 5 mm in diameter occurring singly or in small numbers.
- **Minor aphthous ulceration**: medium-sized ulcers approximately 2–5 mm in diameter occurring in crops around the mouth.
- **Herpetiform aphthous ulceration**: not related in any way to the primary herpes infection as described above, but presents as a very similar clinical appearance with numerous small ulcers. The differential diagnosis is that, unlike the primary herpes, there is usually no pyrexia and ulcers do not appear on the hard palate.

The appearance and location of major and minor aphthae are described in Chapter 3.

The main features of all three types of aphthous ulceration is that the aetiology is unknown and that they are

Table 12.3 Topical medicaments which are commonly used in the treatment of recurrent aphthous ulcers.

Method of administration	Active ingredients	Proprietary names
Mouthwashes	Benzydamine hydrochloride	Difflam Oral Rinse Difflam Oral Spray
	Chlorhexidine gluconate	Corsodyl Mouthwash
Lozenges	Hydrocortisone lozenges	Corlan Pellets

recurrent. Often a group of ulcers heals and there may be a lesion-free period before the next crop of ulcers appears. There are also patients in whom it is a continuous process where one cycle of ulcers merges into the next cycle, resulting in the individual never being free from ulcers.

Treatment will entail the diagnosis of the causative factors, if any, by blood tests, etc. and elimination of any systemic causes. The ulcers are painful but heal in about 10–14 days, although the larger major aphthous ulcers may take much longer. There may be difficulties in eating and it may be particularly distressing for children as sleep may be disturbed. Topical treatment may be given in severe cases and, although it does not prevent ulcers from occurring nor make them heal any faster, it does alleviate symptoms (Table 12.3).

Anxiety and pain control

Behavioural management

General considerations

The ability to be receptive of dental treatment depends on many factors, and this includes the degree of co-operation and the type of treatment that needs to be carried out. Children and adolescents comprise a group of individuals representing a large variation in age, psychology and personality, temperament and emotion, dental experience and welfare. All these factors influence the child's behaviour in the dental environment. Many young patients are deemed 'anxious' or 'unco-operative' and carry this stigma for many years. It has to be remembered that, generally, as children get older they become more mature and are able to accept potentially unpleasant events such as dental treatment. In addition, for the same child, some procedures will be accepted more readily than others. For instance, non-invasive treatment, such as fissure sealing, will evoke a greater degree of co-operation than invasive procedures, such as extractions.

Very young children of 3 years and under are termed '**preco-operative**' in that they do not have a sufficient level of maturity and understanding to tolerate even the simplest of procedures. By the time they have attained 4 or 5 years of age, children may be attending nursery or primary school and will begin to listen with interest. They have lively minds and will ask questions. Their fear of strangers is also lessened. From 6 years of age onwards, a child becomes increasingly independent of parents and may be separated from their parents if well prepared. Their dental fears are often successfully resolved because they can be influenced by reason and explanation and also, as they become more mature, they develop tolerance to unpleasant situations.

It is essential that the surgery environment should be as non-threatening as possible and should be child-friendly. It may be worth considering using an office or oral health room for the initial part of the first visit as this would provide the child with a little more confidence to go into a dental surgery at a later stage. Surgery clothing is essential as a barrier against cross-infection, but to a young child, this may evoke fear and distrust. It may be advantageous to temporarily abandon the clinical uniform, certainly for the initial stages whilst the child is familiarising himself or herself with this new environment.

Communication

Communication skills are the most important tools to achieve confidence with dental treatment for children. Good communication allows the clinician to entrust the child with a positive outlook to dental care and reassure the parents' confidence within the dental environment, thus proving a better dental experience for both child and parent.

Basic communication skills may be verbal and non-verbal communication. Verbal communication entails questioning, listening and explaining. Non-verbal communication is based on body language, eye-contact, and tone and pitch of speech, all of which should occur all the time throughout the appointment. Language should always be age appropriate in order to provide a good level of understanding.

Acclimatisation

Children need to be introduced to new events in a gradual way. Acclimatisation or **behavioural shaping** is a procedure used in everyday activities in order to teach children to cope. The stage-by-stage exposure to dental procedures, starting with the very simple and building up to more complex procedures over a series of visits, increases confidence and enables a child to become accustomed to routine dental care. The least traumatic of procedures is an oral examination with the child seated in the dental chair, but with some younger children this may prove to be difficult and the starting point in this case would be perhaps with the child sitting on the parent's lap. From examination, a prophylaxis using a polishing rubber cup in a slow speed handpiece would be the next stage. This is the first introduction to the use of rotary instruments in the child's mouth and a procedure which may be described to the patient as using an 'electric toothbrush'. This may be followed on a subsequent appointment with fissure sealing/topical fluoride treatment and, thereafter, a small simple restoration without local analgesia and then later a restoration with local analgesia.

Over a series of appointments the child will gain sufficient confidence and develop trust in the operator such that most procedures can be carried out successfully. However, how many visits it takes depends on the progress a child makes at each appointment. For some the goal can be achieved in relatively few visits; for others the process will take longer. There is no doubt that it is a time-consuming technique and may take several visits before even the first restoration is completed. However, once this has been achieved, treatment can proceed quickly with the patient's full co-operation.

Tell-show-do

Many dental anxieties are generated because of the fear of the unknown. It will be a new experience for the child and they do not know what to expect. Tell-show-do serves to overcome this problem to a certain extent. It is exactly as the name suggests in that a simple explanation of what is to be done is given, followed by a demonstration, and finally carrying out the procedure. To give an example, a child can be introduced to a prophylaxis by first describing an 'electric toothbrush', which can then be demonstrated on the child's finger nail. After this has been accepted, the labial surfaces of the upper central incisors may be polished with the patient observing with a face mirror. This is then followed by polishing all the other surfaces of the rest of the teeth. This same technique can be applied to other treatments and it is important that the transition through the three stages of tell-show-do occurs as a continuous procedure.

Enhancing control

When a child requires dental treatment, it is usually not through their own choice nor decision to go and seek help. This decision is usually made by parents or guardians. The child is then taken to the surgery and required to sit in the chair and undergo treatment accordingly. All these actions are generally not of the child's own free will. The technique of enhancing control gives the child some degree of control over the clinician's actions through the use of a stop signal. Such a signal has been shown to reduce stress during routine dental treatment.

The stop signal, usually by raising an arm, should be rehearsed and the clinician must respond quickly when it is used, even if the child is only testing the clinician! This also helps the child to gain trust and build a rapport with the clinician, as the child knows that the clinician is responding to their actions.

Modelling

Children can observe other children in order to imitate their actions. Thus a child can watch a child ascending a climbing frame and then be more confident in imitating those actions. If a child dental patient can observe another patient receiving treatment then this may provide the encouragement for him/her to respond in the same way. In the absence of a 'live' model, photographs or drawings may be used instead. It is important that the patient can identify with the 'model' and therefore the model needs to be of the same or similar age and gender. There is sometimes a temptation to use a model who is younger in an attempt to embarrass the young patient into co-operating. However, this is likely to have a negative effect as the patient cannot identify with the model and sees no reason to attempt to behave in the same way.

Reinforcement

This is a technique by which a pattern of behaviour may be enhanced by reward (positive reinforcement) or by punishment (negative reinforcement). Whilst the former has important significance in altering and controlling child dental behaviour, the latter has no place in the dental care of children. The behaviour change may include a wide range of activities from diet modification, tooth brushing, etc. to operative procedures, such as the delivery of local analgesia and restorative treatment. Verbal praise from the dental team for good effort on the child's part will provide encouragement for continued similar behaviour. More tangible rewards, such as badges, colouring posters, etc., may also have the desired effect. On occasions it may be that little has been achieved during the session owing to negative behaviour by the child, but it still may be prudent to provide positive reinforcement in the usual way in an effort to encourage the child to try harder on the next visit.

Desensitisation

This is a behavioural management technique that has been developed and used by psychologists in helping to overcome fears by gradual exposure to the cause. It is not too dissimilar to acclimatisation or behavioural shaping as described above, except that it focuses on a particular phobia or dislike. If for instance a child has a fear of the 'drill', then over a series of visits this may be introduced in stages until it is accepted. Initial visits would entail explaining and demonstrating the equipment. Subsequent appointments would allow the patient to handle the handpiece and become accustomed to the feel and the noise it emits and, finally, to accept its use in his/her mouth.

Sedation

Occasionally normal behavioural management techniques are insufficient alone to gain co-operative behaviour for adequate dental treatment and sedation may be required. Whilst the mode of administration of sedative drugs can be via various routes, the most commonly used technique is that of inhalation sedation using nitrous oxide.

Nitrous oxide

Nitrous oxide has been used for many years as a general anaesthetic agent but because of its low potency, it has been superseded by other more efficient inhalational agents for this purpose. At lower concentrations it has been shown to be an effective sedative agent in children and, over the past 30 years, it has become the sedation method of choice in paediatric dentistry. The advantages of this technique are that it is non-invasive and does not require the use of injections for its administration which is often the major problem perceived by anxious children. The onset of sedation is fast and the peak clinical effect occurs in about 10 minutes. The recovery period is usually equally fast and patients are commonly fully reversed within 15 minutes of the end of the procedure. The disadvantages are that it requires the use of a nasal mask, which some children find unpleasant and it also limits access, particularly if upper anterior teeth are being treated. The equipment is expensive and the capital outlay for an average dental practice is prohibitive unless it is used on a regular rather than an occasional basis. A further problem is the pollution of the surgery atmosphere with nitrous oxide which, if excessive, would pose potential health and safety issues for the staff involved.

Indications for nitrous oxide include:

- Mild or moderate dental anxiety.
- Pronounced gag reflex.
- Intellectually impaired.
- Ineffective local analgesia (see below).

Contraindications include:

- Extreme unco-operative behaviour.
- Preco-operative children.
- Nasal obstruction, e.g. common cold.
- Chronic obstructive pulmonary disease.
- Patients with psychiatric disorders.
- Pregnancy.

As well as sedative properties, nitrous oxide also provides a degree of analgesia (hence the term often used for this method of sedation – **relative analgesia**). This attribute can be useful where local analgesia is not very effective (e.g. the presence of acute infection) or contraindicated (e.g. a history of haemophilia). Nitrous oxide sedation may provide sufficient analgesia for the restoration of small or moderate cavities, but would be insufficient for procedures such as extractions and pulp treatment.

Other forms of sedation

Oral sedation using tablets or medicines provides a convenient method of administration but, whilst its effectiveness has been demonstrated in adults, there are few studies that have shown similar success in children. The main problem is the slow and unpredictable absorption of the drug from the digestive tract which in turn leads to an unpredictable sedative effect. Similarly, the unpredictability of intravenous sedation in younger children has meant that this method is contraindicated, although it may have a place in the treatment of adolescents.

Sedation is a specialist subject beyond the scope of this book. A more extensive review of sedation may be found in *Advanced Dental Nursing* (Ireland, 2004).

Local analgesia

The question often arises as to whether or not a local analgesic is required for restorations in children. The simple answer is 'yes' unless you can be sure that your procedure is going to be painless. Therefore, bearing in mind that primary teeth (except when approaching natural exfoliation) may be just as sensitive as permanent teeth, a local analgesic will ensure a comfortable procedure. Not giving a local analgesic, on the other hand, can lead to pain which in turn reverses the trust and confidence that the child may have had, and more often than not the treatment is abandoned. Although it may take time and patience on the part of the clinician, patient and parent or guardian, by using the behavioural management techniques previously described in getting children to accept a local analgesic, the end result will provide much more satisfactory conditions for successful treatment.

The administration of the local analgesic is very similar to that for adults but with some important differences. As well as proper psychological preparation (appropriate explanation, using terms such as 'sleepy juice', etc.), the use of a topical analgesic prior to the injection is extremely important. There are numerous proprietary topical analgesics but the most popular one is 20% **benzocaine** which may be flavoured in order to disguise the unpleasant taste. This should be applied to the dried mucosa for at least 2 minutes in order to have the optimal effect. Not only is the trauma of the injection lessened by the pharmacological effects of the topical application, but it also provides valuable psychological support.

In young children, **infiltrations** can be effective in providing analgesia for mandibular restorations, whereas in older children or in adults an inferior dental nerve block will be required for at least the molar teeth. The reason for this is that a successful infiltration injection relies on the local analgesic solution permeating through the bone and reaching the periapical areas. This is achieved in the younger child, but as she or he gets older, the cortical layer of the mandible becomes more dense and less porous, thus preventing the local analgesic reaching the teeth. A 'rule of ten' has been described which provides guidance as to when an infiltration will suffice and when a block is required and this is outlined below:

- The tooth to be anaesthetised is assigned a number according to its position. A central incisor is 1; lateral incisor is 2; canine is 3 and so on.
- This number is added to the age of the child.
- If the result is 10 or less, then an infiltration will be appropriate.
- If the summation is over 10 then a block is required.

Thus if a 5-year-old child requires a restoration in the second primary molar (tooth number 5), then an infiltration is fine. However, if a 7-year-old requires similar treatment for a first primary molar (tooth number 4), then an inferior dental nerve block is required. Thus in younger children an inferior dental block, which is usually more unpleasant and causes a much greater area of soft tissue anaesthesia with potential problems of inadvertent lip biting, etc., can be obviated.

In the maxilla, as in adults, infiltration local analgesia is usually effective. The region that may have inadequate analgesia is the upper permanent first molar area. The reason for this is that the **zygomatic arch**, which forms the cheek bone, is attached to the maxilla just above this tooth and anatomically the bone is thickened and more dense than elsewhere in the maxilla, thus preventing penetration of the local analgesic solution. This is more likely to be a problem in children in the 6–8-year-old age group, as this denser bone lies over the apices of the permanent first molar tooth at this age. As the child becomes older, growth of the maxilla takes place and, in particular, downward alveolar growth moves the teeth and the apices away from the zygomatic arch. Where there is a problem securing adequate anaesthesia, this is usually overcome by injecting slightly mesially and distally, allowing a sideways spread of the local analgesic solution.

The amount of local analgesic solution used should be enough to provide adequate analgesia for the procedure to be carried out comfortably: generally speaking, half a cartridge for pre-school children; three quarters for 5–8-year-olds; and a whole cartridge for 9-year-olds and over (see also Chapter 10). Giving less than these quantities runs the risk that analgesia may be inadequate and the child becomes agitated and less co-operative as a result. Furthermore, to have to give a second injection under these circumstances may meet with a refusal.

It has to be borne in mind that, as with all drugs, the maximum dosage is weight dependent and in a small child that limit may be easily reached by extractions in different quadrants at the same visit. A very simple way of calculating the maximum dose for a child is to use 70 kg as the average adult body weight and the proportion of this figure in terms of the child body weight is the maximum dose for that child. Thus a child who weighs 35 kg would be half the average adult body weight and therefore the dose would be half the adult maximum. The three main types of local analgesic solutions used are:

	Maximum dose (mg/kg body weight)
2% lidocaine with 1:80 000 epinephrine (adrenaline)	4.4
3% prilocaine (Citanest) with felypressin	6.0
4% articaine with 1:100 000 epinephrine (adrenaline)	7.0

Thus the solution that has the lowest maximum dose in terms of mg per kg body weight is 2% lidocaine with 1:80 000 epinephrine (adrenaline), which, in fact, is the commonest local analgesic used in both adults and children in the UK. As one cartridge of this solution contains 45 mg, then approximately one tenth of a cartridge equates to the maximum dose per kg body weight. Thus a whole cartridge is the maximum for a child weighing 10 kg. For accuracy we should weigh our child patients but a good guide to the weight may be derived from the following formula:

$(Age + 4) \times 2 = $ weight of child in kilograms

Thus, a child aged 5 would, by this calculation, weigh $(5+4) \times 2 = 18$ kg and the maximum dose would be 1.8 cartridges. This method of estimating a child's weight is a good guide up to 10 years of age.

Other methods of providing local anaesthesia

Intraligamentary injections apply a small amount of solution into the periodontal ligament. A short fine needle is used and is inserted through the mucosa so the point rests at the alveolar crest. A conventional local anaesthetic syringe may be used but it is usually better to use a syringe designed specifically for intraligamentary use. By the use of a lever mechanism, higher pressure may be applied which is usually required for this technique. Only a very small amount of local anaesthetic solution is injected into the periodontal membrane and provides profound analgesia to the area. It has the advantage of giving rise to local analgesia confined to a much smaller area and of limited duration thus avoiding extensive soft tissue numbness for a long period. Unfortunately, as the solution is injected with a considerable amount of pressure, its administration can be somewhat uncomfortable and, owing to the site of the injection, it can lead to transient damage to the periodontal membrane making the tooth tender to percussion for a day or so after the injection.

Perhaps the most significant obstacle to local analgesia in children is that it usually involves 'needles'. Recently a system (**Injex**) has been developed which does not require the use of a hypodermic needle. This needleless system relies on a jet spray of local anaesthetic solution being applied to the mucosa under pressure. The pressure delivers such a force that the solution penetrates not only the mucosa but also the alveolar bone to provide analgesia of the tooth and surrounding tissues. It is a technique which is acceptable to many children as it does not require the use of a needle. On the other hand the sudden release of pressure of the local analgesic solution provides a jarring or a 'kick' which children may find unpleasant.

The use of general anaesthesia in children

In the past, general anaesthesia for exodontia in children was considered to be standard practice, but in the last decade the appropriateness of this method of pain control was brought into question in the light of the number of anaesthetic deaths that occurred each year. The mortality rate in respect of general anaesthesia was 1 in 200 000 and resulted in four or five deaths per year. Whilst this is a relatively small number, by limiting general anaesthesia to cases where the procedure is fully justified on the grounds that other alternatives have been considered, then the number of deaths can be reduced to an absolute minimum.

In 1999, the Royal College of Anaesthetists put forward three criteria for dental anaesthesia in children. These are where:

- Local analgesia is inappropriate or unlikely to be effective, e.g. the presence of an acute abscess.
- The age/maturity of the child will mean that local analgesia cannot be administered safely.
- The procedure will lead to long-term dental phobia.

The ability of a child to cope not only depends on age and maturity, but also on other important factors, such as past dental experience and the dental procedure that needs to be carried out. If a child has had regular treatment over the years, then she or he is likely to be acclimatised and is more likely to be able to cope with treatment under local analgesia, including extractions. On the other hand a child who has never had any treatment before may not have the confidence to undertake treatment without general anaesthesia. It is ironic that children who have regular dental care are less likely to need extractions, whereas those whose attendance is infrequent are the patients that often require extraction. The dental procedure also needs to be taken into consideration. For instance, a simple extraction of a primary tooth may be tolerated reasonably well but the more difficult extraction of a permanent first molar tooth for the same patient may well be beyond the degree of tolerance. Also multiple extractions involving different quadrants or several visits increase the degree of surgical trauma and are less likely to be tolerated. It is not unusual for extractions under local analgesia to be successful on the first visit but, if the child needs to return for additional extractions, then the degree of co-operation is much less.

Dental general anaesthesia can only be performed where there are adequate facilities and personnel for the procedure to be carried out safely. The anaesthetist must be on the anaesthetic specialist register and must have ready access to critical care facilities. Most dental general anaesthetics are therefore carried out in a hospital environment, although there are a number of health centres and community clinics that are able to provide this service. Most dental general anaesthetics are outpatient procedures, but where children require more complicated surgery or if patients are medically compromised then admission to hospital with inpatient facilities is more appropriate. The American Society of Anesthesiologists (ASA) have produced a table that categorises patients according to the medical status (Table 12.4). ASA I and II patients can be adequately treated in an outpatient facility but it is clear that ASA III and IV require inpatient care and intensive pre- and postoperative monitoring.

Table 12.4 The American Society of Anesthesiologists categories of medical status risk.

ASA status	Description	Example
I	Patients who are healthy with no systemic disease	
II	Patients with systemic disease which is controlled and not affecting lifestyle	Controlled asthma, diabetes, epilepsy
III	Patients who have severe systemic disease that limits activity but is not incapacitating	Congenital or acquired heart disease, severe asthma, obesity, poorly controlled diabetes and epilepsy
IV	Incapacitating disease that is a constant threat to life	Uncontrolled diabetes, uncontrolled hypertension, severe cardiopulmonary disease
V	Moribund patients not expected to survive 24 hours	

Trauma in children

Accidental injuries

There are two peak ages for dental trauma: 2–3 years of age when, at the 'toddler' stage, the child is prone to falling, tripping or running into obstructions, and 9–10 years of age when, particularly with boys, there is an increase in boisterous activity, contact sport and playground accidents. In the younger age group the alveolar bone is less well calcified and is more elastic. This less rigid arrangement leads to the traumatised primary teeth becoming displaced or avulsed, which are common injuries. This is in contrast to the older age group, who, by the time they have the permanent upper anterior teeth erupted, have much denser supporting bone, which has a tendency to hold the teeth much more rigidly and the type of injury experienced is, therefore, one of tooth fracture of either the crown or root. Statistics indicate that anterior teeth are much more prone to damage and that upper teeth are ten times more susceptible than lower teeth. In addition, where children have a Class 2 division I anterior malocclusion, characterised by protruding teeth, it is not surprising that the anterior teeth are also many times more likely to be damaged.

Non-accidental injuries

It is prudent to consider this topic because, as health professionals, we need to be in a position to recognise that there may be problems and in so doing put into motion appropriate help not only for the child, but for the whole

Table 12.5 Most frequent areas of non-accidental injuries in children.

Site of bruising		% of children
Head	Scalp	79
	Forehead	52
Face	Cheek	48
	Upper lip	45
	Lower lip	48
Neck		59

family. Non-accidental injury is one of the many categories that come under the heading of **child abuse**, the other main ones being sexual, deprivation and neglect, and poisoning. Whilst its existence has always been recognised, it was not until 1975 that the formal definition below by Cameron and Rae was adopted to describe what was then termed 'the **battered baby syndrome**'.

'A clinical condition in young children, usually under 3 years of age, who have received non-accidental wholly inexcusable violence or injury on one or more occasions, including minimal as well as severe or fatal trauma, by an adult in a position of trust, generally a parent, guardian, foster parent, or co-habitee.'

Three important points are highlighted by this definition:

- It usually involves very young children below the age of 3 years.
- It can have occurred on a number of occasions.
- The injuries are usually inflicted by someone known to the child.

The commonest type of injury is bruising, and this occurs in more than 80% of the non-accidental injuries. A bruise may take many weeks to heal and disappear and as it does it changes colour. Therefore a child who has suffered bruising on a number of occasions may display several lesions at different stages of healing. Furthermore, a survey of children diagnosed as having had non-accidental injuries showed that head, face and neck were the most frequent areas for bruising (Table 12.5). It is interesting to note that accidental injury to certain areas such as the ears, side of the neck, and top of shoulders, is an unusual event and for this reason it is sometimes referred to as the 'triangle of safety' and trauma arising in this locality should be viewed with some suspicion.

It can be seen from Table 12.5 that, with a child sitting in the dental chair, any member of the dental team is likely to see evidence of a non-accidental injury and, in addition, without arousing suspicion. There are other features which may add weight to the diagnosis of non-accidental injury. Questions which may aid a diagnosis include:

- Were these injuries caused by an ordinary accident?
- Was there an inexplicable delay between the injury and seeking treatment?
- Are the injuries compatible with the explanation given?
- Is the explanation unduly vague?
- Is the explanation likely given the child's age and development?
- Is the general care of the child satisfactory?
- Is the child's behaviour normal?

Local authority social services departments in each area will have protocols in place for dealing with suspected cases and it is important that the dental team is aware of the appropriate procedure. The **NSPCC** have produced four short training modules for the dental team (**educare**) as part of a child protection training exercise. They are designed to help staff to act appropriately if a patient approaches them with child protection issues (www.talktilitstops.org.uk).

References

British Society of Paediatric Dentistry (2000) A policy document on fissure sealants in paediatric dentistry. *International Journal of Paediatric Dentistry*, **10**, 174–177.

British Society of Paediatric Dentistry (2001) A policy document on the use of amalgam in paediatric dentistry. *International Journal of Paediatric Dentistry*, **11**, 233–238.

Chadwick, B. (2002) Non-pharmacological behaviour management – Clinical guidelines. Faculty of Dental Surgery Royal College of Surgeons (England), London.

Field, E.A., Brooks, V. and Tyldesley, W.R. (1992) Recurrent apthous ulcers in children: a review. *International Journal of Paediatric Dentistry*, **2**, 1–10.

Ireland, R.S. (ed.) (2004) Sedation (Chapter 4). In: *Advanced Dental Nursing*. Blackwell Munksgaard, Oxford.

Office of Population Censuses and Surveys (1993) *Children's Dental Health in the United Kingdom*. Office of Population Censuses and Surveys.

Ranly, D.M. and Garcia-Godoy, F. (2000) Current and potential pulp therapies for primary and young permanent teeth. *Journal of Dentistry*, **28**, 153–161.

Further reading

British Society of Paediatric Dentistry (2001) A policy document on management of caries in the primary dentition. *International Journal of Paediatric Dentistry*, **11**, 153–157

Cameron, A.C. and Widmer, R.P. (eds.) (2003) *Handbook of Pediatric Dentistry*, 2nd edn. Mosby, St Louis.

Heasman, P. (ed.) (2003) Paediatric dentistry (Chapter 6) and Special situations (Chapter 7). In: *Master Dentistry*. Churchill Livingstone, Edinburgh.

Klinberg, G., Freeman, R., *et al.* (2006) European Guidelines on behavioural management in paediatric dentistry. European Academy for Paediatric Dentistry, Winterthur, Switzerland.

Sinha, S., Acharya, P., Jafar, H., Bower, E., Harrison, V. and Newton, T. (2005) *The Management of Abuse: A Resource Manual for the Dental Team*. Stephen Hancocks Ltd, London.

Welbury, R.R., Duggal, M.S. and Hosey, M.-T. (eds.) (2005) *Paediatric Dentistry*, 3rd edn. Oxford University Press, Oxford.

13

Adult restorative dentistry

Ann C. Shearer

Summary

This chapter covers:

- Treatment plans
- Dental charting
- Classification of dental diseases
- Tooth preparation and restoration techniques
- Restorative treatment options
- Impression taking
- The working environment

Introduction: the importance of the treatment plan

The treatment plan is the end stage of a process that has involved gathering information from the patient, making a diagnosis, deciding treatment options and working out the care priorities.

The information that is gathered will include the patient's concerns, medical history, dental history and social history. The next important information gathering stage is the clinical examination. This should be carried out extraorally and intraorally for both the soft and hard tissues and must be methodically completed. Special investigations such as sensitivity (vitality) tests, radiographs and diet analysis may also be required. All of these will help with making the diagnosis and formulating an appropriate treatment plan.

Priorities in treatment

This may be a balance between patient and operator as both may have different priorities. This should be established before treatment is started. Normally the relief of pain is the first priority for the patient *and* the operator. Pain is often the reason for initial attendance at the dental surgery. Fortunately, the relief of dental pain is normally possible assuming the correct diagnosis has been made. There may be rare cases when this is not achieved but normally this is due to misdiagnosis or to the pain not being of dental origin.

After the relief of pain, the next stage is usually the control of active disease. This will allow further assessment of the patient, including their attitude towards care and their management and maintenance of their oral health. If active disease control is not a priority for the patient, then the options are either to explain your reasons for managing disease or to accept the patient's point of view. If the patient is going on holiday the next week and has fractured a central incisor, the caries in their molar teeth is not a priority to them – not unreasonably.

Control of disease may involve a number of treatment items. It should certainly include an appropriate preventive regime. This may include dietary advice, oral hygiene instruction or smoking cessation therapy. At this stage any teeth that are of hopeless prognosis should be extracted. Initial periodontal therapy including removal of plaque traps such as ledges on restorations should be completed. This phase, which is termed the **stabilisation phase**, may also include root canal treatment, simple direct restorations and the provision of interim dentures or indirect restorations.

On completion of this stage, it is essential to review what has been achieved and re-assess the treatment plan. Assuming an appropriate level of oral health has been achieved and maintained over a suitable time period, consideration may then be given to the appearance and functional needs and wishes of the patient.

Clinical Textbook of Dental Hygiene and Therapy, Second Edition. Edited by Suzanne L. Noble.
© 2012 John Wiley & Sons, Ltd. Published 2012 by John Wiley & Sons, Ltd.

Therapist/hygienist to see for

1. Dietary analysis and advice
2. Oral hygiene advice–interdental cleaning and toothbrushing
3. Ultrasonic scale, fine scale and polish
4. Fluoride varnish to white spot lesions LL6 buccal, LR6 buccal
5. Composites UR5 mesial, UR4 distal, UR2 distal, UL4 occlusal, LR5 distal
6. Amalgam UL6 MODB

Figure 13.1 An example of a treatment plan.

An important aspect of a treatment plan is that it acts as a scheme that the clinicians involved in the patient's care can follow. It shows the order of treatment and can also indicate who is carrying out each item. See Figure 13.1 for an example of a treatment plan.

Order of treatment provision

- Relief of pain.
- Stabilisation phase – the control of active disease:
  ○ prevention and motivation
  ○ extraction of unrestorable teeth
  ○ direct restorations
  ○ interim restorations.
- Reassess.
- Restorative phase – managing appearance and function:
  ○ indirect restorations
  ○ removable prostheses
- Review and maintenance.

Charting the adult dentition

Tooth notation

Several systems of tooth notation are available, but the systems commonly used in the UK are the FDI (Federation Dentaire International) and Palmer systems.

Federation Dentaire International (FDI) notation

The mouth is divided into four quadrants and each quadrant is given a number: starting with the upper right quadrant and working in a clockwise direction. For example the upper left quadrant is 2. The teeth are then allocated a number starting from the midline, so all central incisors are 1 and all third molars are 8. Therefore the lower right second premolar is 45.

Permanent teeth

Right 18 17 16 15 14 13 12 11 21 22 23 24 25 26 27 28 Upper

Lower 48 47 46 45 44 43 42 41 31 32 33 34 35 36 37 38 Left

Palmer system

In this system, sometimes called the Zsigmondy–Palmer system, the dentition is divided into quadrants and the teeth in each quadrant are numbered 1 through 8 starting at the midline. Each quadrant is separated by a vertical line for right and left and by a horizontal line for upper and lower. Thus |6 is the upper left first molar in the permanent dentition.

Permanent teeth

Right 8 7 6 5 4 3 2 1 | 1 2 3 4 5 6 7 8 Upper

Lower 8 7 6 5 4 3 2 1 | 1 2 3 4 5 6 7 8 Left

This system works well for hand-written notes but is more difficult for computerised notes and printed letters and therefore the lines are sometimes replaced by two letters describing the quadrant, for example UR8 is the upper right third molar tooth.

Universal system

A further system is used in the United States, called the Universal System. This is also a two digit system but the teeth are numbered from 1 through to 32 in a clockwise direction starting with the upper right third molar.

Right   1 2 3 4 5 6 7 8 9 10 11 12 13 14 15 16 Upper
Lower 32 31 30 29 28 27 26 25 24 23 22 21 20 19 18 17 Left

For the charting of primary teeth, see Chapter 12, p. 245.

Charting the teeth

The teeth present and absent, teeth unerupted or partially erupted, the presence of caries and other defects of the teeth and the restorations present are recorded on a chart. The chart shows the buccal/labial, palatal/lingual, mesial, distal and occlusal surfaces of all the teeth (Figure 13.2).

How to examine teeth

The teeth should be examined in a systematic manner, making sure that each surface of each tooth is carefully inspected. A probe is used to remove plaque from the fissures and to detect ledges and deficiencies in existing restorations. The probe should not be pressed firmly into the fissure pattern as this could damage demineralised enamel. Good eyesight and lighting is essential if caries is to be detected. It is also important that the teeth are examined dry and free from plaque as caries is more likely to be detected.

Classification of cavities

Black's classification

G.V. Black was an American dentist who wrote textbooks on dentistry in the early twentieth century in which he outlined principles for cavity preparation. He

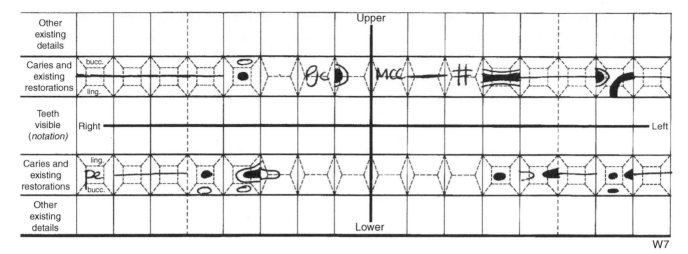

Figure 13.2 An example of a dental charting.

also described a classification for carious lesions. This was based on the knowledge and evidence available at the time and is still used by some people today despite its limitations: namely it only refers to primary carious lesions and does not include root or secondary caries.

Black's classification:

Class I   Caries affecting pits and fissures: commonly used to refer to caries affecting the occlusal surfaces of premolars and molars.
Class II   Caries affecting the proximal surfaces of posterior teeth.
Class III Caries affecting the proximal surfaces of anterior teeth.
Class IV   Caries affecting the proximal surfaces of anterior teeth and also including the incisal angle.
Class V   Caries affecting the cervical surfaces.

Current methods of cavity classification

Cavities or lesions in teeth are described by the cause of the cavitation or lesion and by the surface(s) affected.

Causes:

- Dental caries.
- Tooth wear.
- Trauma.
- Developmental defects.

Dental caries

Carious lesions may be described by the type of caries that is present:

- **Primary:** caries affecting the coronal part of the tooth, on a surface that has not previously had caries.

- **Secondary:** caries around an existing restoration. Also referred to as recurrent caries.
- **Rampant:** occurring quickly; it is soft and pale in colour. Sometimes referred to as **bottle caries** as it may be seen in infants who are given bottles containing sugary drinks.
- **Root surface:** affecting the root surfaces. Seen in patients with gingival recession, namely those with periodontal disease and the elderly.

Tooth wear

For tooth wear, the lesion is described by the type of tooth surface loss:

- **Attrition:** the gradual loss of hard tooth substance as a result of chewing activity. Essentially this is the result of tooth to tooth contact.
- **Erosion:** the loss of hard tooth substance owing to a chemical process not involving bacteria. Usually caused by acid from dietary sources such as carbonated drinks, citrus fruits or by acid from the stomach in patients with regurgitation problems or an eating disorder.
- **Abrasion:** friction from a foreign body, such a toothbrush with toothpaste, independent of occlusion between teeth.
- **Abfraction:** thought to be caused by tooth flexure. Occlusal loading results in loss of cervical enamel.

Developmental defects

Developmental defects may be classified as relating to:

- **Number:** The most common teeth to be absent are lateral incisors, second premolars and third molars.

Absence of one or more teeth is called **hypodontia**. Absence of all teeth is called **anodontia**.

Extra teeth may also occur. These are referred to as **supernumerary** teeth.

- **Shape:** Teeth may be larger than normal (**macrodontia**), smaller than normal (**microdontia**), have extra cusps or be joined together to give a double tooth (**geminated**).
- **Tooth tissue involved:** Defects of enamel and dentine may be described as inherited or acquired. Amelogenesis and dentinogenesis imperfecta are inherited defects.

Fluorosis is an example of an acquired defect. Fluorosis is classified by the extent of mottling of the enamel (see Chapter 11, p. 226).

Trauma

Dental trauma is classified according to the extent of damage to the tooth: from an enamel chip to a fracture involving the pulp. See Table 13.1 for the World Health Organization (WHO) classification of dentoalveolar injuries.

Cavity classification by surface affected

- Pit and fissure – the occlusal surfaces of molars and premolars and pits on the buccal surfaces of molars and cingulum pits in incisors.
- Posterior proximal – adjoining surfaces of molars and premolars.
- Anterior proximal – adjoining surfaces of incisors and canines.
- Smooth surface cervical/necks of teeth.

Preparation of cavities

Instruments for cavity preparation

Conventionally, cavities are prepared using a combination of hand instruments and rotary instruments.

Hand instruments (Figure 13.3)

Examination of teeth

- Mirrors: used for indirect examination of teeth, to retract tissues and to direct light to specific areas of the mouth.
- Straight probe: used to check the margins of restorations and to carefully examine for dentine caries.

Table 13.1 WHO classification of dentoalveolar trauma.

Injury	Description
Injuries to the hard dental tissues and the pulp	
Enamel infraction	Incomplete fracture crack of enamel without loss of tooth substance
Enamel fracture	Loss of tooth substance confined to enamel
Enamel–dentine fracture	Loss of tooth substance confined to enamel and dentine, not involving the pulp
Complicated crown fracture	Fracture of enamel and dentine exposing the pulp
Uncomplicated crown root fracture	Fracture of enamel, dentine and cementum but not involving the pulp
Complicated crown root fracture	Fracture of enamel, dentine and cementum and exposing the pulp
Root fracture	Fracture involving dentine, cementum and pulp; can be subclassified into apical, middle and coronal third
Injuries to the periodontal tissues	
Concussion	No abnormal loosening or displacement but marked reaction to percussion
Subluxation (loosening)	Abnormal loosening but no displacement
Extrusive luxation (partial avulsion)	Partial displacement of tooth from the socket
Lateral luxation	Displacement other than axially with comminution or fracture of the socket
Intrusive luxation	Displacement into alveolar bone with comminution or fracture of the socket
Avulsion	Complete displacement of tooth from the socket
Injuries to supporting bone	
Comminution of alveolar socket wall	Crushing and compression of alveolar socket
Fracture of socket wall	Fracture confined to buccal or lingual socket wall
Fracture of alveolar process	Fracture of the alveolar process: may or may not involve the tooth sockets
Fracture of mandible or maxilla	May or may not involve the alveolar socket
Injuries to gingiva or oral mucosa	
Laceration	Wound in the mucosa resulting from a tear
Contusion	Bruise not accompanied by a break in the mucosa
Abrasion	Superficial wound produced by rubbing or scraping the mucosal surface

- Briault probe: used to detect deficiencies and ledges on proximal surfaces.

Cavity preparation

- Excavators: used to remove soft dentine caries, particularly from the floor of the cavity. Excavators may also be used to remove temporary dressing materials. Small excavators may be employed for carving fissure patterns in plastic materials such as amalgam.
- Chisels: used to remove unsupported enamel.
- Gingival margin trimmers: used to remove unsupported enamel at the base of proximal cavities.

Material placement

- Flat plastic: used to place plastic restorative materials (i.e. those that are soft on placement and subsequently set and harden in the cavity). They can be used to place temporary dressings, linings, glass ionomers and composites. Flat plastics are not suitable for carving amalgams as their blades are too thick and the amalgam is smeared rather than cut and removed.
- Round-ended plastic: used for placing and shaping plastic materials such as temporary dressings and composite.
- Amalgam carrier: used to carry amalgam to the cavity.
- Amalgam plugger: used to condense the amalgam into the cavity.

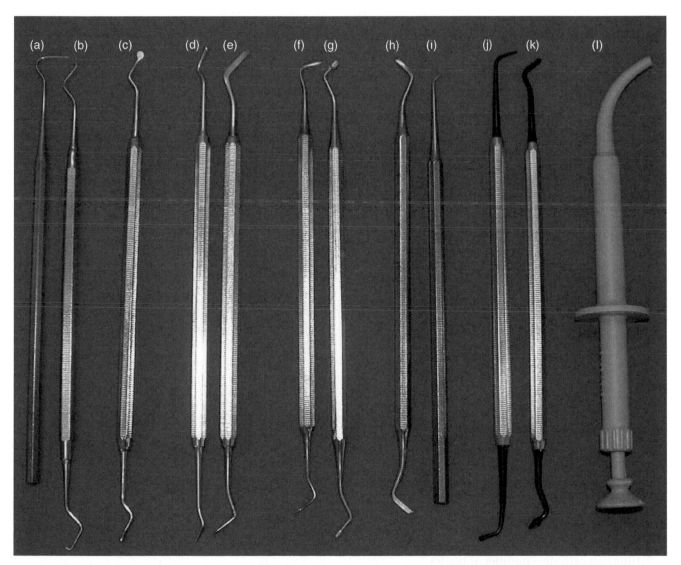

Figure 13.3 Hand instruments: (a) straight probe; (b) Briault probe; (c) excavator; (d) ballended plastic; (e) flat plastic; (f) ½ Hollenbach; (g) amalgam plugger; (h) gingival margin trimmer; (i) hatchet; (j) Teflon coated composite instrument; (k) Teflon coated composite instrument; (l) amalgam carrier.

Material shaping

- Amalgam carvers: examples include Ward's carvers and the ½ Hollenbach. These instruments have thin cutting blades that cut through the amalgam.
- Composite instruments: specific instruments with non-stick coatings, such as Teflon or titanium-nitride, have been developed for placing and shaping composite resins.

Rotary instruments

Slow speed

The slow speed handpiece is driven either by compressed air or directly by an electric motor. The speed of the handpiece ranges from 0 rpm to 40 000 rpm. The most efficient cutting is achieved with a straight handpiece, but this is difficult to use in the mouth and is therefore restricted to extraoral use such as adjusting temporary crowns and dentures. The contra-angle handpiece is used for the removal of caries, polishing and finishing.

High speed

The high speed handpiece is driven by compressed air and is sometimes referred to as an air-turbine or airotor. It is used for cutting through enamel and dentine and removing previous restorations. It has a speed of 250 000–500 000 rpm and to keep it cool, a water spray is directed at the cutting part of the bur which is held in the head of the handpiece by friction. A fibre-optic light in the head of the handpiece aids visibility.

Burs

Burs are described by:

- The method of retention in the handpiece:
  - latch grip for slow speed
  - friction grip for high speed.
- Shape:
  - round
  - football (like an American football or a rugby ball rather than spherical)
  - flame
  - tapered fissure
  - straight fissure
  - pear
  - inverted cone.
- Size.
- The material on the cutting end:
  - diamond – grit size
  - tungsten carbide – number of blades
  - stainless steel.

Figure 13.4 shows examples of a selection of burs.

Removal of caries

Amount of caries removed

Conventionally, in cavity preparation, all caries is removed from the enamel–dentine junction. The reasons for this are the ease with which caries spreads along this junction between the two tissues and the risk of fracture of unsupported enamel that has been undermined by caries. The judgement about whether all caries has been removed from the enamel–dentine junction is based on the colour and hardness of the junction. The area of the enamel–dentine junction should feel hard to a straight probe and staining should normally be removed unless this compromises the tooth structure. Caries in the dentine on the pulpal floor should be removed if it is soft as this will be heavily infected with bacteria. Stained but firm carious dentine may be left in place, especially if there is a risk of pulp exposure, as this dentine will be demineralised but not infected. It is obviously important to prevent further bacterial contamination of the cavity by good isolation, such as rubber dam. A setting calcium hydroxide lining is then placed in this deep area of the cavity to encourage reparative dentine and kill the remaining bacteria. This is described as an **indirect pulp cap**.

If a small pulp exposure occurs in a symptom-free tooth then a **direct pulp cap** may be indicated. Again, a small amount of setting calcium hydroxide lining material is applied to the area of exposure. If a larger pulpal exposure occurs during cavity preparation, then removal of the pulp and root canal treatment, or extraction of the tooth, may have to be carried out.

There is currently a debate about whether dental caries should be removed fully or partially from a cavity or whether it should be sealed in place. Evidence suggests that sealing over caries will arrest the process. Fissure sealants placed over occlusal caries extending into the middle third of dentine will arrest the lesion. However, such techniques are only suitable for patients who are regular attenders so that the restored lesions can be regularly reviewed.

Stepwise excavation

For grossly carious occlusal cavities, stepwise excavation may be used. Caries is removed in two steps, 6–12 months apart. At the first visit access is gained, caries is removed from the periphery only and soft caries is left on the cavity floor. The cavity is lined with calcium hydroxide and restored with glass ionomer. It is important to achieve a good seal with the glass ionomer. At the subsequent visit, on re-entry into the cavity the dentine is found to be harder and drier with fewer

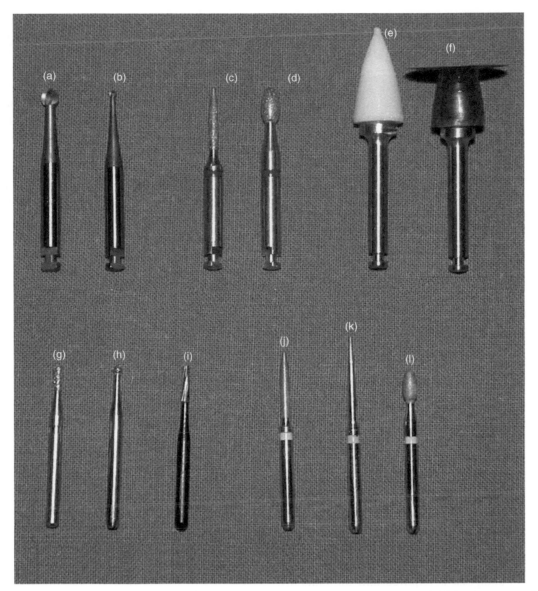

Figure 13.4 Burs: (a) latch grip stainless steel large round; (b) latch grip stainless steel small round; (c) latch grip superfine diamond flame; (d) latch grip superfine diamond football; (e) latch grip composite finishing point; (f) latch grip abrasive disc; (g) friction grip diamond fissure; (h) friction grip diamond round; (i) friction grip diamond pear; (j) friction grip superfine diamond flame; (k) friction grip superfine diamond tapered fissure; (l) friction grip superfine diamond football.

microorganisms present. A conventional restoration may then be placed.

Ultraconservative caries removal

Another technique is ultraconservative caries removal. This involves preparing the tooth minimally by cutting a 1 mm bevel in the sound enamel surrounding the cavitated lesion. No further preparation is carried out and the tooth is restored with acid-etch retained composites and fissure sealant. This technique has been used successfully to arrest occlusal caries (Ricketts, 2001).

Methods of caries removal

Conventionally, caries is removed using a round bur in a slow-speed handpiece or with a sharp round excavator. The roundness of the bur and the excavator mimics the shape of the spread of caries in dentine. A round bur in a slow-speed handpiece is used to remove caries from the enamel-dentine junction. This combination will easily remove soft carious dentine but will cut through sound dentine and enamel more slowly. This means that the operator can feel the difference between carious and non-carious tissues and distinguish between them.

A sharp excavator should be used when removing soft dentine overlying the pulp as the tactile sensation is better than with a handpiece. Excavators are often preferred by anxious patients.

Alternative techniques

Dental caries may be removed in a number of ways other than the conventional use of burs in a handpiece or by hand instruments.

Chemomechanical removal

Chemomechanical removal is an alternative technique for removing caries. It involves the use of a chemical solution, which softens carious dentine thus allowing easy removal. Local analgesia is not usually required. A current product is a red or colourless gel (**Carisolv®**) which softens the collagen in the carious tissue through chlorination of amino acids. This softened tissue can then be removed mechanically with specially designed hand instruments, which have the appearance of multi-bladed hand excavators.

Clinical situations where this technique may be preferred include:

- Root caries.
- Cervical caries.
- Cavitated carious lesions.
- In needle-phobic patients.
- Where local analgesia is contraindicated.
- In countries where there is a limited availability of rotary instrumentation.

Air abrasion

Air abrasion units employ aluminium oxide particles in a high velocity stream of air to remove tooth substance. Again no local analgesia is required and the units are quiet, which may help anxious patients. The cavities produced are saucer shaped and are suitable for restoration with adhesive techniques. However, there are some disadvantages of this technique, namely the dust produced, limited tactile sensation, poor removal of soft caries and the need to protect adjacent teeth from damage by the alumina particle spray.

Lasers

Lasers for removal of enamel and dentine have yet to achieve full acceptance despite their use for soft tissue surgery.

Pulp protection

Introduction

Following cavity preparation and prior to restoring the tooth, protection of the pulp must be considered. The pulp comprises nerves and blood vessels and damage to the pulp can result in inflammation of the pulp (**pulpitis**) and dental pain for the patient (see Chapter 4, p. 88). This inflammation may be reversible or irreversible; in the latter case if the pulp is not removed, either by extraction of the tooth or by removal of the pulp tissue, then the pulp will become necrotic and the patient may develop periapical periodontitis or an acute abscess. The pulp can be damaged by dental caries, tooth wear, trauma and by cavity preparation. The best protection for the pulp is dentine but in the absence of a thick layer of dentine then additional pulp protection must be provided. A lining material may also act as a therapeutic agent by providing active protection of the dentine.

Objectives of pulp protection

- Therapeutic:
  - Stimulate odontoblasts to lay down reparative dentine
  - Encourage remineralisation of dentine
  - Act against any remaining bacteria.
- Protect from chemicals.
  These may come from the oral cavity, bacteria or from the restorative material.
- Protect from temperature.
  Metal restorative materials such as amalgam and gold will transmit changes in temperature from the oral cavity and in the absence of a suitable layer of dentine additional protection must be provided.
- Seal the dentinal tubules. This will prevent fluids containing bacteria, molecules and ions entering the dentinal tubules and as result prevent pain and possible further caries.

Methods of pulp protection

- Minimal cavities: Either a dental adhesive to seal the dentinal tubules or no pulp protection.
- Moderately deep cavities: A layer of a resin modified glass ionomer to give thermal and chemical protection.
- Deep cavities: A thin layer of setting calcium hydroxide as a therapeutic lining, followed by a layer of resin modified glass ionomer.

Techniques for placement

A small ball-ended instrument is used to place the setting calcium hydroxide material. The calcium hydroxide should be placed in a thin layer on the deepest part of the cavity. For the glass ionomer, a flat plastic or ball-ended plastic is used and the material is applied to the pulpal floor and/or pulpal wall depending on the cavity shape. The lining material should not extend to the cavity margins.

Moisture control

Why is moisture control important?

The water spray of the high speed handpiece and three-in-one syringe and the patient's own saliva result in large volumes of fluid accumulating in the mouth. This needs to be removed for the following reasons:

- Patient comfort.
- Visibility for the operator and assistant.
- Avoid contamination of dental materials.
- Reduce or prevent bacterial contamination of cavities.
- Overall operating efficiency.

Methods of moisture control

- **Aspiration:** Suction is used to remove fluids from the mouth. High volume suction is used with high speed handpieces and ultrasonic and sonic scalers. Low volume suction, such as a saliva ejector, is used for smaller volumes of fluid such as patients' saliva.
- **Air:** The air spray from the three-in-one tip is used to blow excess moisture from cavities and the surfaces of the teeth. It can also be used to keep water off the mouth mirror to improve vision for the operator.
- **Absorbent materials: Cotton wool rolls** are a common method of moisture control. They may be placed in the buccal and lingual sulcus to absorb saliva. They also act to retract soft tissues, such as the lips and tongue. Care should be taken when removing cotton wool rolls from the oral cavity. The cotton wool roll must be soaked with water before removal as otherwise the mucosa may be damaged, resulting in a 'burn' of the soft tissues.

  Dry guards are flat triangular pads of absorbent material that are placed inside the cheeks over the parotid duct to absorb saliva and water.
- **Rubber dam.**

Rubber dam

A rubber dam is used for a number of reasons:

- Moisture control: the teeth are isolated from saliva, blood and gingival fluid. Control of water from the handpiece and the three-in-one is easier to manage.
- Dental materials: many dental materials or techniques will be compromised by moisture and a rubber dam is important for successful restorations.
- Protects and retracts soft tissues: the rubber dam keeps the lips, cheeks and tongue out of the way and can help prevent damage of these tissues during treatment.
- Good visibility: by keeping tissues and moisture out of the operating field, visibility for the operator is much improved.

- Airway protection: a rubber dam prevents patients from inhaling or swallowing restorations such as crowns, small instruments such as burs and pieces of filling material such as amalgam.
- Infection control: by keeping saliva from the operating field, contamination is controlled. This is especially important in the management of deep carious cavities.
- Patient comfort: a rubber dam keeps fluids, materials and instruments out of patients' mouths and this can increase their comfort.

Reasons against:

- Time: it takes time to apply the rubber dam, but with experience this decreases. Time is saved during operating by the advantages of rubber dam use.
- Learning curve: the technique of using a rubber dam improves with time and practice.
- Patients' concerns: some patients may feel claustrophobic under the rubber dam. Patients can only talk with difficulty and this makes operator–patient communication more demanding.
- Latex allergy: a non-latex rubber dam is now available so this should not be a difficulty.

How to place the rubber dam

- Assemble the required instruments and equipment (see Figure 13.5).
- Select the appropriate type of rubber dam.
  Rubber dam is made of either latex or a non-latex material and the latter should be selected for patients with a latex allergy. Rubber dam is supplied in different weights and colours and these are usually a personal preference.
- Punch hole(s): First decide how many holes are to be punched on the basis that one hole is punched for each tooth projecting through the rubber dam. For a single buccal, palatal or occlusal restoration only one hole is required. For all other situations, more than one hole is required. Next decide the positions of the holes on the dam. There are a number of methods of doing this:
  - Hold the dam in position over the patient's mouth, checking that the dam does not cover the nose; ask the patient to open wide and locate the tooth/teeth to be isolated. Punch the holes in the dam in these positions.
  - Use a rubber dam stamp. This is an inked stamp with all the teeth in both arches. Stamp the rubber dam and punch holes as required.
  - Use the paper template supplied by some dam manufacturers. Place the template over the rubber dam sheet and mark the holes required with a pen.

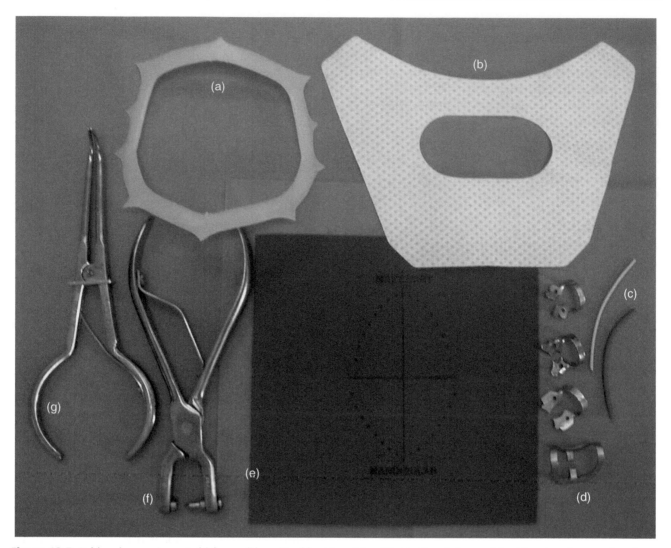

Figure 13.5 Rubber dam equipment: (a) frame; (b) napkin; (c) rubber strips; (d) selection of clamps; (e) rubber dam: latex and nonlatex; (f) hole punch; (g) clamp forceps.

Choose an appropriate size of hole (if the punch has different hole sizes) for the teeth to be isolated. Space the holes allowing a tooth's width between each hole.

- Select method(s) of dam retention.
  Rubber dam may be retained in a number of different ways (Figure 13.6):
  ○ Clamps: Many shapes and sizes of clamps are available. Winged clamps should be used if the dam and clamp are to be placed at the same time, whereas wingless clamps should be placed either before or after the dam.
  ○ Rubber strips: Strips can be cut from a sheet of rubber dam and used to retain the dam interdentally. Commercial strips of rubber in different diameters are also available to retain the dam.

○ Floss: Dental floss may be used to floss the dam between the teeth and as a ligature tied around a tooth to retain the dam.
  ○ Contact areas: Additional forms of retention are not always necessary as the dam may be retained by the contact areas.
- Place dam and method of retention.
  ○ Dam first: This technique should be used where more than one tooth is to be isolated. Stretch each area of dam between the holes and using a flossing movement work between the teeth. The dam may then be retained with any of the methods mentioned above.
  ○ Dam and clamp together: This technique is only suitable for single tooth isolation. A winged clamp is chosen and the dam stretched over the wings. The

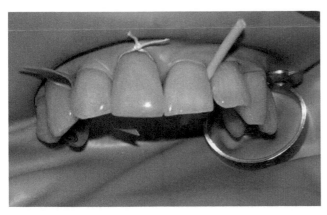

Figure 13.6 Rubber dam in place, showing various methods of retention.

tips of the rubber dam forceps are placed in the holes of the clamp and the dam and clamp are placed on the tooth. In placing the clamp, slide the clamp over the buccal/palatal surfaces of the tooth until the clamp engages the cervical constriction of the tooth. Remove the forceps and, with a flat plastic, flip the rubber dam over the wings to give a tight seal.

○ Clamp first: If this technique is used then a length of floss must be tied to the clamp in case it springs off the tooth prior to the placement of the dam.
- Napkin: An absorbent napkin or paper towel should be placed between the dam and the face for patient comfort.
- Place frame: The frame stretches the dam away from the isolated teeth and holds it in place.
- Saliva ejector: A saliva ejector should be placed if the patient finds swallowing difficult under the dam.
- Removal: To remove the dam, stretch the dam away from the teeth and cut interproximally. Remove the clamp, dam and frame.

Direct restoratives: clinical properties, handling and placement

Teeth may require repair as the result of dental caries, tooth wear, trauma or developmental defects. Despite decreases in the occurrence of primary dental caries in most industrialised countries, the restoration of teeth continues to be necessary. Maintenance and replacement of existing restorations represent a large component of this dental treatment, particularly in the older adult.

A number of factors have to be taken into account when choosing the most appropriate restorative method and material for a clinical situation. The limiting factors include:

- Patient motivation and suitability.
- The number of remaining teeth and their relative positions.
- The condition of their supporting tissues.
- The amount of remaining tooth structure.
- The restorative materials available, and their longevity as restoratives.
- The occlusion and opposing teeth and restorations.
- Aesthetic and other wishes of the patient, including cost factors.

When any method or material is chosen, it must be used in the most appropriate clinical situation.

Available materials

The direct restoratives in current, general use are amalgam, composite, glass ionomer and combinations of the last two groups.

Dental amalgam

Dental amalgam is a mixture of mercury and an alloy containing silver and tin with added copper and zinc. The alloy particles may be lathe cut or spherical in shape: some alloys have a combination of the two shapes. Clinically, spherical alloys are easier to pack but a small diameter instrument will sink through the mix. Lathe cut alloys require more condensation pressure. The alloy and mercury are held together in a capsule, with the two components separated by a plastic diaphragm. When the diaphragm is broken and the capsule is placed in the mixing machine (**amalgamator**), the two components are mixed together (**triturated**) to form a silver-coloured paste. This paste is then condensed into the cavity. This is a very important stage: well-condensed amalgams are stronger than poorly condensed ones as more of the weaker mercury-rich γ_2 phase is removed during carving (see Chapter 9, p. 182).

Amalgam is weak in thin section so cavities have to be cut suitably deep (2 mm) and because amalgam does not adhere to tooth tissue, the cavity must be undercut.

Dental amalgam continues to be used despite concerns about health and the environment because it has high clinical success, known performance, relatively low cost and is easy to manipulate. Despite the high usage of this material it is not ideal and suffers from several problems including marginal breakdown, fracture and poor appearance. Secondary caries is the most common reason given for the replacement of amalgam restorations but this diagnosis may not necessarily always be correct. There is a well-recognised need for effective alternatives, not only because of its less than ideal properties but also because of public and political concerns about its use, the changing patterns of dental disease and patient expectations of dental care.

Dental amalgam has been in use since the nineteenth century. Mercury is toxic but there is no credible scientific evidence to suggest that the small amount of mercury released from dental amalgam restorations on chewing contributes to disease or has any toxicological effects in humans. True amalgam allergy is extremely rare. A number of investigations specifically related to the health problems associated with dental amalgam have been carried out. In these studies no link has been shown between amalgam and such complaints as headache and fatigue or between amalgam and cancer. It has also been shown that no symptoms among dental staff and their children can be related to the use of dental amalgam, assuming that correct hygiene measures are employed. Some studies have found other organic causes for the patients' complaints and this possibility should not be overlooked (Eley, 1997).

Resin composites

Resin composites used in dentistry have several components:

- Resin matrix: commonly a fluid monomer Bis-GMA.
- Filler particles of silica-based glass.
- Silane: an agent that allows the resin and filler particles to bond together.
- Activator for the setting reaction: normally camphorquinone.
- Pigments.

Direct resin composites are the material of choice for anterior restorations and they are increasing in use and popularity for posterior restorations, mainly because of their appearance. Composites do not adhere directly to tooth tissue and rely on the acid-etch technique and the use of dental adhesives for adhesion to enamel and dentine.

The physical characteristics of resin composite materials are much improved from their initial forms, and methods of handling them have developed considerably and are no longer copies of amalgam techniques. However, it can be more difficult to generate good proximal contour and contact with these materials than with amalgam. Polymerisation shrinkage of the resin during curing (in the order of 2–3%) still occurs with most resin composite materials and may contribute to marginal defects, cuspal distortion, crack formation in the enamel or dentine and may therefore contribute to postoperative pain or sensitivity for the patient. There are, however, a number of clinical techniques available to overcome these problems and the longevity of restorations using the newer resin composites is much improved over that of the original materials. Reducing the effect of polymerisation shrinkage may be achieved by incremental packing of the composite. Each

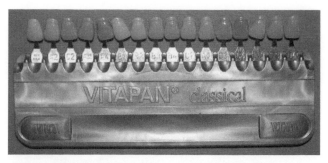

Figure 13.7 Vita shade guide.

increment should touch as few walls of the cavity as possible. The stress induced by polymerisation shrinkage is highest in cavities with more bonded than unbonded surfaces: the occlusal cavity has the potential for the most stress. This is referred to as the configuration or C factor of the cavity.

Resin composites are not suitable in the following clinical situations:

- Deep subgingival preparations.
- Lack of peripheral enamel.
- Poor moisture control.

How to choose a shade

Shades are described as comprising of hue, chroma and value. **Hue** is the colour (e.g. red or green), **Value** refers to the lightness and darkness and **chroma** is the strength of colour.

The most common shade guide for dental materials is the **Vita shade guide** (Figure 13.7), originally a shade system for porcelains but now also used for other tooth-coloured materials such as resin composites. The shade guide is divided into four groups A, B, C and D, which have the following hues:

A	Orange–brown
B	Yellow
C	Grey–brown
D	Red

Each letter group is further divided into four: A1, A2, A3, A4, for example. The value decreases from 1 to 4 (the shade gets darker) whilst the chroma (saturation of colour) increases from 1 to 4.

Choosing a shade:

- Take the shade in a neutral coloured environment.
- Take the shade at the beginning of a clinical session before eyes are tired and before the teeth become dehydrated and become lighter if they are isolated with rubber dam, for example.
- Do not look at the shade tabs for more than five seconds to avoid fatigue of the eyes. First impressions are often more accurate.

- Colours can change appearance under different lighting conditions. This effect is called **metamerism**. Shades should be chosen in natural daylight or under 'daylight corrected' artificial lighting. Do not use the operating light as it is heavily filtered.
- The canines are a good guide to the hue, but have greater chroma than incisors.
- Include the patient and dental nurse in the shade selection.

Light curing

Light curing of resin composites is initiated by light in the wavelength range 450–500 nm. This blue light can damage the eyes so an orange filter should be used when the light is in use. The tip of the light source should be placed as close as possible to the surface of the restoration and each increment of composite should be cured for 40–60 seconds. Under-cured composites will readily absorb stain and will rapidly degenerate.

Types of curing lamps:

- **Conventional quartz halogen** bulbs are present in some curing lights. It is important to check that the output of such lights remains above 400 mW: otherwise the composite will not cure fully.
- **LED** (light emitting diode) light curing units are very energy efficient and are small, portable units. The narrow band width of 460–480 nm means that they will work well with composites containing camphorquinone but will not cure those resins not containing this initiator.
- **Plasma** (xenon) arc lamps produce rapid conversion of the resin but this can produce high shrinkage stresses and the narrow bandwidth means some composites will not cure.

Glass ionomers

Glass ionomers contain poly(alkenoic) acid and fluoroaluminosilicate glass which set by an acid–base reaction to give a cement. They adhere directly to tooth substance and to base metal casting alloys. They release fluoride after placement giving the materials cariostatic properties, although this may only be short term. They also have a low tensile strength, which makes them brittle and unsuitable for use in load-bearing areas in permanent teeth. They are used as lining and luting materials and to restore abrasion and erosion lesions, cervical lesions, and deciduous (primary) teeth and as interim restorations. It must be appreciated however that they are less translucent than resin composite restoratives and therefore their appearance is less acceptable.

Resin modified glass ionomers

Resin modified glass ionomers have a resin (monomer) component as well as the poly (alkenoic) acid and fluoroaluminosilicate glass of conventional glass ionomers. They set by two mechanisms: namely an acid–base reaction and curing of the monomer (chemically, by light or both). They have improved appearance and physical properties compared with conventional glass ionomers. They are used in similar situations to glass ionomers and may also be used for small core build-ups prior to provision of a laboratory-made crown.

Polyacid modified resin composites

Polyacid modified resin composites are also known as **compomers**. Their properties are more like those of composites than glass ionomers. They have limited fluoride release but are stronger and have a better appearance than glass ionomers. Their wear resistance is less than that of composite restoratives. They do not adhere directly to tooth substance without the use of a bonding system. They may be utilised to restore cervical and anterior proximal cavities and for primary teeth.

Material retention

Several techniques may be used to aid the retention of the restorative material.

Retention has to be developed in the shape of the cavity for non-adhesive direct restorations such as amalgam and for indirect restorations such as gold inlays. The removal of primary caries usually creates an undercut cavity that aids retention of direct materials. Additional retention for non-adhesive materials may be gained by cutting slots or grooves in the dentine.

Dentine pins

Pins have been used extensively in the past for retaining large amalgam restorations but they have many disadvantages. They are difficult to place and seat and their incorrect placement can result in perforation, either through the root side into the periodontal ligament space or in to the pulp, resulting in a pulpal exposure. They can also cause tooth fracture. Their use has decreased substantially with the increased use of other methods of retaining restoratives. Pin retention is currently outside the remit of the dental therapist.

Acid etching

Acid etching with phosphoric acid creates pores within the enamel into which resin flows to create tags. This micromechanical retention is very reliable unless there has been contamination of the etched surface by saliva or blood. This technique is used to retain fissure sealants, composite restorations, orthodontic brackets, resin-retained bridges, veneers and other tooth-coloured restorations.

Dental adhesives

Bonding to dentine is more difficult than bonding to enamel as unlike enamel, dentine contains water and has a greater proportion of organic material. Bonding to dentine may be achieved reliably with current systems which involve between one and three steps and which either remove or modify the **smear layer** (this is a layer of debris created by cutting through dentine). The bond to dentine is a combination of chemical and micro-mechanical bonding.

Current systems are classified as follows:

- Total etch (or etch and rinse):
  - 3 step – comprising etch, prime and bond.
  - 2 step – etch followed by a single application of primer mixed with bond.
- Self etch:
  - 2 step – etch and prime step, followed by bond.
  - 1 step- etch, prime and bond in a single application.

Amalgam bonding

Amalgam can be bonded to the cavity using adhesive resins. The *potential* advantages of this technique are reduced sensitivity and marginal leakage, the reduced need for mechanical cavity retentive features and improved strength of the restored tooth.

Stages in cavity preparation and restoration

The stages in cavity preparation and restoration are as follows:

- Gaining access: This is conventionally achieved using a diamond or tungsten carbide bur in a high speed handpiece although alternative methods such as air abrasion may also be employed.
- Removing caries: Methods of caries removal include hand and rotary instruments and chemo-mechanical methods.
- Choosing the restorative material: The choice of material relates to a number of factors that may include:
  - the skill of the clinician to manipulate the material
  - the personal preference of the patient
  - any allergies a patient may have, for example to Bis-GMA in composite
  - occlusal factors
  - the size and position of the cavity
  - the patient's caries disease risk levels.
- Making the cavity retentive: The method of retention relates to the material chosen and the cavity design.

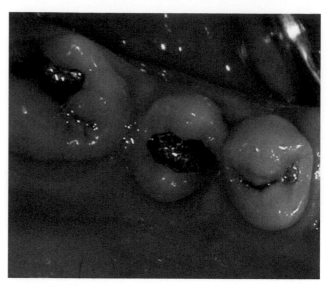

Figure 13.8 Occlusal caries in UR4.

Treatment of pit and fissure lesions

Caries occurs in the pits and fissures of the teeth as plaque collects in these stagnation areas and is not easily removed by toothbrushing or by saliva (Figure 13.8).

Fissure sealants

Fissure sealants are a preventive technique for the management of pit and fissure sealants. They work by closing over the fissures and thus preventing the accumulation of plaque in pits and fissures: areas of the teeth which are difficult to keep plaque free.

Indications:

- High caries risk patients.
- Deep fissures.
- Special needs patients.

Fissures may be sealed with either glass ionomers or resin composites but the failure rates for glass ionomers are much higher. The fissure sealing technique is described in Chapter 11, p. 229–231.

Preventive resin restoration/sealant restoration

In this technique the carious lesion is restored and the rest of the fissure system is sealed. It is indicated for small, discrete carious lesions within the pit and fissure system. Such lesions would be detectable clinically and probably visible on bitewing radiographs (Figures 13.9a and 13.9b).

Technique:

- Consider local analgesia.
- Shade selection.
- Isolation: Ideally a rubber dam should be placed but where this is not possible, cotton wool rolls or dry guards and suction must be used.

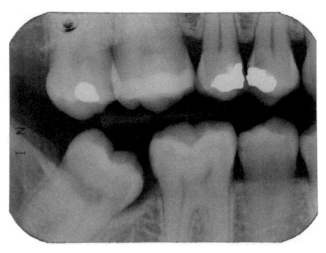

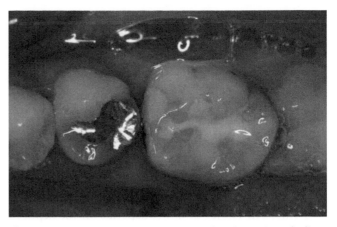

Figure 13.10 Preventive resin restoration in LR6 and disto-occlusal amalgam in LR5.

Figure 13.9a Bitewing radiograph showing occlusal caries in LR6, distal caries in LR5, recurrent caries in UR4 distal and UR5 mesial.

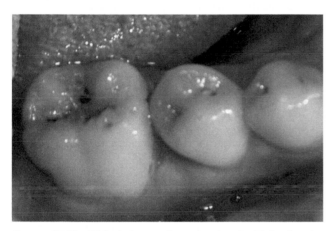

Figure 13.9b Clinical picture of same patient in 13.9a showing occlusal caries in LR6 and distal caries in LR5.

- Cavity preparation: Clean the tooth as for fissure sealants using pumice and water. Open into the area of caries using a small round or pear-shaped diamond or tungsten carbide bur in the high-speed handpiece. As little enamel should be removed as possible. The dentine caries is then removed with a round stainless steel or tungsten carbide bur in a slow speed handpiece. Excavators may also be used for caries removal if the cavity is more extensive. This should result in a cavity shape that is round or oval when viewed occlusally and has rounded internal line angles.
- Lining: The choice of lining depends on the depth of the cavity. In minimal cavities no lining will be necessary, in medium depth cavities a lining is indicated and this may be achieved using a resin modified glass ionomer. The lining should be placed on the pulpal floor.
- Dental adhesive: The technique depends on the dental adhesive system being used (see above).

- Filling the cavity: Composite resin should be placed in small increments of less than 2 mm in depth and each increment fully cured. Ideally each increment should touch the minimum number of walls possible to reduce the effects of polymerisation shrinkage. Composite resin materials should not be handled directly with fingers and excess material should not be wiped on gloved hands as there is a high risk of allergy developing.
- Fissure sealant placement: The occlusal surface is re-etched and a fissure sealant applied to cover the composite and the fissure pattern of the tooth (Figure 13.10).
- Check the occlusion: Once the rubber dam is removed, it is important to check the occlusion using articulating paper, looking at the occlusion of the teeth and by asking the patient.

Occlusal restoration

Technique:

- Check the occlusion: Use articulating paper to mark the occlusal stops (where the upper and lower teeth occlude together). These should be preserved if at all possible during cavity preparation.
- Consider local analgesia.
- Shade selection.
- Isolation: Again, ideally a rubber dam should be placed but where this is not possible, cotton wool rolls or dry guards and suction must be used.
- Cavity preparation: Open into the area of caries using a small round or pear-shaped diamond or tungsten carbide bur in the high-speed handpiece. Enough enamel should be removed to give access to the caries in dentine. This caries is then removed with a round stainless steel or tungsten carbide bur in a slow speed handpiece. It may be necessary to use the high speed handpiece again if the caries is extensive and

more enamel has to be removed to gain access to the carious dentine. Caries should be removed from the enamel–dentine junction first. Check that all the soft dentine has been removed by running a probe along the enamel-dentine junction. Only when this area is clear, should caries removal from the floor of the cavity be carried out, either with a round bur in the slow speed handpiece or with an excavator. When the caries removal stage is complete, the cavity should be reassessed. For cavities that are to be restored with resin composite, it is not necessary to remove unsupported and undermined enamel.

- Lining: The choice of lining depends on the depth of the cavity. In minimal cavities no lining will be necessary, in medium depth cavities a lining is indicated and this may be achieved using a resin modified glass ionomer. In very deep cavities a sub-lining of calcium hydroxide should be placed.
- Dental adhesive: This technique depends on the dental adhesive system being used (see above).
- Filling the cavity: Composite resin should be placed in small increments of less than 2 mm in depth and each increment fully cured. Ideally each increment should touch the minimum number of walls possible to reduce the effects of polymerisation shrinkage.
- Shaping the occlusal surface: The final increments should be shaped to mimic the shape of the occlusal surface of the tooth. Following final curing, check all the margins with a probe to look for deficiencies or ledges.
- Polishing: Once the rubber dam has been removed the occlusion should be checked by asking the patient whether the restoration feels high or not and by using articulating paper. Any high spots should be adjusted and the restoration polished (see section on polishing).

Treatment of posterior proximal lesions

Caries on the proximal surfaces of posterior teeth occurs because plaque can collect cervical to the contact area, resulting in a stagnation area (or plaque trap). The diagnosis of proximal caries requires careful clinical examination of the marginal ridges; this area may appear darker or more opaque than surrounding tooth tissue. Bitewing radiographs are essential for the diagnosis and assessment of posterior proximal lesions.

If the lesion is confined to enamel, as assessed radiographically, then it may be possible to arrest, or even reverse, the progress of the caries. Appropriate dietary advice and interdental cleaning instruction should be given and fluoride, either as an operator-applied varnish or in toothpaste, should be used.

If the lesion has cavitated and spread into dentine then operative intervention will normally be necessary to restore the surface integrity of the tooth.

Access to caries on the posterior proximal surfaces may be gained in a number of ways:

- Through the marginal ridge from the occlusal aspect. The most common technique to gain access to the caries is through the marginal ridge from the occlusal surface of the tooth and this technique will be described in detail.
- From the occlusal surface (**tunnel preparation**), preserving the marginal ridge. The tunnel preparation is difficult to execute unless there is a pre-existing occlusal restoration, which is removed and access to the proximal caries can be gained from the occlusal cavity, without removing the marginal ridge. This technique is not suitable if there is extensive proximal caries as the marginal ridge will collapse.
- From the buccal (or lingual) aspect. This technique is only suitable where there is no risk of marginal ridge collapse and in situations where resin composite can be used as the restorative material.
- Directly, if the adjacent tooth is absent.

Technique for posterior proximal restorations through the marginal ridge

- Local analgesia is usually required.
- Check occlusion and mark occlusal stops with articulating paper.
- Ensure effective isolation.
- Protect adjacent teeth: Some operators like to place a matrix band on the adjacent tooth to prevent damage of this tooth during preparation of the box component of the cavity. This is no guarantee that the tooth will not be damaged and care should always be taken in the preparation of proximal cavities to protect the adjacent tooth.
- Gaining access: Access is gained through the marginal ridge using a pear-shaped diamond or tungsten carbide bur in a high speed handpiece. Start slightly away from the marginal ridge and direct the bur downwards and towards the contact area. The bur should drop down into the caries. Try and leave a thin wall of proximal enamel to protect the adjacent tooth. This can be removed subsequently with gingival margin trimmers. This creates a shape described as a box, but it should not be square: it should have round internal line angles and should be wider cervically than occlusally. If there is also occlusal caries then the cavity should be extended into the occlusal fissure (Figs 13.10 and 13.11). If there is no occlusal caries then the cavity does not need to extend into the fissure (see Figure 13.12).

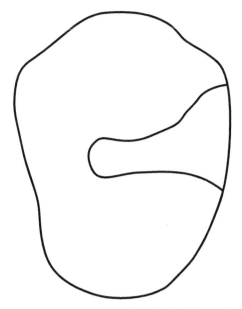

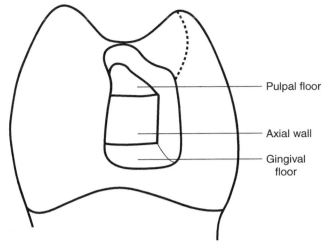

Figure 13.13 Posterior proximal cavity.

Figure 13.11 Posterior proximal cavity involving the occlusal fissure.

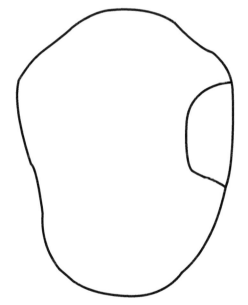

Figure 13.12 Posterior proximal cavity: box only.

- Caries removal: Caries should be removed with a round stainless steel or tungsten carbide bur in the slow speed handpiece. Remove the caries from the enamel dentine junction first before moving to the axial wall (and pulpal floor if the cavity has been extended into the occlusal fissure). An excavator may also be used to remove soft dentine caries.

  This should result in a cavity that clears the contact area cervically and is wider cervically than occlusally.

- Retentive features: Additional retentive features are only necessary if amalgam is to be used as the restorative material. If the cavity has extended into the occlusal fissure then this will act as a key or dovetail

to retain the amalgam and prevent its displacement. If there is no occlusal key and amalgam is to be used, then small grooves should be cut at the junctions between the axial wall and the buccal and lingual walls.

- Lining: If the cavity is suitably deep to require lining then this should be placed on the pulpal floor and on the axial wall (see Figure 13.13).

- Matrix band: A matrix band is placed to help retain the restorative material during placement, to give shape to the proximal surface of the restoration and to allow close adaptation of the restorative material to the cavity. The band should be closely adapted to the cervical margin and should be burnished against the adjacent tooth to help formation of a good contact.

  There are many types of matrix bands and holders (Figure 13.14), but commonly used ones are:

  ○ **Siqveland**. This system uses a straight band and the holder and band are removed from the tooth simultaneously. This can sometimes result in removal of part of the newly packed amalgam.

  ○ **Tofflemire**. This system has the advantage that the holder is removed before the band and this may prevent removal of the restoration with the band. The bands are curved (in a boomerang shape) so that when in the holder the diameter is greater occlusally than cervically; resulting in a better shape for the final restoration. Bands are also available to deal with deep boxes.

  ○ **Circumferential**. A number of systems exist that have no retainer/holder. The band is tightened by a spring mechanism.

  ○ **Ivory**. This has a holder which engages into a selection of holes in a metal band. The metal band replaces only one proximal wall and therefore cannot be used for cavities involving both proximal walls.

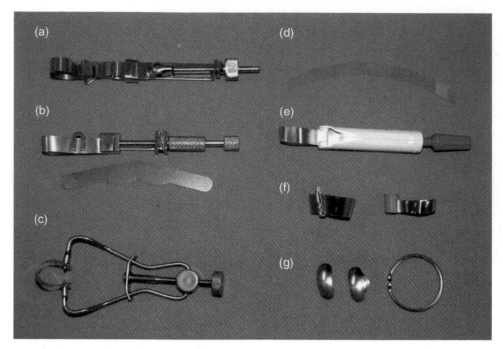

Figure 13.14 Matrix bands and holders: (a) Siqveland; (b) Tofflemire and separate shaped band; (c) ivory; (d) cellulose strip; (e) disposable; (f) circumferential matrix; (g) sectional matrices and ring holder.

- Wedge: The next stage is to place a wedge at the cervical margin of the band, normally from the buccal aspect. The wedge has several functions:
  - It separates the teeth slightly so that when the matrix band is removed there is no space between the adjacent teeth and a tight contact is formed. Wooden wedges swell slightly by absorbing moisture in the mouth so are preferable to plastic wedges.
  - It prevents excess material at the cervical area of the cavity forming a ledge.
  - It shapes band at the cervical margin of the tooth.
  - It can help retain the band in place.
- Material placement (amalgam): Once the amalgam has been mixed, it starts to set so the operator must work quickly to pack and carve the restoration. The amalgam is transferred in increments from the amalgam carrier to the deepest area of cavity - usually the base of the box. It is condensed first with the wider end of amalgam condenser and then with the narrower end. It is important to condense the amalgam well to adapt the material to the cavity walls and to reduce porosity. Place the next increment, condense and continue until the cavity is over-filled. The cavity is over-filled to allow removal of the weak, mercury-rich (γ_2) layer that is at the surface of a well-condensed amalgam. Run a straight probe around the inside surface of the matrix band to remove gross excess of amalgam and to start to shape the marginal ridge. Carefully remove the wedge, matrix retainer and band.

Check the cervical margin for excess amalgam with a straight probe and remove any excess, either with the probe or an amalgam carving instrument, such as a ½ Hollenbach. Use an instrument designed for carving as it will cut through the amalgam, rather than smearing it (as would be the result if a flat plastic were used). Using the tooth as a guide, rest the blade of the carver against the tooth and carve through the amalgam to recreate the cuspal shapes of the tooth. Check that the marginal ridge is a similar height to that of the adjacent tooth.

Check the occlusion by asking the patient to close gently on the restoration. Listen for the sound of the teeth coming together and any impact on the amalgam. Look for any high spots and adjust. Should the amalgam fracture at this stage, it is better to remove the partially set material and start again, rather than try and add to the fractured amalgam.

- Material placement (resin composite): Dental adhesive should be applied to all the surfaces and margins of the cavity. The first increment of restorative material may be placed either at the base of the box or to form the proximal wall. Light cure for the recommended time, then place the next increment, ensuring that this increment only touches either the buccal or lingual wall but not both. Light cure and continue with incremental packing and curing. Carefully shape the marginal ridge by running a straight probe round the inside of the matrix band and finally recreate the cusp shapes to give the correct occlusal contour.

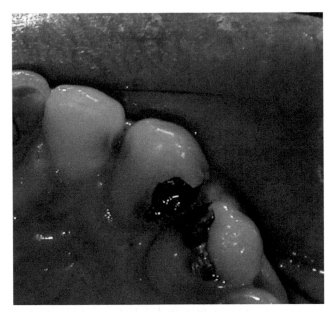

Figure 13.15 Anterior proximal carious lesions in UL2 and UL3.

Remove the wedge, matrix holder and band and check cervically for excess material. Check the occlusion by asking the patient and by the use of articulating paper. Shape and polish as required.

Treatment of anterior proximal lesions

Caries occurs on the anterior proximal surfaces owing to the accumulation of plaque gingival to the contact area (Figure 13.15). Detection of these lesions is by direct vision or by transillumination: reflected light in the mouth mirror.

- Gaining access: Access to the lesion should be from the palatal or lingual aspect if at all possible as this will allow preservation of the labial enamel. A small round diamond in the high speed handpiece is used to drop into the caries.
- Removal of caries: A round bur in the slow speed handpiece is used to remove the caries, trying to preserve the labial enamel. Additional preparation to create a retentive cavity will probably not be necessary as the shape of the carious lesion will result in an undercut cavity. With adhesive restorations, an undercut cavity is unnecessary and amalgam restorations are contraindicated in anterior proximal cavities primarily because of their poor appearance.
- Lining: A lining should be placed as required. Beware that calcium hydroxide lining materials are opaque and can look unsightly through thin labial enamel.
- Matrix: A clear cellulose matrix strip should be placed before use of the dental adhesive to prevent bonding the adjacent teeth together. The strip should be placed so that it is cervical to the gingival margin of the cavity.

- Dental adhesive: Apply the adhesive to the cavity and the cavity margins.
- Material placement: Place the resin composite in the cavity in small increments and light cure. After the final increment has been placed, pull the matrix band tight cervically to prevent formation of a ledge, and light cure.
- Finishing: Check the occlusion as before and finish as required.

Treatment of incisal edge lesions

Incisal edge restorations are the result of trauma, failure of a proximal restoration or extensive proximal caries.

- Access: Access to the lesion is not normally difficult: the difficulty is creating good bonding potential. A labial bevel or chamfer will increase the area of tooth tissue for bonding and will improve the appearance of the final restoration as it will allow the composite to merge gradually with the tooth, rather than having a butt joint. Palatally, a small shoulder will increase the strength of the restoration in this area of occlusal loading. The lack of cavity walls has the advantage of reduced stress from polymerisation shrinkage.
- Lining: In trauma cases, direct or indirect pulp capping with setting calcium hydroxide may be necessary.
- Composite placement: Composite can be built up freehand or by using a matrix. The types of available matrices are:
  - Custom-made: An impression of the palatal aspect of an intact tooth can be used to aid formation of this aspect of the final restoration. To achieve an intact tooth, a temporary restoration can be placed, or a laboratory wax-up used.
  - Preformed: The main types used are clear cellulose strips, incisal corners and complete crown forms.
  To achieve optimal appearance composites of different opacity, such as "dentine", 'body', 'enamel' and translucent should be built up in incremental layers.
- Shaping and finishing: The adjacent teeth may be used as a guide to the shape of the final restoration. Care should be taken not to damage the remaining tooth tissue in the polishing of incisal edge restorations when it may be difficult to distinguish between tooth and restoration.

Treatment of cervical lesions

Lesions occur on the smooth, cervical surfaces owing to enamel and root caries, erosion and abrasion.

- Access: This is not normally difficult unless the lesion is on the lingual surface of a molar tooth. The amount of cavity preparation depends on the cause of the lesion: abrasion and erosion lesions may only require the cutting of a bevel and cleaning of the cavity with a pumice and water paste whereas carious cavities may require access with a high speed round diamond bur and caries removal with an excavator or round stainless steel slow speed bur.

- Material placement: Resin composite is generally the material of choice for such restorations but amalgam may be placed in posterior teeth, and in difficult, subgingival cavities glass ionomer based materials may be used. Glass ionomers should be protected with either varnish or an unfilled resin for the first few days after placement to protect them from moisture contamination (see Chapter 9, p. 190). The material may be shaped freehand or with a matrix.

Polishing and finishing restorations

Restorations should be shaped, finished and polished to a high standard for a number of reasons:

- **Patient comfort.** A restoration left high will result in pulpitis and pain for the patient. A rough restoration is uncomfortable and possibly painful.
- **Aesthetics.** Well polished restorations will reflect the light, minimising the dark appearance of amalgam and making composite restorations more tooth-like.
- **Reduce plaque accumulation.** The smoother the restoration, the less plaque will collect, with subsequent effects on caries development.
- **Restoration longevity.** A restoration with good marginal finish, appropriate contour and high polish will be less likely to fail and be replaced.

Methods

Any polishing regime involves starting with a coarse grit and working through to a fine grit.

Amalgam restorations should not be polished until at least 24 hours after placement. The following sequence may be used:

- Amalgam finishing burs (multi-bladed stainless steel burs for the slow speed handpiece) to develop a smooth surface.
- Silicone points for final polishing.

For resin composite restorations:

- Superfine diamond burs or multi-bladed tungsten carbide burs in the high speed handpiece for the removal of ledges and excess material.
- Superfine diamonds in the slow speed handpiece may also be used where access is more difficult.
- For occlusal surfaces, silicone points may be used to give a smooth finish. This may also be achieved with abrasive discs and strips for other surfaces.
- Finally, a diamond polishing paste will give a high shine to the restoration.

Replacing and repairing restorations

Much time is spent replacing restorations that are considered to have failed. Common reasons given for restoration failure are:

- Secondary caries.
- Marginal defects.
- Fracture.
- Discoloration/staining.
- Ledges.

Each time a restoration is replaced the cavity gets larger, stressing the dental pulp and making the subsequent restoration more difficult to place and shape. It is important therefore to look closely at the reason for failure and assess whether it is necessary to remove all the previous restoration or whether it is possible to repair the existing restoration by cutting a small cavity in the area of the secondary caries or marginal defect and restoring this with an adhesive restoration. Stained and discoloured composites can be refurbished by removal of a thin top layer and replacement with a further layer of resin composite.

Management of heavily restored teeth

Large direct restorations can be difficult to carry out well as access to deep boxes may be awkward and handling a large bulk of material is not easy. Additional means of retention such as slots or the use of bonded amalgams may be necessary (Figure 13.16). It can be difficult to recreate the dental anatomy, especially the contact areas,

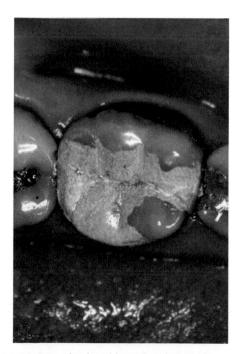

Figure 13.16 Recently placed large bonded amalgam.

occlusal contour and the marginal ridges. Failure rates for large restorations are higher than for small restorations and once one cusp of a posterior tooth has been replaced, an indirect restoration with cuspal coverage should be considered.

Temporary restorative materials and their placement

Why are temporary restorations placed?

- To improve patient comfort by:
  - preventing sensitivity
  - preventing food-packing
  - restoring appearance
  - covering sharp margins of a cavity.
- To provide a sedative effect on an inflamed pulp.
- As an interim restoration before placing the final restoration: perhaps to allow improvement in gingival condition or to assess the patient's response to diet and oral health advice.
- As a planned procedure prior to placing a laboratory-made restoration.
- To assess the prognosis of the tooth and/or pulp.
- To prevent drifting, over-eruption, tilting or gingival overgrowth.
- For caries prevention:
  - By using a fluoride leaching material such as glass ionomer.

Choice of material

This depends on:

- The size and shape of the cavity: a self adhesive material such as a glass ionomer may be required if the cavity has no inherent retentive form.
- The position in the mouth: tooth-coloured material should be used for anterior teeth. Stronger materials should be used for the occlusal surfaces of posterior teeth.
- How long the temporary restoration is to be in place: this depends on the wear characteristics of the material used.
- The choice of eventual restoration: eugenol plasticises composite resin restoratives so there is a risk that any eugenol remaining from the temporary restoration could adversely affect a subsequent composite resin restoration although recent research suggests this is not a problem.

Ideal temporary material

The ideal temporary material should be easy and quick to mix, place and shape. It should set quickly and have appropriate strength and wear characteristics. The material used should be non-toxic and be non-irritant to the pulp, preferably with a sedative effect on the pulp. It should also have an acceptable colour, taste and smell and be cheap and readily available. It is essential that it is easy to remove and is compatible with other materials.

Available materials

- Zinc-oxide eugenol based materials: these are quick and easy to insert and remove but are unaesthetic, lack compressive strength and the taste is sometimes considered unpleasant.
- Polycarboxylates.
- Glass ionomers.
- Light cured polymers.

Temporary crowns

Why are temporary crowns placed?

Temporary crowns are usually placed following preparation of a tooth for a permanent crown. They offer the following advantages:

- Patient comfort, as the temporary crown covers the dentine exposed in the preparation of the tooth for a crown.
- Improved appearance.
- They prevent movement of the adjacent and opposing teeth.
- They prevent overgrowth of the surrounding gingivae.

Types of temporary crowns

- Resin replica technique: In this technique an impression of the tooth is taken in silicone putty or alginate before the crown preparation is started. After the tooth has been prepared the impression is filled with a temporary crown material, commonly a resin composite. This is then replaced in the mouth, removed when almost set and finally trimmed to shape.
- Preformed: Ready-made temporary crowns are available in aluminium and stainless steel for posterior teeth and tooth-coloured polycarbonate for anterior teeth. These crown forms usually need to be trimmed and lined with a temporary crown material to ensure a good fit.
- Temporary post-retained crowns: Posts may be required to retain the temporary crown if the definitive restoration is to be a post-retained crown. Such posts should fit the prepared post-hole and are normally made of metal, such as aluminium.

Cementation of temporary crowns

Cement designed for temporary use should be used as this will allow easy removal of the temporary crown and of any excess cement without damage to the tooth preparation.

The clinical aspects of taking impressions

An impression is a negative imprint of the oral cavity that is used to construct a positive replica of the mouth. Impressions are used to give a permanent record of the dentition for planning treatment (study models) and for the production of appliances, such as dentures and removable orthodontic appliances, and for the construction of indirect restorations, such as crowns and bridges.

Clinical technique for taking impressions for study models

- Assemble materials and equipment which should include:
  - Alginate
  - Trays
  - Adhesive
  - Disinfectant e.g. sodium hypochlorite.
- Prepare the patient: explain the procedure to the patient and seat them in the correct position. Impressions may be recorded with patients sitting up or in a supine position. If a patient is anxious about impressions, then sitting up is more appropriate.
- Selection of tray: trays should be wide enough to allow an adequate thickness of impression material but not too wide so as to make insertion difficult.
- Try in the tray – mandibular arch: work from in front of the patient. Retract one cheek and insert the tray with a rotary motion. Centre the tray over the teeth and ask the patient to lift their tongue.
- Try in the tray – maxillary arch: work from behind the patient. Retract one cheek and insert the tray with a rotary motion. Centre the tray over the teeth and seat at the back first.
- Apply adhesive: a thin layer of adhesive should be applied to the inside of the tray and to the lip of the tray. It is important to wait until the adhesive has set before loading the tray with alginate as otherwise the alginate will slide on the tray rather than adhering to it. The adhesive has set when all the solvent has evaporated off: the adhesive should no longer have a strong smell.
- Mix alginate: the alginate powder and water should be spatulated for about one minute to allow the chemical setting reaction to proceed uniformly throughout the mix. It is important to try and eliminate all air bubbles in the mix. The setting time of three to four minutes can be reduced by increasing the temperature of the water.
- Load the tray: the alginate should be placed in the tray up to the level of the tray lip. Push the alginate down well to ensure no air bubbles.

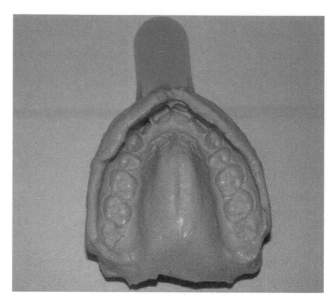

Figure 13.17 Maxillary alginate impression.

- Record the impression: insert the trays as before, manipulating the lips and cheeks to allow the alginate to flow into the sulci, and hold gently in place until the alginate has set. This usually takes 3–4 minutes. To remove the alginate, lift the cheeks away from the borders of the impression, then remove the tray from the mouth in a swift 'snap' movement. If difficulties are encountered in removing the impression, ask the patient to purse the lips and blow. Alginate impressions that are removed from the mouth too early will tear.
- Check the impression: the impression should record all the teeth, the buccal sulci and the palate or lingual sulci as applicable. There should be no air blows, deficiencies or tears in the impression (Figure 13.17).
- Disinfect the impression: the impressions must be disinfected to prevent cross-contamination during laboratory procedures. Various solutions are available to disinfect alginate impressions.
- Send the impression to the laboratory: the alginate impression should be wrapped in a damp tissue and sealed in a polythene bag with the patient's name and date. If alginate is left to dry it distorts (**syneresis**) and if it is soaked for too long it absorbs water (**imbibition**). Ideally, alginate impressions should be poured within one hour of recording.

The management of discoloured teeth

Discoloration is usually classified as **intrinsic** (within the tooth tissue) or **extrinsic** (on the external surfaces of the teeth). Extrinsic staining has a number of causes such as nicotine staining from smoking, red wine, coffee, tea, chlorhexidine or chromogenic bacteria. The common causes of intrinsic staining or mottling in teeth with intact pulps are tetracycline staining, fluoride mottling and inherited or acquired disorders. In non-vital teeth discolouration is usually the result of pulpal haemorrhage following trauma, pulpal necrosis or root canal treatment. The options for management depend on the diagnosis but include prophylaxis of the teeth, bleaching, microabrasion and veneers.

Bleaching vital teeth

This technique involves the use of an agent that contains or produces hydrogen peroxide, a bleaching substance. It is commonly delivered in a gel form that is applied in mouth guards and worn at night for a few weeks, hence the term **night guard bleaching**. The gel is normally 10% carbamide peroxide, although increased strengths may be used for a quick start to the bleaching process. Patients may report dentine hypersensitivity using this technique and the outcome and prognosis is unpredictable. It is more likely to work in patients who have teeth that are towards the darker end of the shade guide. Tetracycline staining will take much longer to lighten.

Bleaching non-vital teeth

Discoloration of non-vital teeth may be due to pulpal haemorrhage following trauma, incomplete removal of pulpal tissue when root canal treatment is carried out, or rarely, root canal cements or restorative materials may cause discoloration. Discoloration is seen in approximately 10% of anterior teeth following root canal treatment. Bleaching techniques include the walking bleach, thermocatalytic bleaching and inside/outside bleaching and is 90% successful over 5 years (Sulieman, 2004). The technique can be repeated if discoloration recurs. Possible complications include cervical resorption and crown fracture.

Enamel microabrasion

This technique uses an acidified abrasive paste to produce removal of superficial enamel layers. It can be used in the management of mottling caused by fluorosis. The technique is unpredictable but can be very successful. Microabrasion uses an abrasive paste that contains hydrochloric acid and therefore a rubber dam must be used to protect the soft tissues. The paste can be bought commercially or can be made from 18% hydrochloric acid and pumice. Use a hard rubber prophy cup at the slowest speed and apply the material to the tooth, rubbing vigorously for 5–10 seconds before washing the tooth. This should be repeated up to 10 times for each tooth. Finally polish the teeth with prophy paste.

Veneers

Teeth may be veneered directly using resin composite or indirectly by laboratory made ceramic or resin composite veneers. Laboratory ceramic veneers can give extremely good results in respect of appearance and tooth shape but will involve some tooth preparation and careful examination of the occlusion is essential. The appearance from composite veneers can be good initially but they will require finishing and polishing on a regular basis and as such may be an interim restoration. Veneers are usually used in the management of discoloured upper anterior teeth as occlusal relationships and the size of the lower incisors may preclude their use in the lower arch.

The management of tooth wear

Preventive advice

Preventive advice is very important in managing tooth wear as it is essential to stop the process that is causing the tooth surface loss. The type of advice given depends on the diagnosis of the type of tooth surface loss and the specific cause. If **erosive tooth surface loss** caused by food or drink is the diagnosis then advice regarding substitution with something less erosive should be given. Carbonated drinks are a common cause of dental erosion and the appropriate advice would be to substitute these drinks with less acidic drinks, such as water, tea, coffee or milk and to restrict the intake of acidic drinks to meal times. If an eating disorder is the cause of the erosive tooth surface loss, it is important to try and ensure that the patient seeks help, as early diagnosis and treatment can alter the course of the disease and the patient's long-term welfare. Other medical conditions such as hiatus hernia may also require medical referral if this is not already in place. There are many other causes of erosive tooth surface loss such as excess vitamin C intake or specific occupations: for example wine tasters. It is difficult to suggest that someone gives up his or her livelihood and advice must therefore be tailored to the individual patient.

The commonest cause of **abrasion** is poor tooth brushing technique. Advice should concentrate on the choice of brush, paste and brushing technique.

Attrition that is pathological, as opposed to physiological (age-related), may be the result of a highly abrasive diet or **parafunction** (a normal movement at an abnormal frequency e.g. grinding or clenching). Making the patient aware of the cause is an important first step. If parafunction (e.g. clenching or grinding) is the cause then careful assessment of the occlusion is important. It may be appropriate to supply a soft splint to prevent further damage to the teeth. In specific cases, attrition may be the result of wear from poorly finished ceramic restorations and these should either be polished or replaced.

Monitoring

This can be an important stage in managing tooth wear as a definitive diagnosis may not have been possible and even if it has been, it is useful to assess whether the advice given has had any affect. Monitoring should involve looking for signs and symptoms of continuing wear. These are not only the amount of tooth surface loss but can include the absence of signs such as tongue scalloping and cheek ridging that indicate a grinding habit or the accumulation of stain on the teeth that may suggest that an erosive habit has ceased. The amount of tooth wear may be monitored clinically by the use of study models, photographs and silicone indices. Mouthguards may be used in the management of tooth wear. If patients grind their teeth they can grind the mouthguard instead. This may also interrupt the habit as well as being diagnostic of the cause of tooth wear and protective of the tooth substance. The mouthguard may be made from soft or hard acrylic for the mandibular or maxillary teeth but should always be full coverage as partial coverage will allow over-eruption of the uncovered teeth.

Restorative treatment

Restorative treatment of tooth substance loss may be required for a number of reasons such as:

- Sensitivity.
- Poor appearance.
- Concern regarding the long-term prognosis, as protection of the teeth may be required to prevent further tissue loss.

The usual concern relating to poor appearance of the teeth is that they are becoming shorter. Short teeth can be difficult to restore as restorations are inherently unretentive. There are, however a number of techniques available to manage such situations. Crown lengthening surgery, orthodontics to extrude the tooth, or elective root canal treatment may be carried out. Appropriate restorations may be chosen and designed to account for the lack of mechanical retention in the remaining tooth structure. Adhesive restorations such as direct resin composites may be utilised or indirect restorations such as composites and ceramics or cast gold, luted with an appropriate composite luting agent, may be fabricated. Alternatively the short teeth may be made into overdenture abutments or restored with an overlay denture.

Lack of space between opposing teeth to allow for restorations may be a problem. Further removal of tooth substance to provide space for restorations may result in pulpal exposure or may reduce the teeth to a height that could not reasonably retain a restoration. Lack of space occurs because of compensatory alveolar growth and the teeth are still in contact despite the loss of inter-occlusal tooth substance.

Space for restorations is therefore required. In general terms, such space may be gained by:

- Increasing the **occluso-vertical dimension** (OVD).
- Orthodontic treatment.
- Using the difference between centric occlusion and centric relation (i.e. the difference between the occlusal position that the patient currently adopts and a reproducible position with the mandible retruded).

Increasing OVD may be achieved in a number of ways:

- Resin composite may be applied to cover worn surfaces and build up incisal edges or occlusal surfaces. Such restorations have the advantages of being relatively simple and quick and of requiring minimal tooth preparation. They are reversible yet provide an immediate improvement in appearance. They are also easy to repair and are relatively inexpensive.
- Extracoronal restorations such as cast metal, ceramic or indirect composite onlays or crowns may be used. These will normally require some form of additional devices to achieve retention to the short clinical crowns. This may take the form of grooves or boxes in the preparation or the use of dentine bonding systems and surface preparation of the restorations.
- Dentures, in the form of partial overlay or **overdentures**, are another method of increasing the OVD. Additions to existing dentures can help the patient adjust to this change.

For anterior tooth wear, the commonest type of orthodontic treatment is the use of an anterior bite plane. This separates the posterior teeth and allows alveolar compensation in the posterior segments and results in space behind the upper anterior teeth that may be used for placing a restoration to cover the palatal surfaces. In restorative dentistry this is known as the **Dahl principle**. Dahl appliances were originally removable and made of cobalt chrome. These have been superseded by fixed alternatives which may be made of cobalt chrome, silver, composite resin or ceramic. Dahl appliances normally work within 6–9 months. The palatal tooth surfaces may subsequently be restored directly with composite or indirectly with gold or ceramic veneers or with dentine bonded crowns.

Another method of obtaining space for restorations is utilising the difference between centric occlusion and centric relation. When teeth or tooth substance is lost posteriorly, patients may posture their mandible forward to a more anterior centric occlusion. If their mandible is allowed to go back towards centric relation, then there may be space available for the restoration of the worn teeth.

Dentine hypersensitivity

In most cases of dentine hypersensitivity, some improvement will be obtained from the use of a desensitising toothpaste containing potassium nitrate or the application of a fluoride varnish. The prescription of a sodium fluoride mouthrinse, once daily for a month, may offer additional relief. If the teeth do not respond to this approach then a resin composite or resin-modified glass ionomer may be applied to the exposed areas of dentine.

Management of trauma

Trauma in the adult dentition usually involves the upper incisors and the loss or damage of these teeth can be very upsetting for patients and can result in the need for extensive dental treatment. Appropriate management of trauma is therefore very important.

Pulpal complications are rare following simple crown fracture without pulpal involvement, but will increase if a luxation injury is involved. (**Luxation** is where the tooth is moved in the socket, but not avulsed.) If pulpal exposure has occurred then treatment with pulp capping or partial pulpotomy will increase the chance of pulp survival. Direct pulp cap is more likely to be successful if pulp exposure is small and treatment is provided within 24hrs of the accident but pulp necrosis is common following luxation injuries to teeth with closed apices.

Avulsion

Ideally, avulsion should be managed immediately by reimplantation of the tooth and the use of a splint. The splint should be a functional (not rigid) splint, such as resin composite, and should be removed after 7–10 days. The aim of the splint is to stabilise the tooth in the bony socket to allow the periodontal ligament to reattach to bone and cementum root surface and for gingival fibres to reattach at the cervical margin of the tooth. The splint should allow some normal tooth movement within the socket to avoid **ankylosis**. The pulp remains vital in 30% of avulsion cases after 5 years. Vitality depends on the size of the apex, the time which the root surface is exposed and how the

tooth was stored (the tooth root should not be handled). The tooth socket is the best storage place for the tooth, but if this is not possible it should be stored in the patient's buccal sulcus or in normal saline or milk until the tooth can be reimplanted. In teeth with closed apices, the pulp should be extirpated and a non-setting calcium hydroxide dressing placed to change local pH and induce osteoblasts to lay down new osteoid material. The canal should be filled with gutta percha 6–12 months later.

Root fracture

The management of root fracture depends on the location of the fracture. If it is close to the gingival margin then the coronal portion should be removed and an assessment made as to whether it is possible to root treat and restore the tooth using a post-retained restoration. It may be possible to extrude the root orthodontically to aid the placement of a crown. Fractures that are in the middle or apical third of the root should be splinted rigidly for 3 months. Root fractures heal by connective tissue, whereas non-healing involves granulation tissue. Pulpal necrosis occurs in approximately 25% of cases, in which case the pulp should be extirpated to the fracture line and managed as for avulsion cases.

The principles of advanced restorative care

Crowns

There are several types of crowns. They may be described by the materials they are constructed from: gold, ceramic or a combination of metal and ceramic, and by the amount of coronal coverage: full, three-quarters.

Gold

Gold is the best of the currently available materials for crowns. The only disadvantage is its appearance and this may not be a consideration for all patients. It is normally used for posterior teeth only. Gold is easy to adjust, can be used in thin section allowing for minimal amounts of tooth substance removal. Gold crowns are adaptable as it is easy to change the shape of tooth or incorporate features such as rest seats or undercuts for clasps to help in the support and retention of a partial denture. Gold has a hardness similar to that of enamel and wears at a similar rate to enamel.

Ceramic

There are several types of all ceramic crowns. The **porcelain jacket crown** (PJC) is the commonest type, although this may be superseded by the dentine-bonded crown. PJCs are only really suitable for anterior teeth as the material is brittle. They require an even amount of tooth substance removal (approximately 1 mm) to ensure support for the crown. High strength ceramics have been used for posterior teeth but these require substantially greater tooth preparation.

Dentine bonded crowns are full coverage ceramic restorations that are bonded to the tooth using a resin composite luting system. Such crowns have good fracture resistance once bonded and require minimal preparation. They can be used where there has already been tooth substance loss or where there is limited remaining crown height. They are often used in cases of tooth substance loss by erosion. Their appearance can be excellent although this may be compromised if care is not taken over the luting stage. This procedure is technique sensitive and time consuming compared with conventional crowns and it should be noted that at present there are no long term clinical results on these restorations.

Metal ceramic

Metal ceramic (porcelain fused to metal) crowns may be used anteriorly and posteriorly. They have good strength and can have excellent appearance. They require more tooth substance removal than cast metal crowns and if tooth reduction is inadequate from the axial walls, appearance and shape can be compromised resulting in opaque, over-contoured restorations. Tooth reduction occlusally can be minimised by designing the crown to have a metal occlusal surface. This improves retention and resistance and is easier to fabricate in the laboratory and to adjust at the chairside and negates the possibility of a rough occlusal ceramic surface damaging the opposing teeth.

Post-retained crowns

A post is used to retain a core which supports a crown. Posts do not strengthen teeth and should be avoided where there is adequate remaining tooth tissue to retain a crown without the need for a post. Parallel-sided posts are retained better than tapering posts; however, in very tapering root canals, a parallel-sided post may result in excess dentine removal. Posts may be fabricated in the laboratory or may be supplied ready made. Laboratory-made posts are made from cast metal and may involve the use of pre-formed elements, such as plastic burn-out posts. Ready-made posts are metal or fibre and require the addition of a core in a plastic material. Cores may be made from amalgam, composite or glass ionomer. The latter is more suitable for small amounts of tooth build-up.

Replacement of teeth

Options for replacing small numbers of missing teeth are:

- Accept the space.
- Orthodontic treatment to close the space.
- A resin retained bridge.
- A conventional bridge.
- A removable prosthesis.
- An immediate denture.
- An implant retained fixed restoration.

Factors to take into account when considering such replacement include the longevity of the different options, the possibility of retrieval if an option fails, the available designs, the patient's occlusion, the condition of the rest of the dentition and supporting tissues and the ability of the patient to maintain the restoration.

Options for replacing a larger number of teeth are:

- Removable prostheses.
- Copy dentures.
- Implant retained removable restorations.
- Bridgework.

Partial dentures/removable prostheses

These may be used as an interim restoration before the provision of a bridge or an implant or may be the definitive restoration. Partial dentures may also be utilised as a transition to over-dentures or complete dentures. There are many different types and designs of partial dentures, but most frameworks are fabricated from either cobalt chrome or acrylic. The choice will depend on the condition of the remaining dentition, the number, position and type of retained teeth, the occlusion and the overall plan for the dentition. Patient preference should also be considered. All-acrylic dentures are light, can have good appearance and can be added to following any further extractions. They need to have bulk for adequate strength and this may result in excessive mucosal coverage. Cobalt chrome dentures are strong in thin section and the design can incorporate clasps (for retention) and rest seats and can cover less mucosa than acrylic dentures. Mechanical interlocking is required for the addition of the acrylic components.

The advantages of partial dentures:

- They can replace teeth, soft tissue and bone.
- There is minimal tooth preparation, if any.
- Other options are still possible as there is little or no tooth preparation.
- They can replace multiple teeth, in different areas of arch.
- They can reduce the occlusal loading on the remaining natural teeth.

- Their appearance can be good.
- They are the least expensive restorative option.
- They can be designed to allow for future additions.

Disadvantages:

- Increased dental plaque can result in caries and gingival problems.
- Coverage of the palate is often unpopular with patients: complaints regarding loss of taste relate to temperature and texture of food.
- The removable aspect is not liked by patients, in general, owing to social concerns.
- The appearance can be compromised by visible clasps.
- There is limited longevity which may negate the lower initial cost.

Resin retained bridges

This type of bridge relies on a metal wing to retain the pontic. The design most likely to succeed is a single cantilever. Double abutments and fixed-fixed designs should be avoided as they are more likely to fail. Before providing a resin-retained bridge the following factors should be taken into account: spacing, occlusion, restoration of adjacent teeth, bone support, the number of other teeth present and the condition of the mouth. There are a number of different surface treatments for the fitting surface of the metal work of resin-retained bridges but the common types are sand-blasted and acid or electrolytic etching (**Maryland bridge**). The **Rochette bridge** relies on mechanical retention from holes in the framework and still has a limited role as an interim restoration, perhaps during implant work. Resin retained components can be used in combination with conventional bridgework but failure in the design by incorporating a movable joint must be allowed for so that when the resin retained component debonds, then that part of the bridge may then be removed and rebonded. The success rate of resin-retained bridges can be high but careful attention must be paid to design, surface treatment and adhesion.

Advantages:

- Minimal tooth preparation is required depending on occlusion.
- Fixed/not removable: patients like this aspect. It is also better for gingival health than a partial denture.
- Appearance can be good but may be compromised by a metal wing showing through.
- Failure due to debonding or caries. This is minimised if a single cantilever is used.

Disadvantages:

- Not feasible in many cases.
- Potential failure of retention (debonding).

- Longevity is limited.
- Technique sensitive.
- Metal work of retainer may compromise appearance.
- Occlusal loading is limited.
- Potential problems when an existing restoration fails under a wing.

Conventional bridgework

Conventional bridgework is often of a fixed-fixed design but may also be a cantilever, fixed-movable or a combination of elements. Common design examples are:

- Cantilever design: e.g. the replacement of an upper lateral incisor from the adjacent upper canine.
- Fixed-fixed: e.g. replacing a lower first permanent molar with the second permanent molar and second premolar as retainers.
- Fixed-movable: where abutment teeth are not parallel, for example a tilted lower molar.

The success rate is higher for short-span bridges involving either the anterior region or the posterior regions of the mouth. Failure increases with the length of span and for bridges involving both anterior and posterior teeth.

Advantages:

- Fixed.
- Appearance can be good.
- Can incorporate changes to occlusion and appearance.
- Predictable.

Disadvantages:

- Tooth preparation.
- Pulpal health compromised.
- Failure – mechanical and biological.
- Long spans have higher failure rates.
- High levels of skill – technical and clinical required.
- Irreversible.

Implant retained prostheses

Modern implants are made of titanium as this material is biologically accepted in bone, allowing for close apposition of the bone to the implant (this is known as **osseointegration**). Most implant systems require two stages of treatment. A hole is cut in the bone and the implant placed into this cavity. This is followed by a period of several months' healing before the implant is uncovered and a crown, bridge or denture provided. Plaque and calculus can attach to implants, resulting in tissue inflammation and possible 'peri-implantitis'.

Implants should be considered as a possible option to replace missing teeth and it is important to be able to outline their advantages and disadvantages to patients when they ask questions about implants.

Advantages:

- Fixed or removable prostheses may be supported by implants.
- Highly predictable, i.e. good prognosis, in experienced hands.
- Longevity of implants is high compared with other restorative techniques.
- Implants maintain alveolar bone following loss of teeth.

Disadvantages:

- Success depends on an adequate amount of high quality bone.
- Surgery is involved.
- Technique sensitive.
- Expensive; in terms of time and money.
- High levels of maintenance are required.
- Smoking can affect success and result in a poorer prognosis.

Overdentures

Overdentures may be complete or partial and are made to cover roots, which support the prosthesis. The advantages of overdentures over conventional dentures are the maintenance of alveolar bone and jaw muscle tone, improved stability and retention from the retained bone, enhanced proprioception from the periodontal ligament and therefore improved masticatory ability for the patient, and the psychological aspects related to the retention of the roots of teeth. Disease control is important in overdenture cases as otherwise the root faces will rapidly decay. The ideal complete overdenture case has a minimum of two roots, symmetrically distributed in the mouth and with a dome shaped crown. They should be at least 50% bone supported and root canal treatment should be possible.

Advantages:

- Bone retained.
- Proprioception enhanced.
- Psychological aspects.
- Transition to complete dentures.

Disadvantages:

- Potential caries on root surfaces.
- Bulky.
- Difficult to maintain.

Risks/outcomes of restorative treatment

All restorations have sequelae for the teeth involved. A number of factors are thought to influence the likelihood of a tooth becoming non-vital following dental treatment. These include the preoperative condition of the tooth, the cutting temperature and duration of any tooth preparation, the use of local analgesia and retraction cord, the length of time of temporisation and the area of exposed root surface. To reduce the risk of loss of vitality following tooth preparation, the following may help:

- Remove infected dentine.
- Use appropriate cooling and preparation design.
- Provide well-fitting temporary restorations.
- Place the permanent restoration as soon as possible.

Loss of pulp vitality can occur following tooth preparation. Histological studies demonstrate pulp reactions in response to dental treatment. The incidence and risk period of pulp deterioration following tooth preparation remains uncertain as a number of cross-sectional studies have shown differing results. From these studies, the approximate mean value for periapical changes on teeth restored with crowns or bridges is 10% at 10 years (Saunders and Saunders 1998). Longevity for crowns is also influenced by other factors such as caries rates, gingival recession, and porcelain fracture. Failure rates are high for post-retained crowns. Loss of retention may occur owing to inadequate post length or design or to vertical root fracture. Perforation is also a risk of post crowns.

Care of instruments and handpieces

Dental instruments and handpieces need regular maintenance if they are to work effectively. Hand instruments designed for cutting enamel or dentine should be kept sharp. Chisels may be sharpened against a lubricated stone or against a stone bur in a slow speed straight handpiece. Excavators and probes are best sharpened against an abrasive disc held in a slow speed straight handpiece.

It is also essential that they are sterilised between patients to prevent cross infection.

- Obvious debris, such as excess dental cement, should be removed immediately after use of the instrument by cleaning with an impregnated wipe.
- Cleaning is a vital step as it removes the nutritive material on which bacteria survive. This may be achieved by manual washing, ultrasonic baths or the use of a washer-disinfector. The washer–disinfector is the most reliable technique for decontamination of instruments.
- Sterilisation is best carried out in an autoclave. Instruments should be clean before they are placed in the autoclave. Sterilisation is achieved by direct contact of the instruments with saturated steam at 134 °C for a minimum of 3 minutes.

- Handpieces must be oiled before being placed in the autoclave and should be maintained according to the manufacturer's instructions.

The ergonomic environment

Working position

It is important to have a good working position to allow efficient, effective working, to maximise patient comfort and to prevent the development of back and neck problems for the operator and dental nurse.

When taking a history or discussing treatment with a patient, the operator should sit facing the patient who should also be in a sitting position in the dental chair. Sitting behind or standing in front of the patient reduces opportunities for non-verbal communication and may intimidate or even distress the patient.

For carrying out treatment, the patient should be put into a supine position and the operator should sit behind the patient. The operator should sit with his/her thighs parallel with the floor, feet flat on the floor, back against the chair support and elbows close to the rib cage. For further details, see Chapter 17, p. 355–356.

Lighting

The operating light should be positioned to give maximum light to the area in which treatment is being carried out: the position is different for the upper and for the lower arches. Additional light may also come from fibre-optic light in the high speed handpiece.

Work surfaces

There are a number of possible positions for work surfaces: beside the operator, beside the dental nurse, behind the head of the chair and as a bracket table over or beside the patient. Instruments, materials and patient records and radiographs need to be placed in appropriate positions around the operator, nurse and patient and therefore a number of surfaces are normally used. Patients' records should be kept well away from instruments to prevent contamination of the notes.

Close support (four-handed) dentistry

An operator and a dental nurse working as a team will result in efficient delivery of dental care in as pleasant a manner as possible for patients with improved safety. The nurse maintains a clear, dry field for the operator by retracting the lip, cheeks and tongue and by aspirating the water from the high-speed handpiece. The dental nurse may also keep the operator's mirror clear of spray by using the air stream of the three-in-one. The nurse passes and collects instruments from the operator.

Instruments should be passed in front of the patient and not over the face, particularly the eyes.

Management of anxiety

Assessment of anxiety

Dental anxiety can be measured both qualitatively and quantitatively. The qualitative measures can be made by observation: the patient may be shaking, sweating and be unwilling or uncertain about sitting in the dental chair. Patients who are nervous often talk incessantly, often avoid eye contact or may even appear aggressive. Important information can also be gained through the dental history that the patient gives. There may have been a previous bad dental experience which has affected the patient's confidence in dental treatment.

Dental anxiety can be measured quantitatively using a questionnaire. There are many dental anxiety questionnaires but the quickest and simplest is the **Modified Dental Anxiety Scale** (MDAS). This questionnaire has five questions relating to different aspects of dental treatment including scaling, drilling and local analgesic injections. The range of scores is from 5–25. The average score is around 11, with those with high anxiety scoring 20+.

Prevention of anxiety

Considerable patient anxiety follows a bad dental experience. It can take only one distressing episode to affect a patient's attitude for many years. It is therefore particularly important to try to prevent any experience that may colour a patient's attitude to dentistry in the future. There are two situations that tend to recur as bad experiences. The first is where a procedure becomes unexpectedly more complex, for example caries removal may result in pulp treatment. The second is where a patient feels pain during a procedure. The key elements to preventing any patient developing anxiety are therefore careful planning and good pain control.

Planning for anxious patients

Good communication skills are vital in planning and carrying out treatment. This is especially so with anxious patients. Many patients, especially when they are anxious, do not remember all that they have been told during dental visits. To take account of this, there are some simple guidelines that can be followed:

- Ensure that the information that you give is in plain, simple, jargon-free language.
- Reinforce your message by repeating it.
- Give your patient control over the procedure by the use of stop signals, e.g. raising the hand.

- Tell the patient what is going to happen as the procedure progresses.
- Ensure that the patient knows what is to happen at the next visit.

This subject is covered more extensively in Chapter 6.

Pain control

Good pain control is achieved through effective local analgesia, which should be given as painlessly as possible. Whatever type of injection has been given, always check analgesia before proceeding. Check for soft tissue analgesia in the area supplied by the nerve that has been blocked, and then ask the patient if he/she is happy for treatment to proceed. The trust between the operator and the patient will be lost if treatment is started before the patient is numb.

Anxious patients often have a low pain threshold. If they use a stop signal to halt the procedure, treatment should stop. If they are feeling pain, additional local analgesic should be administered. If the primary injection (i.e. infiltration or block), is not effective, then the use of intraligamentary or intraosseous anaesthesia is indicated. The fact that treatment has stopped and efforts are being made to gain more effective analgesia is reassuring to patients and will reinforce their trust.

References

Eley, B.M. (1997) The future of dental amalgam, parts 1–7. *British Dental Journal*,; **182**, 247–9, 293–7, 333–8, 373–81, 413–7, 455–9; **183**, 11–14.

Ricketts, D. (2001) Management of the deep carious lesion and the vital pulp dentine complex. *British Dental Journal*, **191**, 606–610.

Saunders, W.P. and Saunders E,M. (1998) Prevalence of per-iradicular periodontitis associated with crowned teeth in an adult Scottish subpopulation *British Dental Journal* **185**, 137–140.

Sulieman, M. (2004) An overview of bleaching techniques 1, 2, 3. *Dental Update*, **31**, 608–616: 2005; **32**, 039–046: 2005; **32**, 101–108.

Further reading

Banerjee, A. and Watson, T.F. (2011) *Pickard's Manual of Operative Dentistry*. Oxford University Press, Oxford.

Brunton, P.A. (2002) *Decision making in Operative Dentistry*. Quintessence, New Malden.

Kidd, E. and JoystonBechal, S. (2005) *Essentials of Dental Caries*. Oxford University Press, Oxford.

Smith, B.G.N. and Howe, L.C. (2006) *Planning and Making Crowns and Bridges*. Informa Healthcare, London.

van Noort, R. (2007) *Introduction to Dental Materials*. Mosby, St Louis.

14

Exodontia

Hazel J. Fraser

Summary

This chapter covers:

- Indications for the extraction of deciduous teeth
- Preparation of the patient
- Obtaining the local analgesia
- Instruments
- Technique
- Postoperative care
- Complications

Introduction

Exodontia is the subject of extraction of teeth or parts of them. It also includes the techniques used in the extraction of teeth.

The current legal position for dental therapists in the United Kingdom is that they are permitted to extract primary (deciduous) teeth only and they can only be extracted using local analgesia. Student dental therapists can extract primary (deciduous) teeth under general anaesthesia with direct supervision from a registered dentist. This is in order to gain practice in extracting primary teeth. If primary teeth are extracted when the patient is sedated then a registered dentist must be present in the room.

Indications for tooth extraction

A study by Alsheneifi and Hughes (2001) showed that first primary molars were the most common tooth type extracted and comprised 30% of teeth removed.

Central incisors were the next most common tooth type extracted and accounted for 25% of extractions.

It may be considered necessary to extract primary teeth because of:

- **Caries**: In a study by Tickle *et al.* (2002) it was found that 44% of primary teeth which were carious or had received an intervention of some kind were extracted, however only 12% were extracted due to pain or sepsis.
- **Pain**.
- **Sepsis**: This may be either chronic or acute e.g. acute abscess with cellulitis.
- **Trauma**: Up to 30% of children up to 7 years of age sustain injury to primary incisors, including crown fracture, root fracture, tooth avulsion, and dental displacement.
- **Failed restorative treatment**: research by Milsom *et al.* (2002) suggests that the risk of carious primary molars being extracted is similar whether these teeth receive restorative care or not.
- **Periodontal disease**: This is an uncommon reason for extraction in children.
- **Altered eruption pattern**: Most infraoccluded and **ankylosed** primary molars with a permanent successor will exfoliate normally; therefore the usual treatment recommendation is to await normal exfoliation and then eruption of the permanent successors. Retained primary teeth can be extracted as part of an orthodontic treatment plan.
- **Misplaced primary teeth, natal and neonatal teeth**: Although rare, teeth present when the baby is born can interfere with the baby's nutrition. The decision

Clinical Textbook of Dental Hygiene and Therapy, Second Edition. Edited by Suzanne L. Noble.
© 2012 John Wiley & Sons, Ltd. Published 2012 by John Wiley & Sons, Ltd.

to extract should take into consideration the trauma to the child's oral tissue or mother's breast, mobility of the tooth, the danger of inhalation and the potential orthodontic effects of tooth loss.

- **Overcrowding**: A study by Kau *et al.* (2004) showed that there was a reduction in lower incisor crowding as a result of lower primary canine extraction. However, arch perimeter decreased more in those patients who had extractions, leaving less space for the eruption of the lower permanent canines.
- **Poor co-operation** of the patient during restorative treatment can lead to extractions as an alternative method to the removal of disease from the patient's mouth.
- **Medical history**: If the patient has a medical condition and the teeth are carious then extractions may be indicated.
- **A negative attitude** regarding restorative treatment from the parent or patient may influence the decision to extract.
- **Insufficient tooth structure** may make satisfactory restoration impossible or impracticable.
- **Pulpal involvement** which might involve more than one tooth could make extraction the preferred treatment option.

Contraindications for tooth extraction

- **Medical history**: Certain medical conditions such as blood dyscrasias or renal disease may be a contraindication to extractions. Healing can be prolonged in diabetic patients or patients suffering from malignancy such that a restorative approach may be the preferred option.
- **Space maintenance**: If a primary tooth is extracted early then the remaining teeth may drift mesially or distally closing the space for the permanent successor. This may prevent its eruption into the correct position resulting in a subsequent malocclusion.

Relevant anatomical structures

The teeth of the primary dentition are situated in the alveolar bone of the maxilla and mandible and as such are not closely related to any major anatomical structures. However, the difficulty of an extraction can be significantly influenced by the presence and position of the developing permanent teeth. This is particularly the case with the developing first and second premolars where the crowns of the teeth are closely related to and enveloped by the roots of the primary molars. Injudicious extraction can therefore result in the dislodgement of the permanent successor.

The eruption dates of primary teeth are described in Chapter 12, p. 245.

Nerve supply

It is important to remember that when extracting primary teeth, the innervation of not only the teeth but also the supporting structures needs to be considered. The relevant nerve supply is described below; however the relationship of the nerves to various anatomical structures in the adult is described in more detail in Chapter 10, p. 209–210.

All the primary dentition is supplied by the **trigeminal (Vth) cranial nerve**; its **maxillary nerve trunk** supplying the maxillary primary dentition and the **mandibular nerve trunk** supplying the mandibular dentition. These two trunks further subdivide as follows:

The **upper anterior primary incisors and canines** and the labial gingivae are supplied by the anterior superior alveolar nerve branch; the palatal gingivae are supplied by the nasopalatine (long sphenopalatine) nerve and the soft palate and uvula are supplied by the lesser palatine nerve.

The **upper primary molars** are supplied by the middle superior alveolar nerve, which also supplies the buccal gingivae whilst the palatal gingivae are supplied by the greater palatine nerve.

The nerve supply to the **primary mandibular teeth** is the inferior alveolar nerve; a branch of the mandibular trunk of the trigeminal nerve. The buccal gingivae and mucosa are supplied by the mental nerve, a branch of the inferior alveolar nerve. The lingual gingivae and mucosa are supplied by the lingual nerve. A more detailed description can be found in Chapter 1, p. 19.

Preparation of the patient

Prior to embarking on the extraction of a primary tooth, it is important to address the preoperative medical and psychological management and care of the patient. The following points need to be considered:

- **Medical history**. This needs to be checked and confirmed particularly with respect to a history of bleeding, blood dyscrasias, etc.
- **Consent**. Consent must be given by both the patient and the parent or guardian before extraction of teeth. The consent must be obtained both orally and in writing.
- **Prescription**. This must be written by a registered dentist who has examined the patient and is included as part of the treatment plan.
- **Confirmation** with the patient and parent/guardian that there is agreement with the tooth or teeth prescribed by the dentist for extraction. Any uncertainty must be clarified.
- **An explanation** to the patient and the parent/guardian as to what the procedure involves and how it will be carried out.

- **Appropriate protection** of the patient. There should be adequate protection of the patient's clothing together with appropriate eye protection. The operator should also have appropriate protective clothing (see Chapter 8, p. 164).
- **Non-pharmacological behaviour techniques** that can be used for the management of an anxious child are: behaviour shaping, tell/show/do, reinforcement, desensitisation, modelling and hypnosis. These and other methods of behaviour management which might apply to any operative dental treatment on a child are fully described in chapter 12, p. 262–263.

Obtaining local analgesia

Topical analgesia

Prior to an injection of local analgesia in children it is wise to use a topical analgesic. Preparations include:

- 10% lidocaine hydrochloride spray.
- 5% lidocaine hydrochloride gel.
- 20% benzocaine gel.

The gel preparation is easier to apply than sprays and can be more easily localised. Sprays can affect unwanted areas in the mouth and because the taste may not be well tolerated by the patient it should be sprayed on to cotton wool before placing in the mouth. Benzocaine gel is flavoured with attractive tastes such as bubble gum, and so is more popular with children.

Topical analgesics penetrate keratinised mucosa poorly. They are much more effective on non-keratinised mucosa. This means that they are less effective on palatal mucosa and attached gingivae. The topical analgesic should be applied to as small an area as possible. This reduces potential toxicity and prevents excessive numbness in the tongue and soft palate which may be unpleasant for the child. Adequate time (approximately 2–3 minutes) should be allowed for the topical analgesic to take effect before embarking on infiltration analgesia.

Infiltration analgesia

The positioning of the local analgesic is crucial to achieving adequate analgesia. Failure to achieve this will result in both loss of confidence and loss of co-operation by the patient. An aspirating syringe should be used for all local analgesia (see Chapter 10).

Maxilla

Buccal infiltration

The needle should be inserted into the free gingivae, just above the attached gingiva of the tooth to be anaesthetised. This is achieved by retracting and holding the cheek or lip taut to improve access and visibility and increase patient comfort. The apices of the primary teeth lie near to the point of needle insertion.

Palatal infiltration

Prior to undertaking a palatal infiltration, it may be necessary to carry out a **transpapillary injection**. The needle is inserted from a buccal approach into the papillae, mesially and distally to the tooth being extracted. The needle is advanced while depositing a small amount of local analgesic solution. Blanching of the mucosa will be seen palatally at the gingival margin.

The palatal infiltration should now be less uncomfortable for the patient. The needle is inserted at right angles to the mucosa at the apex of the tooth to be extracted. This is approximately 5–7 mm from the gingival margin.

Mandible

Buccal infiltration

Infiltration techniques are generally used, (unlike block injections which would normally be necessary in adults) as the alveolar plate is perforated by many vascular canals. The same principles apply as to the maxilla. If analgesia cannot be obtained with a buccal infiltration then an inferior dental block injection may be necessary (see Chapter 10, p. 213).

Lingual infiltration

This may be achieved using a transpapillary injection followed by lingual infiltration if necessary.

The most common choice of analgesia for children is 2% lidocaine hydrochloride with 1:80 000 epinephrine (adrenaline), 3% prilocaine (Citanest) with felypressin or 4% articaine with 1:100 000 epinephrine (adrenaline). The dosage is influenced by age and body weight as described in Chapter 12, p. 265. Epinephrine (adrenaline) and felypressin are added as vasoconstrictors to reduce the dispersion of the local analgesic and thereby localise and prolong the analgesia. They also reduce postoperative bleeding and systemic toxicity. The manufacturer's instructions and current clinical guidelines should always be followed.

Clinical assessment

Prior to embarking on the extraction of a tooth or root, the operator should attempt to assess the degree of difficulty which is likely to be anticipated. Therefore the following factors should be considered:

- **Ease of access.** Children have small mouths and primary molars can present greater access problems than teeth in the anterior part of the mouth.
- **Degree of mobility.** Anterior teeth are generally easier to remove than primary molars. **Ankylosis** (the

fusion between cementum and/or dentine and alveolar bone) is more common in the mandible than the maxilla and more common with first molars than second molars. An ankylosed tooth tends to appear less erupted and tends to occupy a more inferior position in relation to the occlusal plane when compared to the adjacent teeth and tooth extraction can be significantly more difficult.

- **Extent of tooth breakdown.** Heavily carious teeth tend to have fragile crowns which can easily fracture during extraction.
- **Co-operation of the patient.** Successful extraction under local analgesia requires a high degree of cooperation by the patient.

Extraction instruments

Forceps and elevators are the two types of instruments used for the extraction of primary teeth. They are all made to conform to **International Organization for Standardization** (ISO) specifications. A surgical approach must be taken when extracting teeth and therefore the instruments used should have been autoclaved and be sterile immediately prior to use.

Forceps

The choice of forceps depends on the morphology of the tooth, its root anatomy, the number of roots (Table 14.1), and its location in the mouth.

The forceps available are shaped to accommodate these factors. Forceps are manufactured specifically for the extraction of primary teeth and are smaller than those used for the extraction of permanent teeth (Figure 14.1).

The upper arch

Forceps used for extracting teeth in the upper arch have the handles in the same long axis as the blades although the handles of upper molar forceps are slightly sigmoid to allow the beaks to align with the long axis of the molar teeth. The blades of forceps used to extract anterior teeth

Table 14.1 Primary tooth roots.

Primary tooth	Number of roots
Upper molars	3
Upper canines	1
Upper incisors	1
Lower molars	2
Lower canines	1
Lower incisors	1

(incisors and canines) and retained roots have rounded tips. Shorter-bladed forceps can be used for the canines since they have bulkier roots than the incisors. The molar forceps have two broader blades, one of which is pointed or beaked. Because of the morphology of the upper primary molar teeth in that they have two buccal roots, it is necessary to have forceps designed specifically for either the left or right molars (i.e. upper right forceps for the patient's right side and left forceps for the patient's left). The forceps have a beaked blade and a smooth blade. The beaked blade is designed to fit into the trifurcation between the mesiobuccal and distobuccal roots (beak to cheek). The smooth blade is designed to closely approximate to the palatal root.

The lower arch

All the forceps used in the lower arch have straight handles set at right angles to the blades. The blade pattern for forceps used for extracting anterior teeth (incisors and canines) and retained roots are the same as for the upper arch (i.e. they have rounded tips to engage the lingual and labial surfaces of the single roots). Forceps used for lower primary molars have two beaked blades designed to fit between the buccal and lingual root bifurcations between the mesial and distal roots.

Successful extraction technique depends on:

- Careful use of controlled force.
- Obtaining adequate access to the tooth.
- Creating an unimpeded path of removal.

The degree of force required is dependent mainly on the amount of bone supporting the tooth. Generally this is greater for molars than for anterior teeth. Care should be taken to ensure that the forceps blades have close contact with the root surface. The intimate contact of the whole of the inner edge of the beaks of the forceps

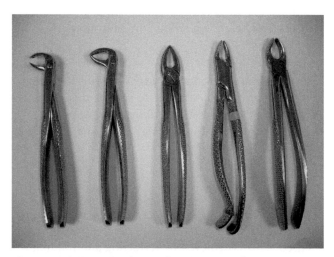

Figure 14.1 Extraction forceps for primary teeth.

on the crown of the tooth is ideal as the same amount of pressure applied to the much smaller area of grip achieved in a single point contact may crush the root or cause the forceps to slip off the crown of the tooth. The cross-sectional shape of the root governs the movements the operator is required to make to achieve extraction with the forceps in correct contact to the tooth. For example, because lower incisors are thinner mesiodistally than they are linguolabially the forceps should be moved in the plane in which the tooth is strongest (i.e. labiolingually).

Elevators

Elevators are single-bladed instruments, which are used to assist in the removal of retained roots. They are usually used when the roots are inaccessible to forceps application. They are designed to elevate a retained root out of its socket so that it can be easily removed or to facilitate the removal of a tooth by widening the periodontal ligament and thereby increasing its mobility. They should be used with great care, as they can cause considerable trauma to adjacent soft tissue and to underlying permanent teeth if improperly handled. They are always applied to the root using bone as a fulcrum rather than another tooth. Using another tooth can result in damage, dislocation or fracture of the tooth being used as the fulcrum.

There are many different types of elevators, but the following are most commonly used in the UK for the removal of retained primary roots.

Warwick James

Warwick James elevators have small operating ends. They are available as left, right and straight (see Figure 14.2). The operating tip is inserted between the tooth root and the socket wall and a rotational movement is applied (Figure 14.3). The elevators should always be used with a finger support on an adjacent tooth (not used as a fulcrum) for stability and great care must be taken not to damage the underlying permanent premolar tooth when extracting primary molars.

Coupland

Coupland's chisels are available in three sizes (1, 2 and 3) and in a straight pattern only (Figure 14.4).

The chisel is used to gently press under the gingival margin of the tooth to be extracted and used in a

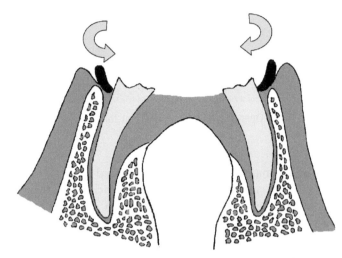

Figure 14.3 Warwick James elevator elevating retained primary molar roots.

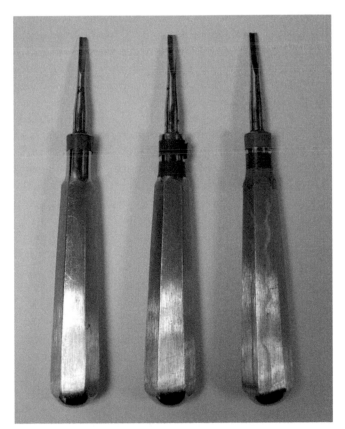

Figure 14.4 Coupland's chisel.

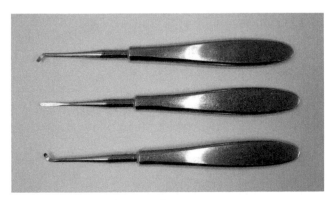

Figure 14.2 Warwick James elevators.

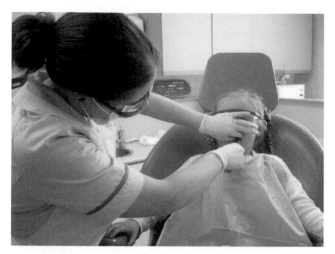

Figure 14.5 Operator and chair position for the extraction of upper teeth.

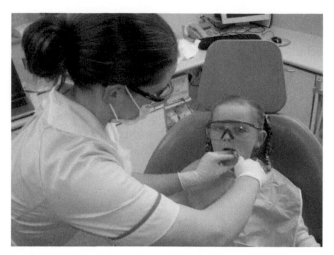

Figure 14.6 Operator and chair position for the extraction of anterior and lower left molar teeth.

rotational manner. This can also be used to release the periodontal membrane and help inform the operator whether effective analgesia has been obtained prior to extraction. Satisfactory analgesia, however, is best checked with a probe on the adjacent gingivae prior to the use of either elevators or forceps.

Extraction technique

Chair position

The chair position is an important factor for both patient and operator. An incorrect position or height will lead to discomfort and muscular stress for the operator, which can result in unnecessary fatigue and possibly to a failed extraction for the patient.

For the extraction of teeth in the two **upper quadrants** the site of the operation should be at elbow height with the chair tipped back at approximately 45° (Figure 14.5).

For the extraction of teeth in the **lower left quadrant** (lower left molars) and lower anterior teeth, the site of the operation should be at or just below elbow height with the chair tipped back at approximately 30° (Figure 14.6).

For the extraction of teeth in the **lower right quadrant** (lower right molars) the site of the operation should be 15 cm (6″) below elbow height with the chair tipped back only slightly (Figure 14.7).

Operator position

Like the chair position, the operator position is important when extracting teeth. Adopting an incorrect posture can not only make the extraction of teeth more difficult but can also lead to long term back problems for the operator. The operator positions described are for a right-handed operator. For a left-handed operator, these positions need to be reversed.

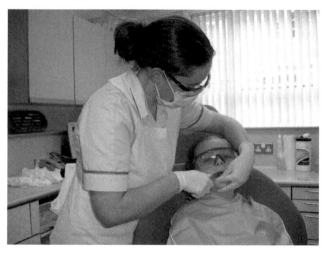

Figure 14.7 Operator and chair position for the extraction of lower right molar teeth.

The extraction of all teeth in the **upper arch** and lower left molars and anterior teeth is carried out with the operator standing facing the patient and standing to the left of the dental chair (Figs 14.5 and 14.6). The extraction of lower right molar teeth is carried out with the operator standing on the right hand side and behind the patient (Figure 14.7).

Extraction of teeth in the maxilla

Upper central incisors: Upper primary straight forceps are used with a primary buccopalatal rotational movement. The final removal is in a buccal direction (Figure 14.8).

Upper lateral incisors: Upper primary straight forceps are used with greater emphasis on a buccopalatal primary movement. The final removal requires a rotational delivery.

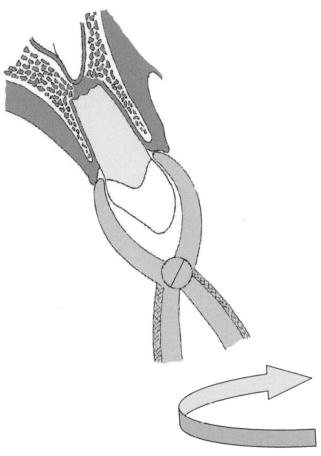

Figure 14.8 Extraction technique for upper primary anterior teeth.

Upper canines: Upper primary straight forceps with shorter blades are used, as the canine root is more bulky than the incisor roots. A buccopalatal primary movement followed by a rotational delivery is employed.

Upper molars: Upper primary molar forceps are used, left or right as appropriate. The forceps are used with the beaked blade on the buccal aspect of the tooth (**beak to cheek**). As previously stated, the handles of the forceps are curved so as to allow the beaks to align with the long axis of the tooth when placed in position on the crown. A buccopalatal primary movement is employed (Figure 14.9).

Extraction of teeth in the mandible

Lower central and lateral incisors, and the lower canines: These teeth have single roots, which tend to be flattened mesiodistally. Lower primary anterior tooth forceps are used. As previously described, lower forceps have the blades at right angles to the handles to enable a vertical downwards force to be applied to the tooth more effectively. The primary movement should be buccolingual with a rotational delivery (Figure 14.10).

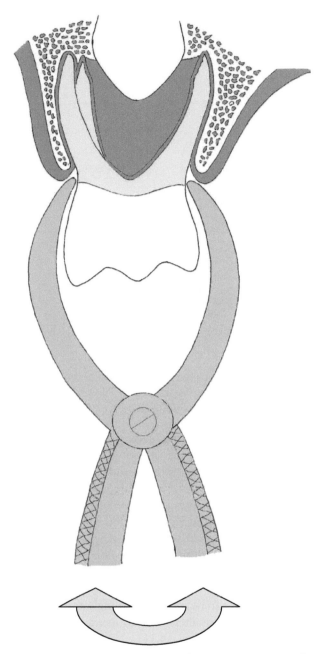

Figure 14.9 Extraction technique for upper primary molars. Buccopalatal primary movement.

Lower molars: Lower primary molar forceps are used. The primary movement is buccolingual with a rotational delivery.

Primary molars have the developing premolars enclosed within their divergent roots, which frequently do not resorb from the apex, as is usually the case with the single rooted anterior teeth, but from the side of the roots. This increases the risk of fracturing the root during extraction. It is undesirable to leave a small piece of root deep in the socket but should fracture occur, leaving the root can be preferable to running the risk of damaging

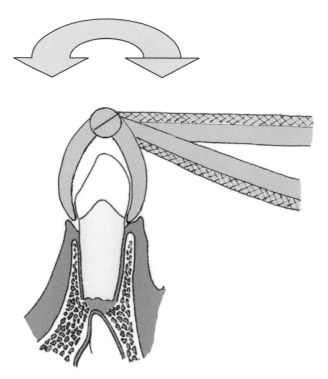

Figure 14.10 Extraction technique for lower anterior teeth. The single root is flattened mesiodistally. Primary movement is buccolingual with rotational delivery.

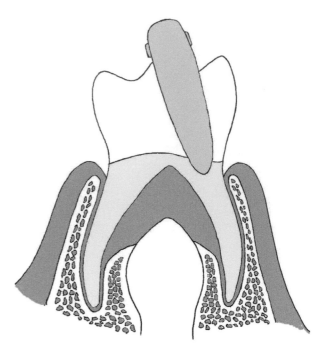

Figure 14.11 Lower primary anterior forceps applied to a single root of a lower primary molar; an alternative to using molar forceps.

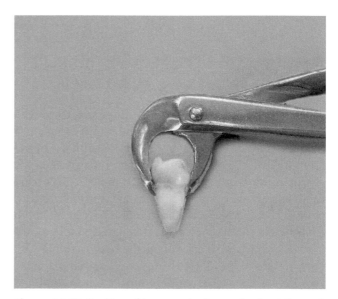

Figure 14.12 Position of lower molar forceps beaks at the neck of the tooth.

the developing underlying successor while trying to remove it. If a small piece of root is retained then the patient and parent/guardian should be informed and the dentist should review the patient after approximately 1 week. The clinical notes should record which root has been retained and how much of it has been left in situ.

Care must be taken when applying lower primary molar forceps. The developing premolar may be damaged if they are applied to the buccal and lingual aspects and then pushed into the soft tissues. Lower primary anterior forceps can be applied to a single root of a lower primary molar as an alternative to using lower primary molar forceps (see Figure 14.11).

With both upper and lower teeth, the blades of the forceps should be pushed over the crown of the tooth so that the beaks make good contact on the root surface at the neck of the tooth (Figure 14.12) and not on the enamel crown where they are likely to slide off when force is applied.

Functions of the non-forceps hand

The extraction of teeth is a two-handed procedure and the contribution of the hand not holding the forceps should not be overlooked. The non-forceps hand has the following important functions during the extraction of a tooth:

- It displaces the tongue, cheek and lips from the site of the extraction, improving visibility and access to the site of the operation (Figure 14.5).

- It protects the patient from damage to the surrounding structures.
- It supports the mandible and gives information to the operator via the alveolar process on the progress of the extraction by the transmission of movements (Figs 14.6 and 14.7).
- On completion of the extraction the fingers on this hand compress both sides of the socket reducing

postoperative discomfort, promoting healing and reducing bleeding.

- It can also be used to distract the patient whilst positioning the forceps on the tooth with such phrases as 'I'm just going to firmly squeeze the sides of your tooth'.
- It holds the child's jaw steady for the operator who can more easily detect any sudden movement he or she may be about to make whilst giving the child a sense of firm control by the operator.

On satisfactory completion of the extraction, all details should be recorded in the patient's clinical record including:

- The teeth/roots extracted.
- The method of obtaining analgesia.
- The quantity and type of analgesic used, batch number, expiry date.
- Any problems encountered e.g. retained roots, excessive tissue damage.
- The postoperative advice given.

Postoperative care

Immediately following extraction, the patient should bite on a gauze pack for 10–15 minutes to arrest the bleeding and satisfactory clotting should be checked before the patient is discharged. It is useful to give the patient some spare packs for home use if needed.

To encourage satisfactory postoperative healing without complications, it is important that the patient and carer are given appropriate aftercare advice. After extraction the following advice should be given both verbally and in writing.

The patient should:

- Avoid any unnecessary exertion for the rest of the day.
- If bleeding occurs, bite on a clean cotton handkerchief (rolled into a 10 mm diameter sausage), not paper tissue or cotton wool. Paper tissues tend to disintegrate and contaminate the wound and cotton wool, if dry, can become entangled within the clot so that the clot is removed with the cotton wool and bleeding will start again. Bleeding will normally cease after 5–10 minutes, but if bleeding does not stop after 20–30 minutes continuous biting then the dental surgery should be contacted, if necessary via the emergency out of hours contact number. It is often helpful to encourage the child to watch their favourite television programme whilst biting partly as a means of distraction and partly so as to measure the time elapsed.
- Avoid swimming pools for 24 hours and until the bleeding has stopped to prevent blood contamination of the pool.

- Take pain killers only if necessary. Calpol paediatric sugar-free medicine may be considered. Aspirin is contraindicated in children under the age of 16 as there is a risk of **Reye's syndrome** (which produces severe effects on the liver and brain). Aspirin also has a detrimental affect on the clotting process. If postoperative pain is considered to be excessive, then the patient should be told to contact the surgery or clinic.
- Consider warm salt mouthwashes after 24 hours and continue for 2/3 days to rinse away food debris and encourage healing. This should consist of a teaspoon of salt in a glass of warm water. The temperature increases vasodilatation and blood flow, which encourages healing. Salt is cheaper than and probably as effective as many proprietary mouthwashes, although chlorhexidine may provide a more acceptable flavour.
- Commence normal twice a day toothbrushing the morning after extraction.

The patient should not:

- Rinse for the first 24 hours.
- Eat or drink for 2–3 hours after extraction and then only on the opposite side of the mouth.
- Drink very hot fluids or eat hard foods for 24 hours.
- Bite their lips, tongue or cheek while they are numb. Patients should be warned of this possibility as this can be a common cause of postoperative trauma.
- Participate in vigorous exercise for the rest of the day.

Complications of exodontia

Complications arising during exodontia

Trauma

Adjacent teeth and soft tissues can be easily damaged when using forceps or elevators and great care must be exercised. Sometimes trauma can unexpectedly occur distant from the site of extraction; for example, when extracting an upper primary molar, the handles of the forceps can inadvertently crush the lower lip against the lower teeth. Sometimes trauma can occur as the tooth or root is being removed from the mouth, particularly if it has sharp edges. Where tissues are anaesthetised, the patient will probably be unaware of any trauma. The operator should take care to check for this prior to dismissing the patient and record any unanticipated trauma in the clinical notes.

If a recently placed class II amalgam is adjacent to the tooth to be extracted then a matrix band can be placed on the adjacent tooth to help prevent damage to the proximal surface of the amalgam during extraction.

Loss of tooth or root

The extracted tooth or root should always be examined carefully to ensure that no part of it is missing.

An extracted tooth may slip from the forceps and be inhaled, swallowed or lost outside the mouth. During exodontia there is a greater risk of objects entering the alimentary tract or lungs via the trachea as there is reduced sensation with local analgesia.

The patient may cough, which suggests the tooth could have been inhaled. If the tooth or root is missing then:

- Check the patient's mouth and clothing thoroughly and the filter/trap of the aspirator if aspiration has been used.
- Check the surrounding area in the surgery.
- Turn the patient onto their side and lower the chair to a 'head down' position; this encourages gravitational forces to bring the object back into the mouth.

If the object cannot be located, inform the patient and their carer and contact the nearest A&E department for chest and abdominal X-rays explaining exactly what has happened and what the radiologist should be looking for. If the object is located in the respiratory tract the hospital will arrange removal as necessary. If the tooth or root is not located, details of this and any subsequent action taken should be recorded in the patient's clinical record and the referring dentist informed.

Fractured tooth or root

If the crown of the tooth is excessively carious or heavily restored then there is the possibility of the forceps fracturing the crown and it coming away from the root during the extraction. The root may be retained in the socket. There is also the possibility of the root fracturing and leaving the apex behind in the socket. This is most likely to occur with curved roots or fine roots. In the event of a tooth fracture:

- Use high volume aspiration if possible to remove the fractured root.
- If the root fragment is visible, use root forceps or an elevator to remove it having undertaken a **risk assessment** of the possibility of damage to a permanent successor.
- If a small fragment is left that is not visible then it is advisable to leave it to exfoliate naturally or resorb because of the risk of damage to the permanent successor. If this action is taken, it should be recorded in the clinical notes.

Haematoma

A haematoma (a collection of blood in the tissues) is a very unusual occurrence when extracting primary teeth in children as there are normally no large blood vessels in the vicinity of the extraction site. It can occur following an inferior dental block injection due to the penetration by the needle of the inferior alveolar vein or due to excessive trauma. Should it occur, the patient and carer should be informed and a note made in the clinical records. Healing is normally uneventful but the condition should be monitored.

Primary haemorrhage

This occurs at the time of or immediately after a tooth is extracted. A blood clot forms to fill the socket. The clot becomes organised initially as granulation tissue, then fibrous tissue with the formation of new capillaries (see Chapter 2, p. 46). Gradually new bone is formed by osteoblastic activity and the socket becomes epithelialised. Bleeding will normally cease after a few minutes and only if this fails to occur can it be considered to be a potential problem.

Excessive primary haemorrhage may be due to:

- An excessively traumatic extraction.
- Existing inflammation of the soft tissues.
- Blood dyscrasias. This highlights the importance of taking a medical history which should normally reveal these. Conditions such as haemophilia A, haemophilia B, Von Willebrand's disease, thrombocytopenia, leukaemia and anaemia may all cause a patient to bleed excessively after tooth extraction.

In the event of continued bleeding, the following action should be taken:

- Reassure the patient.
- Remove the excess blood clot with suction or clean dry gauze.
- Get the patient to bite on a clean gauze sausage shaped pack for 10 to 15 minutes.
- The patient should not be dismissed until all bleeding has ceased.

If bleeding continues then local measures will have to be employed by the dental surgeon. This may involve the use of a haemostatic agent placed in the socket or the use of sutures to approximate the walls of the socket. In the event of an undiagnosed blood dyscrasia, the patient would need to be referred to an appropriate hospital unit.

Complications arising after exodontia

Reactionary haemorrhage

This has the following characteristics:

- It occurs within 24 hours of the extraction.
- It is usually as a result of inadequate home care resulting in disturbance of the blood clot. This can be as a result of vigorous or frequent mouthwashing with hot

fluids, strenuous exercise, or poking with the fingers or a foreign body such as a pencil. Alcohol consumption can also be an uncommon but possible cause, but not usually found in young children.

- It is rarely serious but can appear to be so to the patient as the blood clot is mixed with a large pool of saliva.

Treatment is by means of:

- Pressure applied to the socket by asking the patient to bite down on a sterile mouth pack or pad of gauze for 20–30 minutes.
- A haemostatic drug such as epinephrine (adrenaline), which can be applied to the part of the pack in contact with the socket.
- Suturing the socket by the dentist if necessary.

Secondary haemorrhage

This occurs 4–7 days after the extraction due to bacterial infection of the socket. It is therefore not often seen in the dental surgery. It can be avoided in most cases with good oral hygiene measures and appropriate postoperative care.

Treatment is the same as for reactionary haemorrhage but, depending on the severity of the infection, it may be desirable for the patient to use antimicrobial mouthwashes such as chlorhexidine or for the dentist to prescribe an antibiotic if there are systemic symptoms such as pyrexia or glandular involvement.

Postextraction haemorrhage due to medical conditions should not occur if an adequate medical history is taken beforehand unless the condition has remained undiagnosed. The medical history should include a previous history of dental or other haemorrhage and any family history of haemorrhage.

Acute alveolitis (dry socket)

This acute inflammatory condition is more common following extractions in adults rather than following primary tooth extraction but when it occurs it is more common in the mandible than the maxilla because of the reduced blood supply. It is caused by fibrinolytic activity, which destroys the blood clot. Disturbance of the blood clot or the failure of a blood clot to form may also give rise to acute alveolitis.

Predisposing factors

There are a number of predisposing factors, the most important of which are:

- **Trauma from a difficult extraction**. Pressure on the bone causes the blood vessels to become crushed and therefore a protective blood clot may fail to form.

- **A pre-existing periapical infection**. Microorganisms invade the socket and overwhelm the leucocytic defence mechanism causing a breakdown of the blood clot and an acute inflammation of the exposed bone results.
- **A reduced blood supply** to the socket, e.g. as a result of post-irradiation therapy.
- **Smoking**: although unlikely in young children, can cause a reduced blood supply to the socket.
- **Premature mouth rinsing** disturbing the clot formation and exposing the alveolar bone.
- **Premature clot removal** by the patient removing it with their fingers.

The clinical features

- The patient suffers pain, usually localised to the socket region which occurs one to three days after the extraction.
- The empty socket is surrounded by red inflamed mucosa.
- There is frequently exposed bone visible.
- There is food debris in the socket.

Management of dry socket

Healing of a dry socket can be prolonged with or without intervention. The following procedures should be undertaken:

- A periapical radiograph should be taken to check for any retained root or bone fragments which could be contributing to the problem.
- The socket should be irrigated with warm saline to remove any food debris.
- The socket should be dressed to cover the exposed bone and prevent any further debris entry. A resorbable dressing, such as **Alvogyl**, which is both antiseptic and obtundent (to relieve pain) may be used. Alternatively a non-resorbable dressing such as gauze with zinc oxide and eugenol may be used. The dressing is packed loosely into the socket and the patient is advised to rinse with hot saline mouth washes. Arrangements will need to be made for the eventual removal of the non-resorbable dressing. A resorbable dressing such as Alvogyl should not be used if the patient is allergic to iodine. This treatment may only be carried out to a written prescription from the registered dentist who has examined the patient and if the dental therapist has had appropriate training in the procedure.
- Severe pain can be relieved with paediatric medication, e.g. junior aspirin (if patient aged over 16) or paracetamol.
- It may be considered advisable for the dentist to prescribe an antibiotic such as metronidazole (Flagyl) if there are systemic symptoms or glandular involvement.

Accidental extraction

An unerupted premolar can unwittingly be extracted while its primary predecessor is being removed. The premolar crown is surrounded by the divergent molar roots of the primary tooth and may be dislodged or extracted together with the primary tooth. In the event of this happening, the extracted premolar should be immediately reimplanted into the socket, taking care to replace it accurately in the correct position. The periodontal membrane should not be allowed to become dried out or contaminated. The premolar has a good chance of success if reimplanted immediately. The patient and carer should be informed and the incident recorded in the patient's clinical case notes.

Trauma

Self inflicted cheek, tongue or lip biting may occur in spite of the warnings previously given, due to the patient having lost sensory soft tissue sensation because of the local analgesic. The patient should be reassured and advised to use warm salt water or antiseptic mouthwashes (e.g. chlorhexidine).

Prolonged analgesia

This is extremely rare and if it does occur it most likely the result of damage to the inferior dental nerve when giving an ID block injection. Since the needles used are siliconised, bevelled and very fine (0.3–0.4 mm diameter) they are highly unlikely to sever the nerve but damage from the needle could result in more prolonged paraesthesia (pins and needles sensation) in the lip or tongue. The paraesthesia is unlikely to be more than transient; the patient should be reassured and warned about possible trauma from lip or tongue biting.

The medically compromised patient

There are a number of medical conditions from which child patients may suffer which can present complications when undertaking exodontia. Most of these patients are unsuitable to be treated by a dental therapist in a primary care setting and would normally be referred for specialist care. This highlights the importance of taking a comprehensive medical history. If there is any doubt about the medical history, the referring dentist should be consulted.

References

Alsheneifi, T. and Hughes, C.V. (2001) Reasons for dental extractions in children. *Pediatric Dentistry*, **23**(2), 109–112.

Kau, C.H., Durning, P., Richmond, S., Miotti, F.A. and Harzer, W. (2004) Extractions as a form of interception in the developing dentition: a randomized controlled trial. *Journal of Orthodontics*, **31**(2), 107–114.

Milsom, K.M., Tickle, M., King, D., Kearney-Mitchell, P. and Blinkhorn, A.S. (2002) Outcomes associated with restored and unrestored primary molar teeth. *Primary Dental Care*, **9**(1), 16–19.

Tickle, M., Milsom, K., King, D., Kearney-Mitchell, P. and Blinkhorn, A. (2002) The fate of the carious primary teeth of children who regularly attend the general dental service. *British Dental Journal*, **192**(4), 219–223.

Further reading

Welbury, R. (ed.) (2001) *Paediatric Dentistry*. Oxford University Press Oxford.

Cameron, A.C. and Widmer, R. (2003) *Handbook of Paediatric Dentistry*. Mosby, St Louis.

Heasman, P. (ed.) (2003) *Master Dentistry*. Volume 2 *Restorative Dentistry, Paediatric Dentistry and Orthodontics*. Churchill Livingstone, Edinburgh.

15

Gerodontology

Fiona Sandom

Summary

This chapter covers:

- Physiological age changes
- Pathological age changes
- Dental and oral conditions in the elderly
- Treating the dentate elderly
- Domiciliary care, equipment and treatment
- Treatment of the terminally ill patient

Introduction

Gerontology also comes under the title of geriatric dentistry or gerodontics and can be most simply defined as dentistry for the elderly. How older people are defined can be problematical. For some it is those who have reached the age when they receive a state pension (65 for men and women, as from 2010), but for those who have just reached that landmark it could be 75 years! It has been suggested that rather than having a defined chronological age, a biological age should be considered to be more relevant.

The UK has an ageing population (Figure 15.1). The population grew by 6.5% in the last 30 years, from 55.9 million in 1971 to 59.6 million in mid 2003. Continued population ageing is inevitable during the first half of this century, since the number of elderly people will rise as the relatively large numbers of people born after the Second World War, and during the 1960s baby boom, become older. The working age population will also fall in size as the baby boomers move into retirement, because relatively smaller numbers of people have been born since the mid 1970s. Current (2007-based) life expectancy of 77.7 years for men and 81.9 years for women compares with the1901-based life expectancy of 45 years for men and about 49 years for women (Office of National Statistics, 2009) (Table 15.1).

There has been an increasing demand for dentistry for the elderly. There are three main reasons for this:

- The population of the UK is ageing. The increased life expectancy along with the falling birth rate means that the proportion of the population aged over 65 is projected to rise from its current figure of 16% to nearly 23% by the year 2034.
- The improvement in general dental health has meant that people are keeping their teeth for longer. In 1988 21% of all adults in the UK were edentulous; in 1998 this had reduced to 13% (Kelly *et al.*, 2000) and to 6% in 2009. This has resulted in a corresponding reduction in the wearing of full dentures.
- This has, in turn, led to a general expectation and a desire in the older age groups to retain teeth for as long as possible.

There are several factors associated with dental care for the elderly. These are:

- Age changes.
- Diseases.
- Medication.
- Delivery of care.

Physiological age changes

An exact dividing line between changes which are physiological and pathological cannot always be drawn.

Clinical Textbook of Dental Hygiene and Therapy, Second Edition. Edited by Suzanne L. Noble.
© 2012 John Wiley & Sons, Ltd. Published 2012 by John Wiley & Sons, Ltd.

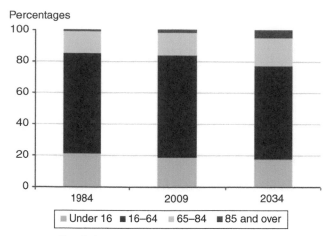

Percentages

| Under 16 | 16–64 | 65–84 | 85 and over |

Population by age, UK, 1984, 2009 and 2034
population: by age, UK

Crown copyright material is reproduced with the permission
of the Controller of HMSO and the Queen's Printer for Scotland.

Figure 15.1 UK population by age.

Table 15.1 Interim life tables.

Life expectancy, 2007–2009	Years			
	At birth		At age 65	
	Males	Females	Males	Females
United Kingdom	77.7	81.9	17.6	20.2
England	78.0	82.1	17.8	20.4
Wales	77.1	81.4	17.2	20.0
Scotland	75.3	80.1	16.4	19.0
Northern Ireland	76.7	81.3	17.1	19.9

Source: Office for National Statistics: Interim Life Tables 2007–09.

General body changes

In general the changes in the elderly are:

- A lengthening in the time taken to repair tissues. This can have important implications when surgery is involved.
- Loss of muscle mass (**sarcopenia**) and strength, which is one of the most obvious effects of ageing.
- A reduction in the metabolic rate. **Basal metabolic rate** (BMR) is the minimal caloric requirement needed to sustain life in a resting individual. The BMR reduces with age. After 20 years of age it drops about 2% per decade. It is generally accepted that decreased **lean body mass** (LBM) with ageing is responsible for a decline in BMR in the elderly.
- Reduction in cellular reproduction. This delays the repair process.

- Reduction in the blood circulation. The elderly tend to restrict their body movements more and more so that eventually, their capacity for mobility becomes markedly reduced and they generally perceive stiffness. Mobility is important to tissue fluid exchange, and so limited mobility seriously reduces blood flow. Blood flow in some circumscribed areas can become so sluggish that the tissues become ischaemic (decreased blood flow).
- Increase in fibrosis. This can occur in many organs, such as the lungs and heart, reducing their function.
- Degeneration of the elastic and nervous tissue. **Ischaemia** can lead to nerve tissue degeneration and loss of sensory input.
- General reduced function of most body systems.
- A loss of cartilage and bone. A loss of cartilage in bone joints can lead to pain, stiffness and loss of function. **Osteoporosis**, which literally means porous bones, occurs when the holes within bone become bigger, making it fragile and liable to break more easily. Osteoporosis usually affects the whole skeleton but it most commonly results in fractures to bone in the wrist, spine and hip. The decrease in the reducible collagen cross-links without an alteration in collagen concentration tends to increase bone fragility. When bone tissue becomes too highly mineralised, it tends to become brittle. One in 3 women and 1 in 12 men in the UK experience osteoporosis over the age of 50. The increased bone turnover following the menopause reduces overall tissue mineralisation. At the time of writing the jury is out as whether there is a link between osteoporosis and periodontal bone loss, but two of the most recent studies; Gomes-Filho *et al.* (2007) and Nicopoulou-Karayianni *et al.* (2009) have shown a link. However, it is worth noting that not all studies have shown a link. In practical terms, the periodontal disease is treated and the osteoporosis is treated and any link is academic.

Patients with oesteoporosis can be treated with bisphosphonates and evidence has emerged that patients taking bisphosphonate drugs are at risk of developing oesteonecrosis of the jaws, sometimes spontaneously, but more usually following dental extractions or oral bone surgery.

Bisphosponates are principally used in the treatment of oesteoporosis, Paget's disease, multiple myeloma, bony metastic lesions and hypercalcaemia of malignancy. The incidence of bisphosphonate-related oesteonecrosis of the jaw (BRONJ) in patients taking oral bisphosphonates for oesteoporosis has been estimated at 1 in 10 000 to 1 in 100 000. Patients taking high dose IV bisphosphonates for cancer are much more at risk (estimated at 1 in 10 to 1 in 100). Other factors associated with an increased risk include dental infection, denture trauma and the risk increases with the length of time the patient has been taking the drugs, with 3 years being the threshold.

Presenting features of BRONJ are:

- Delayed healing.
- Pain.
- Swelling.
- Loosening of teeth.
- Paraesthesia.
- Purulent discharge via intra- or extraoral sinus.

If any of these features develop, early referral to an Oral Surgery or Oral Maxillo Facial Surgical Department is important.

Oral

Oral soft tissues

- Decrease in taste bud function.
- Increase in the size and number of **Fordyce spots** (enlarged ectopic sebaceous glands in the mucosa of the mouth, lips, cheek and tongue), lingual varices and foliate (leaf-like) papillae.
- Decrease in the thickness of the epithelium and mucosa.
- Decrease in saliva flow (xerostomia) and changes in its composition.

Dental hard tissues

- Tooth wear is a natural age-related factor. There is a loss of tooth tissue due to **attrition**, resulting in a loss of occlusal morphology. **Abrasion** can be excessive at the cervical margins as a result of prolonged incorrect toothbrushing techniques. **Erosion** may be more evident as a result of prolonged intake of acid-based or sugary medication.
- Enamel is less permeable.
- Cementum undergoes continuous deposition with age. This is mainly functionally induced and is more pronounced in the apical third of the root.
- The volume of secondary dentine increases, although the rate of deposition decreases with age. The amount of sclerotic root dentine increases with age, proceeding from the apex towards the crown of the tooth. There are obvious optical changes in the dentine, which becomes translucent (dentine is normally opaque). The dentine of older people is characterised by the continuous narrowing of the lumen of the dentinal tubule, increased calcification, a reduction in the amount of peritubular fluid and reduced sensitivity. As a result, dentine tends to be able to take on the function of enamel as it wears.

- There is a reduction in cellularity in the alveolar bone and the surface in contact with the periodontal ligament appears more jagged.

Dental pulp

- Increase in fibrosis and a decrease in vascularity result in the pulp's defensive properties being reduced, but the pulp does not suffer any appreciable loss of vitality. Circulation in the pulp is affected by deposition of mineralised tissue in the apical part of the root canal.
- Increase in pulp calcification. Pulp stones are more evident.
- The volume of the pulp decreases with age, owing to the deposition of secondary dentine.

Periodontium

- An increase in fibrosis. It is generally agreed that the degree of periodontal breakdown increases with increasing age. The extent to which ageing of periodontal tissues plays a part in this respect poses a question which has yet to be answered. Ageing is accompanied by a variety of periodontal changes. The periodontal tissues themselves show evidence of ageing; there are indications that the composition of the plaque changes, and the reaction of the periodontium to the presence of plaque probably changes as well. In plaque there is a decrease with age in the number of viable microorganisms, an increase in the number of spirochaetes and a reduction in the number of streptococci (Milward and Cooper, 2005). There is as yet no significant evidence of a physiological apical migration of the epithelial attachment. It seems plausible that periodontal breakdown can occur only in the presence of plaque, or as a result of trauma with consequent inflammation of the periodontium. Whether changes in plaque composition with age exert any influence on the course of periodontal breakdown is uncertain: the data available are not yet sufficient to warrant definite conclusions. The same applies to the influence which a changing reaction of the periodontium to the presence of plaque may have on the course of periodontal breakdown. Research findings do suggest that the degree of periodontal breakdown increases with age; that with increasing age inflammation of the periodontium tends to develop more rapidly; and that in the process of ageing the periodontium shows a slower rate of wound healing. However, these phenomena are overshadowed by the patients' susceptibility to periodontal disease. This implies that firstly, the susceptibility to periodontal disease is more significant for the rate of periodontal destruction than the length of time plaque is present (the age effect) and secondly, the greater the susceptibility to periodontal disease, the slower the rate of wound healing and the more rapidly inflammation of the periodontium tends to develop (Van der Velden, 1984).

- A decrease in cellularity, vascularity and cell turnover is found with an increase in age.
- Collagen and protein synthesis decrease.

Pathological change

Systemic

There are several systemic conditions which are not uncommonly seen in the elderly, which may have an effect on treatment planning and delivery of care. The reader is referred to a more comprehensive text addressing the large number of pathological conditions affecting patients of all ages and having an impact on oral health care (Nunn, 2004) but the conditions more specifically related to the elderly are described below.

Endocrine disorders

Hypofunction of the adrenal glands (Addison's disease)

This can produce symptoms of tiredness and confusion and lead to a greater incidence of heart attack. Patients may feel dizzy on getting out of the dental chair and do not respond well to the stress of dental procedures. It may be advantageous to keep appointments short.

Hyperfunction of the adrenal glands (Cushing's syndrome)

This can be due to, for example, a pituitary tumour, or the symptoms may be simulated by high steroid dosage. Patients on steroid therapy are susceptible to a steroid crisis and their physician may advise an increase in dosage when undergoing stressful dental treatment.

Diabetes

This is due to a lack of insulin and can occur in several forms. Type 2 diabetes is the most common type seen in older people. These patients may exhibit signs of decreased salivary flow, increased caries if uncontrolled, periodontal problems due to microvascular changes and slow wound healing.

Hyperparathyroidism

Excess of parathyroid hormone (PTH) is usually as a result of a tumour. It results in demineralisation of the bone, causing possible bone fractures, and renal calculi may develop because of the excretion of high levels of phosphate and calcium.

Hypothyroidism (myxoedema)

This is a condition in which the body lacks sufficient thyroid hormone (thyroxine). Since the main purpose of thyroid hormone is to maintain the body's metabolism, people with this condition will have symptoms associated with a slow metabolism. Its incidence increases with age and such patients appear lethargic and slow, have cold dry skin and may have an enlarged tongue. They respond poorly to stress.

The immune system

A reduction in the cell-mediated response and a decreased number of circulating lymphocytes results in an increased incidence of autoimmune disease, combined with a reduced defence against infection with age. As stated above, steroid treatment for autoimmune disease can influence dental treatment because of the suppression of the patient's natural adrenal activity.

Cardiovascular disorders

Hypertension and ischaemic heart disease become more common with an increase in age. Anaemia is also more common in the elderly. Generally, the greatest problems with patients with cardiovascular disorders are associated with general anaesthesia.

Pulmonary system

Lung capacity is decreased with age and chronic obstructive airway diseases are more common.

Muscular system

There is a number of muscular dystrophic diseases which are associated with a decrease in the bulk of the muscle, with slower contractions and less precision of control.

Neurological disorders

There is a physiological decline in function associated with age-related disease.

Parkinson's disease

This is a condition seen mainly over the age of 50 years. Parkinson's disease occurs when a group of cells, in an area of the brain called the substantia nigra, that produce a chemical called **dopamine**, begin to malfunction and eventually die. Dopamine is a neurotransmitter, or chemical messenger, that transports signals to the parts of the brain that control movement initiation and co-ordination. When Parkinson's disease occurs these cells begin to die at a faster rate and the amount of dopamine produced in the brain decreases. The symptoms include tremor of the hands and arms, drooling due to swallowing difficulties, postural instability and speech difficulties.

Dental treatment can be improved by the provision of mouldable head supports and mouth props. Patients are best treated upright in the dental chair because of the difficulty in controlling the airway. Treatment can usually be more successful if undertaken within 2 hours of taking anti-Parkinsonian medication.

Dementia

Dementia is due to a wasting of nerve fibres in the brain. Alzheimer's disease accounts for half of all cases of dementia in older people (5% of people over 65 years; 20% of those over 80 years of age). Patients may be treated by a variety of drugs, although older people tolerate these less well. Some of these drugs have xerostomia as an important side effect. Dental treatment can become increasingly challenging as the condition degenerates. Teeth with a poor prognosis, such as those with a furcation involvement, are probably better removed.

Cerebrovascular accident (stroke)

In older patients this can be due to high blood pressure, the use of anticoagulants (e.g. warfarin), or following heart surgery. Tolerance of dental treatment may be reduced and therefore short appointments are advisable. Patients may have difficulty in swallowing and may tolerate treatment better in an upright position. They may have to be treated in their own wheelchair or in a domiciliary setting.

Psychiatric disorders

Depression

This condition is not specifically related to age but is not uncommon in the elderly. These patients may exhibit signs of oral neglect through lack of self-motivation and low self-esteem. They may have symptoms of xerostomia due to drug therapy. They usually require extensive oral hygiene instruction and supervision with plenty of positive encouragement combined with a high dosage of topical fluoride. Appointments are best kept short.

Schizophrenia

These patients demonstrate thought disturbances, sometimes experience bizarre delusions and have difficulty in communicating with other people. Antipsychotic drug therapy tends to increase the heart rate and patients are generally restless when having dental treatment. They don't respond well to sudden movements of the dental chair. The drug therapy also causes xerostomia with the added problem of an increased risk of extensive dental caries.

Oral

These conditions are covered in more detail in Chapter 3 but there are several mucosal diseases which are more common in the elderly. Some examples are given below.

Leukoplakia

This presents as white patches on the oral mucous membranes, which cannot be removed by scraping. The condition does not reverse with the removal of local irritants. It most commonly occurs between the ages of 40 and 70 and is more common in males (65%). It is usually located around the buccal gingivae or the floor of the mouth. It can be associated with tobacco, alcohol, candida infections or chronic persistent irritants, such as ill-fitting dentures. It requires investigation since these lesions can be considered to be pre-malignant until proven otherwise.

Oral cancer

Whilst oral cancer is a relatively uncommon condition it does increase in occurrence in older adults. If it is not detected early, the survival rate in the elderly is poor. The most common sites are the lips followed by the tongue. Depending on the stage of the disease, survival can be as low as 50%. Approximately 90% of oral carcinomas are squamous cell carcinomas.

If an ulcer with a raised, rolled edge with hardening around the periphery of the lesion is detected, then a thorough history of the ulcer should be taken and the patient referred back to the prescribing dentist as soon as possible.

Candidal infection

This can be either chronic or acute. **Acute candidosis** (**candidiasis**) or **thrush** is most common in the young, elderly and the immunosuppressed. It presents as a creamy white slough, which can be gently removed to reveal a raw red mucosa, usually on the palate, oropharynx or cheek. The patient often complains of discomfort on eating, but it can be painless.

Chronic candidosis (**candidiasis**) or, more commonly **denture stomatitis**, is usually symptomless. It is commonly seen on the palate underneath a full or partial upper denture, as a reddish area with some white patches.

Lichen planus

This is a skin and/or mucosal disorder that is reported to affect about 2% of the population of the UK. The skin lesions usually resolve within about 18 months, but involvement in the oral cavity may last for many years. The intraoral presentation can be bilateral and/or symmetrical white patches affecting the buccal mucosa, tongue and attached gingivae.

Based on its clinical appearance lichen planus has been divided into erosive, plaque-like, reticular, atrophic or bullous. In reality it is difficult to categorise sufferers into these groups as often the patients can have different types of lichen planus not only at different sites in the mouth, but also at different times during the presence of the condition (see also Chapter 3, p. 56–57).

Herpes zoster

This is more common with the increase in age. The virus causes chickenpox as a primary infection and shingles, more commonly seen in the elderly, as a reactivation of the virus. Shingles can be very painful for the patient and can make long dental appointments uncomfortable.

Pemphigus

This is an autoimmune chronic skin disease that affects the mucous membranes. The first identifiable lesions are found in the mouth and are more common in females than males.

Dental conditions

Periodontal disease

Destructive periodontal disease has been consistently associated with ageing, such that many have come to see it as an inevitable consequence of growing old. A number of early studies found a close association between age, periodontal disease and tooth loss. However, more recent research has questioned the association between age and periodontitis (Burt, 1994). With age, some gingival shrinkage and loss of periodontal attachment and bony support are expected, but age alone in a healthy adult does not lead to a critical loss of periodontal support. Severe periodontitis should not be regarded as a natural consequence of ageing. Periodontal disease, although seen more often in older patients, is not actually part of the physiological ageing process, but is as a result of the disease progression in susceptible individuals. Susceptibility is, however, greater in older people because of increased gingival recession, poor oral hygiene, poor diet and potentially reduced salivary flow.

Gingival recession is frequently seen in the older patient. This can result in:

- Exposed root surfaces increasing the susceptibility to root caries.
- Abrasion lesions as a result of poor toothbrushing techniques.
- Thermal sensitivity.
- Exposure of root furcations in molar teeth, leading to increased plaque accumulation.

Age alone should not diminish an individual's right to care because the clinician has reservations about the patient's longevity. Successful treatment of periodontitis by surgical and non-surgical methods has been extensively documented and older patients can benefit from these treatments as much as younger patients. Age is therefore not a barrier to effective periodontal therapy.

Root caries

Root caries has been described as the adult dental problem of the future because of the increasing ageing population and the increased retention of the natural dentition into old age (Figure 15.2).

In many dentate mouths in the elderly, the root surfaces become exposed due to gingival recession and these root surfaces can become susceptible to root caries. Gingival recession is a requirement for exposure of a root surface and, therefore, it is not surprising that root caries is more commonly seen in the elderly. Root caries is associated with periodontal disease, as this is the major cause of gingival recession. It does not mean, however, that all patients with exposed root surfaces will experience root caries. The root surfaces are more vulnerable to caries than enamel since the critical pH of demineralisation for dentine is 6.0–6.5 whereas it is 5.2–5.5 for enamel caries.

The primary causative factors for root caries are:

- A **susceptible root surface:** gingival recession is the predominant factor but, as root caries can occur in a pocket, it is more accurate to use the term loss of attachment.
- **Fermentable carbohydrates:** these are metabolised by the oral bacteria to produce acid. They can be intrinsic

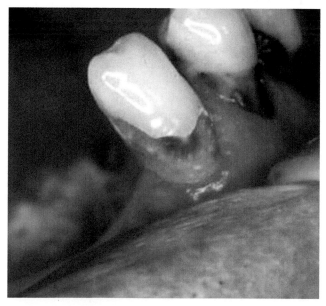

Figure 15.2 Root caries.

(found naturally within the food) or extrinsic (added to foods).

- **Dental plaque biofilm:** the microflora and in particular the levels of *Streptococcus mutans*, which are very effective at acid production and making intra- and extracellular polysaccharide, are important. The concentration of *Actinomyces* is of particular importance in relation to root caries. The amount of fluoride in the plaque fluid and the nature and quantity of plaque are all relevant to the prevalence of root caries in an individual.
- **Time:** as previously stated, the pH level at which enamel starts to demineralise is between 5.2 and 5.5 and for dentine it is between 6.0 and 6.5. The resting pH of the saliva is from 6.8 to 6.9. Therefore, when the pH decreases, the root surface is more susceptible than enamel to demineralisation over the same period of time.

Secondary factors are:

- **Saliva:** the saliva has a protective effect by neutralising the pH and providing an antibacterial and buffering effect. It influences the rate of clearance of acid and sugar. There is a wide individual variation in the viscosity and composition of the saliva.
- **Fluoride:** fluoride is toxic to bacteria; it also inhibits **glycolysis** (the production of acid from sugar by bacteria) as well as increasing remineralisation of the root surface.
- **Root surface factors:** the surface roughness can influence plaque formation.
- **Location:** maxillary teeth are believed to be more susceptible to root caries due to the resting root pH of the maxilla being 6.0 and that of the mandible being 6.4. Incisors are the least vulnerable followed by canines, premolars and molars.

Xerostomia (dry mouth)

It is often assumed that with increasing age there is a normal physiological reduction in saliva flow, but studies have shown this to be very small in healthy individuals who are not taking any medication. The normal unstimulated salivary secretion rate in adults is between 0.3 and 0.5 ml per minute. The normal stimulated secretion rate is 1–2 ml/minute. However, in patients suffering from xerostomia, these rates may be reduced to between 0.7 and 0.1 ml and to less than 0.1 ml/minute in patients with severe salivary gland malfunction.

Xerostomia, as a result of reduced salivary function, can be caused by:

- Radiotherapy: radiotherapy for neoplasms in the head and neck area usually results in a significant reduction in salivary flow. Radiotherapy also has a detrimental effect on the periodontal clinical attachment level (Marques and Dib, 2004).
- Systemic disease, e.g. diabetes, Sjögren's syndrome, liver disease, immunodeficiency diseases.
- Chronic sialadenitis.
- Sialoadenoma.
- Therapeutic drugs: there are several therapeutic drugs commonly used that alter salivary flow and composition. There are about 400 of these medications that are used to treat disease in the over-50s. Some examples are: angiotensin-converting enzyme inhibitors, beta blockers for hypertension, diuretics for hypertension and chronic heart failure, calcium channel blockers for hypertension and stable angina, hypnotics for anxiety, anti-Parkinsonian drugs and antidepressants. It is always wise to check the current *BNF* for oral side-effects of the medicines thepatient is taking.
- Non-therapeutic drugs: illegal drugs, such as ecstasy.
- Hormonal disturbances.
- Dehydration: the elderly tend to have a lower fluid intake.
- Atrophy: a physiological decrease in cellular function with age.

Tooth wear

Tooth wear in the older patient is prevalent, especially where partial tooth loss has occurred. Some tooth wear during life is inevitable and, unless the patient complains of pain, poor aesthetics, sensitivity or problems with function, the condition may not require restorative treatment. Tooth wear is not necessarily a pathological process.

Loss of tooth substance is caused by:

- Attrition, caused by tooth-to-tooth contact.
- Erosion, caused by non-bacterial acid attack of the teeth, i.e. not due to caries.
- Abrasion, caused by wear due to physical contact with an agent other than teeth (e.g. tooth brushing).
- Abfraction, cervical tooth surface loss thought to be caused by flexure of the cusps.

The clinical presentation of these conditions is more fully described in Chapter 3. It is important to identify the aetiology of the condition and assess the amount of tissue loss and the rate of wear before treatment and advice can be given. Unfortunately, tooth wear usually has a multifactorial aetiology and the treatment and management are therefore complex. In cases of attrition an occlusal splint may be used for night time wear. Where erosion is the cause, a detailed diet history should be taken and possible causes highlighted. If a gastric cause is suspected then it may be one of the first clues to gastric disease. Another cause may be bulimia, but this is rare in the elderly. For both these instances further care should be sought from the patient's general medical practitioner (GMP).

Where abrasion is thought to be the cause of wear, advice should be given to appropriately modify any habits.

In cases of abfraction the occlusal contacts may need to be modified. The two treatment options are either to review or to restore. The reasons for restoration are:

- Sensitivity.
- Aesthetics.
- If the tooth is not restored, it could become unrestorable in the future.

Tooth loss

In recent years there has been a marked reduction in edentulousness in adults aged 65 and over in the UK.

There are anatomical changes that take place with the extraction of a tooth, which are both intraoral and extraoral. These changes vary in those who are edentulous and partly dentate. As people age, the loss of alveolar bone is inevitable, but the amount of loss is increased in the edentulous. As well as the anatomical changes, there are other potential problems as a result of tooth loss. These include:

- **Speech problems**: loss of the anterior teeth not replaced by dentures, bridges or implants can have a deleterious affect on speech.
- **Mastication problems**: masticatory efficiency may be reduced but a reduction of tooth arches with maintenance of function and aesthetics of the dentition will not necessarily lead to a decrease in dental health (Kayser and Witter, 1985).
- **Appearance**: in addition to preserving bone, the loss of teeth means that there is also loss of support for the soft tissues which can result in a change in facial appearance.

Nutritional disturbance

A poor diet leading to nutritional problems can be the result of poverty, impaired mobility, loss of taste, reduced masticatory function, lack of transport (to and from the shops to obtain fresh produce) or the lack of motivation to prepare fresh foods, especially for patients living alone. The elderly have lower energy requirements but have a need for a diet high in nutrients and an increased requirement for antioxidant nutrients. There is a dietary requirement for vitamin D; however, in the UK National Diet and Nutrition Survey (Food Standards Agency, 2003), it was found that people aged 65 and over had a diet that was high in saturated fat, high in free sugars, low in fibre, low in fruits and vegetables and low in vitamin D.

The dentate elderly

It is now reasonable to expect the majority of the population to remain dentate throughout life. However, the expectations of the elderly present specific challenges to the clinician in trying to maintain or improve oral health. In general, these challenges do not differ from the rest of the population and are dealt with elsewhere in this book; however, there are several factors that are potentially more specific to the elderly. In addition to the physiological and pathological conditions described earlier, these include:

- **Reduced manual dexterity**: a generalised loss of dexterity, as seen in such conditions as arthritis, can make oral hygiene maintenance both difficult and time consuming. This should be taken into account by setting realistic maintenance goals.
- **Reduced mobility**: as well as providing appropriate access facilities, such as wheelchair access, it is often advisable to allow extra appointment time.
- **Poor visual acuity**: this should be taken into account both with respect to oral hygiene maintenance and to the provision of written information.
- **Heavily restored teeth**: uneven contour and possible ditching can encourage plaque formation and make its removal more difficult.
- **Maloccluded and misaligned teeth**: these make access for maintenance more difficult.
- **Exposed root surfaces**: these provide a more extensive tooth surface to maintain.
- **Communication difficulties**: these can be due to reduced hearing ability or problems in understanding.

Domiciliary care

Physical and mental disability or chronic disease may make it difficult or impossible for elderly patients to attend a dental surgery or clinic for their routine or emergency care. The **Disability Discrimination Act 1995** states that it is the duty of an employer not to place the disabled person concerned at a substantial disadvantage in comparison with persons who are not disabled. It is usually the case that treatment undertaken in the surgery is both more convenient and more cost effective, but there are many patients who find the experience too physically or psychologically traumatic. As a result, there is a large number of people requiring care in their own home, in a residential care setting (temporary or permanent), day centre, nursing home or within a day hospital environment. Although the number of people receiving domiciliary care under NHS regulations in England and Wales is decreasing it is still significantly large.

Table 15.2 Assessment of eligibility criteria for domiciliary oral healthcare (Reproduced by kind permission of the All Wales Special Interest Group/Oral Health Care).

Has patient/carer contacted a local dentist?

      Yes ☐   No ☐   Don't know ☐

Does the patient attend her/his doctor?

      Yes ☐   No ☐   Don't know ☐

If the patient has a hospital appointment, how does he/she get there?

      Ambulance ☐   Taxi ☐   Car ☐   Other ☐

When was the last time the patient was able to leave the house?

Does the patient have someone to bring them to the surgery?

      Yes ☐   No ☐   Don't know ☐

Does the patient use a taxi for other activities?

      Yes ☐   No ☐   Don't know ☐

Does the patient attend a hairdresser/chiropodist?

      Yes ☐   No ☐   Don't know ☐

Mobility:

Walks unaided ☐   Needs assistance ☐   Wheelchair user ☐   Housebound ☐

Additional comments:

The aim of domiciliary care is to provide comprehensive dental care to patients who are unable to access a dental clinic, surgery or mobile dental unit for their dental care. However, it is useful to make an initial assessment of a patient's eligibility and some relevant questions are listed in Table 15.2.

Domiciliary care excludes dental screening. The provision of operative care in a domiciliary setting is challenging in view of the often limited or less than ideal facilities that locations such as a kitchen or living room can provide. For the very anxious or phobic patient there is an important opportunity for the hygienist or therapist to reduce this anxiety and hopefully enable the patient to develop enough confidence to be able to accept further treatment, which may be more complex or in a more conventional surgery setting. The advantages of providing domiciliary care include:

- Better access to dental care for patient.
- Providing a better understanding of a patient's home/living environment.
- Giving access to medication and patient-held documentation, e.g. medical notes.
- Providing a better understanding of a patient's ability to carry out oral hygiene advice.
- Reducing the likelihood of failed appointments.
- Frequently achieving better patient compliance because the patient is usually very appreciative of the individual care provided.
- Providing added interest for the operator.

The disadvantages are:

- It can disrupt the patient's normal routine.
- Appointment times may not be convenient for the patient.
- The patient may consider there to be an invasion of privacy.
- Appointments tend to be much longer and may not be considered economically justified.
- The hygienist/therapist may have to make compromises with treatment.
- The scope of the treatment may be limited.
- Poor working conditions can lead to frustration.
- The clinician may feel more vulnerable because of the lack of emergency back-up and due to working in a non-clinical environment.

As domiciliary care can take place in a variety of environments it is important to consider:

- Confidentiality.
- Privacy.
- Access to services, e.g. water and electricity.
- Health and safety issues.

Domiciliary patients

It is recommended by the **British Society for Disability and Oral Health** that referral criteria for patients to access domiciliary dental care are agreed and an appropriate referral form used (Table 15.3).

Table 15.3 A model referral form for domiciliary oral healthcare (Reproduced by kind permission of the All Wales Special Interest Group).

Name: _____   Next of kin, relationship: _____

Address: _____   Name: _____

_____   Address: _____

DOB: _____ Hosp No: _____   _____

Tel: _____   Tel: _____

GMP: Dr _____   **Contact:** Social/Key worker/Community nurse (please specify)

Address: _____   Name: _____

_____   Address: _____

Tel: _____   _____ Tel: _____

Medical/social history: _____

_____

_____

_____

_____

_____

Dental complaint:	Pain: Yes	☐	Urgent:	☐	Non-urgent:	☐
Dental status:	Edentulous:	☐	Dentate:	☐	Dentures worn:	☐

Sensory impairment:		Mobility:		Services:	
Hearing	☐	Walks unaided	☐	Comm Nurse	☐
Vision	☐	Needs assistance	☐	Meals on wheels	☐
Communication	☐	Wheelchair user	☐	Home Care	☐
		Bedfast	☐	Day Centre/Hosp	☐
		Own transport	☐	Mon/Tues/Wed/Thurs/Fri	☐

Action requested: _____

_____

Domiciliary assessment please: ☐   Please arrange continuing dental care: ☐

Signature: _____ Status: _____ Date: _____

Name: _____ Address: _____

Tel: _____ Fax: _____ Email: _____

Special skills and knowledge are required for provision of domiciliary care. It is essential to have an understanding of the conditions leading to impairments and disabilities, and the effect these conditions have directly and indirectly on oral health. The skills and knowledge include:

- An understanding of mental conditions and associated problems.
- An appreciation of the specific requirements of dental care for the elderly.
- A familiarity of the use of domiciliary equipment.
- Causes and management of medical emergencies.

Table 15.4 Skills required for domiciliary care.

Mandatory	Recommended	Developed
Basic life support	Planning	Time management
Manual handling	Navigation	Flexibility
	Driving	Improvisation
	Liaison	Assertiveness
	Empathy	Anticipation

The skills required for domiciliary care are outlined in Table 15.4. It is important that training is provided in order to develop and maintain the required skills and knowledge to deliver domiciliary care.

The domiciliary visit

Planning

Forward planning is the essential ingredient for the domiciliary visit as this will, one hopes, highlight potential problems and maximise time and resources. Most domiciliary visits are not undertaken as emergencies. It is therefore more cost effective to schedule visits at specific times of the day rather than booking them on a random basis. Generally it is better to arrange visits at the end of a clinic session in view of the unpredictability of the time requirement, which is so dependent on the facilities and working conditions available.

Before the visit:

- The dental hygienist and therapist should check they have a written treatment plan signed by the referring dentist, check that the medical history and the consent forms are complete and up to date.
- Establish if there are any special requirements, e.g. a carer.
- Telephone if possible to clarify the dental problem and the need for a domiciliary visit.
- Check full and correct address and directions.
- Send out a written appointment.
- Undertake a risk assessment. Guidelines are given in Table 15.5. Having a third person present is a legal requirement when making a home visit (Fiske and Lewis, 1999). The hygienist or therapist should have another member of the dental team to accompany them in a patient's home. When making a visit to a residential home or a hospital either a member of the dental team or a member of staff should be present. A mobile telephone or a personal alarm should be carried in case of an emergency. Patients should only be moved or lifted using the correct methods, again in accordance with training and manual handling procedures.

The assessment outcome may change. The risk assessment should be amended and updated when there is a significant change in the treatment to be provided or in the assessed environment.

Domiciliary equipment

The equipment that is required for a domiciliary visit depends on the clinician, the type of treatment and the resources available to purchase it. It is always best to have a kit ready prepared. A babycare box or compartmentalised toolbox can make an excellent domiciliary care kit (Figure 15.3). After each visit the contents should be decontaminated, it should be checked that the materials are in date and the kit restocked as necessary. This means that the kit will always be ready, which is particularly important should there be an emergency.

It is possible to undertake comprehensive restorative and periodontal care in a domiciliary setting but this does involve a considerable cost investment in view of the equipment required. Treatment must therefore be planned according to the resources available. Portable lights, chairs, aspirators, turbines, handpiece motors and ultrasonic scalers are currently available on the market and some examples are illustrated (Figures 15.4–15.7). The instruments, equipment and materials required for a domiciliary visit will also depend on the number and type of visits planned. The checklists given in Tables 15.6–15.9 may be helpful in acting as an *aide mémoire*. The lists are by no means prescriptive and requirements may vary according to individual preference.

Treatment of the terminally ill

Patients in intensive care units can be more vulnerable to oral disease and discomfort than the general population; therefore mouth care is of prime importance to the critically ill. Mouth care is an essential part of the overall care of the patient. It is wise to draw up a care plan for each individual and take into consideration the following factors:

- General health.
- Medical condition.
- Prognosis.
- Medication.
- Previous standard of oral hygiene and care skills.

Whenever possible the cooperation of the patient, the carers, and/or relatives should be considered.

Nurses and carers should be advised and shown how to maintain oral health. Where care is undertaken on a shift rotation basis, it is a good idea for written instructions to be kept at the bedside. All the necessary oral and denture hygiene aids should also be kept close by and be easily available.

Table 15.5 Guidance notes for an environmental risk assessment for domiciliary oral health care (Reproduced by kind permission of the All Wales Special Interest Group).

Personal and location details	Example of information required
Name of assessor	Name of person completing assessment
Discipline	Job title/position held
Patient's name & ID number	As in patient's record
Address	Address of premises being assessed
Telephone	Telephone number of location being assessed
GMP contact number	Name and telephone number of patient's GMP
Number of persons living in premises	Number of individuals living at the address
Examples of hazards	
External access	Difficulty in reaching premises due to location, e.g.:
	• Access gained via back streets or alleyways
	• Items stored on entrance steps or corridors
	• Steep stairs, poorly laid paths
	• Lift frequently out of action
External lighting	Unsafe parking due to lack of, or inadequate street lighting
	Dimly lit stair wells
Internal access	Steep steps, items stored in corridors
Internal lighting	Poorly lit households, insufficient light to carry out procedure
Pets	Pets within treatment area (cats, dogs, birds, etc.)
Obvious fire hazards	Smokers at the location
	Children with access to cigarettes, lighters, matches
	Use of chip pans, electric blankets, portable gas heaters
	Broken flexes, faulty plugs and sockets
	Storage of oxygen cylinders
	Lack of smoke detectors
Slips, trips and falls	Any items that have a potential to cause slips, trips or falls, e.g.:
	• Ill fitting carpets and floor coverings
	• Slippery kitchen/bathroom floors
	• Flooring stained with bodily matter (environmental hazard)
	• Broken furniture
	• Lack of space due to furniture/other clutter
Furniture	Low seating causing manual handling problems
Space availability	Sufficient space to enable treatment of the patient in an appropriate manner with privacy and dignity, e.g. exclude smokers from treatment area and any other person not required for support with agreement of patient
Manual handling assessment	Complete according to trust policy/local rules
Additional comments and actions required	Identify control measures to deal with identified hazards
	Any other information to be noted, e.g. experience of personal aggression or suspicion of abuse
Assessment outcome	An overall measure of assessment as categorised by assessor
→ Green flag	→ Assessment did not highlight any significant problems
→ Amber flag	→ Assessment includes additional comments which must be read by any individual visiting premises or patient
→ Red flag	→ Anyone visiting premises must contact assessor or case manager to discuss hazards
Signature/date	Risk assessment must be signed and dated on completion

Oral care

The frequency and nature of oral care will depend on the medical condition and the oral hygiene of the patient. A satisfactory level of oral health may be maintained, with minimum discomfort to the patient, by the use of small toothbrushes or foam sticks. If brushing is not possible, the mucosa and tongue can be cleaned by using a gloved finger wrapped in gauze. The oral health and effectiveness of the oral care provided should be kept under constant review.

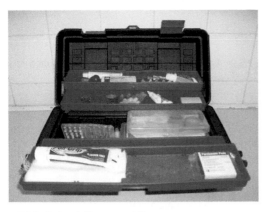

Figure 15.3 A domiciliary care kit.

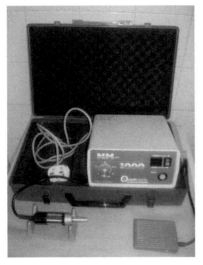

Figure 15.4 A portable motor in carry case. (Reproduced by kind permission of J&S Davis.)

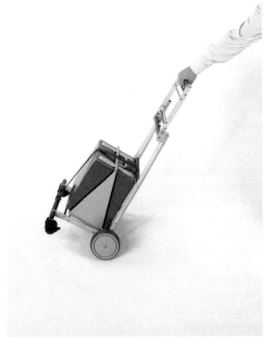

Figure 15.6 Portable domiciliary equipment (Mini-dent) in transit. (Reproduced by kind permission of J&S Davis.)

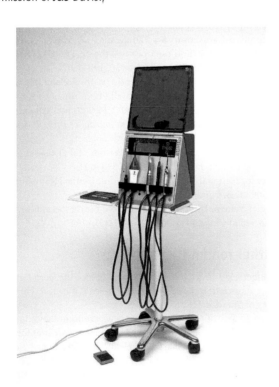

Figure 15.5 Portable dental equipment (Mini-dent). (Reproduced by kind permission of J&S Davis.)

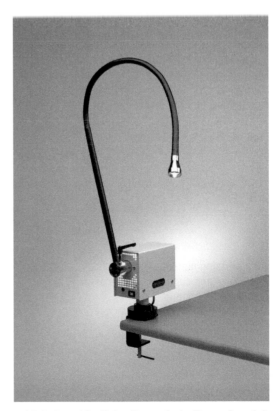

Figure 15.7 Portable light (Dentrolux). (Reproduced by kind permission of J&S Davis.)

Table 15.6 A checklist of general items required for a domiciliary visit.

Items	Tick
Portable light	☐
Gloves	☐
Sharps box	☐
Liquid soap	☐
Waste bags	☐
Box to carry contaminated instruments	☐
Resuscitation pocket mask	☐
Protective clothing for clinician and nurse	☐
Portable suction	☐
Masks and/or visors	☐
Disinfection solution	☐
Paper towels	☐
Protective glasses for patient and staff	☐
Emergency drugs kit and oxygen	☐
Portable handpiece	☐
Basic examination kit	☐

Table 15.7 A checklist of administrative items required for a domiciliary visit.

Items	Tick
Identification badge	☐
Appointment diary	☐
Record card	☐
Laboratory forms	☐
Consent forms	☐
British National Formulary (BNF)	☐
(to check on current medication)	☐
Mobile phone	☐
Writing materials	☐
Health promotion literature	☐
Route map	☐

Table 15.8 A checklist of restorative items required for a domiciliary visit.

Items	Tick
Temporary dressing materials	☐
Filling materials (and curing light if necessary)	☐
Matrix retainers and bands	☐
Handpieces and burs	☐
Gauze, cotton rolls and pellets	☐
Vaseline	☐
Local anaesthetic cartridges	☐
Topical anaesthetic spray/cream	☐
Portable unit	☐
Conservation hand instruments and tray	☐
Syringes, needles and needle guards	☐

Table 15.9 A checklist of periodontal items required for a domiciliary visit.

Item	Tick
Light source	☐
Mirrors	☐
Hand scalers	☐
Portable ultrasonic scalers	☐
Toothbrushes, therapeutic agents, e.g. mouthwash	☐
Oral hygiene aids	☐

References

All Wales Special Interest Group/Oral Health Care. www.sig wales.org/.

Burt, B.A. (1994) Periodontitis and aging: reviewing recent evidence. *Journal of the American Dental Association*, **125**, 273.

Fiske, J. and Lewis, D. (1999) Domiciliary dental care. *Dental Update*, **26**, 396–404.

Food Standards Agency (2003) National Diet and Nutrition Survey. Vol. 3. [Online.] Available from http://www.food.gov. uk/multimedia/pdfs/ndnsv3.pdf (accessed 4 October 2011).

Gomes-Filho, I.S., Passos, J.de S., Crus, S.S., *et al.* (2007) The association between postmenopausal osteoporosis and periodontal diease. *Journal of Periodontology*, **78**(9), 1731–1740.

Kayser, A.F. and Witter, D.J. (1985) Oral functional needs and its consequences for edentulous older people. *Community Dental Health*, **2**, 285–291.

Kelly, M., Steele, J., Nuttall, N., *et al.* (2000) *Adult Dental Health Survey – Oral Health in the United Kingdom, 1998*. The Stationery Office, London.

Nicopoulou-Karayianni, K., Tzoutzoukos P, Mitsea A, *et al.* (2009) Toothloss and osteoporosis: the OSTEODENT *study Journal of Clinical Periodontology* **36**, 190–197.

Nunn, J. (2004) Special care dentistry. In: Ireland, R. (ed.) *Advanced Dental Nursing*. Blackwell Publishing, Oxford.

Marques, M.A. and Dib, L.L. (2004) Periodontal changes in patients undergoing radiotherapy. *Journal of Periodontology*, **75**(9), 1178–1187.

Milward, M. and Cooper, P. (2005) Periodontal disease and the ageing patient. *Dental Update*, **32**, 598–604.

Office for National Statistics (2009) Adult Dental Health Survey 2009.ONS, London.

Van der Velden, U. (1984) Effect of age on the periodontium. *Journal of Clinical Periodontology*, **11**(5),–294.

Further reading

Gerodontology. Journal published on behalf of the Gerodontology Association. Editor-in-Chief: James P Newton, University of Dundee, UK.

British Society of Gerodontology: www.gerodontology.com

British Society for Disability and Oral Heath Guidelines for the Delivery of a Domiciliary Oral Health Service. August 2009.

Famili, P., Cauley, J., Suzuki, J.B. and Weyant, R. (2005) Longitudinal study of periodontal disease and edentulism with rates of bone loss in older women. *Journal of Periodontology*, **76**(1), 11–15.

16

Medical emergencies and their management

Lesley Longman and Colette Balmer

Summary

This chapter covers:

- Avoidance of a medical emergency
- The ABCDE approach to management of the sick patient
- Medical emergencies and their management
- Basic life support in adults and children

Introduction

Medical emergencies by their very nature can occur at any time, without warning and not necessarily in the clinical environment. It is therefore essential to be able to recognise the nature of an emergency as soon as it occurs and to have the knowledge, proficiency and confidence to be able to undertake the appropriate remedial action.

The General Dental Council (GDC, 2009) state that hygienists and dental therapists must:

- Be competent at carrying out resuscitation techniques.
- Have knowledge of how to identify medical emergencies and provide immediate management of anaphylactic reaction, hypoglycaemia, upper respiratory obstruction, cardiac arrest, fits, vasovagal attack, inhalation or ingestion of foreign bodies, and haemorrhage.

Management considerations

Dental therapists and hygienists treat patients of all ages and it is inevitable that some of these patients will have significant medical conditions and take medication, both of which may necessitate a modification to dental treatment. In addition many patients will experience anxiety associated with their treatment. It is to be expected that acute medical conditions will occur in a dental practice, albeit rarely. It is worth remembering that friends or family who often accompany patients, other visitors to the practice and staff may become unwell and require urgent attention. Medical emergencies can therefore occur anywhere on the premises, not just in the surgery. It is essential that all dental health care workers should have the knowledge and skills to recognise and provide appropriate immediate medical care for emergencies that might present in dental practice. In some instances this will require the provision of life saving measures prior to the arrival of specialist help.

A medical emergency can be described as a situation in which a patient's life may be at risk. The medical emergencies that are likely to be encountered in dental practice are shown in Table 16.1. This list is not exhaustive but it represents the commonly accepted conditions for which the dental team should be prepared. The individual management strategies used for these conditions are discussed in more detail later in this chapter.

It is the professional responsibility of hygienists and therapists to ensure that:

- They know the location of, and have easy and prompt access to, all emergency equipment and drugs (see Table 16.2).
- The equipment and drugs conform to contemporaneous standards recommended by respected bodies.
- All equipment is well maintained and all drugs are checked regularly and replaced prior to their expiry date.

Clinical Textbook of Dental Hygiene and Therapy, Second Edition. Edited by Suzanne L. Noble.
© 2012 John Wiley & Sons, Ltd. Published 2012 by John Wiley & Sons, Ltd.

- They are trained regularly in the use of the above.
- Regular 'in-practice' simulation of the management of medical problems including the preparation and administration of emergency drugs. This is in addition to training in cardiopulmonary resuscitation (CPR).

Regular in-house training in cardiopulmonary resuscitation is mandatory for the dental team. These sessions can be easily modified to include a rehearsal of managing other acute medical emergencies that do not necessarily need to progress to a cardiorespiratory arrest, although

Table 16.1 Medical emergencies that can occur in the dental surgery.

• Vasovagal attack (faint/syncope)	• Myocardial infarction
• Hyperventilation (panic attack)	• Anaphylaxis
• Epileptic seizures	• Airway obstruction (including chocking)
• Hypoglycaemia	• Respiratory arrest
• Asthma attack	• Cardiac arrest
• Angina	• Adrenal crisis

this remains a possible outcome. Several scenarios can be devised around an unwell patient who has the potential to progressively deteriorate; such as a patient with angina who may develop severe chest pains or a patient who experiences breathing problems. Regular rehearsal identifies problems that can then be rectified in a non-judgemental and constructive manner. Simulation training undertaken in a familiar working environment allows staff to clearly understand their role and the role of other members of the team, so helping to reduce confusion and panic when faced with a real emergency.

It is also important for members of the team to be cognisant with the different methods of preparation of the emergency drugs. This extends from turning on the oxygen supply and attaching the different types of face masks, to the opening of drug ampoules, and the drawing up and mixing of medications presented as powders with solvents (e.g. glucagon). Epinephrine (adrenaline) is available in several presentations from glass ampoules to preloaded syringes and staff should be confident in preparing the drugs available in their workplace. Preloaded syringes are more user friendly, although there are still training issues to be addressed in assembling many of these presentations. It is not unusual for hygienists and therapists to work in more than

Table 16.2 Emergency equipment and drugs required in the dental surgery[a].

Equipment	Drugs
Pocket mask with one-way valve and oxygen inlet	Oxygen (portable) with pressure reduction valve and flowmeter
Self inflating 1 litre bag, valve and mask with reservoir in various sizes with appropriate tubing to connect to the oxygen (face masks should be in variety of sizes for children and adults)	Epinephrine (adrenaline)
Oropharyngeal airways[b] (sizes 1,2,3,4)	Glyceryl trinitrate (GTN)
Oxygen therapy masks with tubing and appropriate connectors for oxygen cylinder	Aspirin
Sterile syringes and needles to deliver emergency drugs by IM routes	Glucose
Independently powered portable suction apparatus with wide bore aspiration tips.	Glucagon
Spacer device for inhaled bronchodilators (eg salbutamol)	Salbutamol inhaler
Automated blood glucose measurement device	Midazolam
Automated external defibrillator	
Additional equipment and emergency drugs	
Pulse oximeter[c]	
Blood pressure monitor[c]	

[a] Equipment should be free from natural rubber latex and resuscitation equipment must be available in suitable sizes for children. Drugs must be available in preparations free from natural rubber latex, whenever possible.
[b] These are also referred to as Guedel's airway.
[c] Essential in a practice that carries out IV sedation. (Adapted from the Resuscitation Council (UK) Guidance www.resus.org.uk 2010.)

one practice and therefore they may need to be familiar with a wider range of drug presentations.

It is imperative that training exercises are aimed at team building and therefore should be non-threatening. Consideration should be given to the management of patients who have collapsed in areas other than the dental chair or surgery. Toilets, with their confined space can be particularly awkward and problematic. Locked toilet doors should be able to be opened from the outside so that emergency access can be obtained. Formal courses using scenario training for medical emergencies are provided by some postgraduate Deaneries. **Immediate life support** (ILS) courses are organised by the **Resuscitation Council** (UK). The authors consider it best practice for all clinical members of the dental team to receive annual training to ILS standards.

When first commencing work in a new practice it should be standard protocol to identify where the emergency drugs and equipment are kept. You should be satisfied that these are adequate and comply with current guidance. Participation in team training for emergencies should ideally be part of the induction process when starting in a new place of work.

The role of the hygienist/therapist

The General Dental Council (GDC) states that dental hygienists and therapists should:

- Be competent at carrying out resuscitation techniques.
- Have knowledge of how to identify medical emergencies and provide immediate management of anaphylactic reaction, hypoglycaemia, upper respiratory tract obstruction, cardiac arrest, fits, vasovagal attack, inhalation or ingestion of foreign bodies, and haemorrhage (GDC, 2009).

Hygienists and therapists are capable of independent practice. When the dentist is present it is probable that he or she will assume the role of *team leader* in a medical emergency; although another more experienced clinical member of the team may assume this role. In the event of an emergency it is hoped that those present would work as a team, with many of the staff making valuable contributions to the management of the patient. However, a dentist may not be on the premises and a therapist/hygienist may be the most senior person and lead the team, in fact you may be the only staff member present. It is therefore important that the hygienist/therapist understands their role fully in a medical crisis and has a clear idea of what actions they would be prepared to carry out. The guidance given by the GDC clearly indicates that you would be expected to perform CPR; it would be unacceptable for any clinical member

of the dental team not to attempt CPR on a patient in cardiorespiratory arrest. There remains some uncertainty from the guidance given by the GDC as to what would be expected from a therapist/hygienist with regard to the administration of drugs. Does *how to provide* mean that *you should provide*? It is the authors' opinion that hygienists and therapists should be able to administer first line drugs for the patient provided that they have received appropriate training. Therefore in this chapter it is assumed that the hygienist or therapist would carry out essential primary treatment in a medical emergency. This includes the use of the following drugs: oxygen, epinephrine (adrenaline), glucose, glucagon, midazolam, glyceryl trinitrate, aspirin and salbutamol. Further post-qualification training may result in new drugs being added to this list.

It must be appreciated that the overwhelming majority of clinical dental personnel are uncomfortable in managing a medical emergency and are unlikely to feel confident in administering emergency drugs, other than oxygen. This is because their experience is likely to be based solely upon their academic knowledge and clinical skills acquired during simulation training (hence its importance). Other than the management of faints, most dental staff will have little (if any) experience of managing medical emergencies for real.

Avoidance of a medical emergency

Whilst it is accepted that all members of the dental team should be prepared to manage a medical crisis, steps should always be taken to try and prevent an acute condition from arising. In essence this involves:

- Having an accurate contemporaneous record of the patient's medical and drug history.
- Having a realistic and appropriate treatment plan.
- Identifying potential medical problems.
- Observing the patient.
- Rehearsing the systematic approach used for the assessment of the sick patient; as described by the Resuscitation Council (UK).

Prior to treating any patient a detailed medical and drug history is essential, and this should be updated at each treatment session. Knowledge of a patient's medical status is part of **risk assessment**. Details of any medical history previously recorded in the clinical records should be read thoroughly and evaluated before the patient enters the surgery. When treating a patient with a significant medical and drug history *all* staff involved in the care of the patient should know of, and understand, the relevance (if any) of the patient's current and past medical conditions. It is always prudent to ask patients if they have taken their medication as usual. Occasionally a patient will have the misconception that they should stop their regular medication on the day of dental treatment. When this occurs the therapist/hygienist should seek advice from the dentist to see if it is safe to proceed with operative treatment. In the absence of any dentists, a member of The **Medicines Information Service,** who advise on drug therapy relating to dentistry, can be obtained by telephoning 0151 794 8206 (in the UK).

Patients (and sometimes guardians or carers) do not always disclose an accurate medical and drug history. When important questions remain unanswered or there appears to be inconsistencies or conflicting information then clarification should be sought from the patient's medical practitioner. Operative treatment should not be undertaken in the absence of a reliable medical history.

When a patient declares a significant medical condition it is often necessary to ask further in depth questions in order to assess potential risks. An example of this is in patients who have **epilepsy** – it is essential to know how well their epilepsy is controlled and when they had their last seizure. The type of epilepsy should be documented and the patient asked for a description of their seizures, it is also helpful to know if they have warnings prior to a seizure. It is important to identify if they have ever gone into **status epilepticus**, and if so, how often. Any triggers that have been identified as precipitating a seizure should be documented in the records. Whilst all types of epilepsy should be recorded, a generalised seizure generates most concern due to the greatest possibility of injury and post-seizure complications. Patients who have frequent seizures should be asked for details about their recovery, for example some patients sleep after a seizure. Ask this group of patients how they would like to be managed post-seizure.

Treatment planning should be sensible, realistic and the medical and social needs of each patient should be taken into account. The timing and duration of appointments are important when treating patients with chronic disease. Table 16.3 highlights some factors that will influence treatment planning. Patients with **diabetes** should not be kept waiting and ideally treatment should not interfere with the timing of the patient's carbohydrate intake or administration of their medication. Patients who have **debilitating illnesses** and who get tired easily should have their dental appointments at a time that is most suited to their lifestyle. Sometimes carers and patients who have severe disabilities are unable to attend for early morning appointments. Patients who receive **kidney dialysis** should usually be treated on a day when they are not dialysed. A patient who has had a **myocardial infarction** within the last 6 months should only undergo simple emergency dental treatment due to

Table 16.3 Considerations when treating patients with a medical history.

When assessing a patient's health record it is helpful to consider the following possibilities:

- Are there any medical conditions that can affect any aspect of treatment? For example, in patients with cardiorespiratory problems is there breathing adversely affected by chair position? In the patient with diabetes the timing and duration of the appointment needs to be taken into consideration and the timing of their antidiabetic drug medication, meals and snacks. Does the patient have an illness that affects blood clotting?
- Is the medication taken by the patient likely to influence/modify the proposed dental treatment? Is the patient on warfarin? Are there any orofacial side-effects associated with their medication?
- Rescue medication: Does the patient self-medicate with a preparation that may be useful in the prevention or management of a medical emergency? Glyceryl trinitrate or bronchodilators such as a salbutamol inhaler should be easily accessible if needed urgently.
- Are there any known allergies, in particular are there any severe allergies to substances – allergens – that the patient may be exposed to in the dental surgery? Does the patient carry epinephrine (adrenaline) for self administration?

an increased risk of dysrhythmias; routine, elective treatment should be deferred.

It is important that therapists and hygienists recognise dental anxiety in their patients. This is of paramount importance in those who have serious medical conditions that are exacerbated by stress (for example angina, hypertension or epilepsy). This group of patients should be asked if they are made anxious by any aspect of dental treatment because pain and effective anxiety control is essential to avoid a crisis. It may be safer to treat this cohort of anxious patients under sedation. Not all patients are suitable for dental treatment in primary care. It is often necessary to refer patients who have severe unstable medical conditions to a specialist unit when operative dental treatment is required. If there is uncertainty about the safety of managing a patient in primary care advice should be sought.

It is always necessary to clinically observe a patient during dental treatment; careful observation will allow early recognition and prompt management of the unwell or deteriorating patient. Table 16.4 lists some of the signs that may be monitored.

It is rare for a medical emergency to occur without warning. When treating a patient there will usually be signs and/or symptoms, which indicate a deteriorating condition. When a patient looks unduly pale, flushed or

Table 16.4 Clinical monitoring.

Level of consciousness – Assess the patient's response to questions and commands and also their level of co-operation.

Respiration – At rest, respiration should be regular, effortless and quiet; breath sounds should not be obvious. When there is obstruction on inspiration, increased respiratory signs are seen such as excessive abdominal movement. The number of breaths can be counted over a 30 second period and the rate calculated for 1 minute. The respiration rate should be around 14–20 breaths per minute for an adult, but may be as high as 30 in a child.

Pulse – Assess the rate, regularity and quality. A pulse results from the intra-arterial pressure transmitted to arteries by the contraction of the left ventricle. A pulse represents the heart rate. The radial and brachial are the commonly used superficial pulses but the carotid and femoral pulses are the major pulses used in the assessment of an unconscious patient. In a baby, however, the brachial pulse is used because the neck is poorly developed making the carotid pulse difficult to feel. An average resting pulse rate for an adult is around 80 bpm (range 60–100). Children's pulse rates are faster. When taking a radial pulse you should place your 2nd and 3rd fingers in the hollow immediately above the wrist creases at the base of the thumb, and press lightly. You should not use your thumb to record a pulse because it has a pulse of its own. Assess the rate (over a minimum period of 30 seconds) and calculate the value for 1 minute.

Colour of the patient – Assess the pallor of the face, the colour of the fingers. Visual signs of central cyanosis will only be detected by a skilled operator when the arterial oxygen saturation falls to below 85%. Hypoxia is therefore not clinically noticeable in the early stages and if hypoxia is a concern then the use of a pulse oximeter may be advisable. Patients will normally have oxygen saturation levels of 97–100%.

General mood, demeanour, composure and body language – Ascertain if the patient is relaxed or agitated. When a patient is receiving dental treatment the operator and nurse should be aware of how comfortable or restless the patient is. A restless patient may fidget and appear tense.

---

ill ask them if they are feeling unwell. It may just be that they had a disturbed sleep, have missed a meal or are recovering from an illness. Such information is helpful in evaluating the patient. Patients who are clearly unwell should have their dental treatment deferred. Early recognition of a distressed or unwell patient can sometimes prevent an acute incident or prepare the dental team for prompt action in the early stages of a crisis. Knowing when to summon expert assistance is also important. A structured and logical approach to assessing a sick patient is invaluable in the early recognition and management of an unwell patient and one such approach is described in the next section.

Assessment of the sick patient using the 'ABCDE' approach

It is helpful to take an overview of the assessment and management of the unwell patient because early recognition of a sick patient may prevent an emergency. The Resuscitation Council (UK) have issued guidance that provides the dental team with a systematic and rational approach to managing the unwell patient, The principles employed can also be used in all medical emergencies that may be encountered in the dental surgery and is equally applicable if the patient is conscious or unconscious. The '**ABCDE**'approach is summarised in Table 16.5. The acronym is an *aide-mémoire*

Table 16.5 The 'ABCDE' approach to assessing the sick patient.

Assess	Consider
Airway patency of the airway	Removing debris Improving airway with head tilt/chin lift, jaw thrust Airway adjuncts Oxygen
Breathing rate and depth of respiration associated sounds/noises use of accessory muscles	Oxygen Chair position Salbutamol for asthma Re-breathing if hyperventilation
Circulation rate, strength, regularity of pulse capillary refill and blood pressure	Chair position GTN if you suspect angina Aspirin if you suspect an MI
Disability level of consciousness (AVPU) response of pupils to light blood glucose levels	if unconscious lie them flat, consider the recovery position if they are breathing spontaneously Glucose/glucagon for hypoglycaemia
Exposure skin rashes ankle oedema	Adrenaline if anaphylaxis Placing a blanket around the patient

for **A**irway, **B**reathing, **C**irculation, **D**isability, **E**xposure. Information obtained during this assessment will assist you in deciding whether or not to call the emergency services. If any life threatening problems are identified they are treated immediately before moving onto the next part of the assessment. A brief description of the methodology will be given below, but more detail relating it to specific medical emergencies can be found under each condition.

When you have recognised that a patient appears to be unwell you should stop all dental treatment, stay calm and ensure that you and the dental team are safe. You then want to assess the level of consciousness of the patient; this can be done simply by asking them 'if they feel ok'. Depending on their response you may wish to call for a colleague to help you.

Airway

A person must have an open airway to allow oxygen to enter the lungs, so the first step in effective management is to assess the patency of the upper airway – the patency is obvious if the patient is talking, however, if the patient is unconscious, are there any obvious obstructions such as fluid, vomit or the tongue?

Breathing

Look, listen and feel for signs of respiratory distress. Is breathing noisy, are accessory muscles (neck and abdominal muscles) being used? Is the patient blue? What is the rate of respiration? A breathing rate of 12–20 breaths per minute is a reasonable range for an adult. Are both right and left sides of the chest rising and falling with every breath? Patients having an asthma attack (recognised by an expiratory wheeze) require a bronchodilator such as salbutamol.

Patients who have respiratory distress that is not relieved by airway manoeuvres, oxygen or bronchodilators need urgent medical help.

If there is no breathing then you proceed to the algorithm for respiratory arrest.

Circulation

An efficient circulation is essential to distribute oxygenated blood from the lungs to the vital organs, thus maintaining the cardiac output. Circulation can be assessed by looking at the colour of the patient, by feeling the pulse and noting if the extremities, such as the hands, are cold or warm to touch. The pulse may be more easily detected if a central point is used. A simple and quick test, the capillary refill time, gives an indication of how good the blood supply is to the peripheral tissues. This test consist of applying pressure for around 5 seconds to a finger tip (positioned at heart level or just above) in order to cause blanching. The pressure is then released and the time taken for the colour of the surrounding skin to return to normal is recorded. The normal capillary refill time is less than 2 seconds; a longer time suggests poor peripheral circulation.

If a patient has a low pulse rate they should be placed flat, preferably with the legs raised to improve venous return. If the pulse rate remains weak, slow or irregular then further medical help is needed. Patients with breathing and cardiac problems may not feel comfortable or well when they are put in a supine position as it may compromise their cardiorespiratory function. It is essential that these patients, when conscious, are put in a position in which they feel comfortable. Poor pulse rates are suggestive of a low blood pressure and it would be helpful to measure blood pressure if equipment is available.

Disability

Under disability the clinician should assess the patient's level of consciousness, see if their pupils are equally responsive to light and measure blood glucose. Unconscious patients should be monitored in the recovery position whenever possible.

A quick method of assessing a person's level of consciousness is the **AVPU** system, where:

A = **A**lert.
V = response to **V**ocal stimuli.
P = response to **P**ainful stimuli.
U = **U**nresponsive to stimuli.

The level of consciousness may be assessed at the start of the assessment when you are assessing the airway.

Exposure

It is helpful to quickly check if the patient has a rash or swollen ankles. A patient in shock will quickly feel cold so a blanket should be placed around them to minimise heat loss.

The unwell patient should be continually monitored using the above approach until help arrives.

Medical emergencies

A summary of the use of emergency drugs is given in Table 16.6 and a separate chart for the administration routes for emergency drugs is given in Table 16.7.

Airway obstruction

The airway may be obstructed by a foreign body (e.g. a tooth, food or denture), blood, vomitus, oropharyngeal oedema, laryngospasm and bronchospasm.

Table 16.6 Indications and mechanism of action of drugs used in medical emergencies[a].

Drug	Indications	Dose and route	Mechanism of action
Oxygen	Most emergencies but not beneficial in hyperventilation	Flow rate is variable – inhalation Supplemental oxygen: masks 4–6 l/min; nasal cannula 1–2 l/min Resuscitation 10–15 l/min	Prevents cerebral hypoxia
Epinephrine (adrenaline)	Anaphylactic shock	0.5 mg of 1:1000 (1 mg/ml), repeated at 5-minute intervals if required, IM For doses in children see Table 16.8	Suppression of histamine release Vasoconstriction which preserves blood pressure An increase in the rate and force of cardiac contraction Relaxation of bronchial smooth muscle which dilates the airways
Glucose	Hypoglycaemia, conscious patient	10–20 g oral	Rapid absorption; elevates serum glucose levels quickly
Glucagon	Hypoglycaemia, unconscious patient	1 mg, IM, SC or IV routes Children under 8 years give 500 μg	This hormone increases serum glucose by converting stored glycogen into glucose
Salbutamol	Asthma	200 μg (2 puffs) – inhalation	Relaxes bronchial smooth muscle so increasing the size of the airways
Glyceryl trinitrate	Cardiac chest pain/angina	400 μg metered dose – sublingual	Improves blood flow to the myocardium by vasodilatation of the coronary arteries.
Aspirin	Myocardial infarct	300 mg – oral (chewed or crushed)	The anti-thrombotic effect of aspirin reduces mortality after a myocardial infarction
Midazolam	Status epilepticus	10 year and adults: 10 mg buccal or intranasal midazolam (transmucosal midazolam) (child dose 1–5 years 5 mg 5–10 years 7.5 mg 200 μg/kg)	Benzodiazepines have anti-epileptic action by inhibiting CNS activity.

[a]Drug protocols are constantly being updated and modified as new scientific information becomes available; it is the duty of the clinician to keep up to date with current guidance.

Table 16.7 Routes of drug administration important in medical emergencies.

Route	Emergency drugs	Onset of action	Comments
Oral	Aspirin, glucose	30–120 min	
Transmucosal sublingual/buccal	GTN, glucose gel, midazolam	1–5 min	
Intranasal	Midazolam	10–20 min	Use a dedicated mucosal atomization device
Inhalation	Oxygen, salbutamol	1–5 min	If the asthmatic patient is not using the salbutamol inhaler properly use a spacer device (see text)
Intramuscular	Epinephrine (adrenaline), glucagon	5–15 min	Use upper outer arm or outer thigh. No need to remove clothing if it is only a thin layer. For adrenaline aspirate to ensure that you do not give an IV injection.

Inhaled foreign body

In dental practice there is always a risk of foreign bodies such as pieces of tooth or parts of restorations being dislodged into the oropharynx and then being inhaled or ingested. If the foreign body has been ingested, it will usually travel through the gastrointestinal tract and be passed normally. If it is inhaled it may stimulate a cough reflex, or indeed choking if it is large enough. A small object can pass directly into the lower airway where it can cause a lung abscess if not retrieved. The best treatment is prevention, and the use of dental dam for restorative treatment is advised. Should an object be lost and the patient is not coughing or choking then the appropriate management is as follows:

- Check the patient's mouth and clothing thoroughly and the filter/trap of the aspirator.
- If the patient is lying flat ask them to turn onto their side and lower the chair to a 'head down' position; this encourages gravity to bring the object back into the mouth.

If the object cannot be located, inform the patient and contact the nearest A&E department for chest and abdominal X-rays. If the object is located in the respiratory tract the hospital will arrange removal as necessary.

Choking

The conscious patient

Airway obstruction in a conscious patient is easily diagnosed. Typically the person will appear distressed, coughing and have difficulty in breathing. They will usually point towards their neck or throat region to indicate the source of the problem. Choking can occur in the dental chair when water or a foreign body blocks the entrance to the trachea. A patient will usually cough to try and expel the blockage. When this happens, sit the patient up quickly and reassure them. The therapist/hygienist will also need to know how to deliver back blows and abdominal thrusts. Figure 16.1 shows the algorithm for the management of choking in an adult patient.

In the event of a partial airway obstruction in the conscious patient, coughing should clear the blockage; the patient should be encouraged to continue coughing. If the patient is starting to tire, deteriorate or show signs of cyanosis, immediate intervention is required and the rescuer should remove any obvious debris from the mouth and commence up to five back blows. If there has been no improvement abdominal thrusts should be carried out (up to five). Check, the mouth for any obstruction that can be removed and repeat the above cycles of five back blows followed by five abdominal thrusts until the obstruction is removed. If

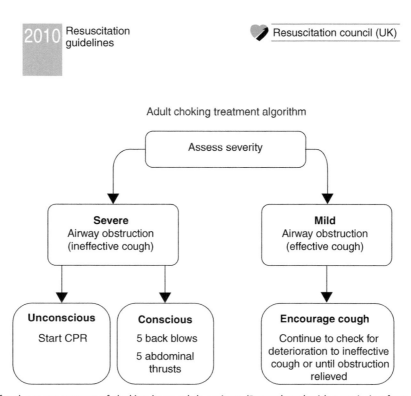

Figure 16.1 Algorithm for the management of choking in an adult patient. (Reproduced with permission from the Resuscitation Council (UK) Guidance website: www.resus.org.uk (2010).)

the casualty has lost consciousness then lay them flat. Check the mouth for any signs of obstruction, open the airway and give two effective breaths. If two effective breathes cannot be achieved within five attempts, start 30 chest compressions *immediately* to relieve the obstruction; there is no need to check the circulation. Check the mouth for blockages and continue to attempt to give cycles of two effective breaths followed by 30 chest compressions. Should effective breaths be given at any time, check for signs of circulation. Undertake rescue breaths and chest compressions as required until help arrives.

The techniques used in a choking adult include:

- **Back blows**. Stand behind and to the side of the casualty. Use one hand to support their chest and lean the victim forwards. Use the heel of your hand to deliver five discrete blows to the casualty's back firmly between the shoulder blades. Do this up to five times then re-evaluate for effect.
- **Abdominal thrusts** (also known as the **Heimlich manoeuvre**) involves the rescuer standing behind the casualty and encircling their arms around their upper abdomen. The rescuer makes a fist with one hand and places it over the casualty's epigastrium (midway between the navel and the xiphisternum) and firmly grasps the back of this fist with their other hand. The rescuer suddenly brings both hands upwards and inwards in a quick sharp movement; hopefully, this will dislodge the obstruction (see Figure 16.2). This motion is repeated up to 5 times. Evaluate between each manoeuvre to see if the foreign body has been expelled or forced into the mouth so that it may be removed by a finger sweep.

The choking child

It is important to remember that you should never try to remove an obstruction blindly by placing your finger in the mouth. Children become hypoxic very quickly so if the obstruction persists the algorithm in Figure 16.3 should be followed.

A baby or small child can usually be held upside down or placed over your knee on to their stomach (head down), and five back blows given. A larger child may be supported in a prone position with the head lower than the chest; five back blows can then be delivered. If the obstruction remains, up to five chest thrusts can be tried. Place the child on their back again with the head lower than the chest if possible. Check the mouth carefully to remove any visible obstruction. Open the airway and check for breathing. If breathing is present then place the casualty on their side and monitor. If the child is not breathing try to achieve two effective ventilations out of

five attempts at rescue breaths. If the obstruction is still present perform five back blows, followed by abdominal thrusts (rather than chest thrusts) and check the mouth again and repeat the cycle (see Figure 16.3); alternating one cycle of chest thrusts with one cycle of abdominal thrusts. Do not perform abdominal thrusts on a baby as these can cause damage to internal organs; use only cycles of back blows and chest thrusts.

The techniques used in a choking child include:

- **Back blows**. Use one hand to support their chest and lean the victim forwards. Use the heel of your hand to deliver five discrete blows to the casualty's back firmly between the shoulder blades.
- **Chest thrusts**. Place the patient on their back with the head lower than the chest. Apply up to five short sharp compressions to the chest (similar to chest compressions in CPR, but deliver in a sharp and vigorous manner at a rate of around 20 per minute).
- **Abdominal thrusts**. The conscious patient is placed in the upright position (you may need to kneel when managing for a small child) and the unconscious casualty is laid on their back. The heel of one hand is placed in the middle of the upper abdomen. Five sharp thrusts directed upwards towards the diaphragm are delivered. Abdominal thrusts are not advised for an infant.

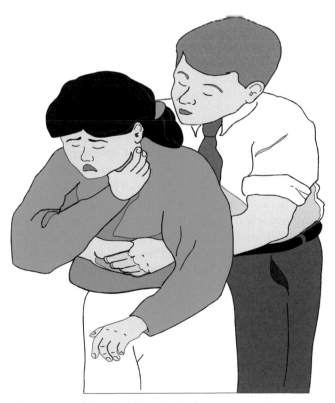

Figure 16.2 Abdominal thrust (Heimlich manoeuvre).

2010 Resuscitation guidelines

Resuscitation council (UK)

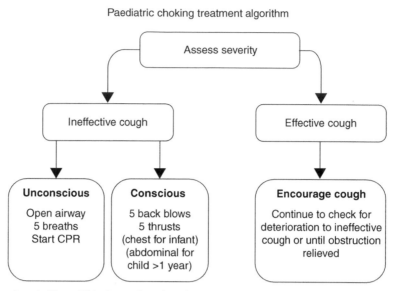

Paediatric choking treatment algorithm

Assess severity

Ineffective cough

Effective cough

Unconscious

Open airway
5 breaths
Start CPR

Conscious

5 back blows
5 thrusts
(chest for infant)
(abdominal for
child >1 year)

Encourage cough

Continue to check for
deterioration to ineffective
cough or until obstruction
relieved

Figure 16.3 Algorithm for the choking child. (Reproduced with permission from the Resuscitation Council (UK) Guidance website: www.resus.org.uk (2010).)

Airway assessment of the unconscious adult patient

The assessment of airway obstruction in an unconscious patient is best achieved using the systematic approach of **Look, Listen** and **Feel**:

- **Look** down the line of the patient's chest and observe for movement.
- Place one ear over the patient's mouth and nose; **listen** for breath sounds.
- Simultaneously **feel** for expired air.

Airway obstruction may be partial or complete. When there is complete airway obstruction, respiration will be silent and there will be an absence of breath sounds from the patient. In a partially obstructed airway, efforts at breathing will be noisy. If inspiration is noisy (**stridor**) this is indicative of obstruction above or at the laryngeal level; for example, semi-solid material may be present in the oropharynx. When expiration is noisy this tends to suggest obstruction of the lower airways, below the level of the larynx, as in asthma. The type of sound can suggest the cause of obstruction, for example:

- **Snoring** – caused by the tongue occluding the pharynx.
- **Gurgling** – suggests the presence of liquids or semi-solids in the airway.
- **Crowing** – indicative of laryngeal spasm.

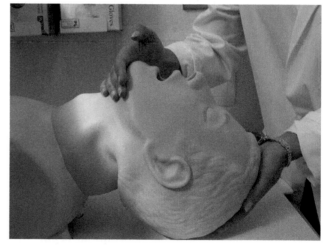

Figure 16.4 Improving the airway using a head tilt chin lift.

The simple positional manoeuvre of a head tilt and chin lift can be successful, especially where the obstruction arises from relaxation of the soft tissues (Figure 16.4).

This method of opening the airway is not advocated in suspected fractures of the cervical spine. Sometimes a jaw thrust is more effective at relieving obstruction of the oropharynx by the tongue. A jaw thrust advances the mandible and this releases the tongue from the posterior pharyngeal wall.

In the case of a partially obstructed airway, a finger sweep may be used in an adult or older child to evacuate solids or semisolid material in the absence of suction apparatus. If the airway has been cleared and adequate spontaneous respiration is taking place, the patient may be placed in the recovery position and their condition checked frequently; this is especially important in patients who are vomiting.

Head tilt and chin lift. A clear airway may easily be achieved by simple backward tilting of the head by pressing on the patient's forehead. Further relief of the obstruction may be provided by supporting the chin. This can be achieved by placing your fingertips under the point of the patients chin and lifting the chin forward.

A **jaw thrust**. The airway can often be improved by advancing the mandible forward. This is done by lifting the mandible upwards and forwards by placing the index fingers behind the angle of the mandible. The thumbs are on either side of the chin ready to depress the mandible and open the mouth slightly.

Airway maintenance using simple adjuncts

In an unconscious patient it may be necessary to maintain the airway using simple adjuncts; all clinical members of the dental team should be trained in their use. Oropharyngeal airways are designed to control backward displacement of the tongue in the unconscious patient but a head tilt–chin lift will usually need to be maintained. These airways come in a range of sizes from newborn to large adult. The most common sizes are 2, 3 and 4 for small, medium and large adults respectively (see Figure 16.5a).

The size required can be estimated by matching the oropharyngeal airway to the distance between the patient's incisors and the angle of the mandible (Figure 16.5b). They are rigid, curved plastic tubes, and are flanged and reinforced at the oral end to withstand pressure from the teeth. They are inserted in to the mouth in the inverted position and rotated through 180° whilst passing through the palate and into the oropharynx. If the patient shows signs of consciousness (coughing, vomiting, retching) remove the airway immediately. There are other airway adjuncts e.g. nasopharyngeal airways, laryngeal masks and endotracheal tubes which can be used by appropriately trained personnel.

Supplemental oxygen

Oxygen should be considered for use in every medical emergency. The only medical emergency where it is not beneficial to the patient is in a hyperventilation/panic attack. Oxygen should be given at a flow rate of 4–6 l/min via an oxygen therapy mask in patients who are breathing. When spontaneous respiration is absent, artificial ventilation is obviously a necessity; this requires a high

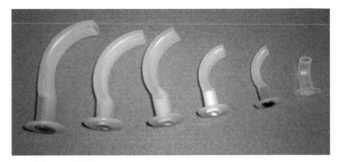

Figure 16.5a Oropharyngeal airways, size 1–4.

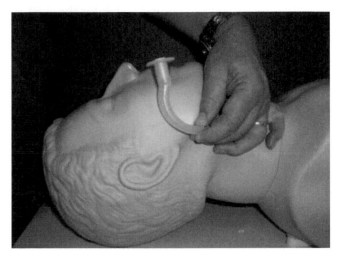

Figure 16.5b Sizing the airway.

oxygen flow rate (10–15 l/min) to be given under positive pressure. The most efficient and secure way of doing this is to intubate the patient with an endotracheal tube. Dental personnel, however, do not usually have the skills to do this. During resuscitation, oxygen can be given to a patient by a variety of methods: the simplest technique is mouth-to-mouth resuscitation. This is not ideal as it uses expired air from the rescuer which contains only 16% oxygen (ambient air contains 21% oxygen) and there are potential cross-infection issues. Some simple adjuncts are available in dental surgeries; the pocket mask, being the most popular device in the UK, has a number of advantages. It eliminates the need for mouth-to-mouth ventilation, which some people find distasteful and unacceptable. The use of a mask also reduces the potential for cross infection. The mask is usually transparent so the rescuer can detect the presence of vomit or bleeding immediately. A non-return valve separates the two airways so the rescuer will not inhale the patients expired air. It is also possible to attach supplemental oxygen, allowing oxygen-enriched air to be delivered to the patient. Whilst resuscitation using expired air with mouth to mask ventilation addresses cross infection problems it still only delivers 16% oxygen, unless oxygen is administered directly into the face mask. When high flow oxygen is delivered to a pocket mask the patient can receive around 40% oxygen. Although effective, the main difficulty with the pocket mask is the maintenance of an airtight seal between the mask and the face of the victim. If other staff are available it is possible for one person to hold the mask in place whilst another delivers rescue breaths. The mask is usually placed on the patient's face using the thumb and forefingers of both hands, lifting the angles of the jaw with the other fingers to obtain an airtight fit. Blow into the port of the mask to inflate the patient's lungs and watch for the chest to rise. Following each rescue breath, watch the chest fall to ensure expiration has taken place. If any leaks are noted, adjust hand position and/or contact pressure. It should be noted that a tidal volume of no greater than 400–500 ml/breath should be used in rescue breathing. Over vigorous breaths can result in **gastric insufflation** (blowing air into the stomach), increasing the risk of vomiting with regurgitation and pulmonary aspiration. In addition, overenthusiastic rescue breathing may also lead to high inflation pressures.

Ventilation using a bag, one-way valve and mask connected to high flow oxygen is a more effective way of delivering oxygen to patients with absent spontaneous respiration; this is shown in Figure 16.6.

The advantages associated with this device are:

- Supplementary oxygen may be given, increasing the oxygen concentration delivered to the patient from 21% to 45%.
- The addition of a reservoir bag (prefilled with oxygen) and the administration of high flow oxygen (10 l/min) will give an oxygen concentration of around 90%.

- This device may be fitted to an endotracheal tube or laryngeal mask airway.
- The patient's expired air is filtered into the atmosphere via a one-way valve.

The most notable difficulty with this system is maintaining an airtight seal whilst delivering ventilations. The percentages quoted above for oxygen depend upon the quality of the seal around the mask to the victim's face. To eradicate this problem, it is advised that a two-person technique is used wherever possible; one to hold the mask, the other to deliver ventilations (see Figure 16.7).

Faints

A faint, also called **syncope** or a **vasovagal attack**, is the most common cause of loss of consciousness in dental practice. Fainting occurs when the blood supply is diminished to the brain (**cerebral ischaemia**) by a transient fall in blood pressure (**hypotension**). The cerebral circulation is not delivering an adequate supply of oxygenated blood. Predisposing factors include hypoglycaemia (low blood sugar), anxiety, fear, pain, hunger, stress, fatigue and a hot environment. Postural hypotension is also a possible cause and this classically occurs when the patient sits or stands up after treatment. A minority of patients have a tendency to faint.

Signs and symptoms

The patient may feel unwell, light-headed, weak, confused, dizzy or nauseous. Obvious signs are usually apparent such as skin pallor and sweating; the skin feels cold and clammy. A vasovagal attack is accompanied by a **bradycardia** (decreased heart rate less than 60 bpm) and loss of consciousness. Muscle twitches can sometimes be seen as the patient is losing consciousness. Convulsions,

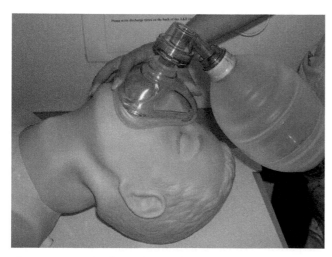

Figure 16.6 Self-inflating bag, valve and mask.

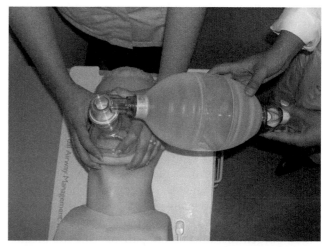

Figure 16.7 Two person technique for bag, valve, mask and reservoir bag.

cyanosis and incontinence can occur in the unconscious patient.

Management

The management of a faint is to lay the patient flat; the legs can be elevated if staff are available and the patient has no known cardiac or respiratory problem, (a pregnant patient should be placed on her side, this prevents the fetus from compressing the inferior venae cavae which would further reduce venous return). If the patient fails to regain consciousness after 3 minutes the diagnosis will need to be reassessed using **A B C D E** approach – give oxygen, call for medical assistance and monitor.

Placing the patient flat improves the venous return, cardiac output and the cerebral blood supply. Alternatively a sitting patient may lower their head by placing it between their knees but this is not as effective as lying a patient down. Loosen tight clothing around the neck. Oxygen can be administered if time allows, but recovery should be quick (within 2–3 minutes). Reassure the recovering patient; a glucose-rich drink may be helpful. When a member of the dental team recognises that a patient is likely to faint, or the patient informs you of this possibility, the patient should be placed in a supine position; this may prevent loss of consciousness.

Enquiries should be made as to the possible cause, for example 'When did you last have something to eat?' 'Are you prone to fainting?' The incident should be recorded in the clinical records and the likely cause noted. When patients have a tendency to faint during dental treatment, treat the patient in the supine position, especially for administration of a local anaesthetic; this will eliminate the majority of vasovagal attacks.

Hypoglycaemia

Hypoglycaemia is a deficiency of glucose in the blood stream. Precipitating factors in a known diabetic are anxiety, infection and fasting. This is sometimes seen in a patient with type 1 diabetes who has taken their insulin as normal but has not ingested a sufficient quantity of carbohydrate.

Signs and symptoms

The patient will feel cold and may have clammy skin, be trembling, confused, have double vision, slurring of speech or show behaviour changes (e.g. they may become excitable, irritable, aggressive or unco-operative). Drowsiness and disorientation and loss of consciousness can occur.

Management

In the first instance the management is aimed at elevating the blood glucose:

- **In the conscious patient:** Administer 10–20 g of glucose in the form of a drink, tablets, sugar cubes or gel (e.g. Hypostop® gel which is absorbed through the oral mucosa). Patients can be given 90 ml of non-diet Coca-Cola® or 200 ml milk which is equivalent to 10 g of glucose.
- **In the unconscious or uncooperative patient:** Give 1 mg (1 unit) of glucagon by the intramuscular (IM) route. This hormone increases serum glucose by converting glycogen stores into glucose. Administer oxygen and monitor – **A B C D E**.

It is unlikely that dental staff would want to administer the alternative therapy to glucagon consisting of a slow IV injection of glucose (25 ml of 50% solution). When the patient has recovered it may be necessary to give oral glucose to maintain blood glucose levels. A child under the age of 8 years or less than 25 kg should be given 500 µg. Call the emergency services if the patient does not recover following the above measures; give oxygen and monitor.

Epilepsy and status epilepticus

Epilepsy is a symptom of an underlying neurological disorder and is characterized by spontaneous, unprovoked recurrence of seizures. Seizures are likely to occur in a known epileptic when they are poorly controlled or do not comply with their drug regime. Some patients, however, have identified triggers that precipitate seizures such as hypoglycaemia, stress, anxiety or odours. Epileptic seizures generally last less than 5 minutes and are not usually considered as an emergency; **convulsive status epilepticus**, however, is an emergency that requires medical intervention. Convulsive (tonic–clonic) status epilepticus is defined as a generalised convulsion lasting 30 minutes or longer, or repeated tonic-clonic convulsions occurring over a 30 minute period without recovery of consciousness between each convulsion. During convulsive status epilepticus there is a risk that the patient may become hypoxic. Hypoglycaemia, brain damage from cerebral hypoxia and cardiac arrest can ensue. This condition carries an acute mortality rate of 10%. Status epilepticus can occur for all forms of epilepsy but non-convulsive status epilepticus is rare and the management is less urgent. A clinician should not wait 30 minutes to confirm a diagnosis of status; any convulsive phase of a tonic-clonic seizure that lasts in excess of 5 minutes, should be treated as status. The incidence of status amongst epileptic patients is around 5%.

Signs and symptoms

The clinical presentation of the seizure will depend upon the type of epilepsy that the patient has; this is a reflection of the area of the brain affected by the excessive electrical activity. Epilepsy may present as a disturbance of movement, sensation or behaviour with or without a loss of consciousness. Patients who have generalised tonic–clonic seizures (previously called **grand mal seizures**) will lose consciousness. The clonic phase consists of jerking movements of the limbs and body; it is during this phase that the patient may bite their tongue and injure themselves. The patient may remain unconscious after such a seizure and may be confused. It can take an individual up to 2 hours for their cognitive function to return to normal.

When patients are accompanied the escort may have a good knowledge of the natural progression of the patient's seizures. Seek their advice about how recovery usually proceeds, for example, does the patient normally have a sleep following a seizure?

Management

Note the time the seizure started. Protect the patient from injuring themselves on any adjacent equipment. Remove potentially harmful objects and if necessary place pillows around the patient to protect them. It is helpful to cover the spittoon with a pillow if it cannot be pushed away from the patient. Administer oxygen if possible and monitor – **A B C**. In the patient who had a convulsive seizure, ensure that they are discharged to the care of an escort in case the patient has post-seizure confusion. If the patient sustained general injuries during a seizure or had an atypical attack they may need to go to hospital.

When the seizure is prolonged or repeat seizures occur over a period exceeding 5 minutes, the patient should be regarded as having status epilepticus. **The emergency services** should be called and oxygen should be given, if possible. **Benzodiazepines** can be administered because of their antiepileptic action. **Midazolam** (10 mg) can be given by a transmucosal route in adults and children over 10 years of age. A preparation for buccal administration is available from and contains 4 ml of 10 mg/ml midazolam in a viscous fluid, complete with four 1 ml syringes for ease of administration. Alternatively undiluted midazolam for injection (the concentrated 10 mg/2 ml preparation) can be administered buccally or intranasally. A dedicated mucosal **atomisation device** can be used; this consists of an atomisation nozzle that attaches to the end of a hypodermic syringe. It should be noted that the use of buccal midazolam and intranasal midazolam for status epilepticus is unlicensed. Children aged 5–10 years require a dose of 7.5 mg of buccal or intranasal midazolam, and those aged 1–5 years a dose of 5 mg. A child's dose regime for midazolam is 200 μg/kg. It is important to realise that benzodiazepines are not always effective in controlling

status epilepticus and other anti-epileptic drugs may be required. The patient should be monitored.

Anaphylaxis

Anaphylaxis is a life-threatening allergic reaction that occurs once the patient has been exposed and sensitized to an antigen, such as natural rubber latex, certain drugs (most notably the penicillins) or additives to drug preparations, insect bites/stings and food (e.g. peanuts). Anaphylaxis caused by modern dental local anaesthetics is *exceptionally* rare; therefore other allergens should be considered in the first instance. In anaphylaxis there is a release of histamine and this causes a peripheral vasodilatation and causes the capillaries to leak fluid into the tissues; this reduces the intravascular circulating volume. The administration of epinephrine (adrenaline) reverses the vasodilatation and restores the circulating volume so increasing venous return. **Bronchospasm** can also occur and cause respiratory distress. Hypotension and/or bronchospasm must be present for a diagnosis of anaphylaxis.

Signs and symptoms

Initial flushing of the skin may occur followed by oedema of the face and neck; the tongue may become swollen. The patient may report altered sensations such as **paraesthesia** around the mouth and fingers. There will be a rapid weak pulse and skin flushing may occur, however severe hypotension may be present and this will result in pallor. **Cyanosis** will accompany acute breathing difficulties with bronchospasm and possible laryngeal oedema. Loss of consciousness, respiratory and/or cardiac arrest are likely to ensue if the patient is not treated. The more rapid the reaction to the antigen occurs then the more severe the symptoms tend to be. Symptoms can develop minutes after exposure to the antigen.

Management

Call for expert assistance. Treatment involves securing the airway and restoring the blood pressure. Administer oxygen via a face mask whilst maintaining the airway. The position that the patient is placed in will depend upon the symptoms and the severity of the reaction. In a breathless conscious patient it may be more comfortable for the patient to be in a semi-reclined position. However, if the patient is hypotensive or loses consciousness, lay them flat. Administer epinephrine (adrenaline) immediately (0.5 ml of 1:1000) intramuscularly (IM), repeat if necessary over 5 minute intervals. Monitor. Patients need to be monitored in hospital to assess their stability even if there is an initial recovery.

The administration of an **antihistamine** and a **steroid** will aid the patient's long-term stability and are second-line drugs that will be administered in by paramedics or hospital staff. The drug regime for epinephrine (adrenaline) in children is given in Table 16.6. Intravascular fluid replacement will be required but usually the paramedics will do this.

Asthma

In asthma there is narrowing of the bronchial airways and this leads to coughing, wheezing and breathing difficulties. Bronchial asthma may be precipitated by exposure to an antigen, drugs (typically non-steroidal anti-inflammatory analgesics), air pollution, anxiety, infection and exercise.

Signs and symptoms

There is breathlessness with wheezing on expiration. In addition there can be restlessness, difficulty in talking (they cannot complete sentences in one breath). Tachycardia (>100 bpm), a fast respiratory rate (>25 per minute) low peak respiratory flow, use of accessory muscles of respiration and cyanosis of the lips and nail beds. If untreated breathing may become increasingly difficult and the patient may develop status asthmaticus; respiratory arrest is also possible.

Management

Administer the patient's bronchodilator (usually **salbutamol** or **terbutaline**) to relax the bronchial smooth muscle; if this is not possible, use the surgery's emergency inhaler to give two inhalations (salbutamol 100 μg/puff). Most patients will respond to this. Give oxygen and repeat the administration of the bronchodilator if there is no improvement. Place the patient in a comfortable position and monitor. If the asthma remains uncontrolled or deteriorates summon the emergency services. Status asthmaticus is a life threatening condition. If a nebuliser is available then use this to administer 2.5–5 mg salbutamol nebules combined with oxygen. When a nebuliser is not available and the emergency services have been called, the salbutamol inhaler (2–10 puffs) should be administered every 10–20 minutes. Salbutamol is more effective in a large volume spacer device and it is advisable for practices that have a large number of asthmatic patients to purchase a spacer device or nebuliser. Alternatively, the salbutamol inhaler mouthpiece can be inserted into a hole made in the base of a plastic/paper cup. When asthma presents as a consequence of anaphylaxis, a bronchodilator (inhaler) may be given initially but adrenaline should also be used.

Cyanosis, a respiratory rate of < 8 breaths per minute a bradycardia (heart rate, 50 bpm), exhaustion, confusion or a decreased level of consciousness are all clinical features of life threatening asthma.

Angina

Angina pectoris is a chest pain produced when the oxygen supply to the myocardium is inadequate. This is usually due to **atheroma** (which causes narrowing) of the coronary arteries. The pain will stop if the myocardium receives sufficient oxygen. Anxiety or exercise can precipitate an attack in patients who are known to have angina.

Signs and symptoms

There is usually an intense crushing chest pain which may travel down the left arm or into the neck and mandible. The patient may experience breathlessness, nausea or vomiting. The heart rate can be variable-slow or fast. The capillary refill time is prolonged.

Management

Administer the patient's own medication for relieving pain caused by angina – a nitrate spray or tablets. When this is not available give **sublingual glyceryl trinitrate** (GTN) spray (400 μg per actuation) and administer oxygen. Ensure that the patient is in a comfortable position, often semireclined as opposed to supine. Ask the patient if they need to sit more upright. Monitor. If the symptoms do not resolve call the emergency services as it is possible that the patient is having a myocardial infarction.

Myocardial infarction (MI)

A myocardial infarction (also called a **coronary thrombosis** or **heart attack**) is the death of a section of the myocardium – usually the ventricle. This occurs because a portion of the heart muscle is deprived of oxygen (**ischaemia**). Arrhythmias frequently occur and ventricular fibrillation may ensue, which may be fatal. A history of angina, cardiac arrhythmias and congestive heart failure will place a patient at risk from an MI. Predisposing factors in at risk patients include stress, pain and infection. It is worth remembering that an MI can occur in patients who have had no previous cardiac symptoms.

Signs and symptoms

The symptoms for an MI are similar to angina, but are more severe and prolonged; in addition the pain is not relieved by GTN. There is severe crushing chest pain that radiates down the left arm or into the neck and mandible. There is an irregular, weak pulse and blood pressure may fall. The patient has an unhealthy pallor, is short of breath, nauseous and may vomit. Loss of consciousness may ensue.

Management

Call the emergency services. Give oxygen, a single dose of oral aspirin (300 mg crushed or chewed). Sit the patient in a comfortable position. Reassure the patient and attempt to keep them as calm as possible. Monitor. Aspirin should not be given if there is a clear contraindication (e.g. a known allergy) or if it distresses the patient. If the patient becomes unconscious and a pulse cannot be detected, follow the protocol for cardiopulmonary resuscitation.

The paramedics will usually give morphine for pain relief, but if you are in a sedation practice with a dedicated inhalation sedation machine and personnel trained in its use, then 50% nitrous oxide mixed with 50% oxygen can be a useful analgesic and anxiolytic. The majority of patients who die after an MI do so within the first hour. This is usually due to ventricular fibrillation.

Hyperventilation

Hyperventilation, or panic attack, occurs when the breathing rate at rest spontaneously becomes abnormally rapid. This causes a fall in the concentration of arterial carbon dioxide which results in an **alkalosis**, giving rise to the characteristic signs and symptoms seen in hyperventilation. Stress, pain or anxiety can precipitate this increase in ventilatory effort. Hyperventilation can be associated with chronic generalised anxiety disorder.

Signs and symptoms

These are rapid breathing (around 25–30 breaths/ minute), decreased depth of respiration, tachycardia, trembling, dizziness, blurred vision, sweating and **paraesthesia** (tingling sensation) in the lips and limbs. Muscle pain and stiffness can lead to muscular twitching and tetanic cramps in the hands and tightness or pain across the chest. Hyperventilation can be prolonged and whilst loss of consciousness can occur it does so only rarely.

Management

Stop treatment and remove all equipment from the mouth. Remove any equipment that may be considered to have provoked the condition (e.g. a syringe or forceps) out of the line of the patient's vision. Ask the patient to breathe slowly. Rebreathing expired air can help restore normal alveolar carbon dioxide levels. This can initially be done by asking the patient to breathe in and out of their cupped hands.

Hyperventilation can be difficult to stop and can be frightening for patients who tend to interpret their symptoms in a catastrophic manner; they often feel they have a cardiac problem or that they are suffocating.

These negative thought processes increase their anxiety. Reassurance is therefore essential and staff should act in a calm and controlled manner. Ensure that the patient is in a comfortable position, usually sitting upright. The patient should be told that their symptoms will resolve once breathing returns to normal. The rationale for the treatment should be explained to the patient so as not to induce further panic. A full facemask can be used, instead of cupped hands, to ensure rebreathing of carbon dioxide. Hyperventilation is an acute condition when oxygen is *not* beneficial to the patient. Rarely would the administration of an anxiolytic, such as intravenous midazolam, be indicated. The long-term management of the anxious patient who is predisposed to hyperventilation attacks may involve relaxation exercises, behavioural therapy and the possible use of sedation for operative dental treatment.

Cardiovascular accident (CVA)

A cerebrovascular accident, also called a stroke, occurs when there is a haemorrhage or obstruction (a **thrombosis** or **embolism**) in one of the cerebral blood vessels. This causes an interruption of the blood supply to an area of the brain. There is a resultant sudden attack of weakness affecting one side of the body. Hypertension, diabetes, renal disease, atherosclerosis of the cerebral arteries and a history of **transient ischaemic attacks** (TIAs, or mini-strokes) will all increase a patient's susceptibility to a CVA.

Signs and symptoms

There is a variation in the onset and severity of symptoms from passing weakness or tingling in a limb to a profound paralysis, coma and death. The patient may complain of a sudden headache; they may have difficulty speaking and speech may be slurred. They may be confused and exhibit muscular weakness or paralysis down one side of their body (**hemiplegia**). There may be loss of consciousness.

Management

Administer oxygen and ensure that the patient is in a comfortable position. Lie the patient in the recovery position if they lose consciousness. Call the emergency services and monitor the patient – **ABC.** If you are uncertain that there is muscle weakness in a conscious patient ask them to smile, raise both arms and say their name or address. These actions should highlight any muscular weakness. Prompt medical care is required as the patient may benefit from **thrombolytic drugs** (clot-busters).

The UK Stroke Association uses an acronym (act **FAST, Face, Arm, Speech Test**) if a member of the public suspects someone has had a stroke.

Facial weakness – can the person smile? Has their mouth or eye drooped?

Arm weakness – can the person raise both arms?

Speech problems – can the person speak clearly and understand what you say?

If a person fails any one of these tests then a stroke should be suspected and the emergency services called.

Local analgesic toxicity

Maximum safe drug values may be considerably reduced in patients with liver or kidney disease. As a consequence, the maximum safe dose of local analgesic agents, as advocated for a healthy patient should be significantly reduced in the elderly, the young and patients with systemic disease (such as heart disease). This is especially important in patients with liver and kidney disease, where drug metabolism and excretion is impaired.

Signs and symptoms

Light headedness, visual or hearing disturbances can occur. Agitation, confusion, seizures and respiratory distress can also develop. Initially, the symptoms are those of central nervous system (CNS) excitation followed by CNS depression in severe toxicity. Loss of consciousness, respiratory and cardiac arrest can occur.

Management

Lay the patient flat and administer oxygen, maintain airway and monitor-**A B C**. Summon expert help and perform CPR if required.

Adrenal insufficiency (Addisonian crisis, steroid crisis)

Addisonian crisis is due to a lack of production of corticosteroid hormones, which are normally produced by the adrenal glands. A patient with adrenal insufficiency may become **hypotensive** under stress and collapse. Adrenal insufficiency can be caused by disease of the adrenal glands themselves or by the use of long-term steroid therapy. In the latter group, patients can still be at risk of adrenal suppression despite having stopped their steroid therapy. A patient who has poor adrenal function and is undergoing a stressful operative procedure, such as surgical removal of mandibular third molars is thought to be at risk from an adrenal crisis. Routine dental treatment is not thought to be important. If a patient is thought to be at risk of adrenal insufficiency whilst undergoing stressful surgery then the patient's routine steroid dose may be doubled on the day of treatment.

Respiratory arrest

A respiratory arrest may result from hypoxia, anaphylaxis, status asthmaticus, airway obstruction, drug or alcohol overdose.

Signs and symptoms

The patient is unconscious and there is no breathing but a central pulse is present.

Management

Follow the basic life support algorithm for rescue breathing; if untreated it will proceed to a cardiac arrest. Expert assistance should be summoned as soon as possible.

Cardiac arrest

A cardiac arrest may result from a myocardial infarction, circulatory collapse, anaphylaxis, hypoxia or respiratory arrest.

Signs and symptoms

The patient is unconscious and there is no central pulse.

Management

Follow the basic life support algorithm. Expert assistance should be summoned as soon as possible to ensure early defibrillation (if indicated) and administration of emergency drugs.

Cardiopulmonary resuscitation (basic life support)

Adult basic life support

All dental health care personnel are trained in cardiopulmonary resuscitation (CPR), which is also commonly referred to as **basic life support** (BLS). The term BLS implies that no equipment, such as airway adjuncts and oxygen are used. In dental practice the term CPR is therefore to be preferred as it is more appropriate to the clinical setting; however, both terms are commonly used synonymously. It is important to emphasise that staff should be familiar with the current guidance from the Resuscitation Council (UK), which is updated from time to time and published on their website (**www.resus.org.uk**).

CPR is the administration of oxygen to an apnoeic patient and the provision of external cardiac massage (to allow circulation of oxygen) to a pulseless patient, after accurately assessing the patient's condition and summoning appropriate medical support. The aim of CPR is to maintain adequate ventilation and circulation in order to prevent irreversible cerebral damage. Deprivation of oxygen in the cerebral blood vessels for 3–4 minutes (or even less if the patient was previously hypoxic) can cause irreversible brain damage.

The stages involved in treating a cardiac arrest can be summarised by Figure 16.8 – the chain of survival; early recognition is important and CPR is essentially a holding operation until a defibrillator arrives. Prompt arrival of a defibrillator and post-resuscitation care are of paramount importance in managing a patient who has arrested. CPR is a very successful holding procedure but will not affect a cure for the patient in cardiac arrest. Well-performed chest compressions give less than 30% of the normal cardiac output and the majority of all primary cardiac arrests in adults present in ventricular fibrillation and the early defibrillation of this problem cannot be over emphasized. The algorithm for BLS in adults is summarised in Figure 16.9 and the sequence of actions is given in detail in the text below. Whilst this is correct at the time of going to press the reader must be aware that this guidance can change.

- **Safe approach:** The safety of the rescuer is of paramount importance; there is no point in you becoming the second victim; check the surrounding area and the patient for signs of danger, and remove or minimise any hazard.
- **Assess for a response:** Gently shake the arm of the patient and and ask 'Are you all right'? Be aware of the possibility that a casualty who has undergone a

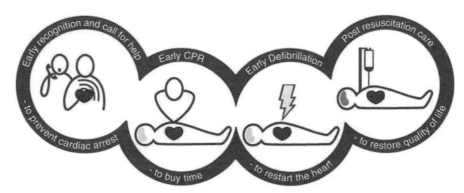

Figure 16.8 The chain of survival. (Reproduced by kind permission of the Resuscitation Council (UK)).

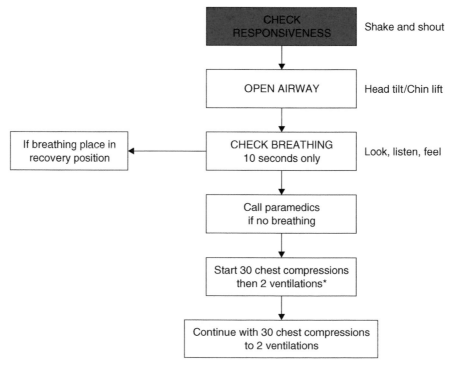

*If you feel confident enough you may also check for a major pulse when assessing for signs of life. If a pulse is identified then rescue breathing only may be undertaken.

Figure 16.9 The algorithm for basic life support in adults. (Reproduced with permission from the Resuscitation Council (UK) Guidance website: www.resus.org.uk (2010).)

fall might have sustained an injury to the cervical spine – although this is more of a theoretical consideration in the context of a dental surgery. Nevertheless it is worth noting in your training sessions because staff may assist in an arrest that has occurred outside of the surgery environment. If there is a response the person should be assessed further using the A, B, C, D, E approach. If there is no response then ideally you need support from someone close by.

- **Shout for help:** Call out to attract attention from people nearby; you will almost certainly require help. You should now proceed with a more detailed evaluation of the casualty.
- **Assess the airway:** This has been described in detail previously. Perform a head tilt and chin lift and examine the mouth for any visible material that could be causing an obstruction; remove any such material. When the patient is wearing dentures and in your judgement they appear to be secure then leave them in place. The advantage is that they can give the face structure and support the lips; it is therefore easier to do *mouth to mouth* rescue breaths. However, you should remove loose and displaced dentures.
- **Assess breathing** and **circulation** with a synchronous breathing and pulse check for 10 seconds. Assessment of breathing has been described previously. To check for a circulation locate the carotid artery by feeling for the Adam's apple and slide your fingers toward you until you meet the sternomastoid muscle (the diagonal muscle that runs down the neck from the base of the skull to the sternum), then check the pulse for no longer than 10 seconds. If the patient is breathing spontaneously, place them in the recovery position before calling for expert assistance. If the casualty is not breathing also call for specialist help and ask for a defibrillator if one is available locally.
- **Telephone for help:** Irrespective of whether someone responded to your initial shouts for help, it is at this point that active measures should be taken to summon specialist assistance. If someone is available ask him or her to call for help, informing the emergency services that the patient has had a suspected cardiorespiratory arrest. Remember that basic life support is only a holding procedure and the casualty's chances of survival will improve with a defibrillator and personnel with advanced life support skills. To call the emergency services and request paramedic support in the United Kingdom you may ring either **999** or **112**. The digits 112 are pan-European digits that can be used within the European Union; also some mobile phone networks may require you to use 122 in the UK. It should be remembered that if you are on an internal telephone network then another digit may be required

to obtain an outside line. If you work in a hospital environment then you should follow the hospital protocol which will involve using a designated priority telephone number to call the local crash/emergency response team. A defibrillator should be brought to the scene as soon as possible.

- **Circulation:** If there is a pulse the patient is in respiratory arrest so rescue breaths should be performed after help has been summoned. The protocol for treatment is to deliver 1 minute of ventilations – around 10 breaths—then the circulation is re-evaluated. If there is no spontaneous respiration, then a loop is effectively created of 1 minute's worth of ventilation with a re-evaluation of the patient's vital signs. This continues until help arrives or the patient is revived. If respiration is restored the patient should be placed in the recovery position and monitored.
- **Chest compressions:** When no central pulse can be felt a diagnosis of cardiorespiratory arrest is made. As a consequence external chest compressions are required in addition to artificial ventilation in a ratio of 30 compressions to 2 ventilations. This ratio must be observed irrespective of the number of rescuers.

Chest compressions are undertaken by placing the heel of one hand in the middle of the lower half of the sternum placing the heel of the other hand on top of the first hand. Fingers should be interlocked to ensure that pressure is not applied over the victim's ribs. All pressure should be transferred to the middle of the sternum (breast bone). Lean over the patient and with your arms straight press down vertically on the sternum to depress it to a depth of 5–6 cm. CPR is performed at a ratio of 15 compressions to 2 ventilations with a compression rate of 100–120 beats per minute, until help arrives.

- **Ventilation:** Ensure that the patient's airway is open and clear, reposition the head if necessary. It is unlikely that mouth-to-mouth resuscitation would be undertaken, as a pocket mask or bag-mask would be available. For completion, however, mouth-to-mouth ventilations are undertaken as follows. Pinch the soft part of the nose to seal off the nostrils with your index finger and thumb. Take a full breath and place your lips over the mouth making sure that you have a good seal. Blow steadily into their mouth for around two seconds, watching their chest wall rise. Take your mouth away and allow the casualty's chest to fall fully as air comes out; expiration takes around 2–4 seconds. Take another full breath and repeat the sequence, all the time maintaining a head tilt and chin lift.

Do not interrupt CPR unless the casualty shows signs of consciousness.

Paediatric basic life support

The reasons for paediatric basic life support are the same as those for an adult.

Paediatric cardiac arrests, however, usually result from the casualty becoming hypoxic and then anoxic. Cardiac arrests in children are normally preceded by respiratory arrests (unless a child has a pre-existing cardiac condition). If this occurs then the outlook for the casualty is bleak, especially outside of a hospital environment. This should not deter the hygienist/therapist from instituting CPR and performing it to the best of their ability. Many of the stages are the same as for adult CPR, for example the safe approach, assessment of responsiveness and the shout for help, and therefore the relevant text will not be duplicated. There are, however, significant differences in the BLS algorithm for children based upon the age of the child, when to call for help, and the rate of chest compressions and ventilations. The age groups for children are defined as follows:-

- An infant is a child under the age of 1 year.
- A child is aged between 1 and 8 years.
- An older child is aged over 8 years.

The algorithm for BLS in children is shown in Figure 16.10.

- **Assess the <u>a</u>irway**: In the child the head may be manipulated like that of the adult into a 'head tilt, chin lift'; however, to efficiently open the airway in the infant the head should be manipulated into the neutral position. The infant's natural position of rest is a position of flexure. If the infant's head were to be hyperextended the airway is in danger of being kinked due to its short conical elastic properties. If there is suspicion of trauma then, like adult patients, the head and neck must be held in a neutral position and a jaw thrust performed in order to open the airway.

Finger sweeps are dangerous in the paediatric patient for a variety of reasons. In the infant, any foreign objects in the pharynx may become impacted. Also, the hard palate is not fully formed and that also may be damaged. By the age of three to four a child may have hypertrophic tonsils. If a rescuer's finger nails inadvertently lacerate the tonsils it may have implications ranging from bleeding to severe mucosal swelling.

- **Assessing <u>b</u>reathing**: Once you have ensured that there is a clear passage from the mouth to the lungs, determine if there is any respiratory effort. If there is, determine the breathing rate and place the patient in the recovery position and go for help. If there is no respiratory effort, ventilate the patient before calling for expert assistance. The way you deliver the ventilations

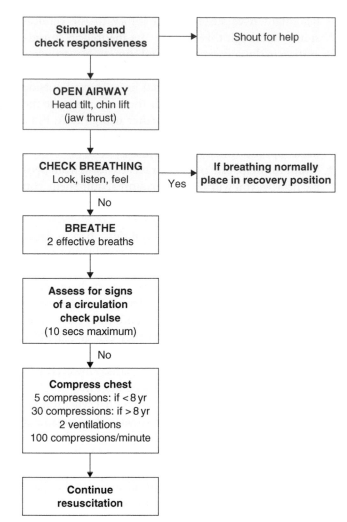

Figure 16.10 The algorithm for paediatric basic life support.

differs from the adult BLS algorithm. If there is no ventilatory effort then five ventilations are given before checking for a pulse. The method of delivering breaths depends upon the age of the casualty. In the infant you should place your mouth over the patient's mouth and nose and using the air in your cheeks get the patient's chest to have a perceptible rise and fall. In a child you may be able to pinch its nose and perform mouth-to-mouth ventilations. Yet again, you aim to have a perceptible rise and fall in the chest.

- **Checking for <u>c</u>irculation**: In children, the neck is reasonably well developed and the carotid artery can be palpated. In the infant you should palpate the brachial artery on the inside of the upper arm, in the antecubital fossa. This is preferable to the carotid artery which is difficult to locate due to infants having short necks. Alternative sites include the femoral artery or palpating in the **fontanelles** (anterior and posterior soft spots on the head) which remain open until around 18 months of age. By palpating the fontanelles, additional information may be obtained. For example, when the tissues at the fontanelles are recessed then **hypovolaemia** (a decrease in the amount of circulating blood) should be considered, if on the other hand the tissues are turgid then there is a suggestion of increased intracranial pressure.

- **Chest compressions**: Once a diagnosis of cardiorespiratory arrest has been made then CPR should be performed. Below the age of 8 years the CPR ratio is 15 chest compressions to2 ventilations, irrespective of the number of rescuers. The ratio of 5:1 tends to favour a higher number of ventilations to the minute, which reflects the likely aetiology of a respiratory arrest in a child. The compressions should be performed with the heel of one hand placed on the lower half of the sternum and the sternum should be depressed to around 1/3rd of the depth of the child's chest. Over 8 years old the adult protocols using a 30:2 ratio may be followed. Irrespective of age, CPR should be performed at 100–120 compressions per minute.

In the infant the land marks for chest compressions are as follows: 1 finger's breadth below the inter-nipple line, placing two fingers below. This system is recommended for single rescue only. The preferred approach is to encircle the chest with your hand and apply pressure with both thumbs. This system works best with two or more rescuers and should be employed wherever possible. In both methods the chest should be depressed between 1 and 2 cm.

In the age category from 1 to 8 years of age the position for cardiac compressions is: 1 finger's breadth off the distal tip of the xiphisternum sliding the heel of your other hand adjacent to your land marking finger. The pressure applied can be achieved by using one arm. The depth of compression is 2–3 cm. Over 8 years of age the land markings and chest compressions are the same as those employed in adults. After having performed a minute's worth of resuscitation, seek help. If the casualty patient is a baby or a small child that you can easily carry, take your patient to the telephone and call for paramedic support.

Defibrillation

The outcome of some cardiac arrests can be improved by the early use of defibrillation. A defibrillator will first analyse the electrical activity of the heart and this will dictate the action required. There are two broad 'categories' describing the rhythms of cardiac arrest according to whether or not they can be rectified by defibrillation.

- **Shockable rhythms** of cardiac arrest occur when the electrical system of the heart has developed a problem and is 'firing' indiscriminately; this uncoordinated electrical activity fails to produce a cardiac output.

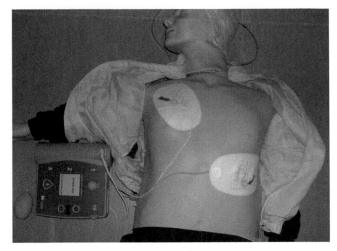

Figure 16.11 Automated external defibrillator.

Ventricular fibrillation and **pulseless ventricular tachycardia** are the shockable rhythms of cardiac arrest and may respond to defibrillation.
- **Non-shockable rhythms** of cardiac arrest occur when the cause is not primarily related to a defect in the electrical conducting system of the heart and therefore applying electric shocks to the heart is not helpful. Asystole and pulseless electrical activity are examples of the non-shockable rhythms of cardiac arrest.

Defibrillators are available that advise the person using them. These **automated external defibrillators** (AEDs) can be used almost anywhere and can be found in shopping centres, large railway stations and on aeroplanes. In these locations non-medical personnel are trained in their use. The machine comes with two electric leads each connected to an adhesive pad. The two pads are applied to the patient's chest (see Figure 16.11). The electrical rhythm of the heart is analysed and if it is a shockable rhythm, the machine can deliver a shock through the electrodes. Voice prompts are provided throughout to allow the operator to know exactly what to do and when. Staff wishing to use defibrillators must attend a formal ILS course and this should be updated annually. AEDs are not routinely recommended for use in children, instead manual defibrillators, which can be adjusted prior to the delivery of every shock are used.

Patient discharge

Following appropriate treatment of a medical emergency there are two possible outcomes:

- The patient recovers enough to be able to be discharged from the dental surgery.
- The patient requires transfer to a hospital for further diagnosis, treatment and/or monitoring of their condition.

There are many occasions when the patient will recover completely, for example after a simple faint, a hypoglycaemic episode, an angina attack or a panic attack. It is always desirable for the patient to travel home escorted by a responsible adult. If the patient is not fit for discharge they will need to be taken to hospital; transfer to the care of the paramedics will therefore be necessary. It is helpful to have insight about what information is required by the paramedics for the patient handover. As the therapist/hygienist may have carried out treatment for the patient, it is essential that the paramedics know exactly what has and has not been done.

Paramedic transfer

Over the past two decades advancements have been made regarding the provision of treatment to the acutely ill patient from the UK Ambulance Services. Paramedics transfer such patients, as quickly as possible, to a secondary care centre that can deliver the necessary definitive care. At the same time the patient's airway and circulatory status are closely monitored and interventions are undertaken, as and when appropriate, prior to the patient's arrival at hospital. Paramedics working within the National Health Service possess many medical skills, some of the procedures that can be undertaken are:

- Endotracheal intubation.
- Intravenous cannulation.
- Administration of IV fluids.
- Manual defibrillation.

When a patient is transferred to the care of a paramedic, relevant information about the patient also needs to be exchanged. The patient handover can be simplified by using the acronym—**S A M P L E**.

> **S**ymptoms
> **A**llergies
> **M**edications
> **P**ast medical history
> **L**ast oral intake
> **E**vents prior to the incident.

Symptoms: This includes the patient's symptoms and signs; for example, did the patient lose consciousness? Was there any pain? Did the patient have a seizure? What was their breathing and pulse like?

Allergies: Any known allergy should be reported to the paramedic team; even allergies that may be unrelated to the current medical crisis may be of relevance to the patient's treatment in both the ambulance and the accident and emergency department.

Medications: A full drug history should be formulated by the dental team ready for handover.

Last oral intake: Dental staff may not always have this information but it can be helpful to the paramedic crew in assessing the potential for the patient to vomit, especially if intubation is required.

Events prior to the incident: A comprehensive history should include those events that took place leading up to the incident that caused the 999 call, e.g. the patient had been given an antibiotic or had undergone surgery.

Conclusion

Medical emergencies occur only rarely in the practise of dentistry. Nevertheless. hygienists and therapists have a duty to ensure that they have the appropriate knowledge and skills to diagnose and manage the common medical emergencies that may be encountered in dental practice. Dental hygienists and therapists should be able to recognise when patients are too ill to receive dental treatment and when expert assistance should be summoned. They should be familiar with the location, preparation and administration of emergency equipment and drugs. It is the authors' opinion that hygienists and therapists should be prepared to use the following drugs: oxygen, epinephrine (adrenaline), glucose, glucagon, midazolam, glyceryl trinitrate, aspirin and salbutamol. They should regularly update their knowledge and refine their skills by scenario training with all members of the dental team; trained colleagues are an invaluable resource in any crisis.

References

British National Formulary 50 (2006) British Medical Association and Royal Pharmaceutical Society of Great Britain, London.

Resuscitation Council, UK website: www.resus.org.uk

Balmer, C. and Longman, L. (2008) *The Management of Medical Emergencies – a guide for dental care professionals*. Quay Books, London.

General Dental Council (2009) *Developing the Dental Team*. General Dental Council, London.

17

Health and safety at work

Hilary R. Samways

Summary

This chapter covers:

- Health and Safety at Work Act
- The Control of Substances Hazardous to Health
- Fire prevention
- Radiation protection
- Personal protection
- Clinical governance
- Risk assessment

Introduction

Dental staff must be aware of and deal appropriately with the health hazards which may occur in relation to dentistry. Responsibilities for health are governed by the **Health and Safety at Work Act 1974**. The Act seeks to protect all those at work (employers, employees and the self-employed) as well as members of the public who may be affected by the work activities of these people.

Under the Act, the employers' statutory responsibilities are to:

- Prepare a written health and safety policy.
- Ensure effective risk assessments are carried out and recorded.
- Ensure the management systems in place provide effective monitoring and reporting.
- Ensure staff are all aware of and comply with health and safety policies and procedures.
- Review health and safety performance at least annually.

- Be aware of and investigate any significant health and safety failures or concerns.

The Health and Safety at Work Act encompasses:

- The provision and maintenance of safe equipment, appliances and systems of work.
- Safe handling and storage of substances or articles which may be potentially harmful to health.
- Maintaining a safe working environment without risks to health including the means of entrance and exit.
- Providing the required instruction, training and supervision to ensure health and safety.

The main responsibility for ensuring the health and safety of staff and for reducing risks to others affected by work activities (including members of the public) rests on employers (section 2 and 3 of the Health and Safety at Work Act 1974). However, failure of employees to discharge the responsibilities laid down by the Act may provide grounds for dismissal and can also lead to prosecution by the Health and Safety Executive.

Working environment

There are specific requirements relating to the environment within a practice or clinic. The **temperature** should reach at least 16 °C after 1 hour and thermometers must be provided in all rooms to check that this has been achieved.

Adequate **ventilation** is essential to minimise any risk of dangerous or irritant vapours from mercury, disinfectants, nitrous oxide and laboratory chemicals. **The Workplace (Health, Safety and Welfare) Regulations 1992** require enclosed workplaces to be ventilated with sufficient fresh or purified air. An open

Clinical Textbook of Dental Hygiene and Therapy, Second Edition. Edited by Suzanne L. Noble.
© 2012 John Wiley & Sons, Ltd. Published 2012 by John Wiley & Sons, Ltd.

window will provide this in most cases, alternatively mechanical ventilation or air conditioning units could be considered. These should provide at least 5–8 litres per second of fresh (not recycled) air per occupant. The working environment normally has a relative humidity of between 40% and 70%.

There should be **washing, toilet and changing facilities** sufficient for all staff and patients. There must also be staff facilities to make hot drinks, heat food and also somewhere for them to eat, drink and relax.

Lighting should be sufficient to work safely without eyestrain and workstations should be arranged so that each task can be carried out safely and comfortably.

Room dimensions of the working environment must also be taken into account, allowing for enough free space for people to move around with ease.

Environmental noise: Noise pollution will depend on intensity and duration. As a simple guide it may be considered to be a problem if speech cannot be clearly heard by someone positioned two metres from the speaker.

Exposure to noise pollution can be minimised by:

- Ensuring that dental handpieces, ultrasonic scalers, aspiration equipment laboratory equipment and compressors are regularly serviced.
- Creating a low emissions working environment by using absorptive materials within the building to reduce reflected sound.
- Limiting time spent in noisy areas.

Materials

Control of Substances Hazardous to Health

The Control of Substances Hazardous to Health Regulations 2002 (CoSHH) provides a legal framework for controlling the exposure of people to hazardous substances, including microbiological hazards, arising from work activity. They impose a duty on employers to ensure safety measures are in place.

Hazardous substances can be liquids, solids, dust, powder or gases and are primarily categorised as irritant, corrosive, flammable, toxic or very toxic and will carry appropriate hazard warning symbols (Figure 17.1). The United Nations Globally Harmonised System of Classification and Labelling of Chemicals (GHS) replaces the European classification. The deadline for substance reclassification in the EU was 1st December 2010.

This information can be found on container labels or in product data. Many chemicals cause specific health effects by targeting various organs or parts of the body. The four main routes of entry are:

- Inhalation, via the bronchial system.
- Absorption, through the skin and eyes.
- Ingestion, through the mouth.
- Injection, via a puncture wound.

Information regarding microbiological hazards can be found in the Control of Cross Infection Guidelines and is dealt with fully in Chapter 8.

Under the CoSHH Regulations it is a requirement to identify and make an assessment of any substances hazardous to health in the practice or clinic. It is necessary to:

- Identify the substances in the practice that may be hazardous to health. These include such substances as mercury, acrylic monomer, volatile liquids, alginate dust and acid etch.
- Assess what the hazard is and who may be affected by its normal use.
- Decide whether the substance presents a hazard in normal use.
- Review the method and frequency of use, storage and disposal.
- Assess the overall risk that each substance poses within the practice.
- Assess the need for health and/or environmental monitoring.
- Compile and implement procedures to control/minimise the risks to health.
- Record the assessment.
- Provide training to ensure that all staff understand the CoSHH assessment and are aware of the appropriate procedures for the hazardous substances in the practice.

After completing a CoSHH assessment for each hazardous substance consideration should be given on how to minimise the risk to health.

Storage

All materials and chemicals should be stored in cupboards with isolated storage for inflammable substances and poisons. Mercury must be stored in a cool environment in sealed containers.

Medicines are required to be stored according to manufacturer's instructions, have restricted and controlled access and stocks regularly checked for availability and shelf life.

Equipment

Electrical equipment

All electrical equipment must be maintained in a safe working order at all times. It is the responsibility of dentists or trained staff to undertake a regular (approximately every 6 months) visual inspection of cables, plugs and fuses and check that wires in the plugs are tightly

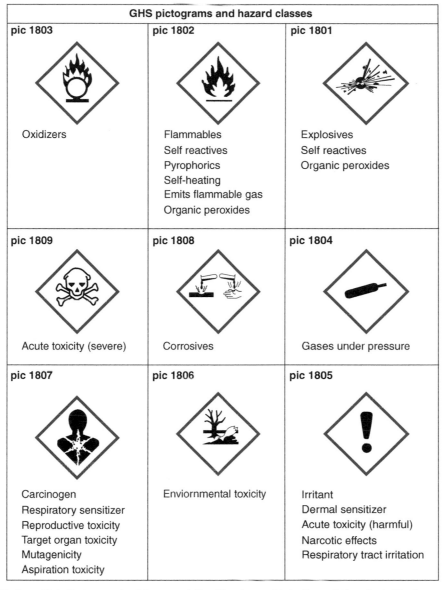

GHS pictograms and hazard classes		
pic 1803 Oxidizers	**pic 1802** Flammables Self reactives Pyrophorics Self-heating Emits flammable gas Organic peroxides	**pic 1801** Explosives Self reactives Organic peroxides
pic 1809 Acute toxicity (severe)	**pic 1808** Corrosives	**pic 1804** Gases under pressure
pic 1807 Carcinogen Respiratory sensitizer Reproductive toxicity Target organ toxicity Mutagenicity Aspiration toxicity	**pic 1806** Enviornmental toxicity	**pic 1805** Irritant Dermal sensitizer Acute toxicity (harmful) Narcotic effects Respiratory tract irritation

Figure 17.1 United Nations Globally Harmonised System of Classification and Labelling of Chemicals (GHS).

attached to the correct terminals. Every 2–3 years all electrical equipment should be checked and tested by an appropriately trained person and records as evidence that this has been carried out must be kept.

Autoclaves and compressors

Before any autoclave or compressor is used, there is a requirement for a written examination procedure to be done, which includes the inspection intervals for defects in function or safety. All staff must be fully trained before operating autoclaves and the manufacturer's recommended safety checks carried out before use.

The Health and Safety Executive has produced guidance to assist in the use of autoclaves, and the safeguards include:

- British Standards design.
- A safety valve to prevent over-pressurisation, a pressure indicator and drainage system.
- A safety door that cannot be pressurised unless the door is completely secured and the chamber sealed.

All autoclaves and compressors must be serviced and maintained at intervals specified by the manufacturer and records of these kept for audit and reference.

Computers/visual display units

Health and safety training is recommended to ensure employees can use all aspects of their workstation equipment safely and know how best to avoid health problems by, for example adjusting the chair, using a wrist pad and foot rest and positioning the desk and screen so that bright lights are not reflected onto the screen.

Computer work stations may be assessed for comfort with respect to operating position, monitor, mouse and keyboard. Lighting must be appropriate and anti-glare screens provided if considered appropriate. Eye tests can be arranged if necessary and corrective eyewear provided.

First aid

Every dental practice or clinic must have personnel trained to take charge of first-aid at all times. There is a requirement for the first-aid box to be easily located and clearly identified and it is a legal requirement for it to have a white cross on a green background.

The contents of the first-aid box should include sufficient assorted dressings, bandages and other suitable first-aid materials but not any medicaments or medicines. Provision of sterile water for eye irrigation must be provided where mains tap water is not available. It must be easily accessible to all members of staff and be regularly checked for out of date stock. A sign indicating the location of the first-aid box is not mandatory although desirable.

Cardiopulmonary resuscitation (CPR)

All members of the dental team are required to be trained and capable of undertaking CPR in the event of a medical emergency. Training should be given on a regular basis, preferably at least once a year, with *ad hoc* rehearsals. This is covered fully in Chapter 16.

Waste disposal

Dealing with sharps

Hazardous instruments, which may comprise of local anaesthetic needles, cartridges, scalpel blades, suture needles, dental burs and metal matrix bands are required to be placed in rigid puncture-proof UN sharps containers (to BS 7320) and filled only three quarters full to prevent personal injury (2010/13/EU Directorate). It is not acceptable practise to intentionally discharge syringes containing residual medicines in order to dispose of them in the sharps bin.

Disposal and use of extracted teeth

The Human Tissue Act 2004 covers the removal, storage and use of relevant material from the living; however, removal of teeth from the living is not included in the Act but once they have been extracted the use of these teeth and the storage of them is covered. The Act is supplemented by regulations, a number of which came into force on 1st September 2006.

Whilst consent may not be always required, any expressed wishes of a patient must be followed; so, for example, if a person expressly states that they do not want their teeth to be used for education or training this must be respected. Extracted teeth can be disposed of in clinical waste if they do not contain amalgam.

Waste segregation system

The management of waste is becoming increasingly complex as environmental issues become more prevalent. New guidelines have accordingly addressed this issue under the **Hazardous Waste (Amendment) Regulations 2009**. Waste must now be segregated in colour-coded bins and sacks. Household waste is disposed of in landfill and clinical waste is dispatched for either treatment or incineration, hazardous waste is stored in a leak-proof container. All categories must be stored in a suitable location prior to disposal. Hazardous waste includes mercury, dental amalgam, cytotoxic and cytostatic prescription only medicines, X-ray developer and fixer solutions. Partially used local anaesthetic cartridges are classified as clinical waste for treatment.

For further information refer to BDA guidelines or see the Department of Health website.

When clinical waste is collected, a transfer note must be completed and a copy retained for two years, by contrast for hazardous waste collection, a consignment note is required and a copy retained for 3 years.

Amalgam and mercury waste, including extracted teeth containing amalgam restorations, is classified as hazardous waste and cannot be incinerated due to the release of toxic mercury vapour. It should be stored separately in rigid airtight containers with a mercury suppressant and then collected by authorised contractors for recovery. It is the responsibility of the dental practice/clinic to ensure that *only* authorised persons collect clinical and hazardous waste. There is an obligation to check licences and registration certificates.

Amalgam separators

Strenuous efforts have been made within the EU since 1997 to reduce the amount of waste amalgam. Following the introduction of the **Hazardous Waste Regulations 2005** all waste amalgam is now classified as 'hazardous waste' and discharge of it into the sewerage system is not allowed. All dental practices must have amalgam separators which comply with BS ISO EN 11143:2000 and ensure that amalgam is collected and disposed of in accordance with the regulations.

Mercury

This is one of the most hazardous substances used in dentistry and all staff must be aware of its potential hazards. Symptoms of chronic mercury poisoning (tiredness, fatigue and lethargy) are difficult to identify but deaths in dental practice from acute poisoning have been reported. There must be good general ventilation (air conditioning systems that recycle air are not recommended). Amalgamators are recommended to be placed on a shallow tray lined with aluminium foil or on a lipped plastic tray. A small funnel must be used when filling the mercury reservoir and a mercury spillage kit available for use if needed.

Using pre-dispensed amalgam capsules eliminates the risk of spillage but the amalgamator should be periodically checked for capsule leakage.

Aspirator tubing and bottles tend to collect mercury-rich amalgam when it is carved away. This type of equipment can thus become a hidden, but persistent source of mercury vapour. Traps should be emptied regularly and tubing cleaned daily with cleaning fluid recommended by the manufacturer.

To reduce the risk to health, all floor and work surfaces should cove slightly up the wall or cabinetry and joins must be sealed. Regular biological health monitoring for staff may be provided. Waste amalgam must be kept in a sealed container with a mercury suppressant.

If hands have been exposed to mercury, they should be washed immediately with liquid soap in a stream of cold water until no stain on the skin is seen. Disposable towels should be used for hand drying.

Mercury spillage

In the event of a spillage, the affected area must be confined to a minimum and protective gloves and mask worn. Increased ventilation is recommended by either opening a window or ensuring that air conditioning is working to maximum potential. The spread of the spill should be reduced as much as possible particularly avoiding mercury dropping onto the floor, however if this has occurred overshoes can additionally be worn.

Mercury spillage kits contain flowers of sulphur and calcium oxide. Using the brush or sponge from the kit, the globules of mercury are moved together to form one large pool and as much of this as possible should be removed using the kit brush and plastic scoop or sponge and placed in the waste container. A paste of flowers of sulphur, calcium oxide and water may be painted on and around the spillage and when dry wiped up using wet disposable tissues and transferred to the waste container. Merconspray is an alternative as this hinders the formation of methyl mercury. This has a shelf life of approximately 1 year.

The cap on the waste container should be replaced tightly, and the container stored in a well ventilated area away from heat sources. The work surface and /or floor can then be decontaminated using the procedure outlined below. The full waste container should be disposed of at a council approved site, where provision for toxic waste is made.

Decontamination procedure

Decontamination using the flowers of sulphur/calcium oxide mixture can be carried out routinely each month to reduce background exposure in the operating room, or after a spillage where the floor or work surfaces are affected. The mixture may be used on carpet if necessary and be followed by spot cleaning with a proprietary cleaner. A vacuum cleaner or aspirator should never be used to remove spilled mercury.

Detection of mercury vapour

If a serious spillage occurs, or there are other reasons for suspecting mercury contamination, equipment is available for determining the amount of atmospheric pollution. Any serious mercury spillage is recorded in the accident book and the Health and Safety Executive informed.

Accident book

This must be used to record all accidents to staff, patients or visitors which have occurred on the practice/clinic premises, regardless of how trivial they may seem. It should be readily available for inspection if required although because it contains personal information consideration should be given to confidentiality under the **Data Protection Act**.

Each entry records:

- Time, date and method of reporting.
- The nature of the accident.
- Where the accident took place.
- Who was involved.
- The action (if any) which was taken.

The accident book is useful for audit purposes and potentially improving the safety of procedures or the environment.

The **Reporting of Injuries, Diseases and Dangerous Occurrences Regulations 1995 (RIDDOR)** came into effect on 1st April 1996. This requires the reporting of work-related accidents, diseases and dangerous occurrences. It applies to all work activities, but not to all incidents.

Reportable accidents

Under the Act, the following accidents and occurrences require reporting:

- Any fatality (to employees and non-employees).
- Major injuries to employees.

- Major injuries to non-employees, which require the person to be taken directly to hospital for treatment.
- Specified dangerous occurrences.
- Accidents causing more than 3 consecutive days' incapacity for work (the day of the accident is excluded, although days off, including weekends, are to be included).
- Certain specified diseases.
- Certain events associated with the safe supply of gas.

Reportable accidents and incidents can be reported directly to the Health and Safety Executive's RIDDOR Incident Contact Centre based at Caerphilly (http://www.riddor.gov.uk/).

The responsibility for reporting cases of work-related disease rests primarily with employers and the self employed. Reports submitted provide information used to target action to improve ill health prevention and control. Further information can be obtained from hse information services@natbrit.com.

Fire prevention

Fire regulations

The **Regulatory Reform (Fire Safety) Order 2005** requires risk assessments to take place within the working environment to determine what fire precautions are needed.

The fire regulations include the following instructions for emergency routes and exits:

- They must be kept free of obstruction at all times and allow employees and patients to evacuate the premises quickly and safely.
- Where possible they should lead directly to a place of safety.
- They need to be clearly indicated.
- Provision of emergency lighting is required where necessary.

The local fire procedures should be clearly displayed in the waiting area where they can be seen by both staff and patients. They may also be included in the practice/clinic manual and referred to in patient information leaflets.

Fire detection

There are three requirements for a fire, namely fuel, oxygen and an ignition source (Figure 17.2) and a number of possible sources of ignition (Figure 17.3).

If there is a fire it is important that everyone is alerted as quickly as possible. Early discovery will allow people to escape before the fire takes hold, possibly blocking escape routes. All workplaces must have arrangements in place for detecting and giving warning of fire or smoke.

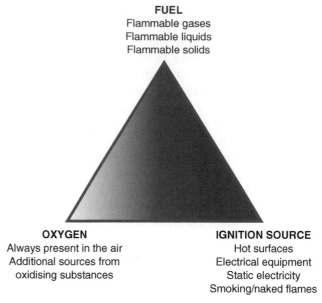

FUEL
Flammable gases
Flammable liquids
Flammable solids

OXYGEN
Always present in the air
Additional sources from oxidising substances

IGNITION SOURCE
Hot surfaces
Electrical equipment
Static electricity
Smoking/naked flames

Figure 17.2 The three requirements of a fire.

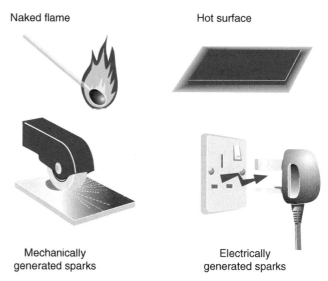

Naked flame

Hot surface

Mechanically generated sparks

Electrically generated sparks

Figure 17.3 Identifying sources of ignition.

In most cases, fires are detected by people in the workplace and no further warning device is needed, but a fire may break out in a part of the working environment that is unoccupied and put people at risk. Fire may also occur when the whole building is unoccupied so some form of automatic fire detection system should be operational.

There are three main types of smoke detectors, which are normally ceiling mounted:

- **Ionisation**. These are the cheapest and are very sensitive to smoke produced by flaming fires.
- **Optical**. Found to be more effective at detecting larger particles of smoke, produced by slow burning upholstery for example.

- **Combined optical and ionisation**. These alarms may be powered by battery or mains electricity or both. They can be connected together so that smoke detected in one site activates all the alarms. Batteries must be checked regularly and normally replaced once every 12 months.

Firefighting equipment

It is a requirement for all workplaces to have suitable firefighting equipment, which must be checked once a year or after use to ensure that they are in effective working order.

Fire blankets

These can be effective for small fires and for wrapping round someone if clothing is on fire. They need to conform to British Standard BS 6575.

Fire extinguishers

No single type of extinguisher is completely effective on every kind of fire. The types available are:

- **Water** (red coloured fire extinguisher). These can be used on burning paper, wood, textiles and solid materials fires. They cannot be used on liquid, electrical or metal fires.
- **Powder** (red coloured fire extinguisher with blue label). To be used on burning liquid, electrical, wood, paper and textile fires, but not on metal fires.
- **AFFF foam** (red coloured fire extinguisher with yellow label). These fire extinguishers can be used on burning liquid, paper, wood and textile fires but not on electrical or metal fires.
- **Carbon dioxide** (red coloured fire extinguisher with black label). These can be used on liquid or electrical fires but not on metal fires.

Fire extinguishers need to be sited near exit routes and staff should be made aware of their locations. They require servicing at least once a year or according to the manufacturer's instructions.

Fire drill

Fire drill regularly practised will ensure that all staff are familiar with the procedure and how to operate the equipment. In the event of fire:

- Shout fire or activate the alarm.
- Identify the source of the fire.
- Phone for the fire services.
- An extinguisher should not be used unless it is considered safe to do so. When using an extinguisher, the operator should stand on the escape route side of the fire.

- Remove patients from danger.
- In the case of disabled patients the Personal Emergency Evacuation Plans (PEEPS) designated first-aider must stay with the patient in a fire-protected area, for example near a designated fire door, for a limited and safe period of time. If the fire reaches the adjacent area, the first-aider and patient must move on to the next protected area.
- Close doors and windows to contain smoke and enable safe evacuation.
- If smoke is seen escaping from behind a closed door, do not open it.
- All persons evacuated from the work place should assemble at the designated assembly point, which must be in a safe area and a check must be made to ensure that everyone is accounted for. The appointment book or day list would be useful in this respect.

Radiation protection

The taking of radiographs has become an integral part of any dental practice or clinic but the use of radiographic equipment introduces the potential for significant health and safety hazards for both staff and patients. Patients therefore must only be exposed to radiation doses which are as low as reasonably practicable (**ALARP**) and the benefit to the patient outweighs the risk. The use of X-ray equipment is covered by the **Ionising Radiation Regulations 1999** and the **Ionising Radiation (Medical Exposure) Regulations 2000**. In order to comply with these regulations, when radiographic equipment is installed it is necessary to:

- Inform the Health and Safety Executive.
- Undertake a risk assessment including action in the event of malfunction.
- Appoint a Radiation Protection Supervisor. This is usually a dentist but it could be a hygienist or therapist.
- Appoint a Radiation Protection Adviser to advise on the installation and choice of equipment which it is intended to install. This adviser is usually the National Radiation Protection Board.
- Make sure all staff who will be operating or involved with the equipment are fully trained.
- Write up local rules which must be visibly displayed for every machine.
- Write a radiation protection file. Local rules and operational procedures are recommended to be included.

The positioning of the equipment requires the operator to be at least 1.5 m from the radiographic tube and as far away from the primary beam as possible. If possible the control switch for the X-ray machine should be outside the controlled zone. Local rules must be displayed for every machine. Servicing of radiographic equipment is usually specified according to the manufacturer's instructions and a radiation safety assessment is usually carried out at least every 3 years by a competent authority.

To keep radiation risk to a minimum for both staff and patients, the following points may be helpful:

- Films should never be held by the operator during exposure. Film holders with beam alignment devices must be used routinely.
- If the workload exceeds 100 intraoral or 50 panoral films per week, personal monitoring badges are required to be used by the operator.
- All staff must be informed about the procedure in the event of accidental exposure to either staff or patient.
- Lead aprons for patients are now no longer considered necessary to be used routinely although they may be used if the patient is known or thought to be pregnant.

Further information on radiation protection can be obtained from The British Dental Association Advice Sheet No. A11.

Personal protection

Medical requirements and occupational health clearance

All clinical dental staff must demonstrate that they are not infectious carriers of hepatitis C, human immunodeficiency virus (HIV), and hepatitis B surface antigen. It is also necessary to demonstrate immunity to hepatitis B. The Occupational Health Unit or prospective employers will require as documentary proof, an authenticated laboratory report.

Prospective staff who have serious health problems or know that they are infected with hepatitis B, hepatitis C or HIV must disclose this. Those members of staff who are HIV or hepatitis C positive would, under Department of Health guidance, be excluded from many clinical activities.

All members of staff are required to have the appropriate vaccination, which is maintained up to date. This subject is covered fully in Chapter 8.

Protective clothing

Uniforms, masks, gloves, glasses and enclosed type shoes reduce the risk of contamination by harmful substances and minimise the transmission of infection from patient or instruments to staff.

Hygienists and therapists are obliged to make sure that they, their nurses and their patients have adequate protective clothing and eye protection at all times during examination or treatment. Clear plastic face visors have been shown to provide better protection for operators than paper face masks. New gloves and masks must be used for every patient.

Hand hygiene

Hands must be cleaned before each episode of dental treatment prior to gloves being used. This prevents contamination of the patient's oral cavity and face with organisms carried on the dental team's hands.

Direct contact is one of the main modes of transmission of the multi-drug resistant pathogenic bacteria methicillin-resistant *Staphylococcus aureus* or of herpes viruses, which cause cold sores and shingles.

This topic is covered in greater detail Chapter 8.

Needlestick injury

Should a hygienist or therapist experience a needlestick injury, the following routine should be adhered to:

- Encourage bleeding by gently squeezing the site – do not suck!
- Wash in warm running water with soap or hand-wash liquid and then dry.
- Apply a waterproof dressing.
- Keep the details of the patient concerned.
- Report the accident to your manager/dentist.
- For your own protection do not delay, act immediately.
- Contact Occupational Health or your medical practitioner or attend Accident and Emergency department/Walk In Centre.
- Complete an incident form.
- Healthcare workers exposed to an HIV-positive source are required to begin post-exposure prophylaxis (PEP) within 24 hours of exposure.

Exposure to blood or body fluid

For a splash in the eye

- Remove contact lens if worn.
- Irrigate thoroughly for at least 5 minutes with eyewash solution or sterile water or tap water if not available.

For a splash in the mouth

- Irrigate thoroughly for at least 5 minutes with drinking water.
- Do not swallow this water.

If there is concern about the source material, the occupational health service or medical practitioner can be contacted. If necessary complete an entry in the accident book.

Latex dermatitis

Latex dermatitis can affect both clinicians and patients. It can present itself as:

- **Irritant contact dermatitis**. A common non-allergic reaction to one or more chemicals found in latex gloves. To avoid this, the hands should be dried thoroughly after washing and a barrier cream or moisturizer can be used to keep the hands supple and prevent chapping.
- **Allergic contact dermatitis**. This involves a T-cell mediated allergic reaction where there is a specific hypersensitivity to proteins in natural rubber latex.

The most common type of reaction to latex is a non allergic contact dermatitis (Figure 17.4). This can be reduced by using powder-free gloves with reduced protein content. After use, the hands should be washed with a mild detergent and then thoroughly dried. Allergic contact dermatitis produces a red itchy rash, which appears about 10–30 hours after the skin comes into contact with latex. Latex does not only come in the form of latex gloves. Rubber dam, prophylactic cups and local anaesthetic bungs can also be made of latex. It is estimated that about 3% of the population and about 10% of regularly exposed health workers are sensitive to latex. Patients should therefore be questioned about a history of latex allergy before treatment. For those patients or staff with a true allergy to latex, non-latex alternatives can be used including Nitrile type gloves and non-latex rubber dam. Good clinical practice encourages working towards a latex free environment.

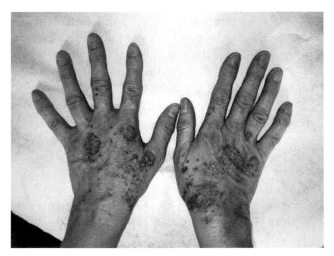

Figure 17.4 Latex hypersensitivity resulting in dermatitis in a female dentist. (Reproduced with kind permission from the Editor, *Norwegian Dental Journal.*)

Pregnancy

The expectant hygienist or therapist may first inform her employer in writing that she is pregnant. Her employer can ask for written medical evidence to confirm this and the employee is required to provide it. This enables the employers to carry out a specific risk assessment for the person concerned. Doctors are required to record advice given to patients about their ability to perform their own type of occupation on medical statements. A sensible risk assessment will take note of the hazards and advice on how to reduce or remove them. The following issues are taken into consideration:

- Restricted spaces and workstations.
- Vibration or excessive noise.
- Radiation (covered by specific legislation).
- Infections. A pregnant woman who catches Rubella during the first 5 months of pregnancy has a high risk of passing the disease on to the foetus.
- Handling of chemicals.
- Inadequate facilities (including rest rooms).
- Excessive working hours.
- Unusually stressful work.
- Exposure to fumes or cigarette smoke.
- Excessively high or low temperatures.
- Handling heavy loads, e.g. patients. During pregnancy, extra care should be taken because the extra weight of the foetus and bulk in the abdominal region leads to an exaggeration of the normal low back curve (lumbar lordosis).

The importance of good operating posture

An estimated 60–80% of people in the UK are affected at some time in their lives by back pain. It is also one of the main reasons for sickness absence, each year, close to 120 million working days are lost in the UK due to back pain. Research indicates that a high percentage of dental operators complain of pain in the upper body and back. This musculoskeletal pain is often the direct result of body positioning and movements made by dental healthcare professionals in their daily work.

Correct operative techniques are essential and require the use of a combination of good posture, effective angulation of the mouth mirror, the best seating position for both the operator and the dental nurse in relation to the patient (Figure 17.5) and the use of direct vision where possible to avoid straining over the patient.

A neutral position is the ideal positioning of the body whilst performing work activities and is associated with decreased risk of musculoskeletal injury. It is generally believed that the more a joint deviates from the neutral position, the greater the risk of strain or injury.

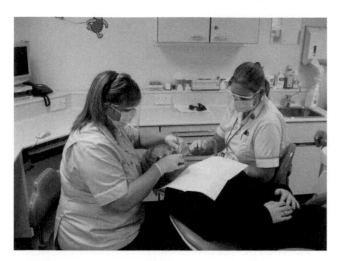

Figure 17.5 Operator, dental nurse and patient position. (Courtesy of Dr Robert Ireland)

Neutral seated operator position

The neutral seated position (Figure 17.6) has the following characteristics:

- The forearms should be parallel.
- The upper arms should be vertical and in contact with the rib cage.
- The head tilted no more than 30° to the vertical plane when operating.
- The weight should be evenly balanced.
- The thighs should be parallel to the floor and splayed no more than 30° to prevent muscular tension.
- The hip angle (the angle between the lower body and the thighs) should be 90°.
- The seat height should be positioned low enough so that it is possible to rest the heels on the floor comfortably.

The operator seats himself/herself so that the feet are flat on the floor, and the abdominal rest of the chair (if there is one) is firmly below the ribcage when inclining forward. A five castor stool will minimise forward tipping as the operator inclines toward the work area. Many stools have backrests and these can be adjusted to provide optimal support for the back.

The height adjustment mechanism for the stool may be a simple screw that moves the seat up or down as the seat is rotated although this is slow and inefficient to adjust. A foot pedal that releases the seat to rise, or a hand lever that raises the seat as weight is lifted from it and lowers the seat if weight is added is an alternative. This mechanism of gas cylinder compression is more efficient particularly when more than one operator is routinely using the stool. Saddle type operator chairs have also recently been introduced where the body weight is gently tipped forward. Regardless of the mechanism, the stool should

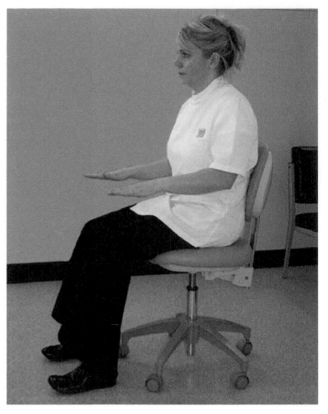

Figure 17.6 Neutral seated operator position. (Copyright Mr. P.F. Gregory.)

be adjusted to the correct operator and assistant height before treatment commences.

The seating position for the dental nurse

- The feet should be firmly on the floor, or on a comfortable foot rest.
- The lower part of the legs, vertical.
- The seating position to be approximately 4 inches (10 cm) higher than the dentist, since this allows for better vision into the oral cavity.
- The upper border of the thighs should be approximately 15° to the horizontal.
- The long axis of the back should be as near vertical as possible and leaning forward should be avoided.
- The thighs parallel to a line drawn from the patient's left ear to the patients left shoulder. This will reduce twisting of the spine.
- The top of the left thigh should be in contact with the left side of the chair. This will reduce the necessity to lean forwards into a stressful and unbalanced position.

In accordance with the General Dental Council publication: *Principles of Dental Team Working* (GDC, 2009), when treating patients, make sure there is someone else, preferably a registered team member present in the room, who is trained to deal with emergencies. It is advised for dental hygienists and therapists to have chairside support; there are many occasions when the assistance of a dental nurse at the chairside will significantly improve patient safety, efficiency and the quality of care.

The patient position

- The chair is positioned near to the horizontal. Many patients will not be comfortable if positioned completely flat, or with the head lower than the feet.
- The patient's head is required to be at the correct focal length for the operator.
- The patient always wears protective glasses.
- The headrest must not impede lateral movement of the patient's head or restrict the wearing of protective glasses. Where possible the patient's head should be moved to give direct vision.

Neither the operator nor the assistant should feel the pressure of the stool against the back of the thighs, as this position inhibits blood circulation to the legs and the possibility of varicose veins developing.

Being mindful that keeping a straight back whilst working will also lessen the eventuality of back and neck tension and aches, which can over a period of time lead to long term back problems.

Hand–arm vibration syndrome (HAVS)

Occupational exposure to vibrating tools can result in hand–arm vibration syndrome (HAVS), which is characterized by finger numbness, tingling or painful finger blanching triggered by cold. There is no effective treatment and sufferers show no signs of recovery after cessation of vibration exposure. Although the prevalence is low there is evidence that dental workers including hygienists are at risk. The **Physical Agents (Vibration) Directive** which came into force in July 2005 requires all those at risk of vibration related disorders to undertake a risk assessment. This should include training on how to minimise the risk and identify the symptoms (Mansfield, 2005).

Carpal tunnel syndrome

Carpal tunnel syndrome (CTS) is also known as **repetitive strain injury (RSI)**, or **cumulative trauma disorder**. It is included under HAVS even though no vibration may be involved. CTS is a common condition that can affect men and women of all ages, but is more common in women. It occurs when a nerve running into the hand becomes entrapped or compressed at the wrist, as it passes through the 'carpal tunnel'. The condition can be precipitated by unaccustomed use of the hands and appears to be more common in individuals whose occupation involves repetitive use of the hands and wrists, and work involving abnormal postures or high forces. Evidence suggests that the prevalence of CTS in dental hygienists is significant (Anton *et al.*, 2002).

To establish a diagnosis, the doctor may choose to arrange a test of the nerves that are passing into the hand. This is called a nerve conduction test and evaluates whether the signals are being transmitted properly along the nerve. Nerve conduction tests are often requested when there is doubt about the diagnosis, to examine other nerves in the arm or when surgery is being considered.

Symptoms

Typical early symptoms include tingling in the hand, which may develop to such an extent that the affected individual can complain of aching, burning, pins and needles (paraesthesia) and numbness in the hand. Some notice these symptoms only in the thumb, index and middle fingers of the hand whilst others have problems over the whole hand. Symptoms are often worse at night, and can interrupt sleep. Weakness of the hand or incoordination (impairment in the performance of precise movement) in the use of the fingers is less common and usually does not occur until symptoms are severe or have been present for some time.

Prevention

Dental hygienists in particular, must be aware of those factors that can aid prevention (Lalumandier and McPhee, 2001). These include:

- Avoidance of over-zealous hand instrumentation and repetitive hand movements.
- Taking adequate rests in between patients.
- Trying not to do the same kind of treatment all day, root surface debridement for example.
- Adopting the neutral body and hands positioning.
- Using sharp hand instruments.
- Adopting a relaxed finger grip to decrease hand muscle tension.
- Using ergonomically designed instruments comprising of a softer, lighter and wider working grip and a dimpled design handle to reduce hand fatigue.
- Vitamin B6 deficiency in humans although unusual has been associated with CTS.
- Various hand exercises can be performed in moderation, some using a compressed ball of foam to prevent problems.

Treatment

Treatment of the condition is either surgical or non surgical. Non-surgical treatment is often adopted while awaiting a surgical opinion. Non-surgical treatment options for CTS involve chiropractic treatment the use of splints, anti-inflammatory tablets and/or a local steroid injection. Rest from activities that exacerbate the problem may help, but this is variable. Those individuals who notice increased symptoms at work should pursue postural alignment through a stretching and strengthening programme which can be performed with the help of a physiotherapist. An occupational therapist may also help to address ergonomic factors and can make suggestions for task modification and suitable resting positions.

Splints can be highly effective and may settle the symptoms on their own. These can either be worn during the day to support the wrist during work, or at night to prevent the wrist from flexing.

Anti-inflammatory drugs are sometimes of use if there is an inflammatory lesion. Local steroid injections may also be useful particularly if inflammation is present.

The control of any underlying disease such as rheumatoid arthritis, diabetes or thyroid complaints is important in restricting the symptoms of CTS.

Manual lifting, carrying and handling

Musculoskeletal disorders, often brought on by lifting heavy objects are the most common occupational illness in the UK, affecting 1.1 million people a year. Any reasonably practicable measures that can be taken to reduce the risk of injury should be implemented. Mechanical hoists should be used wherever possible, especially when transferring disabled patients for treatment in areas with restricted working space. This would be particularly useful when working in mobile dental units for example.

In normal lifting, the back is kept straight but relaxed and the lift achieved by the leg muscles. Snatching, twisting and over reaching must be avoided. Anyone engaged in manual handling as part of their job should undergo appropriate training.

Management of the violent patient

Violence within the workplace is becoming increasingly common. According to the **National Institute for Health and Clinical Excellence** (**NICE**) (www.nice.org. uk), all service providers should have a policy for training employees in relation to the short-term management of disturbed/violent behaviour. This policy should specify who will receive what level of training (based on risk assessment), how often they will be trained, and also outline the techniques in which they will be trained.

The most effective management tool is anticipating a potentially violent situation and adopting a preventive approach by:

- Staying calm.
- Avoiding confrontational body language.

- Adopting a friendly approach.
- Empathising with the patient.
- Recognising potential conflict.

In the event of a patient becoming violent or aggressive, the operator should:

- Attempt to establish a rapport and emphasise co-operation.
- Offer and negotiate realistic options avoiding threats.
- Show concern and attentiveness through non-verbal and verbal responses.
- Listen carefully and show empathy, acknowledging any grievances, concerns or frustrations, and not being patronising or minimising the patient's concerns.
- Ensure that their own non-verbal communication is non-threatening and not provocative.
- Pay attention to non-verbal cues, such as eye contact and allow greater body space than normal.
- Adopt a non-threatening but safe posture.
- Appear calm, self-controlled and confident without being dismissive or over-bearing.

If the situation fails to resolve or starts to escalate the help of a colleague should be sought.

Stress

The influence of physical and mental stress

Work-related stress is an increasing concern for employers and is currently the second most common cause of ill health associated with work. Stress can be defined as the adverse reaction people have to excessive pressure or other types of demand placed upon them: it is the mismatch between the demands placed on people and their ability to meet those demands. Potential causes of work related stress include:

- Time pressures.
- Poor communication.
- Dealing with anxious or abusive patients.
- The repetitive nature of work.
- Physical and psychological demands of the job.
- Level of control over the task being undertaken.
- Relationships with managers or peers.
- Individuals not knowing what their role is, what their work entails or what their responsibilities are.
- Lack of managerial or professional support.

Stress sufferers often demonstrate well-recognised physiological symptoms, which include headaches, aching muscles (particularly neck and shoulders), rashes and increased sweating. Common psychological and behavioural signs include:

- Depression or general negative outlook.
- Increased anxiousness.

- Increased irritability.
- Lack of concentration.
- Loss of aptitude.
- Poor work performance.
- Increased sickness absence.
- Inability to cope with normal tasks.
- Poor time keeping.
- Increased intake of alcohol, caffeine, nicotine, or other forms of drug abuse.

Work related stress is not an illness, but it can lead to increased problems with ill health including heart disease, back pain and gastrointestinal disturbances.

Managing stress

In the working environment stress may be reduced or eliminated by:

- Time management: maximise the benefits and minimise the stress.
- Improving communication skills: dealing with difficult patients is a very common cause of stress.
- Talking to your employer or other representative to raise the issue on your behalf.
- Discussing with your manager/dentist the possibility of redefining your work role to make your work less stressful.
- Channelling your energy into solving the problem rather than worrying about it. Consider what would make you happier at work.
- Speaking to your general medical practitioner.

Outside the working environment stress may be reduced by:

- Eating healthily.
- Stopping smoking.
- Trying to keep within Government recommendations for alcohol consumption.
- Watching your caffeine intake. Tea, coffee and some soft drinks including cola may contribute to anxiety.
- Being physically active. It stimulates and generates energy.
- Trying to learn relaxation techniques. Some people find it helps them cope with pressures in the short term. Taking time out from the work environment at lunchtime can be very beneficial.
- Talking to family and friends about what you're feeling. They may be able to help you and provide the support you need to raise your concerns at work.

Clinical governance

Clinical governance is both an ethical and a health and safety issue. It is therefore additionally referred to in Chapter 20, p. 392. The Department of Health has already introduced policies to enhance patient-centred treatment, which not only includes employing qualified, occupationally competent staff participating in continuing professional development CPD, but also clinical governance. Clinical governance is defined by the Department of Health (2005) as a 'framework through which NHS organisations are accountable for continuously improving the quality of their services and safeguarding high standards by creating an environment in which excellence in clinical care will flourish'. Clinical governance does, however, also apply to dental care provided outside the NHS. It may be stated more simply as ensuring that patients and their carers get the best possible deal out of the health care service provided. This encompasses risk management and appropriate attention to health and safety issues.

Clinical governance aims to safeguard the provision of quality care and management and includes:

- Clear lines of responsibility and accountability for the quality of clinical care.
- A comprehensive programme which improves quality.
- A means by which all members of the dental team can be involved in the development of good practice.
- A means by which patients can be involved in the development of dental care services as well as being appropriately informed about their proposed treatment.
- Clear policies for managing risk. Risks and hazards to patients should be reduced as low as possible by creating a safety culture.
- Procedures for all members of the dental team to identify and remedy poor performance.
- A programme of continual quality improvement including CPD and audit.

Risk assessment

A risk assessment entails considering any potential hazards that could take place within the working environment and then taking the necessary action to prevent harm. Legally employers and the self-employed are required to carry out risk assessments.

There are five simple but important steps to assess the risks in the workplace:

- Look for the hazards.
- Decide who might be harmed and how. Special consideration should be given to the very young, pregnant and nursing mothers (specific risk assessment requirements apply), the elderly and disabled.
- Evaluate the risks and decide whether the existing precautions are adequate or whether more should be done.

- If inadequate, take the necessary action to prevent or minimise the hazard.
- Record your findings.
- Periodically review your assessment and revise if necessary.

The identification, assessment and management of risk is discussed further in Chapter 20, p. 293.

References

Anton, D., Rosecrance, J., Merlino, L. and Cook, T. (2002) Prevalence of musculoskeletal symptoms and carpal tunnel syndrome among dental hygienists. *American Journal of Industrial Medicine*, **42**(3), 248–257.

Department of Health (2005) *Providing Assurance on Clinical Governance: a practical guide.* [Online.] Available from http://www.dh.gov.uk/prod_consum_dh/groups/dh_digitalassets/@dh/@en/documents/digitalasset/dh_4108392.pdf (accessed 6 October 2011).

General Dental Council (2009) *Principles of Dental Team Working.* British Dental Association, London.

Lalumandier, J.A. and McPhee, S.D. (2001) Prevalence and risk factors of hand problems and carpal tunnel syndrome among dental hygienists. *Journal of Dental Hygiene*, **75**(2), 130–134.

Mansfield, N.J. (2005) The European vibration directive – how will it affect the dental profession? *British Dental Journal*, **199**, 575–577.

Further reading

British Dental Association Advice sheets on Health and Safety available to members. (www.bda-dentistry.org.uk)

British Dental Association (2007) Working with dental therapists in general dental practice. Advice sheet D5 British Dental Association, London.

British Dental Association (2008) Health and Safety Law for Dental Practice. Advice sheet A3.British Dental Association, London.

British Dental Journal (2006) **201**,790–791 The implications of the Human Tissue Act 2004 for dentistry.

Ellis Paul, J. (1991) *Team Dentistry*. Martin Dunitz, London.

Fisher, I. (2007) *Intermediate Health and Safety*. Trafford Press, Manchester.

Gibbons, D.E. and Newton, J.T. (1998) *Stress Solutions for the Overstretched*. BDJ Books, London.

Health and Safety Executive. CLP Regulation: Implications and guidance. [Online.] Available from www.hse.gov.uk/ghs/implications.htm (accessed 6 October 2011).

Nield-Gehrig, J.S. (2004) *Fundamentals of Periodontal Instrumentation and Advanced Root Instrumentation*. Lippincott Williams & Wilkins, Baltimore.

Rattan, R. and Tiernan, J. (2004) *Risk Management in General Dental Practice*. Quintessence, New Malden.

18

Complementary and alternative medicine

Philip Wander

Summary

This chapter covers:

- The major complementary/alternative therapies used in dental practice
- Efficacy, efficiency and evidence
- Integrating 'alternative' treatments into dentistry
- Biological dentistry for the 21st century?

Introduction

The **General Dental Council** (GDC) guidelines indicate that student dental hygienists and therapists should be aware of the many complementary and alternative therapies available for patients. In addition, they should be sensitive to the patient's right to choose such methods of treatment (General Dental Council, Learning outcomes: www.gdc-uk.org). Complementary and alternative medicine (CAM) usually involves those types of treatment that are not part of orthodox medical services. It is a definition that sets these treatments apart from the dominant system of healthcare.

- **Complementary therapy**: works *alongside* orthodox healthcare in an attempt to achieve benefits that conventional medicine cannot deliver alone.
- **Alternative medicine**: usually implies a therapy used *instead* of more conventional types of treatment.
- **Integrative medicine**: attempts to *combine* orthodox approaches with complementary treatments so that a new form of medicine is developed combining both forms of medicine.

More and more patients are seeking and using complementary and alternative remedies, and looking to healthcare professionals to understand these treatments for medical and dental problems.

Over the past 20 years there has been a shift away from labelling complementary therapies as fringe or alternative, to regarding them as integrated medicine. It is also a reflection of the impact of eastern philosophies upon the west. Also, over the last two decades a strong movement towards the idea of taking responsibility for our own health has resulted in a huge demand for methods of healing which take a look at the whole person – emotionally and mentally, as well as physically. There has been a subsequent growth in the popularity of complementary medicines, which has resulted in a much wider availability of remedies in healthfood shops, pharmacies and supermarkets.

Much of complementary medicine is based on the quantum perspective that everything, including our bodies, is energy and the effects of energy meridians on the mental, emotional and physical elements have to be considered. Health is more than an absence of disease; it is a state of balance of the spiritual, emotional, mental and physical aspects of the body. Good oral hygiene and a healthy diet protect teeth and gingivae, as well as helping to prevent systemic disease (Krall, 2001). The basis of holistic care relies on encouraging the body's own health balance and reducing noxious stimuli.

The holistic (from the Greek *holos*, meaning whole or complete) dental practitioner, while recording the dental health of each patient, will also look at nutrition, muscle tone and joint function, and assess stress and the effect of toxic materials on the immune system. Above all, by

Clinical Textbook of Dental Hygiene and Therapy, Second Edition. Edited by Suzanne L. Noble.
© 2012 John Wiley & Sons, Ltd. Published 2012 by John Wiley & Sons, Ltd.

listening to the patient, thinking laterally and looking to other complementary practitioners for support, the patient's health will be seen as a whole, not as just a set of teeth – a truly holistic approach.

One of the major problems of evaluating the evidence base for alternative therapies is that non-pharmacological treatments such as acupuncture, physiotherapy, chiropractic, etc. are not best evaluated by randomised double-blind controlled trials (RCTs) because the treatment integrates both specific elements (such as needling in acupuncture) with incidental effects such as talking and listening, normally categorised as part of the placebo effect in RCTs. Therefore the use of RCTs for complex interventions may lead to false-negative results (Paterson and Dieppe, 2005).

The patient's right to choice

Since the **Medical Act of 1512** and the **Herbalists' Charter of 1543**, orthodox and complementary medicines have worked side by side. Even today the public have a choice between a medical doctor and a lay practitioner. This choice has allowed patients to seek alternative methods of treatment in spite of the fact that many of the therapies are not as yet integrated into the National Health Service (NHS).

It is not within the scope of this book to cover all the many kinds of complementary therapies available but some of the more widely used are described below.

Acupuncture

Acupuncture is one of the paramount 'alternative' treatments used for pain relief. It is one facet of traditional Chinese medicine and is based on an acupuncture **meridian system**. This is a network of energetic pathways that run through the body (Figure 18.1) carrying invisible energy (ch'i) which nourishes and vitalises the organs and body tissues. The theory is that any impediment in this circulation leads to an imbalance in the proportions of the Yin and Yang, and thus ill health. Blockages to the flow of the ch'i occur at specific points on the meridians, the acupuncture points. Needling the blockages at these sites would free the flow of the ch'i, allowing this to nourish the organs again, returning normally to the Yin and Yang, and improving health. Function improves, and pain is controlled or cured.

Dental applications of acupuncture include the control of gagging (Figure 18.2), which is startlingly effective, nausea, treatment of temporomandibular joint (TMJ) disorders, stress related headaches linked with TMJ problems (indeed there is increasing evidence for the management of post-operative pain, and even as an adjunct or in some cases alternative to the use of local

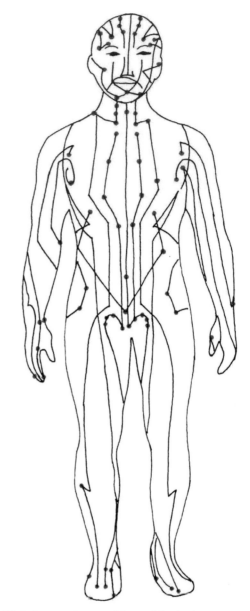

Figure 18.1 Acupuncture meridians of the body.

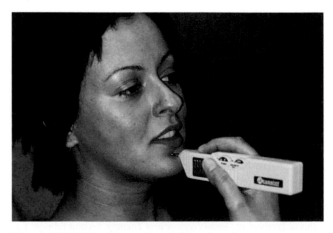

Figure 18.2 Relieving gagging reflex using electro acupuncture.

anesthesia (Figure 18.3). The anesthetic effect is difficult to achieve, however, in the orofacial region.

Acupuncture also has an excellent reputation for the treatment of such conditions as chronic back and neck pain, tennis elbow, period pain, and chronic headache. Research now tends to show that one of the important aspects to appreciate with acupuncture is that the outcomes are generally no different to conventional therapies, but the approach may be more acceptable, and the side effect profile superior.

How does acupuncture work?

The gate control theory

This theory suggests that when body tissues are damaged there are two separate sets of nerve fibres carrying pain signals. In the body, most pain signals are carried by one type of nerve fibre – the 'C fibre'. These signals can be interrupted in the central nervous system during transmission to other nerves. This occurs when other signals from a different type of sensory nerve fibre effectively 'get in the way' of C fibre transmission – or close the transmission gate. The other nerve fibres may be other pain (A-delta) sensory fibres, or non-painful ('B' – touch) sensory fibres. If there are enough alternative sensations travelling, the pain messages will not get through. (This is the principle that **TENS** (transcutaneous electrical nerve stimulation) operates on, and an approach that has been used in dentistry as a local anaesthesia device, reducing the need for local anaesthetic, adrenaline and analgesics.)

The neuroendocrine theory

This suggests that by utilising acupuncture or acupuncture pressure points Endorphins and serotonin are released. These are part of the body's own pain control mechanism. There is increasing evidence for this following magnetic resonance imaging (MRI) of the brain during acupuncture treatments.

Other forms of acupuncture

Acupressure works on the same principle as acupuncture, but pressure from the hands or fingers replaces needle stimulation.

Electro-acupuncture uses a device to pass a small electrical current across acupuncture points, enhancing the stimulus (Figure 18.2). Laser acupuncture uses low wattage laser light to stimulate the acupuncture sites instead of needles. The basic principles are similar, but the theory and application is complex.

Further information about acupuncture can be obtained from the **British Medical Acupuncture Society** (www.medical-acupuncture.co.uk).

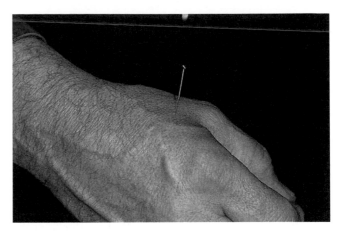

Figure 18.3 Acupuncture being used to relieve pain.

Herbalism

Herbs are used as a major part of treatment in traditional Chinese medicine and have been used in applications in dentistry, including strengthening the immune system in debilitated patients, and the treatment of periodontal disease both systemically and by the use of herbal mouthwashes. For example, 'Plaque Off' tablets containing a dried seeweed (*Ascophyllum nodosum*) are claimed to reduce the formation of plaque and calculus. **Echinacea**, prescribed to support the immune system, may have potential in the treatment of periodontal disease. There are reports of ginger and peppermint being effective for nausea, gagging and travel sickness.

There is some concern, however, about the quality and safety of the largely untested ingredients in Chinese medicine. The adverse interactions and dosage of herbs are also a potential problem. For example, **St John's wort**, commonly prescribed by herbalists for mild depression, interacts with **warfarin** and can render the contraceptive pill ineffective. For these reasons, herbs can be harmful and should be prescribed by a dentist only with appropriate training. Further information is available from the North American Institute of Medical Herbalism at http://medherb.com.

Aromatherapy

Aromatherapy uses the smells of natural herbs and flowers as therapeutic agents. These agents are reduced to essential oils, usually diluted in a carrier oil and massaged into the skin or inhaled. **Lavender**, for example, may be useful in the reception or surgery because of its calming properties. Other examples of conditions which have been treated with aromatherapy oils include abscesses (bergamot, lavender), anxiety (camomile, jasmine, lavender), gingivitis (camomile, myrrh) and halitosis (lavender, peppermint). However, essential oils must be treated like medicines and since the evidence base for treating dental conditions by aromatherapy is lacking, claims about its efficacy should be interpreted with considerable caution unless supported by validated research studies. Further information can be obtained from AromaWeb (www.aromaweb.com/articles/default.asp).

Chiropractic

This term is from the Greek *chiro* (hand) and *praktikos* (to perform). Chiropractic is a primary healthcare profession that specialises in the diagnosis, treatment and overall management of conditions that are due to problems with the joints, ligaments, tendons and nerves of the body, particularly those of the spine. Treatment consists of a wide range of manipulative techniques designed to improve the function of the joints, relieving pain and muscle spasm, for example, **carpal tunnel syndrome** (a pinched nerve in the wrist causing tingling and numbness in the hand) which has been reported as a problem by some hygienists (Figure 18.4).

Other instances where chiropractic treatment can help are neck and lower back problems which are all too common in the dental profession. It must be remembered, however, that chiropractic does not involve the use of any drugs or surgery. Further information can be obtained from the **British Chiropractic Association** at www.chiropractic-uk.co.uk.

Osteopathy

This term is from the Greek *osteon* (bone) and *pathos* (to suffer). Osteopaths primarily work through the neuromusculoskeletal system, mostly on muscles and joints, and pay special attention to how the internal organs affect, and are affected by, that system. Relevant psychological and social factors also form part of the diagnosis. Another important principle of osteopathy is that the body has its own self-healing mechanisms, which can be utilised as part of the treatment. Osteopathy can help relieve chronic or minor problems, such as upper and lower back pain and repetitive strain injury. It can also provide one-off relief from pain and dysfunction or contribute to the management of long-term complaints.

Further information can be obtained from the **British School of Osteopathy** at www.bso.ac.uk.

Hypnosis

The use of hypnosis in dental settings can be traced back to the mid nineteenth century, a time when medics were discovering the powerful effects that could be achieved through hypnotic suggestion. Mainly used during these early days as a form of analgesia or anesthesia, there was a clear role for hypnosis since chemical anesthetics and analgestics were not yet available. Around the turn of the twentieth century the work of Freud was famously linked to the psychological use of hypnosis in his study of the unconscious. The scientific study of hypnosis began in the 1930s and has continued ever since. A particular development in contemporary research has been the use of neuroimaging techniques that enable scientists to examine brain functions during hypnosis and this has led to a new wave of interest in the subject. Whilst there is still need for more studies to be carried out in the use of clinical hypnosis there are increasing numbers of well-designed studies, relevant to dentistry (but not necessarily carried out in dental settings) that have gained empirical support. For example studies have demonstrated the efficacy of hypnotic techniques in treating pain, anxiety and phobias as well as in influencing physiology to the benefit of the patient.

One major area of concern for dental professionals is the significant number of people who fail to seek treatment for a considerable period of time due to severe dental anxiety or phobia. An advantage of being able to offer hypnosis is that his may in itself encourage fearful patients to attend. The use of hypnotic techniques can then calm the patient and enable them to engage with treatment. Following this, hypnotic techniques can be used to comfortably desensitise the patient to their specific fears. It is also possible to use hypnotic techniques to address the underlaying reason for the fear since very often clinical problems are maintained by beliefs and habitual responses that can be difficult to break. Hypnotic suggestions can directly influence such beliefs so that the person experiences change.

The extensive literature supporting the use of hypnosis in pain management and procedural discomfort has increased confidence in using such techniques

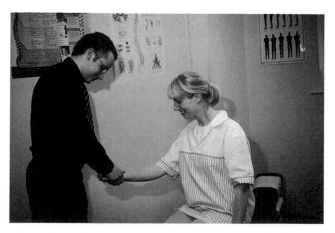

Figure 18.4 Chiropractor treating carpal tunnel syndrome.

in dentistry. Hypnosis can be used to reduce, or even replace chemical analgesics and anaesthetics (if there are medical or psychological reasons for this), and can also be used to complement the use of nitrous oxide. Use of dissociative techniques during uncomfortable procedures can be highly effective. Typically suggestions are given to promote an experience of 'being somewhere else' resulting in a type of 'virtual reality' experience in which the person feels as if they had 'gone away' from the dental surgery.

There are, in addition, a wide range of common dental problems that hypnotic techniques can be used to treat effectively such as gagging, bruxism, and chronic facial pain. Likewise hypnosis can be used to control salivary and blood flow and in stopping unwanted habits relevant to oral health such as thumb sucking, nail biting and smoking. It is also possible to use hypnosis to enable compliance with good oral hygiene regimes.

How does hypnosis work?

Researchers have investigated brain processes involved in the experience of hypnosis and psychological models have been presented by academics in order to explain response to suggestion. However, in order to understand hypnosis at a very basic level it is useful to deconstruct it by examining its components.

There are two main components of hypnosis **trance** and **suggestion**. 'Trance' is the experience we have when we get absorbed such as when we focus on our work or get lost in a day dream. In these situations we attend only to the focus of our attention. Importantly, studies have shown that the trance increases our response to hypnotic suggestions.

Suggestions can influence emotions, thoughts, behaviour and physiology. Individuals respond to suggestions in various ways but most of the population will be able to experience hypnosis to some extent. However the practitioner's understanding of hypnotic phenomena, and skilful application of the knowledge to hypnotic techniques, can aid a person's responsiveness and increase the success of interventions. Children between 8 and 12 years are particularly responsive to hypnosis and quickly become engaged in imagery, especially if the clinician takes into consideration the child's interests and stage of development.

Inducing hypnosis involves taking the patient into a trance by strategically narrowing their focus of attention. Once they are focused and absorbed (and thus more receptive) suggestions are given, usually in the form of imagery, to set up experiences that the person engages with that have been carefully designed to enable the person to overcome their problem. It is possible for the patient to respond verbally during hypnosis or with finger signals. The patient is then alerted by gradually orientating them 'back' into the dental office. During hypnosis, the mind is calm yet alert and focused, and whilst suggestions of relaxation are frequently given when inducing hypnosis, hynosis does not actually require relaxation, as has been demonstrated in studies where subjects are hypnotised on exercise bikes. Post-hypnotic suggestions can be made during hypnosis with the intention of having an effect later, when the person is no longer in hypnosis, a phenomena that is particularly useful in the case of habit control and anxiety.

Hypnosis can be used, after appropriate training, by doctors, dentists, psychologists and other health care workers. It should only be used within the boundaries of the range of problems the clinicians is trained to treat.

For further information about hypnosis research and training visit the website of **HUUK** (formerly the UCL Hypnosis Unit) www.hypnosisunituk.com.

Homeopathy

In the fourth century BCE, the Greek physician Hippocrates found that there were two distinct approaches to illness: one by **opposites** and the other by **similars**. Orthodox medicine, or **allopathy**, heals by opposites (e.g. anti-inflammatory, antibiotic), and homeopathy heals by similars.

Homeopathy originated in the late eighteenth century following Dr Samuel **Hahnemann**'s research into a cure for malaria. He found that cinchona bark (Peruvian bark, from which quinine is derived) activated a fever symptomatic of the disease, and deduced that substances triggering the symptoms in a healthy person could be used to treat similar signs of sickness in an ill person. He then discovered that by diluting remedies, their medicinal powers were not diminished, but rather enhanced. Hahnemann then investigated the effects of different medicinal substances on himself and other healthy volunteers by taking small doses of various substances and noting the symptoms produced. These were called **provings**.

Minimum dose

Because of Hahnemann's efforts to reduce the poisonous effects of large doses of medicines in use at that time (such as mercury in the treatment of syphilis), he investigated diluting them. During this process he discovered that if the medicines were mixed vigorously by striking the bottle against a firm surface (**succussion**) they became stronger in their effects, even though there was less of the original substance because of dilution. This led to the establishment of the major principle of homeopathy, namely that of the **minimum dose**.

Single remedy

Homeopaths normally give one remedy at a time. This tradition dates back to the principles that Hahnemann laid down. His experience showed that it was impossible to assess the outcome accurately if several medicines were given simultaneously. Much information in the homeopathic materia medicas comes from data gathered over the last 150–200 years, mainly from provings of single substances and chemical compounds.

Totality of symptoms

Homeopathic medicines are prescribed individually by the study of the whole person, according to basic temperament and responses. The physical, mental and emotional make-up and lifestyle of the sufferer are of vital importance when prescribing. Symptoms represent the body's attempt to heal itself and are a way of saying that something is out of balance: they are an expression of lack of ease ('disease'). If health is to be restored, symptoms need to be welcomed rather than ignored or suppressed in some way.

Homeopathy is used to enhance a state of health rather than simply to treat disease in a patient, often complementing other aspects of holistic dentistry, such as acupuncture, acupressure, kinesiology, amalgam-/mercury-free fillings and replacement. Other considerations would be the use of non-epinephrine (adrenaline) local anaesthetic, dietary analysis and nutritional supplementation, hypnotherapy and even cranial osteopathy for jaw/joint imbalances.

Principles of homeopathy

These are:

- *Similia similibus curentur* – let like be treated with like. A substance that causes symptoms in a healthy person can be used to treat these same symptoms occurring in an ill person.
- Diluting the homeopathic medicine increases its potency; the curative powers are enhanced and the undesirable side effects lost.
- Homeopathy treats the whole person and not just the illness. The remedies are prescribed individually by studying the whole person, according to basic temperament and responses.
- Single remedy.

How does homeopathy work?

Research is being undertaken to understand how and why highly diluted remedies have a profound influence and curative effect. Studies have shown that homeopathic remedies, when correctly used, are significantly more effective than a placebo (Linde *et al.*, 1997). It is suggested that during **potentisation**, an energetic change occurs in the remedy substance and its medium of dilution (usually water), enabling them to stimulate a person's system to deal with stress and illness more efficiently.

Evidence base

Homeopathic remedies do not have a chemical action in the body, and thus work differently compared to nutrients or drugs. This has made it difficult for some researchers, accustomed to assessing drugs, to consider them adequately. Since the body is clearly affected by many forces that have no chemical content (electricity, radiation, thermal energy, etc.), it is reasonable to think that research designed to observe non-chemical effects will yield more useful information.

As described in the introduction, some therapies, by virtue of their techniques, are more amenable to traditional forms of research such as randomised controlled trials and researchers have been able to substantiate health claims more rapidly. It is therefore understandable how these therapies have become more readily absorbed within the biomedical ethos. These therapies are also more likely to be researched because the use of standard research tools allows results to be measured, evaluated and understood within the biomedical perspective. Results obtained traditionally may encourage more funding and thus further research. As a result, some therapies are now perceived as 'integrated medicine' and afforded greater acceptance in western medical practice.

In contrast, therapies such as therapeutic touch, healing, aromatherapy or reflexology, by virtue of their philosophy and technique, may demand a more challenging research approach. We may still not be asking the right research questions. New research methodologies need to be explored. Measuring the effects of healing can be difficult as there can be so many variables and it can be difficult to establish conclusively which aspect of a therapy initiated an improvement in health. It is very important, however, that further research is undertaken to develop credibility within the medical and dental communities.

Homeopathy is about individualisation; each person is treated with the remedy tailored to their symptoms, personality, lifestyle, nutrition and other influences, which makes application of the parameters of conventional research/trials difficult. However, there is a growing body of evidence demonstrating the safety, benefits and clinical efficacy of homeopathy.

The safety of homeopathy

Homeopathy was recognised by Act of Parliament in 1948, and accepted as a safe alternative form of medical treatment. Doctors who are fully qualified through conventional medical training and recognised by the **General Medical Council** practise it. Homeopathic medicines are not harmful because they are so greatly diluted. They are safe, non-toxic and non-addictive. They are prepared in laboratories licensed by the Department of Health, to stringent standards of quality.

In theory it is possible that a proving could occur whereby the remedy produces the full symptoms of the drug picture and the advice would be to stop taking the remedy. Homeopathic medicines can be taken with ordinary drugs, by children and during pregnancy (however, medicine manufacturers are forbidden by law from claiming that any medicine is safe during pregnancy).

Homeopathy in dentistry

Dental hygienists and therapists are only permitted to practise homeopathic dentistry under the prescription of a dentist and after appropriate training. However, it is important that they are aware of the scope of homeopathy, in view of the increasing number of patients who are taking homeopathic remedies. The scope for homeopathy in dental practice is broad. At the most basic level homeopathy can be used as an effective adjunct to dental surgery to help alleviate associated pain, bleeding and inflammation. At a more advanced level homeopathy can be used in dental practice to:

- Prevent or inhibit the development of morbid processes in the oral cavity.
- Provide adjunctive treatments for a number of defined oral pathologies.
- Prevent, limit or ameliorate complications and sequelae of surgical intervention.
- Ameliorate dental and soft tissue pain.
- Assuage dental phobias and anxieties.
- Improve patient tolerance of medications, agents, prostheses and instrumentation.
- Facilitate recovery from dental trauma, restorative treatments and anaesthetic agents.

Homoeopathic prescribing may be either pathological or constitutional, or a combination of these:

- **Pathological prescribing** is a treatment specifically for the disease or ailment.
- **Constitutional homoeopathic prescribing** involves analysing a person's body type, temperament, disposition and behavioural tendencies.

Homeopathy in holistic dentistry offers a combination of these. It is possible to prescribe one remedy to suit the general temperament or psychological state of a patient and another for the particular problem the patient is experiencing. This is of particular value when using homeopathic remedies as an adjunct in the treatment of periodontal disease. However, prescribing for periodontal disease is complex and should be undertaken only by experienced homeopaths.

Periodontal disease and homeopathy

Homeopathy is a complement to orthodox treatment, not an alternative. It is absolutely essential to the health of the periodontal tissues that the patient understands oral hygiene procedures and appropriate prophylaxis is undertaken. Smoking is known to be particularly detrimental to periodontal health, and negates homeopathic remedies. Homeopathic treatment in periodontal disease involves considerable motivation and patient cooperation. Periodontal treatment can be made more comfortable and topical applications of tinctures and toothpastes can be efficacious.

Some examples of remedies used in dental homeopathy

Arnica is given for any trauma which could cause bruising or when giving an injection and for root surface debridement or subgingival scaling. It is given routinely before and after extractions or operations. The dose is one tablet to be dissolved under the tongue before and after treatment.

Some examples of dental conditions and their homeopathic treatment remedy include:

- **Dental abscess:** for an acute tooth abscess that is red, swollen and throbbing, **Belladonna** is used. For less serious or chronic abscesses, **Hepar sulph** is prescribed and **Silicea** is recommended when the abscess starts to drain.
- **Bleeding:** in a case of dental haemorrhage, **Phosphorus** is the primary remedy.
- **Anxiety:** a certain amount of excess apprehension is sometimes present in patients facing dental procedures and several remedies can be of value. **Aconite** is used where a state of fear and anxiety is present (there is mental and physical restlessness but fright is the predominating feature). **Gelsemium** (yellow jasmine) is used when feeling anxious, fearful and lacking in energy (a hypokinetic picture). **Argenticum nitricum** (silver nitrate) is given where there is a hyperkinetic picture, hurried actions, trepidation, incessant speech and diarrhoea. Other remedies are **Arsenicum** (homeopathic preparation of arsenic trioxide), **Coffea cruda** and **Ignatia**. The remedies can be used the night before and on the day of treatment to give a relaxing effect.
- **Dental trauma:** before and after a tooth is extracted, **Arnica** reduces shock, soreness and bleeding. **Hypericum** is useful should nerves be injured, e.g. endodontics.

- **Mouth ulcers: propolis tincture** is used neat, or as a mouthwash to relieve symptoms while healing occurs. Healing has been shown to reduce from the average of 5–7 days to 2 or 3 days. It is also very useful for alleviating pain and accelerating healing of dry socket and pericoronitis. **Feverfew** is a useful homeopathic remedy for aphthous ulcers.
- **Painful injection** sites: relieved with **ledum** (marsh tea).
- **Toothache** caused by exposed dentine and cementum may be relieved by **Plantago** tincture.
- **Teething:** use **Chamomilia**. This is also beneficial postoperatively after a local anaesthetic.
- **Calculus: Fragaria** (wood strawberry) has been used for discouraging the formation of dental calculus, causing existing calculus to soften and even helping to induce its spontaneous disappearance! (It is used extensively by homeopathic veterinary surgeons.)

Mouthwashes

A range of **homeopathic** mouthwashes is available. Hypercal (Hypericum and Calendula), myrrh, propolis and Weleda medicinal gargle are useful.

Tinctures

- **Plantago** (*Plantago major*) – homoeopathic greater plaintain. The mother tincture, applied locally, is an effective therapy for cervical sensitivity, giving immediate and long-lasting relief after just a few applications. It has been shown in clinical practice to be useful for sensitive cementum and exposed dentine, giving immediate and long-lasting relief after just a few applications.
- **Phosphorus** tincture is useful as an astringent to control gingival haemorrhage in restorative procedures prior to impression taking.

Toothpastes

Toothpastes should contain no injurious components. Such things as **foaming agents** (sodium lauryl sulphate, SLF) are known to be harmful. Most homeopathic patients will not use a toothpaste containing fluoride, sweeteners, brighteners, artificial colouring or flavourings, particularly peppermint. There are a number of companies providing 'alternative' toothpastes (e.g. Weleda, Hollytrees and Kingfisher). A wide range is available. Salt, myrrh and krameria toothpaste is said to be beneficial for gingival health. Sanguinaria (blood root) is another favourite botanic ingredient. Plant tooth gel (http://www.weleda.co.uk) has no abrasive in it at all, the base is vegetable glycerine and it is especially recommended for children. Calendula toothpaste is claimed to have healing properties and is for patients taking homeopathic medicines where their homeopath has instructed them to avoid peppermint. It contains essential oils of fennel and cinnamon as a breath freshener. All the flavourings are natural and not chemical substitutes. Other toothpastes are aloe vera and coenzyme Q10. Most promising is propolis containing myrrh and aloe vera, which suggests efficacy after initial trials.

There is a range of toothpastes and mouthwashes that combine natural and homeopathic ingredients. They also contain soluble salts to stimulate salivation and herbal extracts, which have antiseptic and astringent properties. These are blended with essential oils, to deodorise the breath, and homeopathic ingredients, reputedly to strengthen the gingivae.

Where patients are not using a fluoride-containing toothpaste, diet instruction, oral hygiene procedures and reduction of sugar intake should be stressed. Where there is a high caries rate patients will often accept a fluoride mouthwash along with a fluoride homeopathic remedy.

How homeopathic remedies are made

Homeopathic remedies are derived from all the kingdoms of nature, including such varied substances as bee stings and snake venoms, arsenic, gold and silica (sand) and even from diseased tissue (**nosodes**). Although over 2000 remedies are known to be useful, a very much smaller number is used in dental practice.

The starting material, usually a plant or mineral extract, is soaked in alcohol and water. A drop of this tincture is then diluted, 1 part to 99 parts distilled water. This is a 1C (one to 100) dilution. Then a method called 'succussing' is employed to agitate and 'energise' the solution. Then one part of *this* 1C dilution is placed in another 99 parts of water, and again succussed. This is 2C (one to 1000) dilution – and so on up. This dilution procedure may be repeated many times, and is called **potentisation**. The dilution arrived at (e.g. 6C) is called the potency. Hahnemann discovered that the more dilute the substance, the more powerful is the remedy but without attendant side effects and toxicity. This is a difficult principle for orthodox clinicians to accept and a major contentious point for many.

Homeopathic pharmacies (e.g. Ainsworths at www.ainsworths.com/site/default.aspx, and Freemans www.freemans.uk.com/index2.html) operate according to strict guidelines to ensure that the remedies and potencies are consistent and reliable. Once the potency has been prepared the blank tablets (composed of 80% lactose, 18% sucrose, 1% talc and 1% magnesium stearate) are impregnated with the desired remedy. The potencies used in dental homeopathic treatment are usually 6C or 30C. Remedies can also be presented as powders, spherical pilules, drops, liquids, tinctures, granules (sucrose) and creams (Figure 18.5).

In general, the selected remedy is given as one tablet under the tongue to be sucked or chewed. The tablets must not be handled as they are surface coated with the remedy. Nothing should have been in the mouth for at least 20 minutes. Smoking, coffee and peppermint should be avoided as they are said to be an antidote to the remedies. Remedies should not be exposed to strong sunlight or microwaves and should be kept away from strong odours such as camphor, eucalyptus, menthol and perfumes.

Training and qualifications in homeopathic dentistry

All members of the Faculty of Homeopathy are bound to practise within the competence of their healthcare profession and their level of training and qualification in homeopathy. Introductory training is provided by the Faculty of Homeopathy (http://www.facultyofho meopathy.org) and can lead to the Primary Health Care Examination (PHCE). These courses enable dentists, hygienists, therapists and registered nurses to acquire a basic understanding of homeopathy and to incorporate simple homeopathic practice into their routine patient care.

All defence unions will cover the practice of homeopathy by those with appropriate Faculty of Homeopathy qualifications within their general indemnification. Further information on homeopathy in dentistry can be obtained from the British Homeopathic Dental Association (www.bhda.co.uk) were described.

Biological medicine for the twenty-first century

Homotoxicology is a modern form of homoeopathy and is the most prescribed form of natural medicine in Germany, where is has been used for over 50 years and is practiced by conventional doctors and natural therapists alike. In fact, 80% of orthodox doctors in Germany prescribe homoeopathic or antihomotoxic preparations for their patients. The efficacy and safety of homotoxicology is supported by close to 100 clinical trials.

Homotoxicology was founded in 1952 by Dr Reckeweg. Expanding on the fundamentals of homoeopathy, as developed by Hahnemann, he integrated them with the new discoveries in biochemistry and embryology that had been made by the 1940s. The low dilution medications, which he formulated, are derived from: the enzyme system of the body, allopathic medicines, extensive nosode preparations (from diseased tissue), herbs, and the more traditional homeopathic remedies.

Low potency medications where there is original product present are used in Complex or Homotoxicology preparations. *These remedies are not available over the counter and have to be prescribed by a health care professional.*

The mixing of different medicines and different potencies in one remedy selected for their combined effect is very popular in France and Germany. It is not uncommon to have 15–20 medicines ranging from very low to high potencies in the same preparation.

One such remedy with a wide range of uses in dentistry is Traumeel (a Heel product available in the UK from Bio Pathica Ltd www.biopathica.com infor@ biopathica.com); it is available as ointment, tablets, drops and injection solution (Figure 18.6). It is well researched and primarily used for acute traumatic

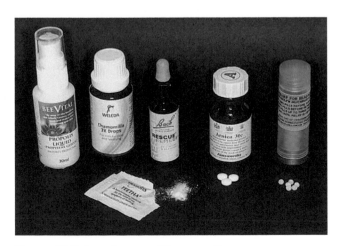

Figure 18.5 Some homeopathic preparations.

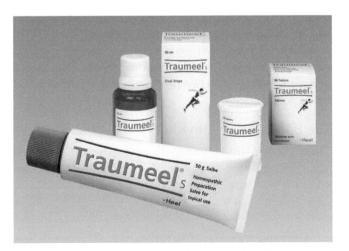

Figure 18.6 Traumeel products. (Reproduced with permission from Bio Pathica Ltd.)

injuries, inflammation and arthritis and an alternative to non-steroidal anti-inflammatory drugs. Specific applications in dentistry are to reduce inflammation, pain and swellings, and accelerate healing.

Traumeel is an excellent adjuct therapy prior to, as well as following dental procedures such as subgingival scaling and surgery.

Other remedies allied to homeopathy

Propolis

Propolis, produced by bees, is a 50–70% mixture of resins and balsams, 30–50% wax, 5–10% pollen and 10% essential oils and mixed with the bee's salivary excretions (beevitalpropolis.com), and is a powerful antioxidant. It has been shown to be of help in patients suffering from periodontal disease (Gebaraa *et al.*, 2003).

Propolis tincture is excellent for the treatment of oral ulcerations, particularly aphthous ulcers, denture trauma, pericoronitis, herpetic lesions, lichen planus and non-specific painful oral ulcerations. The tincture can be applied to areas where other preparations are not so effective in staying in place. It is applied initially on a pledget of cotton wool and then as required by the patient on a cotton wool bud. A residue or film of resin appears over the ulcer almost immediately, relieving pain and providing a healing barrier to further irritation. Propolis is of value in periodontal treatment and can be applied to periodontal abscesses. Propolis can also be used as a mouthwash or gargle and breath freshener (a few drops in warm water) and for the temporary relief of sore gums and throats. Propolis is available as capsules, lozenges, tincture, cream and toothpaste. Propolis tincture can be placed directly into carious deciduous teeth to act as a **mummifying agent**. The cream is excellent used prophylactically, applied round the corners of the mouth before extensive restorative procedures and scaling to prevent cheilitis and for cracked lips and cold sores. The tincture can be useful as a steam inhalation to relieve sinusitis.

Allergy and sensitivity to propolis are uncommon but patients should be questioned about adverse reactions to bee stings, allergies to bee products, honey and sensitivity to pollen.

The Bach flower remedies

These are similar to homeopathic remedies but prepared in a different way. They were discovered by Dr Edward Bach in 1930 and are derived from flowers selected to match a patient's usual and individual moods. The most useful in dentistry is 'Rescue Remedy'. This combination of five flower remedies (impatiens, cherry plum, clematis, rock rose, and star of Bethlehem) is used for collapse, faint, shock, anxiety and stress. The dose is three to four drops in the mouth, every few minutes if necessary.

Coenzyme Q10

Coenzyme Q10 (ubiquinone) is a vital catalyst to the provision of energy for all cells. A feature of chronic gingivitis or periodontitis is a local deficiency of coenzyme Q10.

As health care professionals our training is designed to make us analytical and critical of unfamiliar techniques. This can have the effect of making us dogmatic and even entrenched. While observing a healthy prudence it is important that we are receptive to unfamiliar techniques otherwise no progress would ever be made.

References

Gebaraa, F.C., Pustiglioi, A.N., de Lima, L.A. and Mayer, M.P. (2003) Propolis extract as an adjunct to periodontal treatment. *Oral Health and Preventative Dentistry*, **1**(1), 29–35.

Krall, E.A. (2001) The periodontal connection. Implications for treatment of patients with osteoporosis and periodontal disease. *Annals of Periodontology*, **6**, 209–213.

Linde, K., Clausius, N., Ramirez, G., Melchart, D., Eitel, F., Hedges, L.V. and Jonas, W.B. (1997) Are the clinical effects of homoeopathy placebo effects? A meta-analysis of placebo-controlled trials. *Lancet*, **350**, 834–843.

Paterson, P. and Dieppe, P. (2005) Characteristics and incidental (placebo) effects in complex interventions such as acupuncture. *British Medical Journal*, **330**, 1202–1205.

Further reading

Breiner, M.A. (1999) *Whole Body Dentistry*. Quantum Health Press, Fairfield CT.

British Homeopathic Dental Association www.dhda.co.uk

Estafan, D., Gultz, J., Kaim, J.M., Khaghany, K. and Scherer, W. (1998) Clinical efficacy of an herbal toothpaste. *Journal of Clinical Dentistry*, **9**(2), 31–33.

Faculty of Homeopathy www.facultyofhomeopathy.org

Lessell, C.B. (2000) *A Textbook of Dental Homeopathy*, revised edition. CW Daniel Co Ltd, Saffron Walden.

A comprehensive review of homeopathy in dentistry is available from the Faculty of Homeopathy. (info@homeopathy.org)

Section 3

Non-clinical

19

Primary care services

Sara Holmes and Leanna Wynne

Summary

This chapter covers:

- The definition of primary care
- Key legislation relating to primary care service provision
- The types of primary care NHS dental services
- The primary care dental team
- Introduction to epidemiology

Introduction

This chapter seeks to introduce the role of primary dental care services (PDCS) and the key role that the primary care dental team can play in the assessment and management of evidence-based practice. When thinking about primary care, whether as a patient or as a service provider, we need to consider what the term 'primary care' denotes.

Since its inception in 1948 the National Health Service (NHS) has aimed to provide care which enables equitable access to provision for all. It seeks to provide a service which is acceptable to communities, providing what they want or need, is responsive to changing population needs, is cost effective and, above all, which can be held accountable. It is therefore not surprising that services based in the primary care setting, where most patients receive care, have evolved. In such a model of provision, care is provided at the 'primary' level, based upon the health needs of the local population. The genesis of 'primary dental care' supports notions that health needs can vary with demography (region to region). It accounts

for influences which are placed upon populations who live and work in different environments and by different cultures, customs and traditions. Primary dental care should be based upon the needs of the local population rather than being solely disease based; it accepts that disease rates are not universal and may be more prevalent in certain communities than others. In such a model of healthcare provision, patient needs can be preventative as well as curative, as care can be based upon both health and ill health determinants.

The *Oxford English Dictionary* defines the word 'primary' as meaning 'occurring first in time or sequence'. Primary dental care seeks to provide the point of contact for local populations through devolved funding regimes. Funding is considered against the needs of local and not regional health trends. Primary care is the first facet of care provision working alongside healthcare services in meeting the needs of the overall health economy. Primary care denotes the provision of services which are funded and resourced at a local level, based upon local community and population needs. By 1995 the NHS had officially adopted the term 'primary care'. The framework of dental healthcare provision in the United Kingdom therefore includes primary, secondary and tertiary care services. Secondary healthcare is defined by the European Observatory on Health Systems and Policies as care provided by medical or dental specialists, usually in a hospital setting, but also some specialist services provided in the community. Tertiary care refers to medical and related services of high complexity and usually high cost. Tertiary care is generally only available at national or international referral centres.

Clinical Textbook of Dental Hygiene and Therapy, Second Edition. Edited by Suzanne L. Noble.
© 2012 John Wiley & Sons, Ltd. Published 2012 by John Wiley & Sons, Ltd.

The framework of UK primary dental care service provision

The provision of care through the NHS is an ever evolving process. This section will describe the current existence of the Strategic Health Authority and Primary Care Trusts and the proposed replacement of these bodies with the NHS Commissioning Board and the General Practitioner Commissioning Consortia (GPCC). These reforms, led by the Coalition Government elected in 2010, follow in the footsteps of work carried out prior to the installation of this Government.

In 2008, a report entitled *High Quality Care for All* was published (DoH, 2008). This report, led by Lord Darzi and co-produced with the NHS, examined the provision of high quality care as opposed to building capacity within the NHS. In 2009, building on the findings of this paper, an independent review into NHS dentistry, led by Professor Jimmy Steele, was published (DoH, 2009). His report, *Dental Services in England*, suggested that if dentistry was to be aligned with the rest of the NHS oral health, rather than dental activity, was the required outcome that all practitioners should be working towards. Furthermore, a change to the contractual arrangements within NHS dentistry would be required if a high quality, accessible service was to be delivered to the population. Since 2006, the local commissioning of dental care has been the responsibility of 10 **strategic health authorities** (SHA). At the current time, Strategic Health Authorities are a key link between the Department of Health and the local NHS. Each SHA oversees **primary care trusts** (PCTs), which commission dental services in order to meet community healthcare needs. Primary care trusts are the 'purchasers' (commissioners or procurers) of primary care services and contribute to the work of other health trusts (e.g. acute hospital trusts, ambulance trusts, care trusts, mental health trusts, foundation trusts, etc.) in meeting the health needs of communities.

The SHAs are tasked with working closely with the PCTs, whose remit is to act as service commissioning and workforce planning advisers. So effectively PCTs are local commissioners of medical and dental care. In this model, PCTs are responsible for assessing and meeting the dental needs of their local community, and reporting these to the SHA.

- The installation of the Coalition Government in 2010 brought with it the promise of change and reform in the NHS. Structural Reform Plans (SRPs) were introduced and an SRP was published for each department within Government that set out measureable objectives. This placed accountability for Government reforms within each of the specific departments, and spending within departments was dependant on the Spending Review carried out by HM Treasury. The priorities of SRPs, *Department of Health Structural Reform Plan, October 2010* (DoH, 2010a) were centred upon a patient led NHS, relocation of resources to promote healthcare outcomes, transformation of NHS accountability and improvements in public health and social care.

Publication of the White Paper; *Equity and Excellence: Liberating the NHS* (DoH, 2010b), set a long-term plan for reforming the NHS. Detailed within the paper were changes to the contractual arrangements within NHS dentistry which included replacing SHAs with an NHS Commissioning Board and PCTs with the GPCC, by April 2013. The quality assurance of the GPCC would be the responsibility of the NHS Commissioning Board, as opposed to the Care Quality Commission (CQC). The CQC is an independent regulator of all health and adult social care in England. All primary care dental providers were required to have registered with the CQC by April 2011 to be able to legally carry out the business of dentistry. Primary Dental Care establishments are accountable to the CQC for standards of quality and safety.

Government policies continue to iteratively shape and change oral care provision. Thus, dental services, and the staff who provide such care, will continue to be engaged in on-going cycles of review and reform that will shape the nature and provision of primary care dentistry.

The provision of NHS dental services

The general dental service contract

The UK has a well established framework of general dental services (GDS)/personal dental services (PDS). Such services are often referred to as 'high street dental practices' or 'providers of family dental care'. Dental practices are independent businesses commonly owned and managed by general dental practitioners, although practices may be owned and managed by dental care professionals (DCPs), corporate bodies and limited dental companies. Practitioners are able to offer private treatment whilst also entering into a service level agreement (SLA) with the PCT for the provision of NHS services. The NHS patient activity expected, in terms of SLA delivery, is measured in units of dental activity (UDAs). Each dentist receives a block fee, in accordance with their SLA/defined UDAs, and payments to the dentist are made monthly by the PCT through the agency of the **Business Services Authority.** The practice owner, if unsuccessful in the delivery of the SLA/UDAs, may be required to repay elements of the funding claimed from the PCT.

The patient receiving the NHS treatment contributes to the monies paid in the form of a set patient charge, depending on the work being carried out. Financial implications are commonly cited by patients along with general access problems, as barriers to their receiving dental care.

The GDS/PDS is delivered through the services of dentists, dental therapists, dental hygienists and dental nurses. GDPs can recruit staff as required, and therefore the skill mix will vary from practice to practice. Following changes to the Dentists Act (1984) in July 2002, dental therapists were legally permitted to work as members of the GDS team, in addition to their former roles in the salaried dental services (SDS). A dental practice may also provide dental care through the appointment of a Foundation Trainee (FT). Foundation Training is mandatory for the first year post qualification and a 2-year Foundation Training course is available. A FT will continue to train and work alongside an experienced general dental practitioner, or FT trainer, during his or her first year (or possibly two years) of practice. FT positions are open for application to those dental students who have qualified at a UK dental school. Salaried Therapist Vocational Trainee posts are also becoming available in certain areas of the country, commonly on a part-time basis of three days per week.

The proposals set out in the White Paper *Equity and Excellence. Liberating the NHS* requires the dentist to employ the appropriate skill mix required to meet the needs of their patients. This vision is reinforced in the consultation document *Liberating the NHS: Developing the Healthcare Workforce* 'creating an environment where talent flourishes and where everyone is able to realize their potential' (DoH, 2010c, p. 13). Whilst practices and the salaried services may wish to keep lists of their patients, the formal requirement of patient registration ceased to exist after April 2006, as did the requirement for registered patients to be seen 'out of hours' in an emergency. The responsibility for out-of-hours emergencies lies with the PCT. From April 2006, all local PCTs were allocated a budget for dentistry within their area, after which their funds became what was termed 'cash limited' (i.e. restricted to the agreed level). The GDP must therefore seek prior approval to set up a new dental practice, to expand an existing practice, or to amend their SLA.

Salaried dental services

The salaried services are made up of the traditional community dental service (CDS) and PDS. These services are PCT led, and structures and remits may therefore vary between trusts, dependent on local population needs.

Typically, services operate via a referral service from GDS and other healthcare services (HCS). However, emergency care can be accessed directly by patients at selected centres, called **dental access centres**, which are part of the PDS.

The community dental service

The CDS is a complementary service to the GDS offered through PCTs to fulfil the remit of:

- Providing dental care requiring specialist skills for individuals referred from the GDS and other health professionals, or, for those who cannot otherwise access treatment. These may include people with special needs or requiring specialised services, such as anxious patients, or, assistance with people who are restricted within their homes or are hospitalised.
- Screening of school children.
- Contributing to epidemiological surveys and data, such as the publication of decayed, missing and filled deciduous teeth (dmft) rates.
- The provision of oral health promotion and education services where needs are identified by the PCT.

The CDS are often located in a medical centre or health centre and are subject to the same treatment charges as in the GDS. The staffing skill mix will vary from one CDS centre to another, but traditionally includes: dentists; surgical dentistry and paediatric dentistry, dental therapists, dental hygienists, dental nurses and oral/dental health promotion teams.

The personal dental service agreement

The PDS was first established in 1998, following the introduction of the **NHS (Primary Care) Act 1997**. The government aims of the PDS scheme included increasing access to NHS dental services, enabling practices to adopt a preventative approach to dental treatment and oral health and providing local solutions to local problems. PDS funding is based on the PCT contract.

Initially PDS schemes replaced some GDS and CDS contracts but later some specialised services and practices (e.g. orthodontics, oral surgery, periodontics, endodontics and sedation), transferred to the PDS scheme.

PCTs work in partnership with PDS practices to address inequalities in oral health locally, seeking to provide dental access to those who need it most. PDS practices are not limited to NHS provision, and may offer a mix of both private and NHS care to patients, as in the GDS. Management of the practice remains the responsibility of the principal dentist who holds the PCT contract. This dentist is known as the '**provider**', and may choose to contract others to do some or all of the work within the practice, and these individuals are known as the '**performers**'. Performers may include, for example, other dentists within the practice, dental hygienists and dental therapists. The skill mix of staff is the choice of the dentist, dependent upon the needs of patients.

Dental access centres

In addition to the GDS, SDS and the personal dental services, primary care dental services are also offered through dental access centres. Dental access centres fall within the PDS to provide emergency care to patients who are not able to access a GDP. The service provided can vary from area to area depending on local needs, resources and patient demand/need. The priority is to treat those with an urgent need initially. An adult or child can seek the full range of NHS dental treatment at any access centre during weekday working hours. Dental access centres are located in areas where the patients' oral health needs are high, and access problems are prevalent. Appointments are not always needed as emergency slots are reserved. Standard NHS patient charges apply. Patients are generally directed to access centres for care by the '**NHS Direct**' helpline services.

Until the reforms led by the current Coalition Government are introduced the PDS will continue to be co-ordinated through PCTs, and contracts will be integrated into new arrangements. Patients in pain may present as dental emergencies outside routine working hours; the emergency dental service supports the work of the dental access centres, by providing 'out-of-hours' emergency care.

Emergency dental services

The aim of the emergency dental service (EDS) is to provide urgent dental treatment, out of normal surgery hours, to patients who cannot wait until the next working day. In addition to this, the EDS scheme, funded (currently) by local PCTs, operates in most regions providing emergency care to patients who are not registered with a dentist. These services are commonly linked to health centres or hospitals, providing cover for evenings, weekends and bank holidays.

The provision of 'out-of-hours' emergency dental treatment is currently the responsibility of the PCTs. Strategic health authorities and PCTs work together to ensure that emergency services are available, and that all PCT regions have service provision. The hours and days of availability of an EDS are likely to differ from region to region. Services may be operated:

- On a 'walk in' basis.
- Through an appointment system.
- Through a triage centre which then books an appointment depending on the needs of the patient.
- Via screening through an 'on call' rotational service.

The funding bodies of primary care dentistry and practitioners need to work together to find the most effective and efficient way of providing emergency cover in their region for their patients.

The Defence Dental Service

In addition to the salaried dental services thus far discussed, the Defence Dental Service (DDS) is part of the primary dental care framework. The DDS is part of the Defence Medical Services (DMS) and exists primarily to deliver dental care to serving personnel of the Royal Navy, Army and Royal Air Force within the Military Health System. A referral system exists for treatment required from specialist DDS located in military establishments. Defence service dental teams may be deployed to a variety of settings at home and abroad. The current skill mix of staff that support the DDS includes dentists, dental nurses, dental hygienists and dental technicians. The DDS is committed to the professional development of dental staff in order to meet the needs of serving personnel. Service-based training programmes are offered in dental nursing and dental hygiene at the military base in Aldershot, Hampshire.

The primary dental care team

Dental care professionals

The **Nuffield Report** (1993) and the subsequent publication of the **Dental Auxiliary Review Group** (DARG) **Report** (1998) identified the need to reform the use of members of the dental team. Amongst the recommendations in the reports were the expansion of the dental therapist's role and the introduction of new classes of professionals complementary to dentistry, now referred to as Dental Care Professionals (DCPs). The General Dental Council document, *Developing the Dental Team* (General Dental Council, 2004), identified the need for additional dental professionals. The orthodontic therapist and clinical dental technician were stated as the initial new members to existing categories.

Legislative changes were introduced, following changes approved by Parliament in 2005, to section 60 of the Dentists Act (1984) which were intended to provide an improved standard of care for patients, whilst offering a structured career pathway for DCPs. The GDC accepted that all groups of DCPs should follow recognised pathways of education and training, leading to qualification and statutory registration with the GDC. Prior to 2006, only dentists, dental therapists and dental hygienists were required to register with the GDC. The dually qualified therapist and hygienist wishing to work in both disciplines are required to hold dual registration. As from September 2005, dental care professionals included dental hygienists and dental therapists, dental nurses, dental technicians, clinical dental technicians and orthodontic therapists, all of whom commenced registration with the GDC in 2006. The GDC agreed to use the term 'dental care professional' to be consistent with the Dentists Act which was amended to give the GDC a range of new powers, including the power to start registering other dental team members.

Curricula frameworks have been developed by the GDC and are detailed in the updated document; *Developing the Dental Team Second Edition (Interim) 2009* (GDC, 2009a). *The Scope of Practice* (GDC, 2009b) establishes the role of each member of the dental team. As a registered member of the GDC all registrants are required to engage in compulsory Continuing Professional Development (CPD). To enable the best provision and care to be provided to the patient, the GDC states the required number of hours in a given time frame to be attained and the core activities that must be covered by the individual.

The dentist – team leader

The dentist has the opportunity to pursue several careers offering academic and practical challenges, including post-qualification examinations and specialisation. Dentists are healthcare professionals who are specifically trained in the diagnosis and treatment of a range of problems that affect the oral cavity. Dentists are leaders of the modern dental healthcare team, and they may choose to work in many areas and specialities, which include general practice (NHS, private or mixed), the salaried dental services, industrial dental practice (usually employees of large business organisations) and the armed forces. They may also choose to follow an academic route working in university teaching hospitals and research establishments. Undergraduate education and training takes place in university dental schools throughout the UK and covers the dental syllabus as defined by the General Dental Council; *Outcomes for registration 2011*. Undergraduate education and training in the UK is undertaken over 5 years, or, a 4-year graduate training programme for Honours science graduates is available in a number of Institutions.

The dental therapist

Historically dental therapists and all members of the DCP team were known as 'dental auxiliaries', and initially their education and training was based upon a model of dental education developed in New Zealand, where dental nurses were trained to undertake routine clinical tasks. After the inception of the NHS in 1948 and in order to meet shortages in dental personnel, the first dental therapy training programme was established, at the New Cross Hospital in London. Students completed a 2-year intensive diploma course, qualifying as a dental therapist on completion. The New Cross School continued to train 60 students per year until its closure in 1983.

In the past, the dental therapist had been restricted to practising within the CDS, the hospital dental service (HDS) and, more recently, the PDS, providing essential care to groups of patients not normally found within general dental practice. Therefore, until legislative changes in July 2002, which developed the therapist remit and permitted them to undertake employment in general practice, training numbers were relatively small.

Changes to legislation, duties and educational frameworks have seen the style and nature of some training courses change, from professional diploma to academic degree (BSc) level provision. In October 2004, the first school in the United Kingdom for DCPs was opened in Portsmouth. Course duration varies typically depending on award outcome (e.g. BSc). It is no longer possible to study for the single dental therapy qualification; all awards are dual hygiene and therapy, although it remains possible to study for a single qualification as a dental hygienist.

As of 1 July 2002, legislation permitted dental therapists to work in any sector of dentistry. To comply with this legislation a registered dentist must examine the patient and indicate clearly in writing the course of treatment that the dental therapist is to carry out. The GDC document *The Scope of Practice* describes the remit of each member of the dental team. The number of Therapists on the register, as published by the GDC in August of 2010, was 1548.

The dental hygienist

The role of the dental hygienist was established under the Dentists Act of 1957, which also defined that the dental hygienist must work to the written prescription of a registered dental practitioner. The dental hygienist's role is that of an educator, helping to give patients the necessary skills to prevent dental disease and effectively maintain their oral hygiene, and a clinical operator primarily involved in the removal of tooth deposits. Under the legislative changes introduced in 2002, hygienists are permitted, subject to appropriate additional training, to take impressions, administer inferior dental block anesthesia, replace dislodged crowns with temporary cement and treat patients under conscious sedation. The number of hygienists on the register, as published by the GDC in August 2010, was 5673.

The dental nurse

Dental nurses are an essential part of the dental team in the provision and support of patient care. The dental nurse supports the patient and the clinician during dental treatment. Currently there are several routes to qualification for dental nurses, including the **National Examination Board (NEBDN) Certificate in Dental Nursing** and the **National Vocational Qualification (NVQ) in Dental Nursing** (level 3). Other routes include training within the armed services and within dental hospitals, which offer their own qualification. The GDC considers and approves 'qualifications of equivalence' which lead directly to qualification and registration, for example, the Certificate in Higher Education for Dental Nursing. There are many career opportunities for the dental nurse within all sectors of dentistry. Post-certification courses are currently offered in dental radiography, oral health education, dental anaesthetic nursing, dental sedation nursing, special care dental nursing and orthodontic nursing.

The dental technician

Dental technicians make a wide range of dental appliances and prostheses, for example implants, crowns, bridges, dentures or veneers. Under legislation (see above) introduced in 2006, dental technicians must be registered with the General Dental Council. The dental technician works to the prescription of the dentist and they may be located in laboratories based within, or external to, dental practices.

Clinical dental technician

A qualified dental technician may choose to train as a clinical dental technical (CDT). A registered professional, the CDT is able to provide services as specified in the GDC document Scope of Practice. A prescription from a dentist is required where natural teeth or implants exist. Should the patient be edentulous the CDT is able to provide complete dentures direct to the patient.

Orthodontic therapist

A qualified dental nurse, dental hygienist or dental therapist may, with post qualification experience, choose to train as an orthodontic therapist. The orthodontic therapist is a registered professional who carries out some orthodontic treatments, as stated in the GDC document the Scope of Practice, under prescription from a dentist.

Team working

The GDC's philosophy, regarding all members of the dental team working together on a collaborative basis, is founded on the positive response received to its publication *Professionals Complementary to Dentistry: A Consultation Paper* (GDC, 1998). In this report, the GDC recommended the registration of all groups of PCDs and the regulation of their work through educational curricula and ethical guidance, rather than through prescribed duties. The dentist is seen as 'team leader', responsible for diagnosis, treatment planning and, together with the other members of the dental team, the quality assurance of the treatment provided. Dentists have the additional responsibility to the GDC for ensuring that colleagues in the teams they lead are not asked to undertake practice beyond their competence. The recommendation to adopt a team approach relies on understanding the concept of team working, and an ability to develop new ways of working together. It is therefore worth considering what constitutes team working in the modern primary care dental setting. The GDC has published guidance on standards for dental professionals. This guidance is supported by a collection of six further publications that outline the key principles, one of which is *Principles of Dental Team Working* (GDC, 2006).

The World Health Organization (WHO) defines teamwork as 'coordinated action carried out by two or more individuals jointly, concurrently or sequentially'. It implies common agreed goals and clear awareness of, and respect for, others' roles and functions. Therefore, in order to work effectively as a team in the delivery of patient care it is necessary to understand and find ways in which to work together. The benefits from working as a team in the delivery of primary dental care include:

- The delivery of a more responsive and patient-sensitive service.
- A more clinically effective and/or cost-effective service.
- More satisfying roles and career paths for primary healthcare workers.
- Improved organisation and planning.
- The avoidance of duplication, fragmentation and working in isolation.
- The development of more comprehensive healthcare plans which meet the needs of individual patients and communities.

To work effectively and efficiently as a team, there is a need to foster the belief that each team member's role is essential and rewarding and that there are clear team goals which all strive to achieve. Teams need support to develop and become effective. There is much literature written on group process and working (Naidoo and Wills, 2004), as well as programmes and courses which are designed to help facilitate team working. Therefore it is essential that team-based education and learning are fostered to enable the modern dental team to be able to both assess and meet the needs of its patients. The modern dental team needs to understand its remit, and work together with other agencies in establishing the oral health needs of the local community. The dental team also needs to understand its role in and contribution to the broader primary care public health agenda.

The public health agenda and an introduction to epidemiology

There are two theoretical domains which converge to support us in considering the assessment of our patients' health needs, namely those related to the field of 'public health', where the field of 'dental public health' is particularly relevant, and the teachings associated with the study of epidemiology. There are many definitions of 'public health' but there is a general consensus that the focus is on protecting and improving the health of individuals, communities and populations. Epidemiology can be described as studies associated with patterns of diseases, and what influences such patterns.

The role of the primary dental care team is therefore integral to both the mission of public health and the aims of epidemiology in order to understand more about the influences which are placed upon patients, and to facilitate the identification of the most effective way(s) of supporting them. The primary care dental team is provided daily with opportunities to contribute to a professional understanding about the health of patients, and the population as a whole. Through exploring the types of routine health data which are available and the types of data that the primary care team can generate and contribute to, it is hoped that evidence-based practice will be further informed and developed.

Knowing your patients

To fully understand the health, or ill health, of a community, it is first necessary to consider what can be learnt about them through data which are available. This process is commonly called '**health needs profiling**', and it is an essential first step for the dental hygienist/therapist to consider when planning any type of public health service or activity (e.g. oral health promotion, smoking cessation, etc.). Health needs profiling can be broadly considered within two categories:

- Positive and negative lifestyle influences.
- Positive and negative health influences.

The first category is commonly assessed through various lifestyle questions (e.g. amount of physical exercise, smoking, alcohol rates, etc.) that the dental team ask during the initial, and on-going, evaluative assessment of patients. These data enable the identification of both positive and negative aspects which may influence a patient's health and well-being, and thus enable us to provide targeted information, support and guidance. The second category is often harder to consider and is frequently neglected by the team, as it addresses the broader influences which are placed upon our patients' health, such as social factors, environmental influences (e.g. pollution rates), physical influences, psychological influences and the influences of policy, for example smoking in public places and alcohol licensing laws. However, whilst local data (i.e. those collated by the dental team) help us to identify the care needs of our patients, it is possible to have access to large amounts of wider 'routine' health-related data (e.g. housing data, employment rates, ethnicity data, etc.) which may help to gain a greater understanding of the health needs of the community from which our patients are drawn. The types of data available and how to access them are summarised in Table 19.1.

Measuring health problems

As described in Table 19.1, diseases are reported upon in relation to the characteristics of the disease and those of the population(s) who suffer from the disease. These are known as '**disease determinants**' and epidemiologists seek to discover if the 'distribution' of diseases differs between populations; for example, do more women aged 30–45 suffer from periodontal disease than men aged 30–45? In order for distribution trends to be considered it is first necessary to determine the type of comparisons which will be recorded; for example, gender, race, age, and what characterises the disease (e.g. pocket depths of more than 2 mm). This enables the 'standardisation' of data, which may enable comparisons to be considered. This type of data is usually collected as a '**rate**'. Rates enable frequency to be measured; for example, how many patients are diagnosed with periodontal disease over a given period.

Rates, incidence and prevalence

A rate determines the number of people with a specific condition. It is a 'ratio' which is usually presented as a percentage (%); for example, the number of male patients over the age of 20 years with cavities in virgin teeth, during 2010. The rate would be calculated by dividing the number of male patients (>20 years) with new cavities in virgin teeth during 2010, by the total number of male patients (>20 years) treated during 2010.

$$\text{Rate} = \frac{\text{Number of events in a time period}}{\text{Total population during the time period}}$$

Table 19.1 Sources of population data.

Type of data	Comments/source
Birth rates	It has been a legal requirement to register all births, deaths and marriages in the UK since 1874. National, regional and local data are available through the Office of National Statistics (ONS)
Death rates	Data are collated on perinatal death rates, infant mortality rates, fertility rates and the specific cause of death (e.g. heart failure). National, regional and local data are available through the ONS
Routine census information	This includes, for example, types of housing, the number of people in occupation, employment rates and the number of people with cars. Information is held by the ONS, public libraries and academic libraries
Population estimates	These are commonly seen in government and local health agency papers which may, for example, predict the cost of treating smoking-related illnesses for growing/changing populations. Examples are available from the Department of Health website (www.doh.gov.uk)
Primary care data	These may include, for example, the number of patients receiving care by a dentist/DCP, the number of patients receiving care by a local general medical practitioner and the number of patients receiving care in their home. This type of data may be national, regional or local and is available through the ONS. It is collated and published locally by primary care agencies, e.g. the PCTs
Hospital episodes/ hospital discharges (secondary care data)	Reports collate, for example, the number of patients seen and the completed number of cases over a given timescale. Diseases are coded according to International Classification of Disease (ICD) codes. Data are published through primary care agencies, for example the SHA and PCT (e.g. community health atlas)
Infectious diseases	Doctors are required by law to inform the Local Medical Officer (LMO) if they suspect that a patient is suffering from an infectious disease, e.g. meningitis, food poisoning, etc. Data can be collated from national reports (see for example www.doh.gov.uk)
Cancer registration/HIV/ AIDS rates	These data are collated by diagnosis, age, sex, residence and type(s) of treatment required. Reports are published annually by, for example, the National Cancer Association and are commonly held in academic libraries and on-line (see www.doh.gov.uk)
Socio-economic data	These may include, for example, the number of road traffic accidents in a given area, pollution levels, crime statistics, unemployment statistics and the number of people claiming benefit support. National, regional and local data are available through the ONS, and through primary care agency reports (e.g. healthcare atlas)

Remember that, as written, we would only know the total number of males over 20 years who presented with cavities in virgin teeth; the data would not tell us the number of cavities (e.g. a single or multiple case) or the type of cavity (e.g. single surface), but these data could be established in the same way, by altering what determinants are analysed within the 'rates' classified. When setting a rate the upper number (i.e. number of cases) is called the **numerator** and the lower number (i.e. the total potential population) is called the **denominator**. The rate can then be multiplied by a convenient number (e.g. 10, 100, 1000) to determine the number of cases per population set (10, 100, etc.).

There are two types of 'rate' which are frequently referred to in health data: **prevalence rates** and **incidence rates**. A prevalence rate determines the total number of the population which have a disease or condition during a period of time (referred to as **period prevalence**), or at a specific point in time (referred to as **point prevalence**).

$$\text{Point prevalence} = \frac{\text{Number of persons identified with disease at a point in time}}{\text{Total number of persons in the group at a point in time}}$$

$$\text{Period prevalence} = \frac{\text{Number of persons identified with disease during a period of time}}{\text{Size of population during the time period}}$$

An **incidence rate** differs from a prevalence rate in that it only reports on new cases in the given period rather than all cases. This rate is useful to determine if trends are increasing, decreasing or generally staying the same.

$$\text{Incidence} = \frac{\text{Number of new cases in a specified period}}{\text{Total population at risk in the specified period} \times \text{multiplier (e.g. 100)}}$$

When calculating any type of rate, it is of paramount importance to define the categories correctly, such as the size of the total population. For example, if determining the number of cases of pregnancy gingivitis diagnosed by a dentist it would be necessary to exclude all males and all females who were not pregnant during the period from the **total population**.

Rates can be defined as **specific**, **standardised** and **crude**. Specific rates usually refer to specific causes (e.g. deaths from lung cancer), crude rates usually refer to all given cases during a period (e.g. the total number of deaths in 6 months) and standardised rates aim to predict rates (e.g. 'standard mortality rates' (SMR), which seek to predict death rates based upon existing data, or rates of smokers who will die from smoking related illnesses).

$$\text{Standardised rates} = \frac{\text{Number of cases}}{\text{Expected number of cases}}$$

This type of data can be used to determine if disease rates within a community are as expected and they can enable comparisons to be made between different groups and populations. From such data **standard rates** can be gauged; for example, the standard decayed, missing and filled rate (dmft) for 5 year olds in region X is 1.

Interpreting data with caution

Whilst data are presented in black and white, there is a need for the dental team to interpret them with caution, by considering the influences which may skew what is presented or how it is interpreted. Like all research studies, all data must be considered against such questions as:

- How were they collected?
- Why were they collected?
- Who collected them?
- When were the data collected?
- For what purpose were the data intended?
- How was the sample drawn?
- How were the data analysed?
- Who analysed the data?
- Were the examiners calibrated?

It is important that the dental hygienist/therapist, whether under training or qualified, applies the rules learnt associated with appraising published research evidence to this task so that they are confident in what they use to establish and determine their practice (useful further information can be obtained from Laverack, 2009; Nielsen Nathe, 2010; Webb and Bain, 2010). Many types of study are undertaken to collate such data, for example, case study analysis, cross-sectional studies, randomised controlled trials, single-blind experiments (placebo effects), double-blind experiments, natural experiments and quasi-experiments. Although it is beyond the scope of this chapter, the dental hygienist/therapist needs to develop an understanding of such techniques and when they should be applied.

It is also important to remember when analysing data on your own practise, or that of others, disease rates will only tell part of the story. For example, consider the number of patients who may have toothache but never attend for treatment, the number of patients who seek alternative help for their problem (e.g. hypnosis to support smoking cessation), and those who the health professions as a whole do not regularly see and will therefore have few data on (i.e. those who are healthy!). This is sometimes referred to as the **iceberg effect**, as it is not just what we see but also what we don't see that paints the whole health/ill health picture. Data are also usually drawn from a negative health model, which captures active disease rates as opposed to promotional interventions, which may have prevented such diseases. It is also important to remember that data when published may by their very nature be out of date, as analysis and publication can take a considerable time, during which the demography of the population continues to change; for example, people die, move house, get married, age by another year or give birth. This raises the question of 'why do we bother to collect data?'.

Why bother collecting data?

This question is easy to address. As populations change so do patterns and prevalence of disease; for example, with growing elderly populations we may see more evidence of root abrasion and root caries. Without both monitoring and understanding of such trends, we, as healthcare providers, will not be able to target resources and our care to where treatment needs (whether preventative or disease-based) can be most effectively managed (see Chapter 6). Without such data it would be difficult, if not impossible, for us even to begin to understand the health needs of our patients and the local community or for funding bodies, such as the PCT, to fund the care required by our patients. All members of the dental team are therefore 'agents' in managing such changes and trends, not in isolation but as part of the total healthcare economy.

Your role in health needs assessment

As described earlier, the dental hygienist/therapist and the primary care dental team are conveniently situated to access and record all kinds of health data, from bleeding indices, radiographic reports, basic periodontal examination reports and findings from conservation screening to the number of smokers, all of which contribute to our understanding of the needs of our patients. Whether such needs are defined by us as healthcare professionals (**normative needs**) or by our patients themselves (**expressed needs**), the primary care dental team plays an important role in establishing the 'health profile' of the local community, and is ideally situated to engage populations in addressing both individual (e.g. smoking cessation, periodontal care) and locality-based health needs (e.g. high dmft rates in 5-year-olds).

Summary

Meeting the health needs of local communities and populations can only be achieved through health commissioners and providers working together to achieve common goals. Without using public health and epidemiological data, the goals that will meet the needs of our patients could not be defined, and funding may well therefore be ineffective in delivering the dental care agenda.

The responsibility of service provision rests at local level, where the commissioners of dental care and primary dental care teams need to work together in meeting the challenges of reducing health inequality. The nature, shape and direction that the modern dental team works is changing and clinicians need to find effective ways of utilising the skills of the whole team in meeting the health needs of patients. In doing this, existing practices and traditions will be brought into question. Ideally the dental patient of the future will have more control and involvement in the services they require, whilst the dental team needs to support this through establishing new ways of working together. In establishing a true model of patient-based care, in which the 'expert patient' is central, the dental team needs to be both involved with, and understand the remit of, health needs assessment, so that services and funding can be accurately targeted. In doing this the team may need to explore and develop new skills and practices, so that the dental needs of the community are considered alongside all other health needs of patients.

Through localised commissioning of care, opportunities for greater interprofessional working occur, eliminating the delivery of dental care in isolation. In being part of the overall healthcare economy, the dental team must continue to establish new ways of working with other professional colleagues, so that the holistic health needs of the patient are both addressed and communicated.

References

Department of Health (2008) *High Quality Care For All, NHS Next Stage Review Final Report.* Department of Health, London.

Department of Health (2009) *NHS Dental Services in England; An Independent Review* led by Professor Jimmy Steele. Department of Health, London.

Department of Health (2010a) *Department of Health Draft Structural Reform Plan.* Department of Health, London.

Department of Health (2010b), *Equity and Excellence; Liberating the NHS.* Department of Health, London.

Department of Health (2010c) *Liberating the NHS: Developing the Healthcare Workforce. A consultation on proposals.* Department of Health, London.

General Dental Council (1998) *Professionals Complementary to Dentistry: A Consultation Paper.* General Dental Council, London. www.gdc-uk.org

General Dental Council (2004) *Developing the Dental Team. Curricula Frameworks for Registerable Qualifications for Professionals Complementary to Dentistry.* General Dental Council, London. www.gdc-uk.org

General Dental Council (2006) *Principles of Dental team Working.* General Dental Council, London.

General Dental Council (2009a) *Developing the Dental Team, Second Edition (Interim).* General Dental Council, London.

General Dental Council (2009b) *The Scope of Practice.* General Dental Council, London.

Laverack, G. (2009) *Public Health.* Palgrave Macmillan, Basingstoke.

Naidoo, J. and Wills, J. (2004) *Public Health and Health Promotion Developing Practice.* Baillière Tindall, London.

Nielsen Nathe, C. (2010). *Dental Public Health and Research.* Pearson Education, Oxford.

Saracci, R. (2010) *Epidemiology.* Oxford University Press, Oxford.

Webb, P.M. and Bain, C.J. (2010) *Essential Epidemiology.* Cambridge University Press, Cambridge.

Further reading

Bowling, A. (2009) *Research Methods in Health: Investigating Health and Health Services.* Open University Press, Milton Keynes.

Cottrell, R.R. and Mckenzie, J.F. (2010). *Health Promotion and Education Research Methods.* Jones & Bartlett Publishes Inc., Burlington, MA.

Ireland, R. (ed.) (2010) *Advanced Dental Nursing.* Blackwell Munksgaard, Oxford.

20

Law, ethics and professionalism

Hew Matthewson

Summary

This chapter covers:

- Regulation of dental practice
- Professional duties and obligations towards patients
- Patient consent to treatment
- Regulations with professional colleagues
- Relationship with the public
- Clinical governance
- Sources of advice

Introduction

Traditionally the public has held healthcare professionals in high esteem. Trust in these professions has been based on the belief that their members are highly trained and competent, that they put the interests of their patients first and that they adhere to high standards of conduct both professionally and personally. While there is some justification for this position, concerns surrounding the delivery and practice of healthcare increasingly attract widespread attention and reduce public confidence in the professions. It is important that all involved in healthcare understand the ethical, legal and professional foundations of their activity, appreciating that these are in an almost constant state of reexamination and development in response to professional, public and political debate.

Regulation of dental practice

In the UK the regulation of the dental profession was first formalised by the **Dentists Act 1878** that introduced voluntary registration of dentists with the General Medical Council. It was not until 1921 that a new act made registration with the Dental Board of the United Kingdom mandatory for newly qualifying dentists. The **Dentists Act 1956** established the General Dental Council (GDC) as the professional statutory body responsible for the regulation of dentistry and the **Dentists Act 1984** and **Dental Auxiliaries Regulations 1986** provided for the enrolment and regulation of dental hygienists and dental therapists.

In 1993 a report on the use of auxiliary personnel in dentistry published by the **Nuffield Foundation** recommended a significant expansion in the membership of the dental team, proposing the introduction of a new range of personnel (Nuffield Foundation, 1999), some with direct clinical duties hitherto only undertaken by dentists, and now known collectively as **dental care professionals** (DCPs). Progress towards the implementation of many of the report's agreed recommendations was hindered by the need for Parliament to debate and amend the Dentists Act and, perhaps not surprisingly, this has not been considered a high priority in the context of wider parliamentary activity. However, the **Health Act 1999** provided a mechanism to make certain changes to the statutory arrangements for professional regulation without the need to open the Dentists Act to full parliamentary debate. As a result the GDC has been able to progress a number of significant reforms, including many that affect DCPs.

The General Dental Council

The GDC is the professional statutory body responsible for the regulation of the dental team. As such its overriding aim is the protection of the public and its recent

Clinical Textbook of Dental Hygiene and Therapy, Second Edition. Edited by Suzanne L. Noble.
© 2012 John Wiley & Sons, Ltd. Published 2012 by John Wiley & Sons, Ltd.

Table 20.1 Composition of the General Dental Council, 2009.

8 dental members
4 DCP members
12 lay members
Total membership – 24
One of the members is elected chair in addition, the Chief
Dental Officers of England, Wales, Scotland and Northern
Ireland are associate (non-voting) members
The GDC is served by a Chief Executive/Registrar and staff

reconstitution has been designed to enable it to undertake this task in a more effective way (Table 20.1). This relatively new structure represents an overall reduction in number with a significant shift in balance in favour of the lay and DCP membership.

In order to fulfil its overall aim of protecting the public, the Council has a number of specific roles.

Registration

The GDC maintains the Dentists Register, the Lists of Specialist Practitioners and the DCP Register Registration has been extended to include dental nurses, technicians, clinical dental technicians and orthodontic therapists. Acceptance on to the registers is through appropriate training and qualification.

It is illegal for anyone other than those whose names appear on the registers to use the job title or to undertake their defined duties.

Recertification

Formerly, once dental professionals were registered they remained so until they chose to remove their name from the register or the GDC found reason to do so. There were clearly risks associated with this situation as there was no statutory obligation to undertake any programme of further education or training, although many saw it as a professional duty and chose to do so. Now there is 5-yearly mandatory recertification of all registrants, making participation in continuing professional development (CPD) a requirement for the continuing registration.

Revalidation

Like all Healthcare Regulators the GDC is currently developing a system of revalidation. The current proposals are that every 5 years after first registration a registrant will need to demonstrate that they are still fit to practise and up to date for the work they are currently doing. This will not mean retaking final exams but it will mean showing that you have completed your CPD, that the CPD is relevant to your current practice,

are participating in audit etc., it is expected that for most people this will simply be a matter of supplying the correct proof of activity.

Educational standards

In order to ensure that the training received, and qualifications gained, by dentists and DCPs are of an appropriate level, the GDC takes a particular interest in educational standards. The Council publishes guidelines on the scope and content of course curricula and undertakes visitations to those educational establishments involved in their delivery, such as university dental schools, DCP schools and hospitals, to ensure that the provision measures up to the high standards it requires. As part of this process, teams of appointed and trained visitors attend institutions to inspect the educational provision to ensure it conforms to the GDC's published recommendations. Visitations result in a report that usually recognises the particular strengths of a course but that may also identify areas where improvements could be made. These reports are now made public. Ultimately, if the GDC had serious concerns about a particular course, it has the power to discontinue its recognition of the resulting qualification, an outcome that is serious enough to ensure that schools implement the recommendations of any report.

Fitness for registration

The GDC is concerned that all registrants are fit to practise dentistry. An individual's fitness for registration may be called into question on grounds of their professional performance, conduct or health. As part of the recent reforms the GDC has revised the way it will approach this issue. The hope and intention is that, through mandatory CPD and the introduction of other approaches to enhancing quality and safety in healthcare, the majority of individuals will remain up to date and competent to practise their particular field of dentistry. However, there will be occasions where for a few, this may not be so. For others, deterioration in their health, for example through the abuse of alcohol or drugs, may put their patients at risk if they were to continue practising. There may also be issues concerning the conduct of individuals, either in association with their professional activity or beyond, that call into question the appropriateness of their continuing registration.

With patient safety as the central concern, the GDC has mechanisms to manage such situations, the overall consideration being whether or not an individual is fit to remain on the register and to practise. The starting point will be a screening or 'pre-hearing' stage to consider the issues that have been raised and, if necessary, to refer the case to a fitness to practise panel. The role of the panel will be to determine whether or not the individual's continuing, unconditional registration is likely to pose a threat to patient safety. The GDC has the power to remove or suspend an individual from its register or to make their continuing registration conditional.

Complaints about individual registrants may be received by the GDC from a number of sources, including patients. The GDC considers all such complaints seriously and has to decide whether the complaint, if it were proven would suggest that the individual is no longer fit to remain on the Register, by virtue of the fact that their fitness to practice is impaired.

Any registrant convicted of a criminal offence will automatically have their conviction examined within these arrangements. It is important to realise that the GDC may also consider convictions, cautions and other episodes of misconduct that took place before an individual was registered for registrants cautions are never considered as 'spent' and must be declared to the GDC. An individual whose fitness to practise is called into question may have their name erased from the Register, preventing him/her from practising.

As we have seen, the GDC is concerned that dentists and DCPs are fit to practise at the time of their registration and continue to be so. Although this section has been primarily concerned with professional competence and health, professional and personal conduct is also important. The public has held an expectation that those in the healthcare professions live up to high standards both professionally and personally, although high-profile events have probably introduced some understandable doubts. The GDC may receive complaints about the behaviour of registrants from members of the public or other agencies. Any criminal convictions will automatically be reported to the GDC and the Council accepts as proven the findings of the court. Indeed, individuals are now obliged to declare any former convictions against them at the time of registration. In each case the GDC has to consider if the conviction or behaviour complained of might compromise the individual's fitness for registration.

Professional duties and obligations towards patients

While the GDC imposes statutory control over dental professionals and the practice of dentistry, there are other legal, ethical and professional duties and obligations on those involved in the delivery of patient care. This is not a new concept designed simply to meet the higher expectations of a modern and increasingly litigious society. Hippocrates (460–377 BCE), considered by many to be the 'father' of medicine, set out ethical principles to

Table 20.2 Key principles for ethical dental practice (General Dental Council, 2005).

Putting patients' interests first and acting to protect them
Respecting patients' dignity and choices
Protecting the confidentiality of patients' information
Co-operating with other members of the dental team and other healthcare colleagues in the interests of patients
Maintaining your professional knowledge and competence
Being trustworthy

govern the relationships between physicians and their patients. Many of these principles were subsequently embodied in the **Hippocratic Oath**, still sworn, albeit in modern form, by many qualifying healthcare students. Since then other groups have proposed principles of ethical and professional behaviour that should be adopted by those in healthcare. The GDC has provided its own set of guidance notes for all Registrants This latest and more general guidance, based around six key principles (Table 20.2), has been supplemented by detailed guidance on a range of specific topics, one of which, *Principles of Dental Team Working* (General Dental Council, 2006), is clearly of particular relevance to DCPs. Those embarking on a career as a dentist or DCP are strongly recommended to acquire and read these documents and remain familiar with them as they will inevitably be revised in the future.

Duty of care

From the moment patients are accepted for care by a dental professional they are owed a duty of care. Patients have the right to expect that those caring for them are appropriately trained and qualified to undertake their treatment and that they are competent to do so. Furthermore, there is an expectation that those delivering patient care will put the interests of their patients before their own. This duty of care extends beyond the execution of specific practical procedures, but applies also to every aspect of patient management, including diagnosis and treatment planning and the giving of advice. Indeed, there is an obligation on healthcare professionals to ensure that patients receive all the information and advice necessary to enable them to understand their condition and contribute to their own management. Failure to offer such advice is likely to constitute a breach of duty of care. It is particularly important to appreciate this in dentistry, as the delivery of, for example, oral hygiene instruction, dietary and smoking cessation advice is central to the prevention and management of oral diseases. Healthcare professionals should appreciate that if they have a conversation with an individual about their health or offer advice, a duty of care is owed – even if the individual is not their patient in the usual sense, and even if the interaction took place outside the professional setting.

Not only must practitioners deliver appropriate elements and items of care, but the care they deliver must also be of an acceptable standard. Failure to achieve an appropriate standard of care is also considered a breach of duty. The standard of treatment clearly varies for a number of reasons, not always under the control of the clinician. While most dental care is delivered to an acceptable standard and much is excellent, some does fall below the standard the patient has a right to expect. It is difficult to give a clear definition of this important threshold, below which the standard of treatment is no longer considered adequate.

For many years the standard of care has been determined in legal terms, using a principle established following a judgement in the case of **Bolam v Friern HMC, 1957**. In this landmark case it was concluded that as long as the standard of care reached that of the reasonably competent practitioner working in similar circumstances then clinicians would not be failing in their duty of care. This became known as the **Bolam principle** or test and has been used for decades by lawyers and the courts. It gave rise to the concept of a 'respectable body of medical opinion' and the belief that if a practitioner could show they had acted in accordance with such a body, they would be defensible in the event of litigation. Although such a line of argument is still used and accepted, it has been challenged on occasions and is no longer associated with the security it once appeared to offer. In particular, the court will need to be convinced that the body of opinion being cited is also logical and up to date, at least for the time of the alleged breach of duty (Bolitho, 1997). Given the greater emphasis on CPD it will no longer be a defence to claim that a practitioner's standard of care was adequate simply because some other practitioners did things the same way. It is important to appreciate that the standard of care delivered by a dental hygienist or therapist is not measured against that expected of a specialist practitioner or consultant, but against that of hygienists and therapists generally.

Court actions for negligence

When patients are in a position to show that a dental professional owed them a duty of care and that there was a breach of that duty either by act or omission, they may be in a position to claim that their treatment was negligently provided and make a claim for compensation. In order to be successful they must show that, as a result of the alleged breach of duty, they suffered loss or damage, the relationship between the breach and the damage being referred to in legal terms as **causation**. If it is accepted or proven in court that all three criteria are fulfilled the patient is eligible to receive financial compensation or damages.

It is rare for a practitioner to be able to contest the claim that they owed a patient a duty of care. When once the patient is in the chair and submitted to examination, that duty exists. While the ultimate arbiter in relation to standard of care and breach of duty is the court, such assessments are made in the first instance on the advice of clinical 'experts' instructed by those advising the patient, who is the potential claimant in the case, and the practitioner who is the potential defendant. Increasingly, patients are seeking legal advice from law firms that specialise in personal injury litigation, even specifically in the dental context. The majority of claims are resolved without the need to go to trial, the outcome being the discontinuation of the claim or a negotiated settlement.

Technically, a claim of negligence must be made, for an adult claimant, within 3 years of the alleged negligence. However, this period is often longer as the 3 years are deemed to start from the date the claimant learnt that the event may have been negligent (the date of knowledge), which may be many years after the event. It is important that accurate dental records are retained for many years as it is increasingly common for patients to claim that 15 or 20 years have gone by without anyone telling them they had periodontal disease.

Indemnity

All registrants must be in a position to pay compensation to a patient and this is done by paying for insurance known as 'professional indemnity'. This is usually done by joining a 'Defence Organisation' Those working in the hospital or community services are automatically indemnified for the work they undertake in the course of that employment and this is known as 'NHS Immunity'. However, such indemnity does not cover clinical activity undertaken outside the employment setting nor does it cover dispute with an employer. It is sensible to consider membership of a defence organisation that offers additional benefits, including access to advice, and is recommended to all dental professionals. DCPs working in practice require indemnity through membership of one of the dental defence organisations or other appropriate insurer. **Professional indemnity** is now required by the GDC and lack of it could lay the individual open to a charge of fitness to practise being impaired.

Confidentiality

The relationship between health professional and patient is based on trust. Patients necessarily impart information to healthcare professionals on the understanding

Table 20.3 Caldicott principles.

Justify the purpose(s) for using confidential information
Only use it when absolutely necessary
Use the minimum that is required
Access should be on a strict need-to-know basis
Everyone must understand his or her responsibilities
Understand and comply with the law

that it is held in strict confidence and shared with others only in very particular circumstances. Such information extends beyond what is obviously medical/dental in nature; for example, the very fact that an individual is a patient at a practice is a confidential matter, as are personal details, such as their address and telephone number. Even in ancient times, Hippocrates recognised the need for confidentiality, considering it an ethical duty of the clinician. This ethical duty remains, but confidentiality is now also seen as the patient's right. It is, for example, enshrined in Article 8 of the **European Convention on Human Rights** and was subsequently embodied in the **Human Rights Act 1998**. The professional duty to maintain confidentiality features prominently in the GDC guidance and an undertaking to that effect appears in many hospital and practice brochures.

Clearly, clinicians concerned with the care of particular patients often have to share information about them and this is exemplified by the necessary communication between members of the dental team. However, even in this context, information should be shared on a need-to-know basis. In 1997 Dame Fiona Caldicott published a report addressing how confidential patient information should be managed within the National Health Service (NHS), in which she established six key principles (Table 20.3). Dentists and others who employ healthcare workers have a duty to ensure that all staff with access to patient information understand this important duty of confidentiality. Where breaches of confidentiality occur patients may be in a position to sue those concerned, although they are more likely to express their displeasure by making a formal complaint, perhaps to the GDC. The GDC views such complaints seriously, as, if proven, they are likely to constitute impairment of fitness to practise.

Breaches of confidentiality often occur unintentionally or unwittingly. Overheard conversations, intercom announcements, video display screens or records left where they can be seen by others are obvious everyday examples. Particular care needs to be taken with technologies such as e-mail, fax, text and voicemail services, where messages may be received or viewed by people for whom they were not intended. Employers and school authorities not infrequently approach practices and clinics to verify an individual's appointment arrangements, but it is inappropriate to provide any information on these occasions without the permission of the patient. Dated and signed appointment cards given to patients may be a useful means of enabling them to provide the confirmation required. Rarely, clinicians may be approached by other agencies, for example the police, seeking information about patients. While there may be particular circumstances when it is appropriate to disclose information, clinicians should view such requests with great caution and it is advisable to seek guidance from a dental defence organisation on how to proceed where any doubt exists. Of course, information may be imparted to any third party with the permission of the patient.

Dental records

Characteristics of good dental records

In order to manage patient care effectively and safely, healthcare professionals keep records of the advice and treatment they provide, notes that also record details of the patient's medical and dental history. Dental notes are still recorded in written format on record cards, although increasingly this is done on computers. Clearly, all the information contained in the records is confidential, along with any associated radiographs, photographs, study models or correspondence (all of which are considered part of the record). To be meaningful and effective, dental records need to be clear and carry an appropriate amount of detail to enable the author and other clinicians to have a clear understanding of the patient's management. Entries should be made at the time treatment is delivered (contemporaneously), dated and the author should be identifiable. It is important that a record is made of all advice given to patients and not restricted to an account of physical items of treatment provided. In dentistry, for example, a note should be made of oral hygiene, dietary and smoking cessation advice given and, if appropriate, the patient's response to it.

Occasionally mistakes are made in dental records. The correction of any such errors should be dated, made clearly and in such a way that the original version remains readable. Dental records should never be fabricated after the event. Even if it becomes necessary to replicate a badly damaged record, that fact should be clearly noted and the original retained.

While there is not usually an expectation that the patient will contemplate suing their clinician, the possibility exists and may arise many years after the treatment was provided. Should such unfortunate circumstances occur, the records take on a new and important significance and their clarity, completeness and accuracy become paramount. In this context, it is particularly important to record any accidents or adverse events that occur during treatment, the action taken and the fact that the circumstances were explained to the patient. This approach extends to recording treatment options that have been discussed with patients, crucial in acquiring their informed and valid consent, discussed later. Likewise, it is essential that any warnings given to patients about possible complications of treatment are also recorded fully.

Retention and destruction of records

There has been a variety of protocols to determine how long dental records should be retained before ultimately being destroyed. Almost by definition, they need to be kept for as long the patient is under the care of the clinician concerned. Advice on how long they should be retained thereafter varies and, in some settings, such as NHS general practice, is drafted in regulatory, rather than clinical or legal terms. As implied above, records become highly significant in the event of a subsequent complaint or legal claim and, as indicated, such a claim might not arise for many years after the event. Therefore, the wisest counsel is to retain records for as long as possible during the lifetime of the patient and, if possible, to arrange for their long-term preservation. Records should be destroyed in a way that ensures there will be no breach of confidentiality – by shredding or incineration. At this point there is merit in reviewing records before they are destroyed to identify any where, perhaps, treatment had been problematic and retention might be advisable.

Access to records

Patients have the legal right of access to their dental records. Previously this was governed by the **Access to Health Records Act 1990** for access to written records and by the **Data Protection Act 1984** for electronic records. However, both these acts have effectively been subsumed into the **Data Protection Act 1998**, the principles of which are listed in Table 20.4, the Access to Health

Table 20.4 Data protection principles.

Personal data must be:
- Processed fairly and lawfully
- Processed for specific purposes
- Adequate, relevant and not excessive
- Not kept for longer than necessary
- Processed in accordance with the rights of data subjects
- Protected by appropriate security
- Not transferred outside the practice

Records Act only having limited continuing application. Under the terms of the Data Protection Act, patients who make written application to see their records must be provided with a copy without unreasonable delay, at their expense, along with an explanation of the content if they so wish. If such a request is made by the patient's legal representative, it is usually accompanied by the patient's signed agreement to disclosure. Dental records should not be disclosed to any other third party without the patient's consent. There are circumstances, rare in dentistry, where disclosure of the records can be resisted, where there are grounds to believe that disclosure would be likely to cause serious harm to the physical or mental health of the patient. With the possibility of disclosure at some point in the future in mind, and in any event, clinicians should resist any occasional temptation to make inappropriate or derogatory entries about their patients, however appealing that may seem at the time.

Patient consent to treatment

Autonomy and paternalism

Individuals have the right to determine what is done to their own bodies and, more specifically, patients have the right to decide what treatment they will accept from healthcare professionals. They have autonomy in this context. However, in the past it was unusual for patients to question doctors and dentists about their treatment; they tended to accept treatment proposals on trust, on the assumption that 'the doctor knows best' – **paternalism**. This unquestioning faith in the medical and dental professions has been challenged in the recent past and patients are now inclined to take a much closer interest in their healthcare.

As far as the relationship between patient and clinician is concerned, there has been a shift from the clinician's duties to the patient, based in paternalism, towards patients' rights based on **autonomy** so lines like 'Trust me, I'm a DCP' are not sustainable and have no place in modern practice. Patients no longer accept without question what they are told. Most want to be involved in planning their treatment and many expect to receive all the information they need to play a meaningful part in the process. This is not to say that clinicians must always or automatically deliver the treatment their patients demand. Clinicians have rights too. It may be that, notwithstanding a detailed consideration of treatment proposals, some patients feel unable to accept the advice on offer and make inappropriate or impossible demands. When this occurs it may be necessary for the clinician to decline to treat the patient.

Patients who are treated without their valid consent may claim to have suffered an assault or battery. While a few pursue such a course, it is more usual for patients to make a claim in negligence in the terms discussed earlier. The GDC provides ethical and professional guidance on consent.

Characteristics of valid consent

It is the discussion between patient and clinician that forms the basis for consent. Readers may have come across a range of expressions – informed consent, implied consent, written consent, express consent, verbal consent, fully informed consent – and may be forgiven for becoming confused. It is accepted now that for consent to be 'valid' it certainly needs to be informed, but there is more to it than that. It is more important for clinicians to understand the necessary criteria that make consent valid, rather than to provide precise definitions for each of the above expressions.

In order for patients to give valid consent to treatment they must first understand what is wrong with them and the possible consequences of leaving their condition untreated. This is, in effect, the 'no treatment' option and may be overlooked, or underestimated, in dentistry. While it would clearly be inappropriate to suggest doing nothing about well established caries or periodontal disease, it may be the wisest course of action for a patient who enquires about possible solutions to a relatively minor aesthetic problem affecting otherwise healthy anterior teeth.

The patient should be presented with all the reasonable treatment options, the execution of which may sometimes require referral to another practitioner with specialist expertise. Discussion should include consideration of the benefits, risks and expected outcome of each option. Failure to include a treatment option may invalidate the patient's consent, especially if they claim later that they would have preferred the omitted option. A classic example would be the recommendation to extract a tooth without telling the patient that there was a realistic chance of conserving it following root canal treatment. A note should be made in the record of the options considered.

The extent to which patients are warned of the risks and possible side effects of each treatment option is potentially problematic. If every possible complication of every aspect of treatment is explained in detail, there would be little time left for its eventual execution and patients may become so worried that they elect not to be treated at all. It is clearly important to warn patients of material risks, especially where they occur frequently or are particularly severe. In the past practitioners were judged in this regard with reference to their peers, the Bolam test referred to earlier in this chapter What warnings would the reasonable and prudent practitioner give to the patient? However, increasing emphasis is now placed on the patient's point of view, the courts asking what warnings the prudent patient might reasonably want to receive.

This issue has been brought to the fore in a recent medical case (**Chester v Afshar, 2004**) in which the House of Lords ruled that a patient could successfully pursue a claim in negligence against a clinician for failing to warn of material risks, even if the claimant might have agreed to the procedure in any event having received the warning. Previously a practitioner who had failed to warn of a risk that materialised could defend a claim by satisfying the court that had the warning been given, the patient would still have agreed to the treatment. In other words, the outcome would have been the same. In such cases, claimants have usually, and not surprisingly, maintained that had they received the warning they would not have had the treatment and so avoided the adverse outcome. In practical day-to-day terms this judgement reaffirms the importance of the duty to warn patients of material risks and of the need to record in specific terms the fact that warnings have been given.

To complete the patient's understanding of proposed treatment they should be given an indication of the likely duration, outcome and prognosis, especially when their own contribution to management is important. It is unwise to paint an over-optimistic picture and to create a level of expectation that might not be met. Where expectations are unrealistically high, disappointments can fuel dissatisfaction and possibly complaints or claims. Finally, patients should understand the costs of treatment and when charges are expected to be paid.

The GDC requires that consent to certain forms of treatment be recorded and some practitioners employ written consent forms more widely. While such documents are helpful, the fact that a patient has signed one does not of itself make the consent valid. It is the information, discussion and resulting understanding that are important. It is now usual practice for patients to be given a written treatment plan and some are asked to sign it. Again, while such practices are useful and help to avoid misunderstandings, they do not, taken in isolation, constitute evidence of valid consent.

It will usually be the case that the dentist with overall responsibility for the care of the patient will acquire their consent to the planned treatment. Nevertheless, it is appropriate for DCPs contributing to the care to confirm that patients understand the treatment they are to carry out and how it fits in to the overall plan. Occasionally, treatment does not go as expected and it becomes necessary to review the proposed plan in the light of events. Similar considerations of consent apply when new options are addressed and DCPs should recognise when it is necessary to seek the further involvement of the prescribing dentist.

The above consideration of consent has assumed that the patient is an adult, competent to engage effectively in the process. Not all patients fall into this category.

Consent for the treatment of children

In law individuals over the age of 16 are considered competent to make decisions about their own healthcare and are able to consent to treatment. However, it is clear that some young people have reached an appropriate level of competence before that age, while some individuals will never do so, even as adults. For the treatment of young children consent is usually given by their parents, or, on occasions, by those who have been legally granted parental responsibility.

Many children, as they approach the age of 16, demonstrate an adequate level of competence to consent to treatment and such consent can be validly acquired in the usual way. The clinician must be satisfied that the young patient is able to understand the issues surrounding the proposed treatment and to weigh them in the balance. Such a child is said to be **Gillick competent**, the name being that of the claimant in the case that established the principle (Gillick, 1985). Although valid consent may be acquired from patients below the age of 16, it is always wise to encourage the involvement of parents in such discussions.

Consent for the treatment of incompetent adults

Nobody is entitled to give consent on behalf of adults who, through severe learning difficulties or other reasons, are not competent to give valid consent for themselves. While it is helpful to engage relatives and carers in a discussion over the best way to manage these patients, it falls to clinicians and, in extreme circumstances, the court to decide how the patient should be treated in their own best interests. In reaching that decision the clinician should take account of any views the patient might have expressed during any previous period of competence. Before proceeding to treat such patients the practitioner should seek a second opinion from a colleague to confirm that the proposed treatment is appropriate and it is wise for both clinicians to sign the plan or a 'consent' form as evidence of the dual consultation.

Healthcare professionals should be careful in their assessment of patients and not be misled by the appearance of some patients with severe physical disabilities but who are completely competent to consent to treatment, although this may present some practical problems.

The treatment of patients under conscious sedation and general anaesthesia introduces particular issues.

Consent needs to be acquired not only for the dental treatment but also for the sedation or anaesthetic, and here the prescribing dentist and the person performing sedation/anaesthesia have particular responsibilities to discuss alternative methods of anxiolysis and pain control. Furthermore, consent should not be sought immediately before treatment commences when patients are likely to be particularly nervous, and certainly not while they are under the influence of the sedative or anaesthetic drugs which impair their judgement.

Relationships with professional colleagues

The DCP and the dentist

Much of what has gone before is concerned with aspects of the relationships health professionals have with their patients. The working relationship between a DCP and the prescribing dentist also has a legal, ethical and professional basis and should be clearly understood. In recent years there has been progressive development of the role and duties of registered DCPs and in some ways a more flexible approach is being adopted to the range of tasks that can be undertaken by any particular category of DCP. The GDC has the statutory power to determine the range of activity for each category of registered DCP. The important principles that always underpin these determinations are that individuals should be appropriately educated, trained and qualified, and be working with an appropriate level of supervision, and in certain circumstances working to the prescription of a dentist.

In December 2005, the GDC agreed that it would welcome proposals to expand the curricula of DCP groups to enable direct access by patients to DCPs, where there was robust training to ensure that patient safety was protected. However, patients should have a full mouth assessment carried out by a dentist, following which the patient would be given an outline or full treatment plan including:

- Recall intervals, dependent upon the patient's clinical needs. These recalls might not be recalls to the dentist, and the dentist might delegate the setting of the recalls to a DCP.
- A date for a full mouth reassessment.
- A referral if required.

The treatment plan could vary dependent on the patient's needs. It could be as simple as a statement that the patient had good oral health, and required no more than routine oral care for the next 3 years, or as complex as a detailed plan and reassessment in 3 months. The setting of recall intervals could be delegated by the dentist to the treating DCP. The only absolute requirements would be a date for full mouth reassessment and

Table 20.5 The basis of DCP practice.

DCPs should understand:
- The legal basis for their practice and employment
- The education, training and qualifications they require
- The scope of their permitted activity
- The locations in which such activity is permitted
- The level of prescription and supervision that is required

that there are arrangements for at least two people to be available to deal with medical emergencies when treatment is planned to take place.

It is inevitable that the scope of activity of DCPs will change in the future and it is therefore important that individuals keep up to date in this respect, to ensure that they are not working beyond the limits of their permitted scope (Table 20.5).

In approaching the treatment of patients, DCPs should ensure that they understand the prescription and seek clarification from the prescribing dentist if they do not. It is possible that, on occasions, the DCP may have reservations about the prescribed treatment and honestly held differences of opinion will arise from time to time. Whether, or to what extent, the DCP should pursue such differences will depend on their significance. A simple discussion may serve to clarify the prescribing dentist's intentions or create the opportunity for the proposed treatment to be reconsidered. While the dentist is ultimately responsible for the patient's care, DCPs cannot claim in defence that they did something they knew to be wrong because they were told to do so, especially where the issue may have a potentially serious outcome.

Generally, differences of opinion can be resolved with a courteous discussion, but where this proves difficult or impossible the DCP should consider seeking advice from their dental defence organisation.

The performance of professional colleagues

A DCP may, at some point in their career, become concerned about the work of a dentist or DCP colleague. It would be unwise to draw conclusions on the basis of a single or small number of incidents, and it would certainly be inappropriate to make derogatory comments about a professional colleague to patients in such circumstances. Not all treatment goes completely according to plan and a range of factors, unbeknown to the observer, may have contributed to the outcome.

However, if the issues giving rise to the concern are potentially serious or occur frequently and it appears that the safety of patients may be compromised, there is a duty to take an appropriate course of action, difficult though it may be. Such problems may relate to the

individual's knowledge and skill, making them a matter of professional competence. At other times deterioration in the clinician's health may be affecting his or her performance, perhaps resulting from alcohol or drug abuse or stress. While the DCP might occasionally feel they know the individual well enough to discuss concerns person to person, it is generally appropriate and certainly wise to seek advice on how to proceed before taking any action. Again, dental defence organisations are probably best situated to provide such advice. Simply ignoring difficult circumstances seldom results in a long-term satisfactory outcome.

Clearly there are messages here for all clinicians in relation to their own behaviour and performance. There is an expectation that health professionals possess a range of skills that they practise to a high standard and this is usually the case. Notwithstanding these expectations, individuals have a duty to ensure that they maintain their skills and competence and to recognise their own limitations. This will be considered further in the discussion on clinical governance. If DCPs think that their professional skills are becoming or have become impaired, for whatever reason, they should seek advice in the context of their continuing professional activity and act upon it. There are sources of advice and support for people in this position and the dental defence organisations provide a useful initial point of contact.

Relationships with the public

Advertising

In the past advertising by the dental profession was considered inappropriate and attempts to do so were even seen as professional misconduct. Times have changed and advertising is permitted by the GDC, provided it complies with advertising standards and is not of a style that might be seen to bring the dental profession into disrepute. Thus, at the very least advertisements must be legal, honest and decent and should not mislead. The GDC provides guidance on the advertising of dental services, both by dentists and DCPs. The essence remains that advertising should be to inform patients and to facilitate choice rather than to imply that services are of a higher standard or quality than those provided by others. Particular care should be taken to ensure that websites are both up to date and accurate. Professional associations also offer detailed advice on advertising.

Public access to information

The **Freedom of Information Act 2000** requires 'public authorities' to provide a list of certain types of recorded information it maintains and gives the public right of access to it. Hospitals and NHS dental practices are considered to be public authorities and must have a 'scheme' setting out the recorded information they make available, the form in which it is presented and any charges made for access. In a dental practice documents such as the practice brochure, list of services provided, list of staff, complaints procedure and other specific practice policies should be included. Professional Associations and defence organisations are able to advise members on how to conform with the provisions of the Act.

Discrimination

The **Declaration of Geneva** that replaced the famous Hippocratic Oath calls upon doctors not to allow considerations of age, disease or disability, creed, ethnic origin, gender, nationality, political affiliation, race, sexual orientation or social standing to influence their approach to their patients – a comprehensive list. In their dealings with the public and patients, members of the dental team must ensure that they do not discriminate knowingly or unwittingly against any particular individuals or groups. In addition to ethical obligations in this respect, it is illegal to discriminate on a number of grounds, including gender, race and disability. The potential for discrimination may arise, for example, in relation to the acceptance and management of patients and in the recruitment, appointment and management of staff.

The **Disability Discrimination Act 1995** is now fully operational and makes it necessary for those offering services to the public, including dental practices, to ensure that disabled people are able to access those services and benefit from them to the same extent as others, as far as is reasonably practicable. This may be facilitated by a range of simple actions, such as providing information sheets in large print format for patients with visual impairment, or by making alterations to practice facilities, for example making wheelchair access possible.

Practical and up-to-date advice on those aspects of discrimination of relevance to the practice of dentistry is available from a number of organisations.

Clinical governance

Clinical governance is designed to promote and ensure, as far as possible, that patients are treated safely and effectively. It is not a single procedure or process, but has brought together a number of approaches, most of which are familiar and have been in use for some time. Clinical governance was introduced by the government and has application in all branches of the NHS, including dental practice and is officially defined as 'a framework through which NHS organisations are accountable for continuously improving the quality of their services

Table 20.6 Principal elements and some contributors to clinical governance.

Quality measurement and improvement
Clinical effectiveness guidelines
Evidence-based practice
Clinical audit

Risk management
Risk identification
Risk analysis and assessment
Risk reduction, elimination, transfer
Complaints procedures
Accident and adverse event reporting

Continuing professional development
General Dental Council mandatory CPD and recertification
Appraisal
Personal development plan/training
Revalidation

---

and safeguarding high standards of care by creating an environment in which excellence in clinical care will flourish'. Although applying initially to the NHS, the provisions of clinical governance have application in other branches of healthcare and this may become formalised in the future.

The processes that collectively make up clinical governance may be considered under three major headings. What follows gives a flavour of each, and is summarised in Table 20.6.

Quality measurement and improvement

Increasingly, the healthcare professions are being challenged to show that the treatments they provide are effective and to possess the evidence for any claims they make in this regard: the emphasis is on evidence-based practise. Although there are techniques and materials that have been used in dentistry for many years and have stood the test of time, new products and methods require a proven scientific basis before widespread acceptance and use.

Practising clinicians are expected to keep abreast of developments and can be assisted in that with reference to published guidelines. Here other agencies have assessed the evidence and produced recommendations on how to manage a wide range of clinical conditions, treatments and processes. For example, there are published guidelines on disinfection and decontamination and the **National Institute for Health and Clinical Excellence** (NICE) has published guidelines on the removal of third molars and dental recall intervals. DCPs should be familiar with accepted guidelines in their field of practice and would generally be expected to follow them or to have good reasons for choosing to adopt an alternative approach.

Clinical audit

All clinicians should, at least periodically, be engaged in clinical audit. This is a cyclical process designed to identify ways in which clinical practice may be improved, to instigate change for the better and to confirm a successful outcome. To illustrate the process with a simple example: there may be concern within a practice that the quality of record keeping is inconsistent, important information not always being recorded. In order to conduct an audit the clinicians need to identify best practise in this regard, referring to the literature and current teaching, and agree on the information that should be recorded. A number of record cards, say 100, are examined and 'measured' against the agreed standard. If the initial concern was justified, failure to meet the agreed standard will arise in a significant proportion of the notes. A course of action is agreed among the clinicians and implemented with a view to ensuring improved record keeping in the future. To complete the audit cycle the process is repeated after an appropriate period of time, to confirm that the desired improvement has been achieved and is being maintained.

Risk management

Risk management is not a new concept; we all practise it every day without thinking, in all sorts of settings. It has very wide scope and application in dentistry, from clinical practice itself to the way in which individuals conduct their professional careers, to the way practices are managed, to matters of health and safety (Chapter 17). The principle is straightforward with three stages: risk identification, risk assessment and risk reduction, elimination or transfer.

The identification of risk

The identification of risks can be undertaken in a variety of ways. Risks associated with clinical techniques are generally widely recognised and reported. Students usually learn about the risks associated with the processes and techniques they are taught and how to avoid, reduce or eliminate them. Dentists and DCPs can establish a checklist of those actions they must take to be sure they are practising legally and securely, while practice principals and managers can develop strategies to ensure that the practice and those working there are complying with the many legal and regulatory arrangements that exist. To do all this and more from scratch as an individual is a daunting task. However, there are several useful sources of advice. Professional associations and dental defence

organisations produce useful material on risk management in a variety of formats to support their members.

Assessment of risk

Such supportive material assists with the process of identifying or highlighting risks but also extends to their assessment and how to cope with them. In assessing a risk it is necessary to consider its expected frequency along with the severity of the consequences that might arise if it materialised. The outcome of this process will point to the most appropriate approach to dealing with it. The more frequently a risk materialises and/or the more severe its consequences, the more compelling is the need to be in control of it.

Dealing with risk

Ideally, appropriate measures should be taken to eliminate risks. Where this is not possible every effort should be made to minimise the opportunity for them to materialise and to reduce the adverse effects should they do so. This necessarily entails the acceptance of some residual risk that is outweighed by the benefits to be gained by use of the process or procedure in question. In some circumstances the effects arising from a materialising risk may be transferred, for example, through insurance. These approaches are illustrated in the following example. There is always the risk that an operator might slip while preparing a cavity for tooth restoration and inflict injury on the oral soft tissues. While such injuries are unpleasant and even alarming, they are seldom serious or leave long-term damage and can be reduced by appropriate handling of instruments, soft tissue retraction and protection. The use of a rubber dam dramatically reduces the risk, effectively to the point of elimination.

If an accident did occur the clinician may be obliged to compensate the patient financially should a legal claim be successfully pursued. This risk may be transferred through membership of a defence organisation who will normally meet the financial liability in the matter. In practice, when something does go wrong with a patient's treatment it is always best to be open and honest with the patient, explaining what has gone wrong, what will be done to put it right in so far as that can be done and what will be done to avoid a repeat for future patients. If this is done then it is rare for patients to pursue a more formal complaint or legal action.

Accidents, adverse events and complaints

The process of risk management can also be informed by events such as accidents, other adverse occurrences and complaints. The emphasis here is on the opportunities that arise to identify why things have gone wrong and, if possible, to take action to prevent their recurrence.

Accident reporting is an important aspect of health and safety provision and there is a legal requirement to report certain adverse events occurring in the workplace to the **Health and Safety Executive**. Within the NHS there is the obligation to report serious adverse events associated with patient treatment so that such reports may be analysed and collated with the intention of making recommendations to improve the safety of patient care. There is also a requirement for every hospital, practice or clinic, including dental practices providing treatment, to operate a complaints procedure. The emphasis is on facilitating resolution of complaints as quickly as possible at the local level and the majority is managed effectively in this way. Where a satisfactory outcome proves impossible, the complaint is referred for independent review and the opportunity exists ultimately for patients who have had treatment carried out under the NHS to put their complaint to the **Health Service Ombudsman** if they remain dissatisfied. These arrangements have recently been the subject of a report by the Health Service Ombudsman and the process has been revised to introduce a more unified and responsive procedure in health and social care. In 2006, the GDC launched a complaints procedure, the **Dental Complaints Service**, for patients who have received private treatment. This service allows patients with a complaint about treatment received from either a dentist or DCP to contact the GDC directly. If the complaint cannot be resolved, the GDC may pass it on to the **Dental Complaints Panel**, which consists of two lay persons and an independent professional (either dentist or DCP as appropriate) who will be required to make a judgement. If the dentist or DCP fails to accept or implement the decision of the Complaints Panel, then it may become a fitness to practise issue for the dentist or DCP. The existence of the Dental Complaints Service does not of course preclude the patient from pursuing their complaint or grievance independently through the courts.

The topic of risk management is clearly an extensive and significant one. Professional associations and defence organisations offer valuable practical advice and guidance.

Continuing professional development

Continuing professional development is a requirement for those registered with the GDC. Recertification for DCPs is conditional upon them undertaking 150 hours of CPD over a 5-year period, averaging out at 30 hours a year. Of these, 10 have to be 'verifiable', being more formalised and complying with criteria set by the GDC. It is important to carefully retain records and certificates of this verifiable CPD. The remaining CPD is described as '**general**' and might include reading, audit, staff training and attendance at relevant meetings not fulfilling the particular requirements of verifiable CPD. A record of this general CPD should be maintained. Individuals are requested to submit an account of their CPD activity to the GDC annually and it is sensible to do so. There is a requirement to submit their record after five years. The GDC may subsequently request evidence of that activity in the form of records and certificates of participation.

It is for individuals, including DCPs, to identify their own CPD requirements and to establish a personal development plan suited to their particular needs and aspirations while taking into account the compulsory elements of CPD as specified by the GDC.

In many work settings the process of appraisal enables individuals to identify areas in which they require further education and training and to plan how that might be acquired. Appraisal is usually conducted in the form of a documented interview with a senior colleague, perhaps the head of a department or principal of a practice. The process is cyclical, usually occurring annually, at which progress towards the attainment of the previous year's objectives is assessed and plans for the coming year agreed. It is meant to be non-threatening and separate from issues of discipline and promotion and the term 'personal development planning' is preferred by some to reflect this.

Employment law

Employment law, as it relates to those in the DCPs, is a large and important topic, but is beyond the scope of this chapter. Important issues relate to the security, quality and safety of employment and some aspects, such as employment status and contracts of employment, are complex and of particular significance to DCPs. Readers are referred to the expert advice provided by the professional associations, in particular the British Association of Dental Therapists (www.badt.org.uk), the British Society of Dental Hygiene and Therapy (www.bsdht.org.uk) and the BDA (www.bda-dentistry.org.uk).

Sources of advice

The ethical, professional and legal aspects of dental practice are demanding and frequently changing. It is every bit as important to keep abreast of these changes as those affecting the clinical aspects of practice. Although many professional and legal issues are encountered and dealt with on a daily basis without any difficulty, others occur only occasionally and may be more serious. DCPs and dentists should not hesitate to seek advice over such matters and where they involve complaints or potential litigation, they should act without delay. Professional associations, and the GDC (www.gdc-uk.org), are in a position to offer advice on general professional and some legal matters, but where complaints or litigation are concerned, the individual's dental defence organisation is usually the best source of advice and support. DCPs should also appreciate the significant benefits of being a member of their own particular professional association.

References

Bolam v Friern Hospital Management Committee 1957; 1 WLR 582.

Bolitho v City of Hackney HA 1997; 4 All ER 771.

Caldicott Committee (1997) *Report on the Review of Patient-Identifiable Information*. Department of Health, London.

Chester v Afshar 2004; UKHL 41.

General Dental Council (2006) *Standards Guidance*. General Dental Council, London.

Gillick v Norfolk and Wisbech AHA and DHSS 1985; 3 All ER 402.

Nuffield Foundation (1999) *The Education and Training of Personnel Auxiliary to Dentistry*. The Nuffield Foundation, London.

Index

Clinical Textbook of Dental Hygiene and Therapy, Second Edition. Edited by Suzanne L. Noble.
© 2012 John Wiley & Sons, Ltd. Published 2012 by John Wiley & Sons, Ltd.